Second Edition

Accident and Emergency

Etiology, Diagnosis and Management

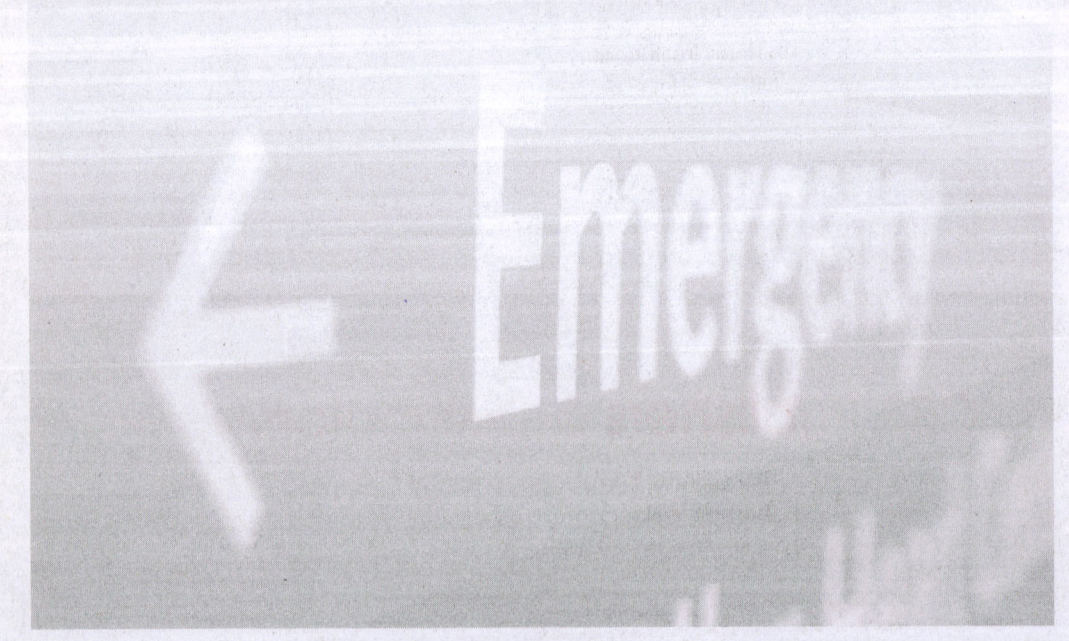

Second Edition

Accident and Emergency

Etiology, Diagnosis and Management

PS Kapoor MBBS, MS (Orthopedics), PCMS (Ex)

Senior Consultant Trauma and Orthopedics
Chandigarh Surgical Centre, Chandigarh

Former
Chief Consultant and Head of Orthopedics, Derna, Libya
Senior Consultant Orthopedics
Fortis Heart Institute and Multispeciality Hospital, Mohali
Surgical Specialist (PCMS), ESI Hospital, Ludhiana

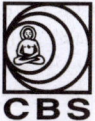

CBS

CBS Publishers & Distributors Pvt Ltd

New Delhi • Bengaluru • Chennai • Kochi • Kolkata • Mumbai
Hyderabad • Nagpur • Patna • Pune • Vijayawada

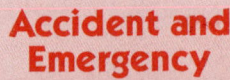

Accident and Emergency
Etiology, Diagnosis and Management
Second Edition

ISBN: 978-81-239-2944-6

Second Edition: 2016
First Edition: 2012

Published by Satish Kumar Jain and produced by Varun Jain for
CBS Publishers & Distributors Pvt Ltd
4819/XI Prahlad Street, 24 Ansari Road, Daryaganj, New Delhi 110 002, India.

Ph: 23289259, 23266861, 23266867   Fax: 011-23243014   Website: www.cbspd.com
e-mail: delhi@cbspd.com; cbspubs@airtelmail.in.
Corporate Office: 204 FIE, Industrial Area, Patparganj, Delhi 110 092
Ph: 4934 4934   Fax: 4934 4935   e-mail: publishing@cbspd.com; publicity@cbspd.com

Branches

- **Bengaluru:** Seema House 2975, 17th Cross, K.R. Road, Banasankari 2nd Stage, Bengaluru 560 070, Karnataka
  Ph: +91-80-26771678/79   Fax: +91-80-26771680   e-mail: bangalore@cbspd.com
- **Chennai:** No. 7, Subbaraya Street, Shenoy Nagar, Chennai 600 030, Tamil Nadu
  Ph: +91-44-26680620, 26681266   Fax: +91-44-42032115   e-mail: chennai@cbspd.com
- **Kochi:** Ashana House, 39/1904, AM Thomas Road, Valanjambalam, Ernakulam 682 016, Kochi, Kerala
  Ph: +91-484-4059061-65,67   Fax: +91-484-4059065   e-mail: kochi@cbspd.com
- **Kolkata:** No. 6/B, Ground Floor, Rameswar Shaw Road, Kolkata-700014 (West Bengal), India
  Ph: +91-33-2289-1126, 2289-1127, 2289-1128   e-mail: kolkata@cbspd.com
- **Mumbai:** 83-C, Dr E Moses Road, Worli, Mumbai-400018, Maharashtra
  Ph: +91-22-24902340/41   Fax: +91-22-24902342   e-mail: mumbai@cbspd.com

Representatives

- **Hyderabad** 0-9885175004   • **Nagpur** 0-9021734563   • **Patna**   0-9334159340
- **Pune**   0-9623451994   • **Vijayawada** 0-9000660880

Printed at Rashtriya Printers Delhi-110095

to
Charlie
....

Preface to the Second Edition

The generous acceptance of the first edition has encouraged me for revision of this textbook. While no changes have been required for this edition, yet a number of additions have been made throughout the volume especially in sections of cardiovascular, gastrointestinal and liver, pediatrics, orthopedics, respiratory, environmental, and emerging disorders.

Hoping that this second edition will be a worthy successor to its predecessor, and will prove useful to the medical student, medical officers and others, especially those working as a team in the department of Accident and Emergency (A&E). Accident and Emergency has emerged as a speciality, stressing on the knowledge and medical skills required for the prevention, diagnosis, and management of the acute and urgent aspects of illness and injury affecting patients of all age groups with the coverage of physical and behavioural disorders. It is a speciality in which time is critical.

This book is intended to serve as a useful reference, on widely accepted techniques currently available for finding causes, clinical diagnosis, investigations, and management of acute medical and surgical emergencies, and other common disorders. The contents of this book are presented as separate sections, any one of which is complete in itself, i.e. management of emergencies/disorders have been described fully, e.g. initial emergency treatment by the A&E staff, followed by further required treatment by the referred specialists, in the A&E/or in their respective departments, depending upon the infrastructure of the hospital.

Specific references are included as a guide to further study. The evaluation of new medical concepts and advances in determining causes, diagnosis, investigation and treatment has been a constant challenge. Medical progress and space limitations are the deciding factors.

This book aims to guide the physician who treats the patient in the A&E department, on how to keep adequate records of history, physical examination, investigation, and management of cases. An attempt has been made to mention the acute emergencies, and at the same time make mention of other common disorders, for which the patients use to visit the department of A&E for consultation and treatment. Special mention has been made about examination and management of acute emergeny cases on priority basis, especially while dealing with multiple injuries.

I have made endeavoured throughout to mention authorities whose work I have made use of, but I should like to express here my appreciation of the fact that it is the work of others which gives this book any value it may have.

My sincere thanks are due to the senior Vice President Mr YN Arjuna, editorial and production staff, and Managing Director of CBS Publishers & Distributors, for their encouragement and generous help, and for excellent work done in printing the book.

PS Kapoor

Preface to the First Edition

This book has been written primarily for the medical students, medical officers and others, especially those working as a team in the department of accident and emergency (A&E). Accident and emergency has emerged as a speciality, stressing on the knowledge and medical skills required for the prevention, diagnosis and management of the acute and urgent aspects of illness and injury affecting patients of all age groups with the coverage of physical and behavioral disorders. It is a speciality in which time is critical.

This book is intended to serve as a useful reference, on widely accepted techniques currently available for finding causes, clinical diagnosis, investigations, and management of acute medical emergencies, and other common disorders. The contents of this book are presented as separate sections, any one of which is complete in itself, i.e. management of emergencies/disorders has been described fully, for example, initial emergency treatment by the accident and emergency staff, followed by further definitive treatment provided with the help of referred specialists in the accident and emergency or by the referred specialists in their respective departments, depending upon the infrastructure of the hospital.

Specific references are included as a guide to further study. The evaluation of new medical concepts and advances in determining causes, diagnosis, investigation and treatment has been a constant challenge. Medical progress and space limitations are the deciding factors.

This book aims to guide the physician who treats the patient in the accident and emergency department on how to keep adequate records of history, physical examination, investigation, and management of cases. An attempt has been made to mention the acute emergencies, and at the same time make mention of the other common disorders for which the patients use to visit the department of accident and emergency for consultation and treatment. Special mention has been made about examination and management of acute emergency cases on priority basis, especially while dealing with multiple emergencies.

Special chapters on pediatric infections, cardiovascular diseases, psychiatric problems, obstetrics and gynecological problems, environmental disorders, acute abdomen, and fractures are intended to serve as medically oriented discussions of these fields with important clinical implications for the patient's care. Recent developments in orthopedic surgery such as interlocking nailing, total joint replacement, revised hip arthroplasty, anterior cruciate ligament replacement, arthroscopic surgery, etc. have received special attention.

I have made endeavour throughout to mention the authorities whose works I have made use of, but I should like to express here my appreciation of the fact that it is the work of others which gives this textbook any value it may have.

PS Kapoor

Acknowledgements

I wish to express my appreciation to Miss Komal Kapoor, Mr Siva Padhi and Ms Anju Malhotra for their skilful assistance with the manuscript and electronic information. Without their help the job would have been many times more difficult. I would like to acknowledge the help received from Ms Rita Kapoor, in the form of useful suggestions and moral support. I am indebted to genius Mr Jagdeep Kapoor for encouragement, criticism and generous help. It is heartening to acknowledge the encouragement gained at each step by the sweet chatting with dearest Isaac.

I am indebted to Dr CN Malla, Dr Abha Gupta, Dr SK Madan, Dr. S Saggar, Dr Vaneet Sharma, Dr Ram Kumar, Dr AP Sanwaria, Dr HV Jindal, Dr Vandana Sabharwal, Dr HK Kheterpal and Dr Rajinder Singh, who have offered special suggestions, comments and corrections.

I am highly thankful to the management of British Library and PGI Library, for access to the medical books and journals.

Last my sincere thanks are extended to senior Vice President Mr YN Arjuna, editorial and production staff, and Managing Director of CBS Publishers & Distributors, for their encouragement and generous help, and for the work done in maintaining a good standard of printing the book.

PS Kapoor

Contents

Part III Accident Emergencies

Part IV Surgical Emergencies

Part V Administrative and Legal Considerations

Appendices

Abbreviations

A&E	Accident and emergency		BAL	Bronchoalveolar
Ab	Antibody		BACTEC	Bacterial culture
ABC	Airway, breathing, circulation		BCG	bacille Calmette-Guerin
ABG	Arterial blood gases		b.d. (bd)	Bis die (twice daily)
ACE	Angiotensin-converting enzyme		b.i.w.	Twice a week
ACEI	Angiotensin-converting enzyme inhibitor		BKPOP	Below knee plaster of Paris
			BLS	Basic life support
ACL	Anterior cruciate ligament		BMD	Bone mineral density
ACLS	Advanced cardiac life support		BMJ	British medical journal
ACTH	Adrenocorticotropic hormone		BMT	Bone marrow transplant
ACS	Acute coronary syndromes		B/L	Bilateral
ADH	Antidiuretic hormone		BP	Blood pressure
ADS	Anti-diphtheritic serum		BSA	Broad spectrum antibiotic
AF	Atrial fibrillation		BUN	Blood urea nitrogen
AFB	Acid-fast bacillus			
Ag	Antigen		Ca	Carcinoma
AHF	Anti-hemophilic factor		Ca+	Calcium
AIDS	Acquired immune deficiency syndrome		CABG	Coronary artery bypass grafting (surgery)
AKPOP	Above knee plaster of Paris		CAD	Coronary artery disease
AMI	Acute myocardial infarction		C1	First cervical vertebra
ANF	Antinuclear factor		C7	Seventh cervical vertebra
A-O (ASIF)	Association for the study of Internal Fixation		CBF	Cerebral blood flow
			CBV	Cerebral blood volume
APH	Ante-partum hemorrhage (hemorrhage)		CCU	Coronary care unit
			CHF	Congestive heart failure
ATS	Anti-tetanus serum		Cl	Chloride
APLS	Advanced pediatric (paediatric) life support		C/I	Contraindication
			CK	Creatine kinase
AP	Anteroposterior		cm	Centimeter (s)
AR	Aortic regurgitation (incompetence)		CNS	Central nervous system
			CO	Carbon monoxide
ARBS	Angiotensin II receptor blockers		CO_2	Carbon dioxide
ARDS	Adult respiratory distress syndrome		COHb	Carboxyhemoglobin
			COPD	Chronic obstructive pulmonary disease
ART	Antiretroviral therapy			
AS	Aortic stenosis		CPR	Cardiopulmonary resuscitation
ASAP	As soon as possible		CPAP	Continuous positive airways pressure
ASD	Atrial septal defect			
ATLS	Advanced trauma life support		CPP	Cerebral perfusion pressure
AV	Atrioventricular		CRP	C-reactive protein
AXR	Abdominal X-ray		CRT	Cardiac resynchronization therapy

CSF	Cerebrospinal fluid
CT	Computerised (axial) tomography
CuSO$_4$	Copper sulphate
CVA	Cerebrovascular accident
CVD	Cardiovascular disease
CVP	Central venous pressure
CVS	Cardiovascular system
CXR	Chest X-ray
D	Dimension
dB	Decibel
DBS	Deep brain stimulation
DBP	Diastolic blood pressure
DC	Direct current
D&C	Dilatation and curettage
DCS	Dynamic condylar screw
DHS	Dynamic hip screw
DEXA	Dual energy X-ray absorptiometry
DFN	Distal femoral nail
D&I	Dilatation and insufflation
DIP	Distal interphalangeal joint
dL	Decilitre
DLC	Differential leucocytic count
DM	Diabetes mellitus
DMARDs	Disease modifying anti-rheumatic drugs
DNA	Deoxyribonucleic acid
DOT	Directly observed treatment
DPL	Diagnostic peritoneal lavage
DSS	Dengue shock syndrome
DT	Delirium tremens
DU	Duodenal ulcer
DVT	Deep vein thrombosis
EBM	Evidence based medicine (journal)
ECF	Extracellular fluid
ECG	Electrocardiogram
Echo	Echocardiogram
ECT	Electroconvulsive therapy
ED	Emergency department
EEG	Electro-encephalography
e.g.	For example
EMG	Electromyogram
ENT	Ear, nose and throat
EOD	Every other day (syn. alternate day)
EPTB	Extrapulmonary tuberculosis
ESR	Erythrocyte sedimentation rate
ET	Endotracheal
ETOH	Exposure to occupational hazards

FB	Foreign body
FBC	Full blood count
FBS	Fastin blood sugar
FH	Family history
FISH	Fluorescence in situ hybridisation
FSH	Follicle stimulating hormone
G	Gauge
g	Gram (s)
GA	General anaesthesia
GCS	Glasgow Coma Score
GERD/ GORD	Gastroesophageal disorder
GI	Gastrointestinal
GIT	Gastrointestinal tract
GP	General practitioner
GTN	Glyceryl trinitrate
GTT	Glucose tolerance test
Hb	Hemoglobin (haemoglobin)
HbA1c	Hemoglobin glycosylated
HBV	Hepatitis B virus
HCG	Human chorionic gonadotrophin
HCO$_3$	Bicarbonate
H$_2$CO$_3$	Carbonate
HDL	High density lipoprotein
Hg	Mercury
HiB	Haemophilus influenzae type B
HIV	Human immunodeficiency virus
HOB	Head end of bed
hr	Hour
HPLC	High performance liquid chronography
HRT	Hormone replacement therapy
HTIG	Human tetanus immunoglobulin
Ib/ibid	In the same place
ICF	Intracellular fluid
ICP	Intracranial pressure
ICS	Intercostal space
ICU	Intensive care unit
i.e.	That is
IDDM	Insulin dependent diabetes mellitus
IDK	Internal derangement knee
Ig A, G, E	Immunoglobulin A, G, E
IHD	Ischemic heart disease
ILN	Interlocking nail
IMN	Intramedullary nail
i.m. (IM)	Intramuscular
Inf	Inferior

IQ	Intelligence quotient		MI	Myocardial infarction
IP	Interphalangeal		min	Minute/minutes
Iu	International unit		mL	Millilitre
IUCD	Intrauterine contraceptive device		mm Hg	Millimetres of mercury
			mmol	Millimoles
IV	Intravenous		mU	Million units
IVI	Intravenous infusion		MR	Mitral regurgitation
IVP	Intravenous pyelography		MRI	Magnetic resonance imaging
IVU	Intravenous urogram		MS	Mitral stenosis
			MSU	Midstream urine
JVP	Jugular venous pressure		MTP	Metatarsophalangeal
			MTP	Medical termination of pregnancy
K^+	Potassium			
KCl	Potassium chloride		Na^+	Sodium
kg	Kilogram		NaCl	Sodium chloride
kl	Kilolitre		$NaHCO_2$	Sodium bicarbonate
KUB	Kidneys, ureters, bladder		NBM	Nothing by mouth
			NG	Nasogastric
LES	Laryngoesophagus sphincter		NHS	National health service
L	Litre		NICU	Neonatal intensive care unit
LA	Local anaesthesia		NMDA	N-methyl-d-aspartate
Lab	Laboratory		N_2O	Nitrous oxide
LAD	Left axis deviation		NPO	Nothing by mouth
LAT	Lateral		NSAIDs	Nonsteroidal anti-inflammatory drugs
LBBB	Left bundle branch block			
LDL	Low density lipoprotein		NSTEMI	Non-ST elevation myocardial infarction
LDL-C	Low density lipoprotein cholesterol			
			N&V	Nausea and/or vomiting
LFTs	Liver function tests		NWBPOP	Non-weight bearing plaster of Paris
LH	Luteinizing hormone			
LMP	First day of last menstrual period			
LMWH	Low molecular weight heparin		O_2	Oxygen
LP	Lmbar puncture		OA	osteoarthritis
LSD	Lysergic acid diethylamide		o.d. (od)	Omni die (once daily)
Lt	Left		OD	Overdose
LVET	Left ventricular ejection time		O&G	Obstetrics and gynaecology
LVF	Left ventricular failure		om	Omni mane (in the morning)
LVH	Left ventricular hypertrophy		on	Omni nocte (at night)
			OPD	Out-patients department
MAOI	Monoamine oxidase inhibitor		ORIF	Open reduction and internal fixation
MAP	Mean arterial pressure			
max	Maximum		ORT	Oral replacement therapy
MC	Metacarpal			
MCH	Mean corpuscular haemoglobin		PA	Postero-anterior
MCHC	Mean corpuscular hemoglobin concentration per cent		PAIDS	Pediatric aids immunodeficiency syndrome
			$PaCO_2$	Partial pressure of carbon dioxide (arterial)
MCP	Metacarpophalangeal			
MCV	Mean cell volume		PaO_2	Partial pressure of oxygen (arterial)
MDO	Medical defence organisation			
mEq/L	Millieqivalents per litre			
mg	Milligrams		PCL	posterior cruciate ligament
MHA	Mental health act		PCR	Polymerase chain reaction

PCV	Packed cell volume	s	Second(s)
PE	Pulmonary embolism	SGOT	Serum glutamic-oxaloacetic transaminase
PEP	Pre-ejection period		
PFN	Proximal femoral nail	SGPT	Serum glutamic pyruvic transaminase
PHN	Proximal humeral nail		
PIP	Proximal interphalangeal	SIDS	Sudden infant death syndrome
PNDT	Prenatal diagnostic techniques	SL	Sublingual
PO	Per os (orally/by mouth)	SLE	Systemic lupus erythematosus
POP	Plaster of Paris	SLR	Straight leg raising
PPH	Post-partum hemorrhage	SNRIs	Selective serotonin and noradrenaline reuptake inhibitors
PPI	Proton pump inhibitors		
PPMs	Pathogenic micro-organisms	SSRIs	Selective serotonin reuptake inhibitors
PPR	Price's precipitation reaction		
P/R	Per-rectum	Stat	Immediately
PRC	Post-resuscitation care	STD	Sexually transmitted disease
PSVT	Paroxysmal supraventricular tachycardia	STEMI	ST-elevation myocardial infarction
PTA	Post-traumatic amnesia	SVCS	Superior vena cava syndrome
PTB	Pulmonary tuberculosis	SVG	Saphenous vein graft
PTCA	Percutaneous transluminal coronary angioplasty	SXR	Skull X-ray
PTMR	Percutaneous transmyocardial revascularisation	TIA	Transient ischemic attack
		TB	Tuberculosis
PUO	Pyrexia of unknown origion	TCADs	Tricyclic antidepressants
P/V	Per vaginum	t.d.s.(TDS)	Ter in die sumendus (three times daily)
q.d.s.(qds)	Quater in die summendus (four times daily)	TFTs	Thyroid function tests
		THR	Total hip replacement
q.i.d.	Quarter in die (4 times a day)	TIA	Transient ischaemic attack
		t.i.w.	Three times per week
RA	Rheumatoid arthritis	TKR	Total knee replacement
RBBB	Right bundle branch block	TLC	Total leucocytic count
RBC	Red blood cell	TNF	Tumor necrosis factor
Rh	Rhesus	TPA	Tissue plasmino activator
RNA	Ribonucleic acid	TSH	Thyroid stimulating harmone
RNTCP	Revised national tuberculosis control programme	THR	Total hip replacement
		TI	Tricuspid insufficiency
Rt	Right	TS	Tricuspid stenosis
RSA	Road side accident	TURP	Transurethral resection of the prostate
RUA	Right upper abdomen		
RVF	Right ventricular failure		
RVH	Right ventricular hypertrophy	u/U/IU	Unit
		UA	Unstable angina
SA	Sino-atrial	U&E	Urea and electrolytes
SARS	Severe acute respiratory syndrome	UFH	Unfractionated heparin
		ug	Microgram
SaO$_2$	Arterial oxygen saturation	UHN	Universal humeral nail
SBE	Subacute bacterial endocarditis	ULQ	Upper left quadrant abdomen
s.c.(S/c)	Subcutaneously	URC	Upper respiratory catarrh
SCC	Spinal cord compression	UTI	Urinary tract infection
SHS	Sliding hip screw	USS	Ultrasound (ultrasonography) study
SCT	Stem cell therapy		
SE (S/E)	Side-effect(s)		

V	Volts	WBC	White blood cell(s)
VA	Visual acuity	WCC	White cell count
VDRL	Venereal diseases research laboratory	WHO	World Health Organisation
		Wk(s)	Week(s)
VF	Ventricular fibrillation	wt	Weight
VNS	Vagal nerve stimulation		
VSD	Ventricular septal defect	X-match	Cross-match blood
VT	Ventricular tachycardia		
VTE	Venous thrombo-embolism	Yr(s)	year(s)
		ZN	Ziehl-Neelsen syndrome

Triage of Medical/ Surgical Emergency Patient

Triage is a French word meaning sorting, selection, choice. It is the process of sorting patients based upon their requirement of immediate medical or surgical treatment as compared to their chance of benefiting from such care. Patients visiting A&E are to be sorted immediately by an experienced triage staff on duty in order to attend to serious patients on priority basis. A strategy must be driven for the detection of the highest risk group in whom immediate intervention can improve outcome. The decision has to be taken upon considering the seriousness of the illness or injury, e.g. critical, serious or alert (Table: Triage).

Triage of Medical/Surgical Emergency Patient			
Risk group	Airway	Priority	Care
Critical (Highest)	Unconscious Breathless Airway obstructed	1st	Immediate
Serious (High)	Semiconscious Breathing noisy Airway obstructed	2nd	Within 2–5 min
Alert (Low)	Conscious Talking Airway patent	3rd	Within 30 min

The A&E staff must have a clear knowledge of the benefit and harm of each therapy, allowing formulation of a simple approach to treatment selection based upon the disease or injury presentation. Properly attended or treated, acute emergency should have low hospital mortality, but if left neglected or untreated, mortality is high. Proper history taking and investigations usually suffice for diagnosis. Careful surveillance and management, including invasive management in selected cases, substantially reduce long-term risks. The clinical question is which patients with acute symptoms have a presentation benign enough to make discharge from the A&E department safe and appropriate.

Part I

Introduction
(History Taking and
Physical Examination)

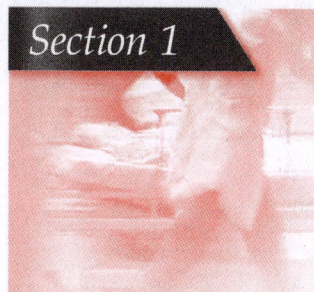

Case Taking

1

- Interrogation of the patient (history)
- General physical examination of the patient

Significance of Case Taking

The systematically interrogation, physical examination of the patient and maintenance of records, are essential for providing a good emergency medical care in the very busy A&E department with doctors and paramedical staff, working under great pressure to handle the serious/sick patients as priorities, besides frequently facing medicolegal problems. The relevance/significance of each criterion is:

Age
Some diseases/disorders are common in certain age groups, i.e.
- *Neonatal:* Heart disease, CNS disorders, meningocele, cleft palate, cleft lip, tongue tie, hydrocephalus, club foot, present at birth.
- *Infancy:* Respiratory infections, CHF, vomiting, jaundice, hiccup, rickets, scurvy, bed wetting, delayed speech, Wilms' tumor, umbilical hernia.
- *Childhood:* Respiratory infections, measles, asthma, diarrhea, malaria, juvenile diabetes, appendicitis, asthma, osteomyelitis, osteosarcoma.
- *Adults:* Rheumatoid arthritis, migraine.
- *Elders:* Hypertension, heart failure, osteoarthritis, Alzheimer's disease, falls, senile osteoporosis, SE prostate, pneumonia, carcinomas.

Religion
- Carcinoma penis less common in those having circumcision.

Sex
- Hemophilia affects males only, although transmitted through females.
- Carcinoma lips, tongue, GI tract, more prevalent in males.
- Hysteria–more in females.

Occupation
Some ailments more common in certain professions (trades), i.e.
- Internal derangement knee (IDK) common in footballers and mine workers.
- Intestinal colic – due to lead poisoning–common in painters.
- Housemaid knee – common in maids.
- Hydated cyst disease – common in dogs, domestic animals caretakers.

Address
- *Travel hazards:* Exposure to infections, e.g. sleeping sickness (African countries), hydated disease (Australia), influenza infection (Prone areas).

Interrogation of the Patient (history): Includes

Particulars of the patient

Surname ....First name .... A&E no ....

Age/DOB ....Sex .... Date ....

Son/daughter/wife of .... Time ....

Occupation ....

Address .... Tel ....

DOA .... DOD ....

Diagnosis ....

A&E consultant/Dr I/C ....

Complaints (Symptoms) and their Duration

Inquire the patient (parents/attendants in case of a child/unconscious patient):

- What are his/her currently troubling (chief) complaints?
- Symptoms recorded in a chronological manner of their appearance, i.e. pain in the chest, dyspnea, swelling of feet.
- Either write down how many (weeks, days, months) last, the complaints started/mention the exact date, e.g.

Patterns:

- Weeks: (no. of weeks/total no. of weeks per year – symbol)

13/52	Pain in the chest
09/52	Dyspnea
05/52	Swelling of feet

- Days: (no. of days/weekly – symbol)

92/7	Pain in the chest
61/7	Dyspnea
31/7	Swelling of feet

- Date:

14.5.2009	Pain in the chest
15.5.2009	Dyspnea
20.5.2009	Swelling of feet

- Months: (no. of months/total no. of months per year – symbol)

3/12	Pain in the chest
2/12	Dyspnea
1/12	Swelling of feet

Pain in the chest	Three months
Dyspnea	Two months
Swelling of feet	One month

History of Present Illness

This covers the period from appearance of first symptom to the present time. Let the patient narrate his/her own history of complaints and do not put any leading questions having their own readymade answers.

Inquire The patient/accompanied person of unconscious/accidental case and the mother/accompanied person in case of a young child, about:
- How did the symptoms start?
- What happened next?
- Whether symptoms started suddenly or gradually?
- Whether any relief from complaints during the whole period?
- What sort of treatment taken and whether any relief or not?

Past History Record any ailments suffered by the patient prior to current one, in a chronological manner, along with their duration.
Child: Record development milestones, e.g. head holding, sitting, crawling, standing, teething, smile, speech, walking.

Personal History
- Whether married or single, number of children and their health condition?
- Habits, diet, appetite, bowl and urinary conditions.
- Any addiction–drugs, smoking, alcohol abuse, etc.
- History of menstrual cycle (female patient) – normal or abnormal, i.e. amenorrhea, epimenorrhea, menorrhagia, metrorrhagia, dysmenorrhea.
- Any history of miscarriage, post menopausal condition, vaginal discharge.

Family History (Inquire)
- About the condition of health of parents, children, and other family members living along with. Anybody suffering from similar ailments.
- Any death in the family and the cause of death.
- Any family history of diabetes, hypertension, congestive heart failure, asthma, tuberculosis, hemophilia, cancer.

Pediatric History (Inquire the mother or accompanying person)
- Number of children in the family, any dead and the cause of death.
- Was it a normal delivery and full time child?
- Was the child breastfed?
- Digestion and bowl habits.
- Any previous illnesses (measles, whooping cough, chickenpox, scarlet fever, fits, nausea, vomiting, diarrhea, sore throat, running nose and ears).
- Immunization status (when were primary/booster/repeat doses given) of BCG, polio, DPT, measles, hepatitis B, hib, MMR, typhoid and tetanus toxoid.

Special Interrogation (Systemic Review)

To inquire about the involvement of a particular organ/system, thought to be affected most and about nature of the disease, i.e.

Cardiovascular System (Inquire about)

- History of rheumatic fever, scarlet fever, diphtheria, or sore throat.
- *Chest pain*: One of the most presenting complaints. *Inquire about its* site, character, localization, radiation, duration, factors which precipitate, or relieve it, any medication.
- *Dyspnea*: Is it present at rest or on exertion–relieved by rest.
- Any history of orthopnea–relieved by sitting.
- *Palpitation:* Inquire about any rapid, forceful, irregular heart beating.
- *Fatigueness:* Is there easy fatigability–relieved by rest.
- *Edema feet:* Is there swelling of feet?

Respiratory System (Inquire about)

- History of tuberculosis, exposure to fumes/dust, smoking
- Sneezing
- *Cough:* Inquire about its character and frequency, is it dry or purulent one, any association with chest pain
- *Expectoration:* Inquire about its quality and quantity
- *Hemoptysis:* Any spitting or coughing of blood
- *Dyspnea:* May appear at rest or on exertion
- *Cyanosis:* More marked, if the patient is cold
- Chest pain
- *Cold:* Running nose, nasal block

Nervous System (Inquire about)

- History of fits/seizure, paralysis, mental disorders, drugs/alcohol abuse
- Headache, giddiness, vertigo
- Memory and concentration
- Sleep
- Weakness of any limb
- Proximal muscle weakness
- Tremors
- Tingling sensation
- Feeling ground like cotton wool
- Urinary bladder sphincter control
- Bowel sphincter control

Blood (Inquire about)

- Any history of bleeders in the family, any passage of blood per rectum, any passage of black coloured stools
- Any breathlessness on exertion, muscular weakness, headache
- Swelling of feet.

Gastrointestinal Tract and Abdomen (Inquire about)

- *Diet:* Quality and quantity of food
- *Appetite:* Decreased or increased
- *Pain:* Site – localised or referred, character – throbbing, dull or aching, duration – any interval of relief from pain, relation to meals
- History of peptic ulcers
- Heartburn (retrosternal burning)
- *Dysphasia:* Any difficulty in swallowing
- *Flatulence and dyspepsia:* Relation to food, any relief to pain
- Nausea
- *Vomiting:* Frequency, quantity, quality, relation to food and pain
- Hematemesis
- *Constipation:* Bowl habits – regular or irregular. Any history of use of purgatives
- *Diarrhea:* Frequency, quality, quantity, relation to meals, passing of blood/slime
- Any history of tenesmus during defaecation
- History of piles
- *Liver/gallbladder:* Any pain in region of liver, any history of jaundice, any change in colour of urine or stools

Genitourinary System (Inquire about)

- History of renal disorders
- *Pain:* Site, character – dull, aching or severe colicky, localized or referral to groin or testicles
- *Urinary symptoms:* Frequency, urgency, hesitancy, dribbling, overflow, nocturia, dysuria
- Nausea, vomiting, drowsiness, headache, fever, puffiness of face, edema ankle
- History of prostate enlargement
- History of hydrocele

Obstetric and Gynecology System (Inquire about)

- *Menstrual history:* Menarche, cycle, loss, pain, IMB, PCB, LMP
- Vaginal discharge, cervical smear, contraception

- Obstetric history
- Gynecological – any bleeding per vaginum, vaginal discharge, pain abdomen

Eye (Inquire about)

- Vision – any disturbance of vision
- Any complaint of halos around lights, flashes
- Pain – irritable, dull-ache or severe
- Headache
- Discharge from eye(s) – watery, or purulent.

Ear, Nose, Throat (ENT) (Inquire about)

- Earache
- Discharge – watery/purulent
- Deafness – any hearing loss
- Tinnitus – any ringing sensation
- Vertigo – any hallucination of movement.

Bones/Joints Disorders (Inquire about)

- History of rheumatism, gout, tuberculosis, syphilis, leucorrhea, diabetes mellitus, shifting joint pains.

Physical Examination (Includes)

- General physical examination (GPE)
- Local examination
- Examination of different systems/parts of the body

Physical examination (preliminary and detailed examination).

General Physical Examination (GPE): Observe

- *Appearance:* Build, nutrition, presence or absence of anemia, jaundice, cyanosis, clubbing, edema
- *Intelligence:* Expression
- *Attitude:* Helplessness, keeping limbs in a particular position
- *Facial expression*: Tense, nervous, toxic, fatigue
- Pulse: Rate, rhythm, volume
- *Respiration:* Rate, rhythm, thoracic or abdominal
- Temperature
- Blood pressure

Local Examination: **The interrogation of the patient leads to the system/organ of the body to be examined first.** Examination include:

Inspection	Looking at the patient's body
Palpation	Feeling the parts of the body

Percussion	Listening the sounds elicited by tapping the part with finger
Auscultation	Listening body's sounds with a stethoscope

Examination of Different Systems/Parts of the Body

Observe	Begin with the head and neck, and proceeds downwards, i.e.
Head	*Skull:* Size, Shape: hydrocephalus, bossing of fore/hind head (rickets)

- *Hair:* Colour, texture
- *Eyes:*
  - Orbits–exophthalmos/enophthalmos/proptosis
  - Eyeballs – strabismus (squint)
    nystagmus (oscillatory movements)
  - Eyelids – ptosis, edema, inflammation (blepharitis), entropion/ ectropion
  - Pupils – size, equally, reaction to light and accommodation
  - Conjunctiva – anemia, jaundice, trachoma, inflammation, tumor
  - Cornea – size – glaucoma
    curvature – conical
    surfaces – corneal reflex, ulcer, opacity
  - Sclera – myopia, scleritis
  - Iris – color, iritis
  - Lens -- cataract
  - Vitreous – fluidity, hemorrhage, foreign body, opacity
  - Visual acuity – testing distant/near vision
  - Ocular tension (IOP) - testing by
    ◊ Palpating eyeball with eyes open, and by
    ◊ Tonometer
  - Fundus examination with an ophthalmoscope
  - Optic disc status, e.g. papilledema, hemorrhage, inflammation
  - Retinopathy (diabetic/hypertensive)
- *Ears:*
  - Foreign body in the ear
  - Discharging ear
  - Audiometry–hearing assessment
- *Face:* Expression, shape, paralysis, puffiness
  - Mouth – shape, cleft lip, lips–pale or cyanotic, fissures (cracks) on lips
  - Tongue – appearance, protrusion (any deviation), tongue-tie, ulcer
  - Teeth and gums–hygiene, no. of missing teeth, any denture worn, any bleeding gums
  - Soft palate – movements
  - Tonsil – normal/swollen

Neck	• Any engorgement (distension) of neck veins
	• Thyroid – normal/swollen
	¨ Lymph nodes – any enlargement

Chest inspection	• Shape of chest – any deformity: Rickety rosary (rickets)
	• Respiration – rate, rhythm, volume
	• Pulsations/dilated vessels
	• Apex beat

Palpation	• Local tenderness
	• Tracheal position, apex beat

Percussion	Cardiac dullness

Auscultation	Heart sounds, murmurs, breath sounds

Spine (Inspection and Palpation)

• *Deformity:* Kyphosis – posterior curvature common in thoracic region.
Lordosis – anterior curvature common in lumbar region.
Scoliosis – lateral curvature–right/or left side.
• Local tenderness.

Abdomen Inspection	• Size, shape, distension, abdominal movements, dilated vessels, umbilicus, any operational or wound scar.
	• Hernial sites – impulse on coughing.

Palpation and Percussion: Local tenderness, any rigidity, (resentment to palpation esp. by a child c/o pain abdomen)

• Any palpable swelling, liver, spleen, kidneys, inguinal glands
• Genitalia
 – Male – penis, scrotum, testicles
 – Female – external genitalia (if indicated)

Auscultation	Peristaltic sounds

P/R (Per rectum) examination
Gynaecology and Obstetrics Examination

Rules	The examiner should explain about the purpose of examination, what is about to be done, and verbal/written consent to be taken in advance. Presence of female staff/attendant is desirable/required as per rules.

Breast Examination	• Any pigmentation of skin, discoloration of skin
	• Any retraction of nipple
	• Any swelling visible/palpable
	• Any discharge from nipples
	• Any enlargement (palpable) of axillary glands.

Abdominal examination: Described in appropriate sections

P/V	If indicated
Limbs	Upper and lower limbs

Inspection	• Appearance – shape and size: deformity, shortning • Nutrition – built, any muscular wasting • Edema – any swelling of feet and thighs
Palpation	• Muscle tone, power, reflexes, sensations • Any pitting edema over ankles and thighs • Local tenderness
Pulsations	Radial, femoral, posterior tibial, dorsalis pedis
Lymph nodes	Any enlargement
Measurements	Shortening, muscular wasting
Movements	Active and passive

Neurological Examination

• *Higher centres:* Mental status, intelligence, emotional status, speech
• Cranial nerves
• Trunk, gait

Upper and lower limbs:

Inspection	Any muscular wasting, skin–pale/cyanotic/red/shining, dry or moist, trophic ulcers, nails–any brittleness
Palpation	Muscle power, tone, reflexes, sensations

Provisional Diagnosis: As a routine, diagnosis of common diseases should be commonly preferred over rare diseases.

Investigations Include

Routine examination: Blood, urine, stools, vomitus, sputum and CSF.

• *Hematology:* Complete blood count (CBC): Hemoglobin, RBC, PCV, MCV, MCH, MCHC, TLC and DLC, platelet, BT and CT, ESR
• *Biochemistry:* Blood sugar – fasting, PP and random.
• *Serum electrolytes:* Sodium, potassium, chloride, calcium, phosphorus, magnesium, iron, amylase, lipase, CPK-MB, CPK-NAC, troponin-T/I.
• *Serology:* Mantoux test, widal test, Coomb's test, pregnancy test, CRP, RA factor, VDRL, HBsAg (rapid/elisa), HIV (rapid/elisa), HAV-IgM, HEV-IgM, torch IgG/IgM, HCV (rapid/elisa), flocculation tests – Kahn test and Price's precipitation reaction (PPR) for syphilis.
• *Liver function tests (LFT):* Serum bilirubin, SGOT, SGPT, serum proteins – total/albumin/globulin, serum alkaline phosphatase.
• *Renal function tests (RFT):* Serum creatinine, serum uric acid, BUN.
• *Lipid profile:* Serum cholesterol, triglycerides, HDL, LDL, VLDL.

- *Hormones and tumor markers:* TSH, FSH, LH, prolactin, testosterone, PSA, AFP.
- *Urine examination:* Colour, reaction, specific gravity, albumin, blood, deposits, electrolytes, Bence Jones proteose, ketones.
- *Stool examination:* Amoebiasis/bacteria
- *Sputum examination:* Any foreign body (AFB)
- *Vomitus examination:* AFB
- *Cerebrospinal fluid (CS) examination:* Bacterial infections
- Microbiology
- Blood culture and sensitivity, pus culture and sensitivity, AFB culture, urine and stool culture and sensitivity, throat swab culture and sensitivity.

Special Investigations: Depending on the system affected, e.g.
- CXR (X-ray chest)
- X-ray of affected part
- Ultrasound, MRI, CT scan, myelography
- ECG, sonography, angiography
- Hysteroscopy, hysterosalpingography, hysterosonography, colposcopy, laparoscope, pregnancy testing, endometrial biopsy
- Bone densitometry
- EEG

Note: **These are described in appropriate sections**

Clinical Diagnosis: Clinical diagnosis at this stage should be complete and precise as much as possible. It is made on the basis of interrogation of the patient, examination, and investigations.

Treatment and Progress: Daily recording of following:
- Treatment given, i.e. medicines, etc.
- Procedures include operations performed.
- *Monitoring:* Daily progress esp. of acute cases, i.e. recording of general condition of the patient, pulse, respiration, temperature, blood pressure, changes in the size of inflammatory swelling, treatment being received. All investigation reports to be recorded in the case sheet. If any surgery performed, then operation notes to be recorded by the doctor incharge of the case.

Completion of Hospital Record (Discharge Summary)

Recording of condition of patient at time of discharge from the hospital (Table 1.1)

Table 1.1: Discharge summary

Surname ....First name .... A&E no ....

Age/DOB ....Sex .... Date ....

Son/daughter/wife of .... Time ....

Address .... Tel ....

DOA .... DOD ....

Diagnosis ....

A&E consultant/Dr. I/C ....

Complaints ....

....

Present illness ....

....

Past history ....

....

GP examination ....

....

Treatment and investigations ....

....

Condition at time of discharge: Fully cured, relieved of symptoms/signs, or any complication/ death. In case of death, postmortem examination report to be entered in the hospital records. Instructions to the patient at time of discharge: Schedule of medicines use, any precaution to be taken, date of check up at the hospital/GP's clinic.

Signature... Date ....

Referral System

Always inform the GP prior to the discharge of a patient for follow-up purpose, instructions/ information to GP about discharged patient (Table 1.2).

Table 1.2: Referral letter to the GP

Dear Dr..

Patient ....Attended A&E department on ....

Diagnosis ....

Investigation ....

Treatment given ....

Aftercare (follow-up) ....

Yours sincerely

Signature.. Date ....

Table 1.3: Proforma

Surname .... First name .... A&E no ....

Age/DOB .... Sex .... Date ....

Son/daughter/wife of .... Time ....

Address .... Tel ....

DOA .... DOD ....

Diagnosis ....

A&E consultant/Dr I/C ....

Case taking

Chief complaint ....

....

....

History of present illness ....

....

....

Past history ....

....

....

Personal history

Marital status: Single/married/widow/widower .... Children ....

Diet ....

Smoking .... Alcohol .... Drugs abuse ....

Physical activity ....

Family history

Father ....

Mother ....

Siblings ....

Interrogation in case of a young child ....

(Inquire the mother or accompanying person) ....

Delivery status .... Normal .... Full time ....

Postnatal .... Cyanosis .... Jaundice ....

Birth weight .... Breastfed .... Diet ....

Habits .... Eating .... Sleep ....

Bowel...Bladder .... Bed wetting ....

Development milestones ....Head holding .... Crawling ....

Sitting ....Standing .... Teething ....

Smile ....Speech .... Walking ....

Immunization status ....BCG .... Polio ....

DPT ....Measles .... Hepatitis B ....

Chickenpox ....

Special interrogation of the patient (systemic review):

Cardiovascular system

History of rheumatic fever, scarlet fever, diphtheria, or sore throat.

Chest pain ....

Dyspnea ....

Orthopnea ....

Palpitation ....

Fatigueness ....

Edema feet..

Respiratory system

History of tuberculosis ....

History of exposure to fumes/dust...

History of smoking...

Cough ....Sneezing ....

Cold ....Running nose .... Nasal block ....

Expectoration ....

Hemoptysis ....

Dyspnea ....

Cyanosis ....

Chest pain ....

Nervous system

History of fits/seizure, paralysis, mental disorders ....

Drugs abuse ....Alcohol abuse ....

Headache..Giddiness .... Vertigo ....

Memory and concentration .... Sleep ....

Weakness of limb/limbs ....Muscle weakness ....

Tremors ....Tingling sensation.............................

Urinary bladder sphincter control .... Bowel sphincter control ....

Blood system

History of bleeders in the family ....

History of malena ....

Dyspnea on exertion ....

Weakness ....

Headache...

Palpitation ....

Edema feet...

Gastrointestinal tract and abdomen system

Diet ....

Appetite ....

Abdominal pain ....

History of peptic ulcers ....

Heartburn (retrosternal burning) ....

Dysphasia ....

Flatulence and dyspepsia ....

Nausea ....Vomiting ....Diarrhea.................

Hematemesis ....

Diarrhea ....

Constipation ....

History of piles ....

Liver/gallbladder ....

Genitourinary system

History of renal disorders ....

Pain ....

Urinary symptoms:

Frequency ....Urgency ....Hesitancy ....

Dribbling ....Overflow ....

Nocturia ....Dysuria ....

Nausea ....Vomiting ....Drowsiness ....

Headache ....Fever ....

Puffiness of face ....Edema ankle ....

Prostate enlargement ....Hydrocele ....

Obstetric and gynecology system

Menstrual history: Menarche ....Cycle ....Loss ....

Pain ....IMB ....PCB ....LMP ....

Vaginal discharge ....Contraception ....

Obstetric history ....

Gynecological:

Bleeding per vaginum ....Vaginal discharge ....

Pain abdomen..

Eye

Vision .... Halos around lights ....

Pain (eye-strain) .... Headache ....

Discharge .... Watery .... Purulent ....

Diplopia ....

ENT

Earache .... Deafness ....

Discharge .... Watery .... Purulent ....

Tinnitus .... Vertigo ....

Sneezing .... Stuffiness ....

Nasal discharge .... Epistaxis ....

Sore throat .... Cough .... Expectoration ....

Bones and joints disorders

History of rheumatism .... Gout ....

Tuberculosis .... Diabetes mellitus ....

Syphilis .... Urethral discharge ....

Leukorrhea .... Trauma ....

Examination of the Patient

General physical examination (GPE)

Appearance ....

Intelligence..

Attitude ....

Facial expression..

Pulse ....

Respiration ....

Temperature ....

Blood pressure: SBP .... DBP ....

Local examination (System/organ of the body to be examined first)

Inspection ....

Palpation ....

Percussion ....

Auscultation ....

Examination of different systems/parts of the body

Head and neck

Skull hydrocephalus .... Bossing of fore/hind head ....

Hair ....

Eyes

Orbits .... Eyeballs ....

Eyelids .... Pupils ....

Conjunctiva ....

Cornea ....

Sclera .... Iris ....

Lens.. Vitreous ....

Visual acuity .... Ocular tension (IOP) ....

Fundus examination with an ophthalmoscope ....

Ears ....

Audiometry..

Face..

Mouth

Shape .... Lips ....

Tongue ....

Teeth and gums ....

Soft palate .... Tonsil ....

Neck ....

Thyroid .... Lymph nodes ....

Chest

Inspection: Shape of chest ....

Respiration ....

Pulsations/dilated vessels ....

Apex beat..

Palpation: Local tenderness ....

Tracheal position .... Apex beat ....

Percussion: Cardiac dullness ....

Auscultation: Heart sounds/murmurs ....

Breath sounds ....

Deformity.. Local tenderness ....

Spine Abdomen

Inspection: Size .... Shape ....

Distension .... Dilated vessels ....

Abdominal movements ....

Umbilicus .... Scar ....

Hernial sites–impulse on coughing ....

Palpation and Percussion

Local tenderness .... Rigidity ....

Swelling ....

Liver .... Spleen ....

Kidneys .... Inguinal glands ....

Genitalia: Male – penis, scrotum, testicles ....

Female – external genitalia (if indicated) ....

Auscultation: Peristalsis sounds ....

P/R (per-rectum) examination ....

Gynecology and obstetric examination

Breast: Skin pigmentation/discoloration ....

Nipple retraction .... Discharge from nipples ....

Swelling .... Axillary lymph nodes ....

Abdominal examination ....

....

....

....

....

P/V examination ....

....

Limbs: Upper and lower limbs

Inspection: Shape .... Size ....

Built .... Muscle wastings ....

Edema feet/thighs ....

Palpation: Muscle tone .... Power ....

Reflexes .... Sensations ....

Edema ankles/thigh .... Local tenderness ....

Pulsations: Radial .... Femoral ....

Posterior tibial .... Dorsalis pedis ....

Lymph nodes enlargement ....

Measurements ....

Neurological examination

Higher centres:

Intelligence .... Emotional status ....

Speech ....

Cranial nerves ....

Trunk .... Gait ....

Upper and lower limbs:

Muscular wasting .... Skin ....

Trophic ulcers .... Nails ....

Muscle power .... Muscle tone ....

Reflexes .... Sensations ....

Examination of a young child

Height .... Weight .... Head circumference ....

Chest circumference .... Midarm circumference ....

Anterior fontanel .... Clubbing .... Koilonychia ....

Immunization status .... BCG scar .... Umbilicus ....

Pallor .... Jaundice .... Cyanosis ....

Provisional diagnosis ....

....

Investigations

....

....

....

....

....

....

....

....

Clinical diagnosis ....

....

Treatment and progress

....

....

....

....

....

....

....

Signature .... Date ....

Table 1.4: Completion of hospital record

Fully cured, relieved of symptoms/signs ....

Complication/death ....

Postmortem examination report ....

Instructions to the patient at the time of discharge:

Schedule of medicines use ....

Precaution to be taken ....

Date of follow-up (check up) at the hospital/GP's clinic ....

Signature.. Date ....

Referral System

Instructions/information to GP about discharged patient:

Table 1.5: Referral system

Dear Dr...

Patient ....Attended A&E Department on ....

Diagnosis ....

Investigation..

Treatment given ....

....

....

....

Aftercare (follow up) ....

Yours sincerely

Signature.. Date ....

References

1. Hunter Donald, Bomford RR: Case Taking. Hutchison's Clinical Methods, Cassel, London; 1963.
2. Das K: General Scheme of Case–Taking. Clinical Methods in Surgery. Lakshman Chander Sil, Calcutta; 1961.
3. Hill, G: A&E risk management. Medical Defence Union, London; 1991.
4. Guly HR: History Taking, Examination, and Record Keeping in Emergency Medicine. Oxford University Press, Oxford; 1996.
5. United Kingdom Central Council (UKCC): Standards for records and record Keeping, pp. 15–16, April; 1993.

General Symptoms (Conditions)

- Fever
- Pain
- Shock syndrome

Fever

Definition	Fever is defined as an abnormal rise in the body temperature, i.e. of > 37.8°C (100°F).
Measurement	*Temperature:* Is measured with an instrument called thermometer. The temperature is recorded normally by inserting the thermometer in the mouth below the tongue or in the rectum in case of a younger child or an unconscious patient. The rectal temperature is about one degree higher than the oral one.
Temperature	Normal body temperature in adult – 37°C (98.6°F) and in child one degree above than that of an adult
Grades	Light – 37.8°C (100°F). Moderate – 38.9°C (102°F). High – 40.0°C (104°F).

Types of fever

Continuous type	Fever does not fluctuate > 1.5°F (1°C) during 24 hrs and does not touch the normal at any time.
Remittent type	Fluctuation >1°C (1.5°F) during 24 hrs.
Intermittent type	Fever present only for few hrs during 24 hrs.

Subtypes of intermittent fever

Quotidian: Fever occurring daily.

Tertian: Fever occurring on alternate days.

Quartan: Fever occurring after 2/7 days interval.

Ending of fever
- Resolve by crisis – fever ending rapidly.
- Resolve by lysis – fever ending gradually.

Etiology of fever
- Traumatic: Head injury, spinal cord injury, crush injuries, surgical trauma.

- Inflammatory: Acute osteomyelitis, acute appendicitis, acute pancreatitis, gastroenteritis, endocarditis.
- Infective: Viral, bacterial, rickettsial, parasitic, and fungal are the main causes of fever.
- Infections without local signs – septicemia.
- Infections with local signs – URC (pharyngitis, tonsillitis).
- Physical/chemical agents: Heat stroke, chemical poisoning, drugs
- Reactions: Anaesthesia reactions, serum sickness, IV fluids/blood transfusion reactions.
- Endocrinological: Hyperthyroidism.
- Neoplastic: Brain and spinal cord tumors, osteosarcomas, primary and secondary neoplasms of lungs, thyroid, liver, genitourinary tract.
- Pyrexia/fever of unknown origin (PUO/FUO) – mostly due to infections.

Diagnosis	History taking, examination, and investigations include X-rays, etc.
Management	
General measures	Rest, fluids – PO or parenteral, cold sponges therapy – ice bags alcohol sponging.
Drugs	Antipyretic drugs – aspirin 0.3–0.6 g 4–6 hrly. PO as per need
	– paracetamol 0.5–0.750 g 4–6 hrly. PO.

Specific measures: Removal of cause of fever.

Pain

Pain is one of the commonest symptom of visiting patients.

Etiology	• Traumatic: RSA, fall from a height, sports injury, surgical trauma.
	• Inflammatory: Appendicitis, pancreatitis, endocarditis, gastroenteritis, arthritis.
	• Cardiovascular: Angina, myocardial infarction.
	• Obstructive: Acute renal colic, acute cholecystitis, acute obstructive hernia.
	• Neoplastic: Primary and secondary neoplasms.
Management	Removal of the primary cause of pain.

Drugs
Analgesics, Antipyretics, Non-Steroid Anti-Inflammatory Drugs (NSAIDs)
A. Narcotic Analgesics (Opioids): Analgesic and sedative:

Morphine	Adult: 10–15 mg IV rept 4 hrly.	
	Children: 0.1–0.2 mg/kg/dose IM, IV, s.c. rept 4 hrly max 15 mg.	
C/I	Respiratory distress	
S/E	Nausea, vomiting, respiratory depression	
Antidote	Naloxone	Adult: 5–10 mg IV
		Children: 0.01 mg/kg IV

Codeine	Adult: 15–60 mg orally or hypodermically
	Children: For pain: 3 mg/kg/day PO. Rept. 4 hrly.
	For cough: 0.2 mg/kg/dose PO. Rept. 4 hrly.
C/I	Respiratory distress.
S/E	Nausea, vomiting, constipation.
Fentanyl	Adult: 50–200 μg/day, then 50 μg/day.
	Children: 0.5–5.0 μg/kg/dose IV or 1–5 μg/kg/hr infusion.
Pentazocine	Adult: 25–100 mg PO and 30–60 mg IM or IV Rept. 4 hrly.
	Children: 0.5–1.0 mg/kg/dose q.i.d. IM.
C/I	Head injury, raised intracranial pressure.
S/E	Nausea, vomiting, constipation.
Pethidine	Adult: 50–150 mg PO, IM or IV Rept. 4 hrly.
	Children: 1–2 mg/kg/dose IM or IV.
C/I	Hepatic dysfunction, raised intracranial pressure.
S/E	Addiction, respiratory depression, coma.
Tramadol	Adult: 50–100 mg b.d. PO and 50–100 mg IV, IM or s.c. Rept. 6 hrly.
C/I	Hypersensitivity, head injury, respiratory depression, CHF.
S/E	Nausea, vomiting, dizziness.

B. Non-narcotic Analgesics: Analgesics, Antipyretics, Anti-inflammatory: Salicylates

Aspirin, salicylamide, sodium salicylate

Dose	Acute rheumatic fever: Adult: 6–10 g/day in 6 divided doses PO.
	Children: 65–130 mg/kg/day in divided doses.
	Analgesic and antipyretic: Adult: 0.3–1.0 g every 3–4 hrly. PO.
	Children: 65 mg/kg/day in divided doses.
C/I	Peptic ulcer, GI tract lesions, lactation.
S/E	Nausea, vomiting, GI bleeding, hypersensitivity.

p-Aminophenols

Acetaminophen

Dose	0.5–1.0 g (up to 4.0 g) per day in divided doses.
C/I	Renal/or hepatic impairment.
S/E	Skin rashes, nausea, dyspepsia.

Paracetamol

Dose	Adult: 0.5–1.0 g 3–6 times/day PO.
	Children: 25–50 mg/kg/day in 4 divided doses.
C/I	Not recommended for infants.
S/E	Skin rashes, hepatotoxicity, renal damage.

NSAIDs Anti-inflammatory:
Propionic Acid Derivatives

Ibuprofen	Adult: 400–600 mg t.d.s. PO. Children: 20–30 mg/kg/day in 3 divided doses
Ketoprofen	Adult: 250 mg b.d. PO Children: 5 mg/kg/dose b.d.
Naproxen	Adult: 250 mg b.d. PO Children: 5 mg/kg/dose b.d.

Aryl Acetic Acid Derivatives

Diclofenac sodium	Adult: 25–50 mg IM b.d. PO. Children: 2–5 mg/kg/day.

Indole Derivatives

Indomethacin	Adult: 25 mg b.d. or t.d.s. PO. Children: 1–3 mg/kg/day orally in 3–4 divided doses.
Nimesulide	Adult:100 mg b.d. PO. Children: 5 mg/kg/day.
C/I	Not recommended for children below 5 yrs of age.
S/E	Hepatic enzyme elevation.
Piroxicam	Adult: 20 mg/day PO. Children: 0.2–0.3 mg/kg/day.
C/I	Not recommended for infants.
S/E	Nausea, vomiting, skin rashes.

Pyrazolones

Phenylbutazone	Adult: 100–200 mg t.d.s. PO. Children: Not recommended for children < 12 yrs.
Indications	Inflammatory conditions, i.e. gout, rheumatoid arthritis.
Colchicine	Adult: 1 mg followed by 0.5–1.0 mg every 2 hrs PO. Children: Not recommended for children < 12 yrs.
Indications	Gout, acute and chronic leukemia (antimitotic).

Muscle Relaxants (skeletal muscle relaxants antispasmodic):

Benzodiazepines	Diazepam and ketazolam.
Diazepam	Adult: 5–50 mg/ day PO, 10–20 mg IM, IV. Children: 0.1–0.5 mg/kg/dose IM, IV or 1 mg/year – max 10 mg. 0.1–0.8 mg/kg/day in divided doses PO.
C/I	Acute narrow angle glaucoma.
S/E	Nausea, vomiting, impaired alertness.
Carisoprodal (Carisoma)	Adult: 125–350 mg t.d.s. Children: Not recommended for children < 12 yrs.

C/I	Porphyria, pregnancy.
S/E	Nausea, drowsiness, headache.
Chlorzoxazone	Adult: 250–500 mg t.d.s.
	Children: Not recommended for children < 12 yrs.
C/I	Hypersensitivity.
S/E	Nausea, headache.
Methocarbamol	Adult: 750–1500 mg t.d.s.
	Children: Not recommended for children < 12 yrs.
C/I	Coma, epilepsy.
S/E	Drowsiness, allergy.

C. Local Analgesic Drugs

- Spinal subarachnoid block (spinal anesthetic): Drug – bupivacaine.
  Indication: TURF Prostate.
- Epidural analgesia:
  Indication: Postoperative pain relief.
  Day care surgery, e.g. circumcision, anal surgery
- Intercostal block
  Indication: Chest injury – for pain relief.
  Nerve blocks (femoral and sciatic nerve).
  Indication : Orthopedic procedures.

D. Inhalation Methods (Nitrous Oxide + Oxygen)

Indication: Postoperative – short procedures, e.g. dressings.
Physiotherapy.

E. Transcutaneous Electrical Nerve Stimulation

Indication: Postoperative pain relief.

F. Cryotherapy

Indication: Short procedures, e.g. removal of cervical polyp, tumours.

Shock Syndrome

Definition	Shock is a complex syndrome caused by many unrecognized factors. It is a threat to existence, and requires top priority (life-saving measures) treatment.
Classification	Depending upon cause and mechanism, shock syndrome is classified into following:

Neurogenic Shock (Vasovagal)

Etiology	Neurological or psychological factors, i.e. fright, pain, violence, spinal cord injury, drugs.
Mechanism	Decrease in the circulating blood volume, resulting in pooling of blood in the skeletal muscles (of limbs) and dilated splanchnic areas, leading to

low cardiac output, hypotension, until spontaneous recovery by peripheral vasoconstriction, but persistence of the condition, may lead to syncope and death.

Diagnosis	Patient may be unconscious.
	Air hunger.
	Skin – cold, clamy, pale.
	Tachycardia.
	Hypotension.
Management	Aim is to increase the circulating blood volume and to decrease the pooled blood volume by restoring it back into active circulation. It is achieved by:

- Position of patient: Trendelenburg position.
- Oxygen therapy.

Drugs   Vasoconstrictor drugs to be given in early stage, if given late, may cause renal and hepatic failure (leading to death) due to prolonged vasoconstriction.

- Methamphetamine (methedrine) 15 mg/L of IV fluid
- Hydrocortisone sodium succinate 100 mg may be added to the IV fluid, if required, as per the response.

Traumatic Shock (Oligemic/hemorrhagic/surgical shock)

Etiology   Direct violence – external injuries.

Indirect violence – internal injuries, i.e. chest, abdominal and pelvic injuries.

Bleeding peptic ulcer – bleeding piles (hemorrhoids).

Burns – loss of plasma.

Mechanism   Hemorrhage results in oligemia, low cardiac output, and compensatory vasoconstriction (preserving the function of vital structures, i.e. brainstem and heart) of splanchnic and hepatic areas along with skeletal muscles and skin. Failure of this compensatory vasoconstriction leads to systemic collapse, hypotension, low cardiac output, followed by systemic disturbances – low RBC count, increase in WBC count, anoxia, and finally death.

Investigation Hemogram – RBCs count, Hb, TLC and DLC.

Serum albumin/globulin – ratio is reduced.

Serum proteins – fall below 5 gm/100 ml – may lead to a critical state.

Serum and chloride – excretion lowered, potassium – excretion increased.

Hyperglycemia.

Urea – excretion increased.

Management
- Position of patient – Trendelenburg position.
- Bed rest.
- Morphine 10–20 mg IV. Contraindicated in head injuries, because of the respiratory depression. Alternatively given:
- Pentazocine (fortwin) 50–100 mg IV.

- Arrest of hemorrhage.
- Blood transfusion.
- Overheating is harmful.
- Oxygen therapy.

Burns Shock Due to plasma loss from the burnt tissues.
Management
- Removal of cause
- Replacement of plasma loss by:
  – Plasma or plasma expanders IV.
- Fluids IV.
- Antibiotics.
- Analgesics.

Septic Shock Due to toxemia, is characterized by vasoconstriction, followed by dilatation.
Organisms
- Gram-negative organisms, e.g. *E. coli*, *Proteus*, *Pseudomonas*.
- Gram-positive organisms, e.g. *Staphylococcus*, clostridia.
Diagnosis   Fever with chills, hypotension, respiratory alkalosis.
Investigation   TLC and DLC: Leukopenia followed by leukocytosis.
                Blood culture.
                Urine culture.
Management
- Antibiotics.
- Analgesics.
- Fluids IV.
- Blood transfusion.
- Debridement of affected tissues.

Cardiogenic Shock Due to inefficiency of the left ventricle, to maintain an adequate cardiac output.
Etiology   Left ventricular failure – due to myocardial infarction (MI).
                Ventricular arrhythmias.
                Cardiac tamponade.
                Pulmonary embolism.
                Congestive heart failure.
Management   Treatment of the cause.

Metabolic Shock Due to disturbed biochemical and hormonal balance.
Etiology   Diabetic acidosis.
                Uremia.
Management   Treatment of the cause.

Anaphylactic Shock Due to induced hypersensitivity.
Etiology   Reaction to drugs or sera or rarely with certain food items.
                Bee/wasp stings.

Mechanism	Laryngeal edema, bronchospasm, and shock.
Diagnosis	Restlessness, chocking sensation, wheezing, cough, fever, urticaria, edema, loss of consciousness, shock, death.
Management	Is a life-threatening emergency – that requires an urgent and energetic care of laryngeal edema, bronchospasm, and hypotension, e.g.

- Airway maintenance.
- Endotracheal intubation.
- Oxygen therapy: 4–6 L/mt.

Drugs	Inj. epinephrine 0.5–1.0 mL of 1:1000 sol IM or IV. Rept. every 10 mts.
	Inj. pheniramine 22.75 (1 mL) o.d. or b.d. IM.
	Inj. aminophylline 250–500 mg IV.

References

1. Chatton MJ: General Symptoms. Current Medical Diagnosis and Treatment. Mauzen Asian Edition, Tokyo; 1975.
2. Goodman LS, Gilman A: The Pharmacology Basis of Therapeutics. 2nd ed. The MacMillan Co. New York; 1960.
3. Hunter D, Bomford RR: Hutchison's Clinical Methods, 14th ed., Cassel, London; 1964.
4. Arora V: Drug Update. Vol 7, No. 2, Jaipur; 2010.
5. Gulhati CM: MIMS. Vol. 30 No. 5, New Delhi; 2010.

Part II   Medical Emergencies

Cardiovascular System Emergencies and Common Disorders

Signs and symptoms (non-specific manifestations)

Cardiovascular disease (CVD)

- Dyslipidemia
- Chest pain
- Angina pectoris
- Acute coronary syndromes (ACS)
- Acute myocardial infarction
- Stokes-Adams Syndrome
- Acute pericarditis with effusion (cardiac tamponade)
- Acute pulmonary edema
- Acute myocarditis
- Arrhythmias:
  - Bradyarrhythmia:
    ◊ Sinus bradycardia
  - Tachyarrhythmias:
    ◊ Supraventricular tachycardia
    ◊ Sinus tachycardia
    ◊ Inappropriate sinus tachycardia
    ◊ Paroxysmal supraventricular tachycardia (PSVT)
    ◊ Ventricular tachycardia (VT)
    ◊ Ventricular flutter and ventricular fibrillation (VT)
    ◊ Atrial flutter
    ◊ Atrial fibrillation (AF)
- Acquired heart diseases
  ◊ Acute rheumatic fever
  ◊ Rheumatic heart disease (syn. rheumatic valvulities)
  ◊ Acute bacterial endocarditis (ABE) (syn. subacute bacterial endocarditis)

Hypertension

- Antihypertensive drugs
- Hypertension crisis (emergencies and urgencies)
- Patient specific antihypertensive selection

Cardiac arrest

- Cardiopulmonary resuscitation (CPR)
- Basic life support (BLS)
- Advanced life support (ALS)
- Resuscitation in trauma

Congestive heart failure

Peripheral vascular disease (PVD)

Deep vein thrombosis (DVT)

Cardiovascular drugs

Practical procedures:

- ECG
- Ambulatory ECG monitoring
- Pericardiocentesis
- Cardiac catheterization
- Angiocardiography
- New imaging techniques:
  - Ultrasonography (US)
  - Computed tomography (CT) scan
  - Magnetic resonance imaging (MRI)
  - Nuclear medicine procedures
- X-ray chest (CXR) – PA view
  - Balloon angioplasty
  - Atherectomy
  - Stent angioplasty
  - Thrombectomy and embolectomy
  - Endarterectomy
  - Bypass surgery
  - Coronary artery bypass surgery

Signs and Symptoms (Non-specific Manifestations)

1. Dyspnea
2. Chest pain
3. Palpitation
4. Fatigue
5. Edema feet
6. Cyanosis
7. Murmurs
8. Growing pains

Dyspnea	Due to cardiovascular disorder, usually associated with heart enlargement and anatomical or physiological changes.
Types	Exertional dyspnea – commonest type, due to exertion, relieved by rest.
Etiology	Cardiovascular disorders.
	Non-cardiac causes: Poor physique, obesity, old age, anemia.
	Deflected nasal septum (DNS).

Orthopnea	Dyspnea in recumbency, relieved by sitting up.
Etiology	Obesity, abdominal distension.

Paroxysmal Nocturnal Dyspnea	Awakens the patient suddenly, forcing him/her to sit/stand up for relief.
Etiology	Cardiovascular disorders – Left ventricular failure (LVF)
	Non-cardiac disorders – Bronchial asthma.
	– Airway obstruction.

Chest Pain	One of the commonest presenting symptoms. May reflect life-threatening disorder. Triage patients with chest pain as urgent, to be examined and managed on priority basis.
Etiology	Cardiovascular disorders.
	Non-cardiac disorders.

Palpitation	Awareness of forceful/irregular thump.
Etiology	Anxiety, anemia, thyrotoxicosis.
Types	Sinus tachycardia – due to exertion, excitement.
	Paroxysmal tachycardia – fluttering sensation.
	Paroxysmal atrial fibrillation – pounding sensation.

Fatigue	Easy fatigue, relieved by rest.
Etiology	Cardiovascular disorders – Congestive heart failure
	– Cor pulmonale
	– Hypertension

Non-cardiac disorders – Anemia
                       – Chronic infections
                       – Diabetes
                       – Neoplastic

Edema Feet Appears in ankles, legs, sacrum, buttocks.

Etiology   Cardiovascular: Congestive heart failure.

               Non-cardiac : Obesity, wearing of garters, stockings, premenstrual syndrome, nephritis, anemia, malnutrition syndrome.

Cyanosis   Types: Central and peripheral.

Central cyanosis Due to low arterial oxygen saturation.

Etiology   Cardiovascular: Right-left shunts, AV fistula

               Non-cardiac: Pneumonia, polycythemia vera.

Peripheral   Appears in the presence of normal arterial oxygen saturation, characterized
cyanosis   by cold clammy hands due to slow peripheral circulation.

Etiology   Cardiovascular: Reduced cardiac output due to:
                            MS, pulmonary stenosis, CHF
               Non-cardiac: Exposure to cold, nervous tension.

Murmurs

Types   Systolic murmurs: AS – mid-systolic ejection murmur
                            MR – pansystolic apical murmur
         Diastolic murmurs: MS – mid-diastolic (short) murmur
                            AR – early diastolic murmur
         Tricuspid murmurs: Tricuspid stenosis and incompetence.

Growing Pains Rheumatic fever.

Cardiovascular Disease (CVD)

Cardiovascular disease (CVD) is a major cause of global morbidity and mortality. Majority of individuals who develop heart attacks and strokes repeatedly every year, have one or more cardiovascular risk factors.

Types of CVD The cardiovascular diseases (CVD) include abnormal conditions of the heart, arteries and veins, which supply oxygen to the vital life-sustaining body organs, e.g. brain, heart itself, and other vital organs.

Common CVD
- Angina pectoris.
- Acute coronary syndrome.
- Acute myocardial infarction .
- Heart attack.
- Hypertension.
- Stroke.
- Transient ischemic attack (TIA).

Risk factors
- Dyslipidemia
- Faulty food, e.g. fatty, fried, fast food, added salt.
- Physical inactivity.
- Diabetes.
- Smoking – tobacco use.
- Alcohol abuse.

Management

Prevention　Most of these CVD events are preventable, if purposeful action taken against these risk factors.

Treatment　Of the cause.

Dyslipidemia

Etiology
- Obesity and over weight
- Physical inactivity
- Diabetes mellitus
- Elevated triglycerides
- Smoking of cigarette
- Alcohol abuse
- High carbohydrate diet.
- Drugs – Bêta blockers, anabolic steroids.

Diagnosis
- Hypertriglyceridemia
- High levels of low-density lipoprotein cholesterol (LDL-C)
- Low levels of high-density lipoprotein cholesterol (HDL-C)
- Diabetic dyslipidemia

Investigation　Lipid profile – triglycerides, cholesterol total, LDL-C, HDL-C, Apolipoprotein. Lipoprotein evaluation. CBC and ESR.

Management

Preventive
- Regular exercise
- Avoid carbohydrate rich diet
- Avoid smoking cigarettes
- Restrict alcohol consumption.

Drugs　Lipid lowering agents:
- Statins – reduce LDL-C and triglycerids:
  - Atorvastatin 40–80 mg o.d. PO, Alt:
  - Simvastatin 5–40 mg o.d. PO, Alt:
  - Pravastatin 10–40 mg o.d. PO, Alt:
  - Others: Lovastatin, fluvastatin

S/E: Headache, constipation, myalgias.

Niacin – reduce LDL-C and triglycerides and increases HDL-C.
Dose: 0.5–1.0 g t.d.s. PO.
S/E: Flushing, nausea.

Fibrates – reduce triglycerides and increases HDL-C.
- Gemfibrozil 0.6 g b.d. PO, Alt:
- Others: Benzafibrate, fenofibrate, clofibrate

S/E: Nausea, vomiting, diarrhea, pain abdomen.

Combination drug therapy: More effective esp. for high-risk patients, e.g. **statin + niacin and statin + fibrate**.

Chest Pain

Chest pain is one of the most common presenting complaints of patients visiting accident and emergency medicine unit of the hospital.

Etiology

1. Cardiovascular disorders:

Angina pectoris
Myocardial infarction
Pulmonary embolism
Aortic dissection or aneurysm
Pericardial effusion or tamponade
Myocarditis.

2. Non-cardiac disorders:

Often associated with chest pain that resembles/indistinguishable from that of cardiac disorder, e.g.
Cervical spondylosis
Periarthritis left shoulder
Costochondritis
Muscle pull, myositis
Prolapsed disc
Neuralgia, root compression
Oesophagitis
Hiatus hernia
Hyperacidity, peptic ulcer
Pancreatitis
Cholecystitis
Pneumonia
Emotional disorders, anxiety
Herpes zoster.

Diagnosis   History of:
- Heart attack
- Angina
- Stroke
- TIA
- Heart failure

- Peripheral vascular disease
- Smoking of tobacco
- Alcohol abuse
- Family history of premature CVD.

Examination   Careful clinical evaluation includes:
- Inquiry concerning its quality, site, radiation, duration, and the factors that precipitate, aggravate, or relieve it.
- Examine for any apex heaving
- Measure BMI or waist circumference
- Repeat examinations are often required.

Investigations
- Complete hemogram
- Serum creatinine
- Serum electrolytes
- FBS
- Total cholesterol
- Low density lipoprotein (LDL-C) cholesterol
- High density lipoprotein (HDL-C) cholesterol
- Urine albumin
- ECG – 12 lead: Normal to ST elevation
- Exercise tests: Tread mill test (TMT) – in a normal ECG case
- CXR
- Ultrasound
- Angiography – is of great value: Diagnostic and therapeutic
- Fundus examination – for hypertensive diabetic retinopathy.

Management   Admit the patient

Refer: The patient to the medical team for management of the underlying cause.

Angina Pectoris

Definition   Is defined as chest pain on exertion (relieves on rest) which might radiate to neck, shoulder, arm, and back.

Types   Stable angina – due to atherosclerotic plaques in the coronary artery
Unstable angina – due to plaque's rupture in the coronary artery.

Etiology
- Coronary artery disease (CAD) due to arteriosclerosis, is usually the cause.
- Aortic stenosis (AS) or aortic insufficiency (AI)
- Syphylitic aortitis
- Pulmonary stenosis
- Hyperthyroidism
- Anemia.

Risk factors
- Fried, fatty, fast food, added salt
- Physical inactivity, obesity and over weight
- Smoking

- Alcohol abuse
- Hypertension
- Diabetes
- Excitement, anger, emotional disorders.

Pathogenesis A disturbed balance between the myocardial requirement for oxygen and the amount supplied by the coronary arteries, resulting in the myocardial ischemia. There may be:

A. Restricted oxygen supply by the coronary arteries due to:
- Blood vessel disorders, e.g. atherosclerotic narrowing, deficient collateral circulation, reflex narrowing – due to stress, fear, cold, smoking, alcohol abuse.
- Blood disorders, e.g. anemia, hypoxemia, polycythemia.
- Circulatory disorders, e.g. hypotension due to arrhythmias, bleeding, aortic stenosis or insufficiency.

B. Increased cardiac output due to:
- Exertion, stress, strong emotions, anxiety, undigestion, anemia, thyrotoxicosis.

C. Increased myocardial requirement for oxygen due to:
- Increased heart work, e.g. aortic stenosis/insufficiency, hypertension, thyrotoxicosis, hypoglycemia.

Diagnosis History: Inquire about:
- Any pain/discomfort/or any pressure/heaviness in the chest?
- Site of pain, e.g. is it retrosternal or slightly to the left?
- Radiation of pain – is it referred to neck, shoulder, arm or back?
- Quality of pain, e.g. is it squeezing or pressure-like pain?
- Exertion (walk uphill/or in hurry) any relation with appearance of pain?
- Any relief – by taking rest?
- Any use of drugs for relief?

S/S Is not a disease but a symptom – chest pain.

Chest pain:
- On exertion
- Relieves on rest
- Squeezing (feeling of constriction in chest) or pressure-like pain
- Retrosternal or slightly to the left
- Radiates to neck, shoulder, arm, and back.

Signs of diseases precipitating arteriosclerotic cardiac disorder:
- Diabetes mellitus (retinopathy or neuropathy).

Investigation
- CBC – to evaluate for anemia
- Hemogram
- Blood cholesterol – hypercholesterolemia

- LDL and HDL
- Serum creatinine
- Serum electrolytes
- Serum proteins
- Cardiac enzymes
- BUN
- Blood sugar
- Thyroid function tests
- Fundus examination – for hypertensive retinopathy, if BP:
    Systolic > 180 or diastolic > 110
- Urine for albumin
- CXR
- ECG: Holter monitoring (continuous monitoring)
    Normal in 25% of angina patients
    Abnormal in 75%, e.g. – AV/or IV conduction defects
        – left ventricular hypertrophy
        – MI (old)
- TMT: Majority of cases have diagnostic ECG abnormalities after mild exercise.
- Echocardiography (ultrasound) is of great value in diagnosing pericardial effusion, valvular disease, cardiomyopathy and estimates sizes of the septum, atrium, and ventricular walls.

Angiography: Is of great value in outlining the anatomical information of heart and coronary arteries, degree of valvular insufficiencies, and assessing left ventricular function. Also it helps in diagnosing the extent of coronary lesion, e.g. whether the stenosis involves 1, 2 or all 3 coronary arteries/or main left coronary artery.

Cardiac catheterization: Is of great value in determining pressures within heart and great vessels, types and origions of arrhythmias, to assess oxygen saturation, to image the anatomy of heart and blood flow in vessels, to perform angioplasty and valvuloplasty, and to perform intravascular ultrasound to assess arterial narrowing.

Management

Treatment of acute attack

- Admit the patient immediately
- Complete rest during the attack (sit/or lie down)
- Avoid work during the attack
- Establish IV lines
- Attach cardiac monitor and pulse oximeter to the patient.

Drugs

Aspirin, nitrates, heparin, beta-blockers, calcium channel blockers.

Anti-anginals:

- Nitrates:
    - Nitroglycerine (glyceryl trinitrate) is the drug of choice.

Acts (coronary vasodilatation) in about 1–2 min.

As soon as the attack begins, place 1 tab (0.5 mg) under the tongue

If little or no relief, then increase the dose to 1.0 mg, Alt.:

IV nitroglycerine – quite effective

Dose: 5 μg/min. Rept. 5 μg/min increments till chest pain relieved

S/E: Headache and hypotension.

- Isosorbide dinitrate – indicated if nitroglycerine not effective.

Dose: 5–10 mg sublingually.

- Amyl nitrite – crush a pearl and inhale the vapor. Acts in 10–30 sec

S/E: Headache, flushes, dizziness, pounding of the pulse.

- Antiplatelets:
  - Aspirin is most preffered choice and to be given ASAP

    Dose: 150–300 mg o.d. PO. Alt.:
  - Clopidogrel – given to aspirin sensitive patients.

    Dose: 75 mg o.d. PO
- Anticoagulants:
  - Heparin – low molecular weight heparin for 3–5 days to maintain PT.
  - Enoxaparin 1 mg/kg (100 units/kg) s.c. b.i.d., Alt.
  - Dalteparin 1 mg/kg (100 units/kg) s.c. b.i.d.
- Beta-blockers: Reduce myocardial oxygen demand (by reducing heart rate and myocardial contractility).
  - Metoprolol 50–100 mg b.i.d. PO

    S/E: Headache, hypotension, fatigue. Alt:
  - Propranolol 40 mg b.i.d., up to 40 mg q.d.s. PO

    S/E: Headache, nausea, hypotension. Alt:
  - Atenolol 50 mg o.d., up to 100 mg o.d. PO

    S/E: Headache, indigestion, hypotension
- ACE-inhibitors:
  - Enalapril 5 mg o.d., up to 40 mg o.d. PO

    S/E: Headache, nausea, hypotension
- Ca-channel blockers:
  - Verapamil 30 mg t.d.s., up to 60 mg t.d.s. PO

    S/E: Headache, nausea, vomiting. Alt:
  - Nifedipine 30 mg t.d.s., up to 120 mg o.d. PO

    S/E: Headache, flushes, edema. Alt:
  - Diltiazem 30 mg b.i.d./or q.d.s. PO

    S/E: Bradycardia, headache, dizziness. Alt:
  - Amlodipine besylate 5.0 mg o.d., up to 10 mg o.d. PO

    S/E: Headache, nausea, pain abdomen.

General measures

Avoid   Fried, fatty, fast food and added salt

Smoking, alcohol

Obesity and overweight, physical inactivity.

Control/treat: Hypertension, diabetes, anemia, hyperlipidemia.

Refer: The patient to the cardiac team for management of the case.

Prognosis   Depends upon:
- Whether single, double or triple coronary artery disease (as revealed by coronary angiography)
- Associated following disorders – if present along with angina, e.g.
  - Ischemic changes (as revealed by ECG)
  - Hypertension – causing myocardial hypertrophy
  - LVF
  - Diabetes mellitus
  - Arrhythmias.

Acute Coronary Syndromes (ACS)

Definition   Acute coronary syndrome encompasses a spectrum of patients who present with chest discomfort or other symptoms caused by myocardial ischemia. This refers to a syndrome intermediate between the angina pectoris of effort and acute myocardial infarction in the spectrum of clinical events that occur in coronary heart disease.

Etiology   Coronary artery disease (CAD).

Risk factors   Family history, smoking, diabetes, hypertension, hyperlipidemia.

Diagnosis   Chest pain – of different character, duration, radiation, severity, or of occurrence at rest or during night.

Dyspnea, diaphoresis, nausea, and/or vomiting

Syncope, mental status change, weakness, stroke

Patients are considered to be in precarious balance between coronary supply and demand.

Triage   Clinical points favoring cardiac pain:
- Retrosternal pain, that may refer to the neck, jaw or arm and wrist, most often on the left side
- Sweating
- Feeling – of tightening, squeezing or constricting across chest
- Provoked – by stress or exertion
- Relieved by rest or NTG

Clinical points favoring non-cardiac pain:
- Myalgia – of chest wall muscles, reproduced by localized pressure
- Localized to region below left nipple or radiating to right lower chest
- Pain – momentary or for few seconds
- Pain provoked – by emotional feelings – sighing or depression.

Investigation   • CBC
- Lipid profile – total blood cholesterol, triglycerides, LDL-C, HDL-C.

- ECG (12 lead): ST-segment elevation, especially if resolves with resolution of chest pain, strongly suggests acute ischemia.

  D/d: ST-segment elevation may be considered for alternative diagnosis, e.g. pericarditis, and left ventricular aneurysm

Biochemical cardiac markers:
- Elevated creatine kinase MB band (CK-MB), troponin I and troponin T,
- Myoglobin: An early cardiac marker of myonecrosis.

Coronary angiography: Early angiography provides a far better delineation of coronary artery pathology and subsequent management.

Management	Risk of mortality rises with delayed treatment.

Clinical opinion must be made immediately as per ECG.

If symptoms have been continuous for > 20 min, then:

UA/NSTEMI/ STEMI, must be considered.

Refer: The patient to the cardiac team for management of the case.

General principles

Urgent admission in CCU

Establish IV lines

Oxygen therapy – for hypoxemia only

ECG monitoring

Aspirin 150–300 mg PO, unless C/I by hypersensitivity

Pain relief – achieved by nitroglycerin, but is mostly guaranteed with morphine.

Medical intervention

Anti-ischemic therapy

Aim	To decrease or abort myocardial ischemia.
Drugs	• Nitroglycerin – reduces preload and myocardial oxygen consumption.

Dose: Three 0.5 mg tablets taken sublingually at 5 min intervals along with beta-blocker IV.

Failure to improve: Continuous infusion IV nitroglycerin 10 μg/mt, with 10 μg increases every 3–5 min.

Partial response: Reduce the dose or lengthen the interval. Alt:

- Morphine (anxiolytic and analgesic) only indicated for patients who fail to respond to nitroglycerin.
- Beta-blockers – reduce myocardial oxygen consumption through their negative inotropic effects.

  To start with IV, followed by oral therapy

  Beta-blocker may reduce progression from ACS to MI by 13%

  C/I: AV block, asthma, LV dysfunction with CHF
- Calcium antagonists may be appropriate for recurrent ischemia. They inhibit myocardial and vascular smooth muscle contraction, and share coronary dilatory properties.

  S/E: Hypotension, CHF, AV block, bradycardia.

Antithrombotic therapy

Aim	Inhibition of clot formation and propagation (clot lysis or destruction).
Types	Anticoagulant, thrombolytic and antiplatelet therapy.

Anticoagulant therapy

Drugs
- Heparin – most used anticoagulant.
  Action: Indirect thrombin inhibitor (antithrombin-III)
  Therapy: Unfractionated IV heparin or s.c. low molecular weight heparin.
- Hirudin – has a predictable dose response. Is expensive.
  Action: Direct thrombin inhibitor (does not require antithrombin-III).

Thrombolytic therapy

Action   Thrombolytic agents can reduce mortality for MI by up to 50% when given during initial phase, e.g. within first hr. of onset of symptoms.

Drugs
- Tissue plasminogen activator (TPA): Superior IRA patency and TIMI flow rates. Dose: 100 mg IV over 3 hrs.
  C/I: Hypertension, CVH, ulcerative colitis.
- Streptokinase 1.5 million units/dL IV over an hr.
  C/I: Pregnancy
- Urokinase 6000 i.u./min IV infusion (saline or 5% dextrose)
  C/I: GItract or Utract hemorrhage.

Antiplatelet therapy

1st generation platelet inhibitors:

Action   Inhibit the activity of cyclo-oxygenase in all body cells.

Drugs
- Aspirin – as an antiplatelet. Aspirin (the first choice) to be given as soon as possible. Aspirin – is an important and inexpensive therapy and to be given in all patients
  Dose: 150–300 mg o.d. PO unless contraindicated, e.g. history of aspirin sensitivity.

2nd generation platelet inhibitors:

Action   Inhibit the ADP receptor on the platelet surface and do not interfere with the cyclo-oxygenase pathway inhibition by aspirin.

Drugs   Ticlopidine – prolongs BT > that of aspirin.
Clopidogrel

3rd generation platelet inhibitors:

Action   Inhibit the fibrinogen receptor on the platelet.

Drugs   Glycoprotein
IIb/IIIa-receptor antagonists.

Surgical treatment

Surgical measures: Coronary revascularization (interventional) procedures:
- Coronary angioplasty

- Percutaneous transluminal coronary angioplasty (PTCA)
- Percutaneous transluminal myocardial revascularization (PTMR)
- Coronary artery bypass grafting (CABG).

Coronary Angioplasty

Strongly improved by the use of better balloon technology, better stents, better antiplatelet therapy.

Indication   Symptomatic ischemic heart disease
Acute myocardial infarction.

Percutaneous Transluminal Coronary Angioplasty (PTCA)

Indication
- As an alternative to thrombolytic therapy in patients with AMI and ST segment elevation or new or presumed new LBBB.
- Patients who are within 36 hrs ST elevation/Q wave or new LBBB MI who develop cardiogenic shock are:
- Age < 75 yrs.
- Recurrent angina
- Spontaneous silent ischemia
- Stress-induced myocardial ischemia.

Percutaneous Transmyocardial Revascularisation (PTMR) with Laser

Indication
- CAD – not amenable to available coronary revascularization methods, e.g. angioplasty or coronary bypass surgery.
- CAD – not controlled by drugs
- Ischemic myocardium
- Severe angina.

Disadvantage   Very few hospitals have the resources to perform PTCA and PTMR.

Coronary Artery Bypass Graft (CABG)

Indications
Clinical indications
- Angina – unstable
- Angina – unresponsive to medical therapy
- Angina – post infarction
- Acute ischemia
- Acute MI (evolving)
- Acute MI – causing cardiogenic shock
- Pulmonary edema–ischemic
- MI – mechanical complication.

Anatomic/physiologic indications
- CAD – left main stenosis > 50%
- Tripple vessel disease – with impaired LV function

- Tripple vessel disease – with normal LV function but inducible ischemia on physiologic testing
- Two vessel disease – with significant proximal LAD stenosis
- PTCA failure
- VSD–severely depressed LV function with reversible ischemia
- Positive stress test–with angiographic abnormalities prior to major
- Non-cardiac procedure.

Technique	Bypass surgery has become very sophisticated over the past decade. The surgery is done on a beating heart through a 15 cm incision with the patient getting back to normal within three weeks. Robotic bypass–is done through three 2.5 cm incisions.
Disadvantage	Cost factor
Conduits	Greater saphenous vein graft (SVG) – conduit of choice for most surgeons, although results of long-term patency of SVG are not encouraging. Other grafts: Internal mammary artery graft – is the current conduit of choice–long-term patency 95% at 10 yrs Radial artery graft – 2nd conduit of choice Right gastroepiploic artery graft 90% at 5 yrs.
Objective	Improvement in long-term survival is the main objective of CABG and has been documented in several studies.

Acute Myocardial Infarction (AMI)

Definition	Acute myocardial infarction (AMI) is a very commonly encountered, life-threatening medical emergency. It is the leading cause of death in western countries. An early and correct diagnosis is important in order to initiate the treatment ASAP. While drugs are beneficial in stabilizing these patients, the crux of matter is institution of early and definitive revascularization of blocked artery. Primary PCI is the preferred mode of achieving revascularization.
Etiology	Coronary artery disease (CAD) due to: Blockage of a coronary artery by – Thrombus formation – Hemorrhage – subintimal.
Pathogenesis	Pathologically, MI reflects death of cardiac myocytes due to prolonged ischemia. CAD results in ischemic necrosis of a localized area of myocardium, may be anterior or posterior infarction. The size and site of infarction depend upon the affected coronary and functioning of collateral circulation. Ventricular remodeling starts immediately after MI.
Risk factors	• Fried, fatty, fast food, and added salt • Physical inactivity, obesity and overweight • Hypertension • Diabetes • Smoking cigarettes • Alcohol abuse.

Diagnosis	• Chest pain:

      – Character: Similar to angina in site and radiation, but more severe

      – Severity: Pain often unbearable

      – Rest: – No relief on rest,

             – Pain appears suddenly or builds up in a short time

             – Nitroglycerin has no effect.

• Dyspnea, orthopnea, cough, wheezing
• Nausea, vomiting, abdominal discomfort
• Fever
• Cold clammy skin
• Cyanosis
• Engorged (full) neck veins
• Tachycardia, or bradycardia
• Pulse – weak
• Hypotension – systolic BP < 80 mm Hg
• Heart sounds – faint
• Shock – due to severe pain
• Sudden death – usually due to ventricular fibrillation.

Investigation
• Hemogram
• ESR – rising
• TLC and DLC – leukocytosis
• Blood grouping
• Platelets count, BT, CT, PT
• AST (SGOT) – elevated
• ALT (SGPT) – elevated
• BUN
• Serum creatinine
• Serum electrolytes
• Blood sugar – fasting, PP
• Total cholesterol, LDL and HDL
• FBS (fasting blood sugar)
• Cardiac enzymes (CK, LDH) rise within 24 hrs and fall by 72 hrs
• ECG: Do not correlate well with severity of infarction
    – Anterior infarction:
      Abnormal Q wave
      Loss of R wave
      Elevation of ST segment and T wave in lead I and chest leads facing right ventricle
    – Posterior infarction:
      Abnormal Q wave
      Elevation of ST segment and T wave in leads III and IV.

D/d
Acute Pulmonary Embolism
- Chest pain – similar to that in myocardial infarction
- Dyspnea
- Hypotension
- Engorged neck veins
- ECG – right axis deviation or right ventricular conduction defect
- SGOT, CPK, LDH, are elevated.

Acute Cervical Spondylosis
- Chest pain – similar in myocardial infarction
- ECG – normal
- X-ray cervical spine – confirms diagnosis.

Hiatus Hernia
- Chest pain – similar in myocardial infarction
- ECG – T wave may be flat or inverted during attack.

Acute Pancreatitis and Acute Cholecystitis
- Findings per abdomen
- Jaundice
- Serum amylase – elevated
- X-ray (plane) abdomen and ultrasound – confirm diagnosis
- ECG – normal

Pneumothorax
Mediastinal Emphysema.
Complications:

CHF and Shock   May be present at the beginning of infarction or may develop following some arrhythmia or pulmonary embolism.

S/S
- Dyspnea, orthopnea – may be marked by sedation and weakness
- Engorged neck veins, edema legs
- Liver – enlarged, tender
- CXR – reveal pulmonary congestion.

Arrhythmias   Occur commonly after myocardial infarction:
- Sinus bradycardia
- Ventricular tachycardia
- Ventricular fibrillation: Main cause of sudden death in MI patients. Mostly ventricular fibrillation appears as a primary event
- Suprventricular tachycardias – sinus tachycardia
- Atrial flutter and atrial fibrillation: Less common and often transient

CVA   May result from:
- Hypotension
- Thromboembolism

Shoulder Hand Syndrome   Early pain and tenderness over the affected shoulder, followed by pain and swelling of the hand.

Oliguria, or Anuria – due to shock's persistence.

Management

Aims
- Main aim in the management of AMI is to prevent death
- Desirable – treatment modalities that aim to minimize the patient's discomfort and distress and to restrict the extent of myocardial damage.

Time frame of treatment divided into 4 phases:

Phase I   Emergency (immediate) treatment includes:

Early diagnosis, relief of pain and preventing and managing sudden cardiac arrest.

Phase II   Prehospital/early in-hospital treatment includes:

Restoring coronary flow and myocardial tissue reperfusion: Restoration of blood flow either with early mechanical/pharmacological reperfusion is the most beneficial intervention.

Phase III   Late in-hospital treatment includes:

Early diagnosis, long-term drug therapy and management of late mechanical complications.

Phase IV   Long-term treatment includes:

Risk evaluation and steps to prevent progression of CAD, development of new infarction, heart failure and death.

Measures:

General:
- Admit the patient to **coronary care unit (CCU)** as soon as possible to reduce the mortality rate, due to availability of pacemaker, suscitation equipment and specially trained staff.
- Rest: Complete bedrest is essential, especially during first week, to control the increasing size of the infarct and for healing of infracted myocardium.
- Oxygen – by facemask or nasal prongs.
  Oxygen (reduces area of ischemia) therapy (2–5 L/mt) for relief of dyspnea, cyanosis, shock, chest pain, and pulmonary edema
- Attach cardiac monitor
- IV access.

Drugs   Analgesics: For severe pain, give:
- Nitrates: Nitroglycerin 0.3 mg sublingual prior to morphine, relives or diminishes chest discomfort.
  C/I: Hypotension
- Morphine: Diamorphine 4–8 mg IV, with additional doses of 2 mg at intervals of 5 mts., if pain is not relieved. Care should be taken of respiratory rate, nausea, vomiting, and hypotension.
- Mepridine hydrochloride (pethidine) 50–100 mg IV. Less nausea and vomiting.
- Aminophylline 0.5 g IV given very slowly, if pain not relieved by morphine, etc.
- Beta blockers: Relieve pain by reducing myocardial oxygen consumption.

- Metoprolol 5 mg IV every 5–10 mts, gradually increasing doses up to 50 mg o.d.
  C/I: Heart failure, heart block, hypotension, LVD.

Revascularization (Reperfusion): Pharmacologically or mechanically:

Pharmacological Revascularization

Thrombolysis Thrombolytic agents: Can reduce mortality for MI by up to 50% when given during initial phase, e.g. within first hour of onset of symptoms.

- Tissue plasminogen activator (tPA): Superior IRA patency and TIMI flow rates
- Streptokinase 1.5 million units/dL IV over an hr.
- UFH 5000 IU as initial bolus IV, followed by continuous infusion of 1000–1500 IU/hr., Alt:. LMWH 5000 units s.c. b.i.d. in patients not getting thrombolytic agents.

Adjunctive anticoagulants and antiplatelets therapy:

- As an antiplatelet, aspirin (first choice) to be given ASAP:
  Aspirin 150–325 mg o.d. PO unless contraindicated (aspirin sensitivity)
  Aspirin – more beneficial, if used along with thrombolytic, e.g. aspirin + clopidogrel – loading dose of both followed by maintenance dose of 150 mg and 75 mg, respectively

ACE inhibitor:

- Ramipril 1.25 mg in gradually increasing doses up to 10 mg o.d. Ventricular remodeling starts immediately after the MI. Thrombolytic therapy helps to improve potency, while the angiotensin converting enzyme (ACE) inhibitors following MI may prevent further ventricular dilatation and reduce the probability of progression to heart failure and mortality from an evolving MI.

Mechanical Revascularization (Interventional)

It is the strategy of choice, in cases of reocclusion/reinfraction with the recurrence of ST-elavation or bundle block. If not available then further thrombolytic therapy (danger of hemorrhage) or better tPA and its variants may be readministered (no Ab formation).

Procedures
1. Percutaneous transluminal coronary angioplasty (PTCA)
2. Percutaneous coronary intervention (PCI)
3. Percutaneous transluminal myocardial revascularisation (PTMR)
4. Coronary artery bypass surgery (CABG).

Percutaneous Transluminal Coronary Angioplasty (PTCA)

Since 1977, PTCA has become the most commonly performed procedure to achieve revascularization of the myocardium in patients with symptomatic ischemic heart disease and CAD – stenosis. Significant advances in technique and technology has been made in the past three decades.

Indications
- Angina pectoris: Stable and unstable
- Patients: With AMI, STEMI and new/presumed new LBBB
- Patients: Within 36 hrs ST elevation/Q wave or new LBBB
- MI: Who develop cardiogenic shock

Complications
- Procedural related MI
- Coronary restenosis
- Acute or threatened vessel closure due to thrombosis and/or embolism
- VF

Percutaneous Coronary Intervention (PCI)

Accepted as an optimal reperfusion strategy for acute STSMI, with its proven superiority over thrombolysis for short- and long-term gains, e.g. survival benefit and diminished risk of hemorrhage. In 1986, coronary stents were first implanted and indicated for threatened/abrupt coronary restenosis following PTCA. In 2003, drug eluting stents (DES) were introduced and since then have become the mainstay of PCI. ACC advocated the use of stents to improve the short- and long-term gains of PTCA. As a matter of fact, the term PCI came to replace PTCA. (Source: American College of Cardiology (ACC)

Types

Primary PCI
Defined as an angioplasty and/or stenting without pre/concomitant thrombolytic therapy.

Indications
- As an alternative to thrombolytic therapy in patients with AMI and STEMI or new/presumed new LBBB
- Patients who are within 36 hrs ST elevation/Q wave or new LBBB
- MI who develop cardiogenic shock
- < 75 years of age.

Advantages
- Superior to thrombolysis in all subsets of patients and in all time frames
- Reocclusion – lesser
- LV – improved residual function
- Mortality rate – low.

Facilitated PCI
Defined as PCI combined with low dose pharmacological reperfusion therapy.

Rescue PCI
Defined as PCI performed on a coronary artery which remains occluded despite fibrinolytic therapy. PTCA remains the only option in this situation.

Indications
- Large inferior MI
- Anterior wall MI
- Poor cardiac reserve due to prior MI.

Method
- Diagnostic angiography done – to demonstrate a blocked artery
- Glycoprotein IIb/IIIa (most potent platelet aggregation inhibitors) antagonists may be instituted as soon as occluded artery is confirmed on diagnostic angiogram and decision to undertake PCI is taken
- Target artery – is intubated with a guiding catheter
- Lesion – is crossed with a guidewire and then dilated with a PTCA balloon catheter
- A balloon mounted stent deployed to cover the lesion.

Complication   Hemorrhage.
Method of hemostasis and timing of sheath removal:
          Manual compression and removal of sheath 8 hrs after giving 1 mg/kg IV
          of enoxaparin.
Approaches   Transradial approach – better approach
               Transfemoral approach – patient handicapped for a day or so.

Percutaneous Transluminal Myocardial Revascularization (PTMR) with Laser

Indications   • CAD – unsuitable for angiography or angioplasty
               • Severe angina: Inspite of optimal medical therapy
               • MI: Inducible
C/I   • MI: Within 3/52
               • Hemorrhage
Future   Trials are ongoing to evaluate short- and long-term procedural success
               and clinical benefits.
Disadvantage   Very few hospitals have the resources to perform PTCA and PTMR.

Coronary Artery Bypass Grafting (CABG)

The number of patients who require CABG in acute MI – is limited.
Indications   • Medical therapy – inadequate
               • PTCA failure
               • Tripple vessel disease
               • LVF
               • VSD
               • MR
               • Acute MI – causing cardiogenic shock
               • Left main stenosis
Objective   Improvement in long-term survival is the main objective of CABG and
               has been documented in several studies.
Management of complications
CHF   • Oxygen therapy
               • Diuretics – furosemide IV decreases pulmonary congestion.
               • Potassium chloride 1 g t.d.s., given along with diuretics
               • Low sodium intake
               • ACE inhibitors
               • Beta-blockers
               • Digitalization with caution.
Shock   • Oxygen therapy
               • Digitalization – for CHF, causing shock of MI.
Arrhythmias (see also management of arrhythmias in this section)
Sinus bradycardia
               • Atropine 600 μg–3 mg IV bolus, given for increasing heart beat. Rept.
                 If the bradycardia persists. If fails then pacemaker inserted.

Ventricular Tachycardia (VT)

Antiarrhythmics:

- Lidocaine 1.5 mg/kg as IV bolus followed by 2–4 mg/min IV infusion. (Lidocaine being given in a non-hypotensive patient). If fails, then Alt:
- Amiodarone 5–10 mg/kg as IV bolus followed by 1 mg/mt IV infusion for 6 hrs and 0.6 mg/min for next 18 hrs. Alt:
- Bretylium 5–10 mg/kg IV, then 1–2 mg/min IV infusion, followed by:
  - Defibrillation: DC (cardioversion) counter shock therapy
  - CPR: Closed chest massage and mouth-to-mouth respiration – pre- and post-shock therapy, and before attempting electroshock again.

Ventricular Fibrillation (VF)

Antiarrhythmics:

- Lidocaine (lidnocaine) 50–100 mg IV is the drug of choice to control irritability of the myocardium.
- Quinidine sulfate – used along with digitalis therapy, for the treatment of persistent ventricular ectopic activity
- Potassium salts – as an alternative, if arrhythmia due to digitalis
- Bretylium 5–10 mg/kg IV. Then 1–2 mg/min IV infusion. It is useful in the treatment of both VF and VT. Followed by:
  - Defibrillation – DC counter shock therapy – given immediately, if lidnocaine or bretyliun fails to control fibrillation
  - CPR: Closed chest massage and mouth to mouth respiration – pre- and post-shock therapy, and before attempting electroshock again.

Thromboembolism: Anticoagulants to be used without any delay.

Oliguria, anuria: Treat accordingly.

Shoulder hand syndrome:

- Analgesics
- Physiotherapy.

Diabetes mellitus	Treat accordingly.
Prognosis:	High mortality during first 24 hrs. Mortality high in presence of above said complications.

Stokes-Adams Syndrome

Definition	Is an acute emergency, having high mortality, usually lasts less than a week. Stokes-Adams attacks with fatal syncope are rare in presence of inferior MI.
Etiology	Inflammatory: Acute myocarditis, rheumatic fever, fibrosed conduction system of cardiac skeletal *Drugs:* Digitalis
Pathogenesis	AV conduction block (AV node, bundle of His, distal to bundle of His) due to transient ischemia of right coronary artery—AV conduction

damage—necrosis of septum and bundle of His or bundle branches—complete heart block.

Diagnosis	Syncope
	Convulsions
	Death–due to prolonged asystole.
Investigation	CBC, ESR
	Cardiac enzymes
	ECG: P-R interval – prolonged (0.21 sec or >)
	CXR
Management	Treatment and prognosis depend on whether block is proximal or distal to bundle of His. Prognosis is better if block is proximal.
	Eliminate or treat the cause: Pacemaker (transvenous)—discharging rate 70/min–life saving

Drugs

- Ephedrine sulphate 50 mg qds PO
- Isoproterenol Hcl 10 mg qds sublingually or IV infusion 10 mg/0.5 L
- Epinephrine (Adrenaline) – (in case uncontrolled with Ephedrine or Isoproterenol), 0.5 mL of 1:1000 sol. tds s/c.
- Epinephrine (Adrenaline) – 0.5 mL of 1:1000 sol. Intracardiac be given in case cardiac arrest persists
- Corticosteroids – may reverse complete AV block (recent onset).

Refer: The patient to the medical team.

Acute Pericarditis with Effusion (Cardiac Tamponade)

Is a serious emergency and demands treatment on priority basis.

Etiology	Myocardial infarction
	Cardiac trauma: Postoperative
	Tuberculosis
	Viral (HIV)
	Rheumatoid arthritis
	Myxedema
	Malignancy (carcinoma breast, bronchogenic carcinoma).
Diagnosis	Chest pain – dull aching/sharp, diffuse, pericardial/substernal
	Dyspnea, cough, orthopnea
	Fever
	Engorged neck veins
	Pulsus paradoxus
	Tachycardia
	Hypotension
	Enlarged liver
	Ascitis
	Edema legs.

Investigation   TLC and DLC: Leukocytosis

ESR: Raised

Aspirate fluid: For bacteriological and cytological examination

X-ray chest (CXR) shows: Cardiomegaly, pleural effusion

ECG: T waves – flat or depressed or inverted in all leads

Echocardiography: Highly diagnostic

Angiocardiography: Confirms diagnosis.

Complications Cardiac tamponade is a serious emergency

Pericardial fluid increases rapidly.

Increased volume raises the venous pressure.

Myocardium efficiency markedly affected.

Cardiac output falls.

Patient feels exhausted, dyspneic, pale, cyanotic.

Shock, renal failure, death – ultimately.

Management

Pericardiocentesis It is a life-saving measure.

Method   The needle (no. 16) is pushed slowly in the epigastric region, between xiphoid and left sternal margin, directing upward at an angle of 30° towards midline, 4–5 cm deeper into pericardium, and aspirate the pericardial fluid, with great relief to the patient.

Refer: The patient to the cardiac team (CCU) for further investigation and management of the underlying cause.

Treatment of underlying cause:

Tuberculosis Pericarditis:

Bed rest

Diet – nutritious diet

Antitubercular chemotherapy.

Rheumatoid Arthritis:

Drugs: Salicylates and anti-inflammatory drugs

Physiotherapy.

Congestive Heart Failure:

Treat accordingly.

Infection   Chemotherapy

Incision drainage.

Acute Pulmonary Edema

It is a serious emergency and demands treatment on priority basis. It is due to increased pulmonary venous pressure, resulting in engorged pulmonary vasculature.

Etiology   Left ventricular failure due to MI

Ventricular arrhythmia

Failure of heart valve prosthesis

	Acute myocarditis
	Hypertension
	Pulmonary infarction
	Anemia
	Hyperthyroidism
	Head injury
	Exposure to high altitude
	Narcotic overdose
	Hepatitis
	Nephrotic syndrome.
Diagnosis	Dyspnea, orthopnea
	Cough, blood-stained frothy sputum
	Chest pain
	Palpitations
	Oliguria, hematuria, renal failure
	Cardiac arrest
	Shock.
Investigation	CXR (X-ray chest): Shows enlarged hila, pleural effusion.
	Attach a cardiac monitor and check SaO_2 with pulse monitor.
	ECG: Sinus tachycardia, cardiac arrhythmia.
	Echocardiography: To assess LV function, VSD, valve disorders, pericardial effusion.
	Blood for U and E, glucose, FBC.
Management	Posture of patient – maintain the patient in sitting position in a chair or semifowler position in the bed. It decreases the venous return to heart.
	Oxygen therapy – to relieve hypoxia and dyspnea.
	Venesection – to reduce venous return to the heart.
	Catheterize the bladder and monitor urine output.
Drugs	• Diamorphine 2.5–5 mg IV
	• Diuretics: Furosemide (lasix) 40–80 mg IV
	• Digitalization
	• Aminophylline 0.25–0.5 g IV. It increases:
	– Cardiac output, renal blood flow, urinary excretion of water and sodium
	• Reserpine 1–2 mg IM. Repeat 12 hrly for acute hypertensive cases
	Caution: Development of hypotension.

Refer: The patient to the cardiac team for management of the underlying cause.

Acute Myocarditis

Definition	Is defined as inflammation of the myocardium (focal or diffuse).
Etiology	Infective:
	• Viral (Coxsackie, Influenza, Rubella, Adenovirus)
	• Bacterial–Diphtheria

	Inflammatory: RA, Rheumatic fever
	Drugs: Chloroquine
	Trauma: Chest injury (crush).
Pathogenesis	Left ventricular hypertrophy
Diagnosis	Nausea, vomiting, dizziness, dyspnea
	Fever, malaise
	Chest pain
	Tachycardia, murmurs, arrhythmias, gallop rhythm
	CHF – right-sided, pericardial rub
	LVF
	Hepatomegaly
Investigation	CBC, ESR
	Cardiac enzymes – raised
	Viral serology
	ECG – ST segment and T- wave abnormalities
	CXR – Heart enlargement.
D/d	Alcoholic cardiomyopathy, SLE, scleroderma, polyarteritis nodosa.
Management	General measures: Supportive treatment.
	Bed rest
	Specific treatment: Treatment of arrhythmias and heart failure.

Refer: The patient to the medical team.

Management of Arrhythmias
Bradyarrhythmias
Sinus Bradycardia

Etiology	Hypothyroidism – myxedema
	Hypothermia
	ICP – raised
	Exercise – athletic heart.
Diagnosis	Heart rate – < 60/min
	Rhythm – regular
	ECG – normal
	Weakness, confusion in elderly patients.
Management	Atropine sulfate 600 μg–3 mg IV bolus. Rpt if necessary
	Isoprenaline 0.5–10 μg/min IV infusion.
Pacemaker	Indicated when other means fail and when it is documented to be symptomatic, device like pacemaker is implanted to treat the bradyarrhythmia.
Technique	Inserted into right ventricle to prevent sinus slowing.

Tachyarrhythmias
Supraventricular Tachycardias
Sinus Tachycardia

Most common arrhythmia of this type.

Etiology	Emotion
	Exercise
	Fever
	Hyperthyroidism
	Anemia
Diagnosis	Pulse rate: > 90–100/min
	Rhythm : regular
	ECG : P waves with sinus contour preceding each QRS complex
Management	Treatment of primary cause, e.g.

- Heart failure: Digitalis and/or diuretics
- Heart failure (absence): Verapamil – also controls ischemia
- Hypoxemia: Oxygen therapy
- Hyperthyroidism: Treatment of thyrotoxicosis
- Electroshock – in case of heart rate persists for > 120/mt.
- Treatment of secondary causes
- Fever: Antipyretics, e.g. aspirin.

Inappropriate Sinus Tachycardia

Sinus tachycardia in the absence of any precipitating factors.

Management
- Beta-adrenergic blockers: Propranolol
- CCB: Verapamil
- Radiofrequency ablation (RFA).
- Treatment of secondary causes: Fever – antipyretics.

Paroxysmal Supraventricular Tachycardia (PSVT)

Is a serious arrhythmia due to fast ectopic impulse formation in the ventricles.

Diagnosis	Heart rate: > 200/min.
	Heart rhythm: regular
	Usually occurs after myocardial infarction
	Chest pain – due to myocardial ischemia
	Hypotension, shock.

Management

General measures
- Carotid sinus massage – in absence of hypotension
- Carotid sinus massage + IV phenylepherine – in hypotension.

Emergency measures
- DC cardioversion – for life-threatening ventricular response. It terminates the rhythm.

Alternatively:
- Lignocaine 1.5 mg/kg IV as bolus followed by 2–4 mg/kg infusion. Alt:
- Procainamide 25 mg/min IV as bolus followed by 2 mg/kg infusion. Alt:
- Quinidine 0.4 g PO, IM, or IV, repeat every 2 hrs for 3 doses. Alt:
- Adenosine 6 mg given very rapidly. Rept 3–6 mg – if not reverted.
- Beta blockers:
  – Propranolol (inderal) 1 mg IV, given in severe cases.
- CCB: Verapamil to control ischemia – in absence of heart failure
- Vasopressor drugs – for shock
- Magnesium 8 mmol IV bolus over 2–4 min. Then 60 mmol IV infusion
- Calcium salts – to counteract magnesium toxicity.
- Cardiac glycosides: Digoxin – in presence of heart failure.

Ventricular Tachycardia (VT)

It is defined as tachycardia that persists for > 30 sec.

Etiology	• Ischemic heart disease associated with a prior MI
	• Cardiomyopathies: Non-ischemic
	• Metabolic disorders
	• Drug toxicity
Types	• Sustained VT: Symptomatic
	• Non-sustained: Non-symptomatic
Diagnosis	• Symptoms as per ventricular rate, duration of tachycardia and underlying cardiac disorder
	• ECG (12-lead): Rate – wide-complex tachycardia at a rate > 100/mt.
	Rhythm – regular
	QRS complex > 0.14 sec.
Management	Of sustained VT with evidence of ischemia, CHF or CNS hypoperfusion:
	• DC cardioversion: To terminate rhythm promptly
Drugs	• Procainamide: Most effective for acute VT, as it slows down the rate. It may/may not terminate the rhythm. If not then:
Pacing method	Anti-tachycardia pacing: To terminate rhythm.
	A pacing catheter passed transvenously into right ventricle and the rhythm terminated by overdrive pacing.

Refer: The patient to the cardiac team.

Ventricular Flutter and Ventricular Fibrillation (VF)

Arises from an irritable focus in the ventricle. The rate of impulse formation is fast and transmission becomes irregular, resulting in ineffective ventricular contractions.

Etiology	Ischemic heart disease
	Drug toxicity – antiarrhythmic drugs
	Accidents – electrical shock.

Diagnosis   ECG shows grossly deformed QRS complexes occurring at a fast rate. It is usually a terminal event.

Management   External cardiac massage

Ventilation

Cardioversion and defibrillation – DC countershock, is treatment of choice

Shock cycles: In groups of 3 : 200J, 200J, 360J.

Rpt. shock cycle every min, if VF persists

Monitoring of patient with acute myocardial infarction

Medical treatment – usually ineffective

Indication: Failed defibrillation:

Inj lidocaine (lignocaine) 1.5 mg/kg IV bolus

Repeat (infusion of 2–4 mg/min) if necessary.

Caution: Reduce the dose by ½ – in CHF, shock or hepatitis.

Refer: The patient to the cardiac team for management of the case.

Atrial Flutter

Heart rhythm is usually regular. More P waves than QRS waves due to 2:1 or 4:1 AV nodal conduction.

Etiology   MS/MR

Alcohol

Postoperative especially in children

ASD.

Diagnosis   Heart rate: 280–320/min

Heart rhythm: Regular.

Investigation   ECG: More P waves than QRS waves

Management

DC cardioversion: 25–50J is the top choice

Overdrive pacing to convert the atrial flutter to sinus rhythm. If not effective then use:

Drugs   IV beta-blockers, calcium channel blockers (verapamil) or digitalis

Indication: To slow AV nodal conduction

Quinidine or like drugs, e.g. amiodarone

Indication: To prevent recurrences of atrial flutter and fibrillation

Atrial Fibrillation (AF)

It is the commonest chronic arrhythmia.

Etiology   Rheumatic heart disease

Ischemic heart disease

Cardiomyopathies

Hypertension

Thyrotoxicosis

Emotional stress

Exercise

	Hypoxia, hypercapnea
	Metabolic/hemodynamic derangements.
Diagnosis	Heart rate: 400–600/min and irregular
	Pulse deficit.
Investigation	ECG: No discernable P waves, broad QRS
	CXR: Shows cardiomegaly, pulmonary edema
	Thyroid function test.
Management	DC cardioversion – is the treatment of choice
Indication	AF <48 hrs duration
Drugs	AF >48 hrs duration
Indications	For slowing of ventricular rate:

- CCB: Verapamil 5–10 mg IV – for most rapid response. Followed by:
- Beta-blockers: May be favored to slow AV node conduction
- Digitalis: Digoxin 500 μg PO/or IV
- Anticoagulants: Started 2/52 prior to and 2/52 after cardioversion, for lowering the chances of embolism associated with cardioversion

Conversion to sinus rhythm: Amiodarone, quinidine and lidocaine.

- IV amiodarone 300 mg over ½ hr. Then IV infusion of 1 g over 24 hrs.

Palliative AV node ablation with pacemaker implantation	
Indication	For refractory AF especially with rapid ventricular response. Alternatively:
Defibrillation	DC shock 20–50J. If DC shock fails then:
Indication	For paroxysmal AF
Other measures	Correct hypokalemia
	Attempt further DC shock.

Refer: The patient to the cardiac team for management of the case.

Acute Rheumatic Fever

Definition	Is defined as an immunological disorder, self-limiting or leading to slowly progressive valvular disorder/deformity. It is the commonest cause of heart disease, next to hypertension and coronary syndrome (atherosclerotic).
Etiology	*Infective:* Group A beta-hemolytic streptococci.
	Latent period: 1–4 weeks after URC.
Predisposing factors	URC-nasopharyngitis, tonsillitis, quinsy, otitis media, caries teeth, unhygienic living conditions, overcrowded places.
Pathogenesis	Fibrinous pericarditis, carditis.
Epidemiology	Peak incidence in childhood (5–15 yrs.of age).
	Most common in developing countries.
Diagnosis	Follows recent streptococcal infection of throat
	Carditis: An early manifestation – within first two weeks of fever onset
	Pericarditis: (fibrinous or with effusion)
	Myocarditis: Cardiac enlargement, congestive failure (right and left sided), murmurs (mitral or aortic diastolic)

Erythema marginatum (marginal erythema with central pallor)

Sydenham's chorea – abrupt appearance (continual, non-repetitive, purposeless jerky movements of facial, trunk, and limbs muscles).

Facial grimaces – common

Arthritis – flitting polyarthritis of abrupt or gradual onset, involving large joints sequentially, inflamed – swollen, red, hot, and tender, arthralgia

Fever – rises progressively, malaise, asthenia, loss of weight, anorexia

Pain abdomen – variable in site and severity

Subcutaneous nodules – firm, non-tender

Investigations	CBC–leukocytosis, normochromic anemia, ESR increased, presence of C-reactive protein
	ASO titres – high titer or increasing anti-sterptolysin
	Throat swab
	ECG – ST segment and T wave changes consistent with pericarditis
	Echocardiogram
	X-ray joints
D/d	Traumatic, rheumatoid arthritis, bacterial endocarditis, osteomyelitis, pulmonary tuberculosis, poliomyelitis
Management	*Preventive treatment:*

To avoid beta-hemolytic infections and treat streptococcal infections promptly with suitable antibiotics.

Bed rest – mandatory during acute phase

Plenty of fluids

Medical treatment:

Antibiotics: Penicillin during acute phase

Analgesics: salicylates, aspirin

Corticosteroids–for reversing the acute exudative phase

Specific (treatment of complications):

CHF: Low sodium diet and diuretics. Digitalis to be given with extreme care, as may accentuate myocardial irritation – producing arrhythmias, thereby embarrassing the heart further.

Pericarditis: Relief from pain by opiates/morphine, removal of fluid by cardiac paracentesis, under coverage of penicillin to ward off infection. Corticosteroids and salicylates have favorable effect.

Chorea: Self limiting, needs reassurance, mental and physical rest, drugs–phenobarbitone, chlorpromazine, promethazine, aspirin, corticosteroids.

Refer: The patient to the medical team.

Rheumatic Heart Disease (syn. Rheumatic valvulitis)

Definition	Single or repeated attacks of rheumatic fever results in rheumatic heart disease, characterized by rigidity and deformity of the cusps, fusion of commissures, or shortening and fusion of the chordate tendineae.

Sequelae of mitral, aortic and tricuspid valves disease – mitral regurgitation, aortic regurgitation and tricuspid regurgitation. Pulmonary valve rarely affected.

Etiology	Rheumatic fever (single or repeated attacks).
Predisposing factors	URC – nasopharyngitis, tonsillitis, quinsy, otitis media, caries teeth, unhygienic living conditions, overcrowded places.
Pathogenesis	Deformed cusps, fused commissures, or shortened, fused chordate tendineae.
Diagnosis	History of rheumatic fever – in majority of cases.
	Physical examination – diagnostic.
	Hemodynamic changes, symptoms, signs, and course.
Investigations	ECG
	X-ray
	Cardiac catheterization
	Angiography
Management	Asymptomatic valvular heart disease:
	Preventive treatment:
	Avoid exposure to streptococcal infections
	Advice: Dental extraction, surgical procedures, urological procedures
	Antibiotics
	General measures:
	Avoid obesity, sedantary life
	Avoid strenuous exercises.
D/d	Mitral stenosis
	Mitral regurgitation (insufficiency)
	Aortic stenosis
	Aortic regurgitation (insufficiency)
	Tricuspid stenosis
	Tricuspid regurgitation (insufficiency).
Valves of heart	*Anatomy:* Heart has four sets of valves. The right atrio-ventricular opening is guarded by the tri-cuspid (three cusps/leaflets) valve, the left auriculo-ventricular opening by the mitral or bi-cuspid (two cusps/leaflets) valve. The openings of aorta and pulmonary artery are guarded by the tri-cuspid (three cusps/leaflets) semi-lunar valves.
	Physiology: The atrio-ventricular valves open towards the ventricles and close towards the auricles. The semi-lunar valves open away from the ventricles and close towards the ventricles. Thus when atriums contract, the atrio-ventricular valves open and blood passes into ventricles. When ventricles contract, the atrio-ventricular valves close, whereas semi-lunar valves open. That prevents regurgitation of blood into the atriums while allowing it to flow out of the ventricles, resulting in one-way circulation.
	Heart works in syncitium – the two ventricles contract simultaneously, so also the two atriums. During systole, the same volume of blood leaves the

ventricles, while during diastole, the same volume of blood enters the atriums. Any discrepancy in the time or quantitative relations may cause heart failure.

Mitral Stenosis

Definition	Is due to the fusion of the two mitral leaflets/cusps along their margins, extending from the periphery of the valvular ring, towards the centre.
	It is less common than mitral regurgitation in younger age group (10%).
	More common in females (> 75%) < age of 45 yrs.
Etiology	Rheumatic heart disease
Predisposing factors	Acute bronchitis, subacute bacterial endocarditis, acute rheumatic carditis.
Hemo-dynamics	The normal valve closed by the apposition of two mobile leaflets, over its length of 3.5 cm, becomes a fibrotic diaphragm with a small central orifice closed by the apposition of 1 cm. or less of leaflet tissue.

Mitral stenosis causes obstruction to blood flow through mitral valve during left ventricular diastole. To overcome this obstruction the left atrium increases its pressure, to maintain normal blood flow across the valve and a normal cardiac output, resulting in a pressure difference between left atrium and left ventricle during diastole. The pressure gradient reflects the severity of the mitral stenosis, persisting throughout diastole when the stenosis is severe or the ventricular rate is fast, whereas the duration is shorter and confined to middle of diastole when the stenosis is slight or ventricular rate is slow. The increased left atrial pressure raises the pulmonary venous capillary "wedge" pressure also, as there are no valves between left atrium and the pulmonary veins.

The pulmonary arterial pressure increases to maintain forward flow from the pulmonary artery to the left side of the heart. The right ventricle hypertrophies and its systolic pressure increases as it is the right ventricle that has to maintain the pulmonary pressure as well as the blood flow, resulting in right ventricular failure.

Mild stenosis: Left atrial pressure and cardiac output normal – patient asymptomatic

Moderate stenosis: On exertion, dyspnea and fatigue appear due to increased left atrial pressure

Severe stenosis: Increased left atrial pressure at rest produces pulmonary venous congestion at rest, worsening rapidly on exertion.

Recumbency at night, further increases the pulmonary blood volume, causing orthopnea, paroxysmal nocturnal dyspnea, resulting in pulmonary edema.

The increased pressure results in hypertrophy of left atrial's wall. The capacity for hypertrophy of left atrium is limited due to its thinner wall.

Complications	Paroxysmal or chronic atrial fibrillation (50–80%): The uncontrolled ventricular rate precipitates dyspnea or pulmonary edema. Emboli (30%): Cerebral, visceral, or peripheral arteries from thrombus formed in the left atrium.
Diagnosis	Male patients twice as common as female patients in young age group.
	Dyspnea on exertion or even at rest (severe)
	Paroxysmal nocturnal dyspnea
	Angina – atypical
	Pulmonary edema
	Malar flush
	Pulse – small amplitude, often complete irregularity (atrial fibrillation)
	Chest – precordial bulge
	Thrill – mid diastolic/presystolic thrill at apex
	Dullness – left 3rd ICS
	Heart sounds – loud snapping M1
	Murmurs – at apex, mid-diastolic, Graham Steell high pitched, blowing
Investigations	ECG: P waves – broad in standard leads, normal axis.
	Pulmonary hypertension – tall peaked P waves, right axis deviation or right ventricular hypertrophy.
	CXR: Left heart border – straight, large left atrium
	Pulmonary hypertension – large right ventricle and pulmonary artery.
	Angio-cardiography left ventricle
	Echo-cardiography – showing decreased closing slope of anterior mitral valve leaflet in mid-diastole with increased reflectance. The leaflets move together.
D/d	Congenital mitral stenosis – opening snap less commonly heard
	Obstructive pulmonary vein
	Neoplastic – left atrial myxoma.
Management	Is essentially surgical
	Closed valvulotomy: Indicated in mechanical obstruction of mitral valve
	Baloon valvuloplasty
	Open valvulotomy: Preferred as better repair under direct vision
	Replacement of valve: Indicated in combined mitral stenosis and insufficiency, and in case of distorted and calcified mitral valve.

Mitral Regurgitation (Insufficiency)

Definition	It is regurgitation of blood through an incompetent mitral valve, back into left atrium instead of being pumped into the aorta. It is the commonest manifestation of acute as well as previous rheumatic carditis.
Etiology	Rheumatic heart disease
Predisposing factors	Acute bronchitis, subacute bacterial endocarditis, acute rheumatic carditis.

Hemo-dynamics	Mitral leaflets during ventricular systole, do not shut normally, thereby force blood back into the atrium as well as through the aortic valve, resulting in increased workload on the left ventricle. The left atrium enlarges, whereas the pressure in pulmonary veins and capillaries rises transiently on exertion, causing dyspnea on exertion and fatigue. Left ventricular failure develops, causing orthopnea and paroxysmal dyspnea, followed by symptoms of right ventricular failure at alarming rate. The course may be more acute when mitral regurgitation caused by other than rheumatic fever. Fully developed heart failure responds inadequately to therapy, and the patient remains incapacitated.
Complications	• Atrial fibrillation • Subacute bacterial endocarditis.
Diagnosis	Pulse pressure: Wide, resting pulse rate increased to maintain cardiac output Respiratory rate: Normal in absent pulmonary congestion Left ventricular failure: Features present in acute, severe cases Apical impulse – forceful/thrusting, to left of MCL Thrill: Forcefull, brisk PMI, systolic thrill over PMI ACD increased to left of MCL Heart sounds :M1 normal or burried in murmur. 3rd heart sound, atrial fibrillation. Murmur: Loudest over PMI, transmitted to left axial or left scapular area BP: normal
Investigations	ECG: P waves broad, prominent or notched in standard leads, left axis deviation or left ventricular hypertrophy CXR: Showing enlarged left atrium and left ventricle Echo-cardiography – showing enlarged left atrium and left ventricle.
D/d	ASD, coarctation of aorta, myocarditis, Marfan and Hurler syndrome
Management	*Medical treatment:* Digitalis, diuretics, vasodilators, and prophylactic penicillin to prevent recurrences of rheumatic fever. *Surgical treatment:* Prosthetic valve replacement – not a permanent cure. Anticoagulant coverage mandatory as long as the patient has the valve.

Aortic Stenosis

Definition	Is due to the fusion of the three aortic leaflets/cusps (semi-lunar) along their margins, extending from the periphery of the valvular ring, towards the centre. The stenosis may be valvular, subvalvular, or supravalvular.
Etiology	Rheumatic heart disease
Predisposing factors	Acute bronchitis, subacute bacterial endocarditis, acute rheumatic carditis.

Hemo-dynamics	Cardinal feature of aortic valve stenosis is a systolic gradient across the aortic valve (systolic pressure difference between left ventricle and aorta). Narrowing of valvular area increases the gradient, the increased left ventricular systolic pressure leads to left ventricular hypertrophy, and low cardiac output. Left atrial pressure increases on exertion, leading to left ventricular failure and low cardiac output.
Complications	Triad of syncope on exertion, left ventricular failure, and angina pectoris
Diagnosis	Dyspnea on exertion, fatigue, palpitation, giddiness, weakness, syncope
	Chest: Localized heaving PMI, left of MCl
	Pulse: Small amplitude, sloping upstroke (plateau pulse), or tidal wave higher than percussion wave (anacrotic pulse)
	Respiratory rate: Normal in the absence pulmonary congestion
	Left ventricular failure: Features present in acute, severe cases
	Apical impulse: Less forceful, to left of MCL
	Thrill: Systolic thrill over aortic area
	ACD increased to left and down
	Heart sounds: A2 normal or delayed and weak 3rd heart sound, atrial fibrillation.
	Murmur: Harsh, over right 2nd ICS parasternally, or at apex
	BP: Normal or systolic normal with high diastolic
Investigations	ECG: Left ventricular hypertrophy.
	CXR: Left ventricular hypertrophy.
	Angiography: Aortic, coronary and left ventricle – to evaluate degree of valvular regurgitation and valvular and coronary stenosis
	Cath-lab: Right and left heart catheterization – to evaluate degree of valvular regurgitation and valvular and coronary stenosis
	Echocardiography – to demonstrate impaired or absent valve motion
D/d	Supravalvular obstruction
Management	*Medical treatment:*
	• Sedation
	• Propranolol
	Surgical treatment:
	Indications: Progressive left ventricular failure, syncope from cerebral ischemia, angina pectoris due to low cardiac output of aortic stenosis.
	Surgery:
	• Myotomy and resection (limited) of hypertrophied muscle.
	• Reconstruction: Valve replacement: Prosthetic or homograft valve – procedure of choice in severe congenital stenosis.

Aortic Regurgitation (Insufficiency, incompetence)

Definition	Pure aortic regurgitation without associated mitral valve disorder is a rare entity (5–10%). Pathologically pure rheumatic aortic valve disorder is an unknown entity.

Etiology	Rheumatic heart disease
	Dissecting aneurysm of aorta
	Infective endocarditis
	Hypertension
	Rheumatoid arthritis
Predisposing factors	Acute bronchitis, subacute bacterial endocarditis, acute rheumatic carditis.
Hemo-dynamics	During diastole, there occurs back flow from the aorta into the left ventricle, resulting in increased blood volume entering left ventricle, thereby enlarging the left ventricle size to accommodate that extra blood volume. The forward flow of blood impaired due to backward flow (leakage), being compensated by peripheral vasodilatation and increased ejection of blood from the left ventricle during initial part of systole. However, low cardiac output occurs in advanced regurgitation, pulse pressure becomes wide due to increased systolic and decreased diastolic pressure. Bradycardia increases the diastolic period, and increases the regurgitant blood volume in aortic regurgitation. Aortic regurgitation is tolerated for long periods, provided the moderate functioning of the left ventricle's myocardium. However, failing left ventricular myocardium, leads to increased left ventricular pressure, resulting in an increased left atrial pressure and pulmonary congestion, mitral valve stressing, inadequate apposition of mitral valve leaflets resulting in mitral regurgitation.
Complications	Left ventricular failure, acute pulmonary edema.
Diagnosis	*Dyspnea:* Recurrent paroxysmal nocturnal, orthopnea, fatigue, weakness
	Angina pectoris or protracted chest pain simulating angina
	Pulse: Great amplitude, abrupt upstroke, rapid fall (water-hammer pulse), wide, resting pulse rate increased to maintain cardiac output
	Respiratory rate: Normal in the absence of pulmonary congestion
	Left ventricular failure: Features present in acute, severe cases
	Heart failure: Sudden death in 10–20%
	Apical impulse: Forceful/thrusting, to left of MCL
	Thrill: Forceful, brisk PMI, systolic thrill over PMI
	ACD increased to left of MCL
	Heart sounds :M1 normal or burried in murmur. 3rd heart sound, atrial fibrillation.
	Murmur: Loudest over PMI, transmitted to left axial or left scapular area
	BP: Normal
Investigations	ECG: Great amplitude, abrupt upstroke, rapid fall, little or no dicrotic wave (water-hammer, collapsing, or Corrigan pulse) deviation or left ventricular hypertrophy
	CXR: Showing enlarged left atrium and left ventricle

Echo-cardiography: Showing fluttering of mitral valve leaflet during diastole.

Angiography : Best quantified by supra-aortic angiography.

Management   *Medical treatment:*
- Sedation
- Propranolol

Surgical treatment:

Indications : Dissecting aneurysm or perforated cusp in bacterial endocarditis

Surgery: • Myotomy and resection (limited) of hypertrophied muscle.
- Reconstruction: Valve replacement: Prosthetic or homograft.

Tricuspid Stenosis

Definition   It acts as a mechanical block to the return of blood to the heart, and the systemic venous engorgement is analogous to the pulmonary venous engorgement caused by mitral stenosis.

Etiology   Rheumatic heart disease

Predisposing factors   Acute bronchitis, subacute bacterial endocarditis, acute rheumatic carditis.

Hemo-dynamics   A diastolic pressure gradient found across the tricuspid valve between the right atrium and right ventricle, with raised pressure in the right atrium and jugular veins, and slow right ventricular filling, low cardiac output, that rises a little on exercise.

Complications   Hepatomegaly, cardiac cirrhosis, right heart failure.

Diagnosis   Hepatomegaly, ascitis, edema, jaundice

Pulse pressure: Wide, resting pulse rate increased to maintain cardiac output

Respiratory rate: Normal in the absence of pulmonary congestion

Giant alpha wave in jugular pulse with sinus rhythm

Thrill: Mid-diastolic thrill between left sternal border and PMI

Heart sounds: M1 often loud

Murmur: Loudest over 3rd–5th ICS, transmitted to apex

BP: Normal.

Investigations   *ECG:* Wide, tall peaked P waves, with normal axis.

Wave (water-hammer, collapsing, or Corrigan pulse) deviation or left ventricular hypertrophy

CXR: Showing enlarged left atrium and left ventricle

Echo-cardiography: Showing fluttering of mitral valve leaflet during diastole.

Angiography: Best quantified by supra-aortic angiography.

Management   *Medical treatment:*
- Sedation
- Propranolol

Surgical treatment:

Indications: Dissecting aneurysm or perforated cusp in bacterial endocarditis

Surgery

- Valvotomy under direct vision for acquired tricuspid stenosis
- Reconstruction: Valve replacement: prosthetic or homograft.

Tricuspid Regurgitation (Insufficiency)

Definition	It is difficult to decide in an individual patient, whether the tricuspid regurgitation is organic or functional. In rheumatic heart disease, the tricuspid regurgitation may be associated with mitral stenosis/or regurgitation (with mitral stenosis – may be organic or functional due to pulmonary hypertension, whereas with mitral regurgitation – mostly organic).
Etiology	Rheumatic heart disease
Predisposing factors	Acute bronchitis, subacute bacterial endocarditis, acute rheumatic carditis.
Hemo-dynamics	Systolic regurgitation of blood from the right ventricle to the right atrium, resulting in a systolic murmur and a volume load of the right atrium as well as the right ventricle, causing an increased size of the right atrium and right ventricle (displaced downwards and outwards).
	Right ventricular angiography reveals a prominent regurgitant systolic 'v' wave in the right atrium and jugular venous pulse, with a rapid 'y' descent and a small or absent 'x' descent, and by regurgitation of blood from the right ventricle to the right atrium during systole. Like systolic murmur the regurgitant wave, increased with inspiration, its size depending as per right atrium size. The right ventricular angiography can estimate the regurgitation volume.
Diagnosis	Dyspnea: Relieved to some extent – in mitral stenosis
	Pain: Right hypochondrium (congested liver)
	Fatigue: Decreased cardiac output.
	Jugular venous pulse: Prominent 'v' waves
	Systolic pulsations of liver
	Right ventricular failure
	Apex beat: Displaced outward and downward
	Thrill: Systolic thrill at lower left sterna edge
	Heart: Cardiac enlargement
	Heart sounds: Atrial fibrillation.
	Murmur: 3rd–5th ICS, along left sternal border to apex (pansystolic)
	BP: Normal
Investigations	ECG: Right axis usually
	CXR: Showing enlarged right atrium and right ventricle

Echo-cardiography: Showing fluttering of mitral valve leaflet during diastole.

Angiography: Right ventricular – to estimate regurgitated volume.

Management   *Medical treatment:*

- Anticoagulants – to reduce the severity of regurgitation
- Propranolol

Surgical treatment:

Indications: Dissecting aneurysm or perforated cusp in bacterial endocarditis

Surgery: Reconstruction: Tricuspid valve replacement: Prosthetic or homograft. Tricuspid regurgitation secondary to severe mitral valve disorder may regress by replacing mitral valve only.

Acute Bacterial Endocarditis (ABE)(syn. Subacute Bacterial Endocarditis)

Definition   Is defined as a rapidly progressive bacterial infection of the endocardium, superimposed mostly on pre-existing rheumatic or calcified valvular or congenital heart disease.

Etiology   Infective:

- Group A beta-hemolytic streptococci.
- Staphylococcal sepsis
- Candidiasis

Incubation period: 2–7 days of fever.

Predisposing factors   URC: Nasopharyngitis, tonsillitis, quinsy, otitis media, caries teeth, UTI Osteomyelitis

Pelvic infections: Septic abortion

Interventions: Dental procedures, genitor-urinary procedures, cardiac catheterization, bronchoscopy

Unhygienic living conditions, overcrowded places.

Pathogenesis   Large, friable vegetations, emboli with metastatic abscess formation, rapid perforation, tearing, damaging affected valves or rupturing chordate tendineae.

Epidemiology   Is rare under 2 years.of age. Peak incidence in childhood (5–15 years of age). Most common in developing countries.

Diagnosis   Fever: Rises progressively, chills, malaise, asthenia, loss of weight, anorexia,

Pain: Abdomen, chest or flanks -- variable in site and severity

Petechiae: Skin, mucous membranes, fundus, nails (splinter)

Clubbing: Fingers and toes – in SBE

Arthritis: Flitting polyarthritis of abrupt or gradual onset, involving large joints sequentially, inflammed – swollen, red, hot, and tender, arthralgia

Carditis: An early manifestation – within first two weeks of fever onset

Pericarditis: (fibrinous or with effusion)

Myocarditis: Cardiac enlagement, congestive failure (right and left sided), murmurs (mitral or aortic diastolic)

Erythema marginatum (marginal erythema with central pallor)

Sydenham's chorea – abrupt appearance (continual, non-repetitive, purposeless jerky movements of facial, trunk, and limbs muscles).

Hematuria, proteinuria, casts – in ABE and SBE.

Note: ABE or SBE may occur during inadequate therapeutic antibiotics, whereby the onset is masked, resulting in sudden embolic episode, petichiae, high fever, and heart failure.

Complications	Hemiplegia, aphasia, renal failure, CHF, hemorrhage, splenic abscess.
Investigations	CBC: Leukocytosis, normochromic anemia, ESR increased, presence of C-reactive protein
	ASO titres: High titer or increasing anti-sterptolysin
	Throat swab: For culture sensitivity
	Urine: Microscopic and culture study
	ECG – ST segment and T wave changes consistent with pericarditis
	Echocardiogram
	X-ray joints
D/d	Hemiplegia, purpura, uremia, anemia, intractable heart failure, leukemia, acute rheumatic fever, DLE, polyarteritis nodosa, tuberculosis
Management	*Preventive treatment:*

To avoid beta-hemolytic infections and treat streptococcal infections promptly with suitable antibiotics.

Bed rest – mandatory during acute phase

Plenty of fluids

Medical treatment:

Antibiotics: Penicillin during acute phase – drug of choice

- Penicillin G 3–5 million units od IM or IV
- Ampicillin 6 g tid IV
- Amoxycillin 10 g od IV
- Cephalosporins 6 g bid IV
- Gentamycin 5 mg/kg/day IM.

Analgesics: Salicylates, aspirin

Corticosteroids – for reversing the acute exudative phase

Specific (treatment of complications);

CHF: Low sodium diet and diuretics. Digitalis to be given with extreme care, as may accentuate myocardial irritation – producing arrhythmias, thereby embarrassing the heart further.

Myocarditis: Digitalization and salt restriction.

Uremia: To be treated until renal function improves.

Surgical: Valve replacement – aortic regurgitation merits top.

Refer: The patient to the medical team.

Hypertensive Cardiovascular Disorder (Hypertension)

Definition   Is defined as high blood pressure. Is an important preventable cause of cardiovascular disorder, and without treatment, it raises the incidence of heart failure, coronary disease with angina pectoris and myocardial infarction, stroke, and renal failure. Hypertension is a lifelong process, known as 'silent killer', thereby deserves mandatory treatment for an effective result.

Pathogenesis

- Essential and renal hypertension: Increased peripheral arteriolar resistance, cardiac output and blood volume normal (unless heart failure or edema present)
- Pheochromocytoma: Increased cardiac output and peripheral resistance, increased release of epinephrine and nor-epinephrine, increased cardiac output and peripheral resistance–hypertension.
- Coarctation of aorta: Constriction forcing left ventricle to eject blood into short chamber (aorta).

Pathology   Sustained hypertension: Initially causes functional (reversible) arteriolar narrowing, that later on results into structural (permanent) changes – intimal thickening, hypertrophic medial muscular coat, and hyaline degeneration.

Malignant hypertension: renal arteriolar necrosis, renal failure.

Dominant manifestations of hypertension: Left ventricular hypertrophy and failure, and arteriolar lesions. Hypertension aggravates coronary and cerebral artery atherosclerosis, MI, and ICH or thrombosis.

Normal blood pressure:

In adults   Systolic blood pressure (SBP): 100–140 mm Hg

Diastolic blood pressure (DBP): 60–90 mm Hg

Pulse blood pressure (PBP): SBP–DBP: 30–60 mm Hg

In children   Lower level in each case

In elderly   Higher level in each case.

Hypertension   Systolic pressure: > 160 mm Hg

Diastolic pressure: > 100 mm Hg.

Categories   As per guidelines from Joint National Committee (JNC) USA:

Reports: JNC IV, V, VI and VII (Table 3.1).

JNC VII: Revised the previous reports (JNC V and VI), related to therapy, classification of hypertension and risk stratification.

JNC VI: Define hypertension at lower levels than previous guidelines and focuses on both systolic and diastolic blood pressure levels as did JNC V.

JNC IV: Focuses on the borderline categories – mild, moderate, severe. It has been abandoned due to inaccurate prediction of complications.

Classification   Primary, secondary, and malignant hypertension.

Table 3.1: Categories of blood pressure in adults and elders

Categories	BP systolic (mm Hg)	BP diastolic (mm Hg)	Check up in
JNC VII:			
Normal	<120	< 80	Yearly
Pre-hypertension	120–139	80–89	Yearly
Hypertension	> 160	> 100	Refer to care 1/52
JNC V & VI:			
Optimal	< 120	< 80	Yearly
Normal	< 130	< 85	Yearly
High normal	130–139	85–90	Half yearly
Hypertension:			
Stage I	140–159	90–99	2/12
II	160–179	100–109	Refer to care 1/12
III	>180	>110	Refer to care 1/52

Primary Hypertension (syn. Essential or Idiopathic)

Etiology	Common type. In majority – the cause is unknown.
Risk factors	Age: > 60 yrs. Younger the patient – poor the prognosis
	Sex: More in women, although they fare better than males
	Race: Common in all races
	Family history of cardiovascular disease, e.g.:

• CVD: Heart failure, MI, hypertension, dyslipidemia

CVA: Stroke

Endocranial: Diabetes mellitus

Respiratory: Asthma

Arthritis: Gout

Obesity

Physical inactivity

Smoking

Alcohol abuse

Target organs damage – sudden death.

Evaluation   To assess the severity of the hypertension based on target organs damage (Table 3.2), in order to administer appropriate treatment.

Secondary Hypertension   Rare type.

Etiology   • Renal disorders:

  – Atherosclerosis of renal arteries

  – Acute and chronic glomerulonephritis

  – Acute pyelonephritis

  – Polycystic kidney

  – Hydronephrosis

Table 3.2: Target organs damage

CVD:
Angina pectoris
Myocardial infarction
Prior coronary revascularization
Left ventricular hypertrophy (LVH)
Heart failure
Brain:
Stroke
Tansient ischemic attack (TIA)
Kidneys:
Renal impairment
Eyes:
Retinopathy
Arteries:
Peripheral vascular disease (PVD)

- Endocrinal disorders:
  - Cushing's syndrome
  - Pheochromocytoma
  - Acromegaly
  - Myxedema
  - Oral contraceptives – containing estrogen

- Miscellaneous:
  - Toxemias of pregnancy
  - Intracranial tumors
  - Intracranial hemorrhage (ICH)
  - Disseminated lupus erythematosus (DLE)
  - Drugs misuse – steroids.

Malignant Hypertension (Acute Hypertensive Crises): DBP >140 mm Hg.

It is a rare but serious emergency and demands treatment on priority basis.

Etiology   Sustained primary or secondary hypertension
                  Associated with papilledema, retinal hemorrhages and exudates.

Diagnosis of hypertension:

S/S   Signs and symptoms of hypertension are of involved target organs, e.g. heart, brain, kidneys, eyes, and arteries.

Symptoms   - Symptomless for many years (hypertension known as silent killer)
                  - Headache, feeling of fullness in the head, blurring of vision
                  - Anxiety, palpitation, perspiration, pallor, temperature intolerance
                  - Nausea, vomiting
                  - Chest pain
                  - Low backache, fatigue, muscular weakness, paresis, hemiplegia

- Polyuria, nocturia, hematuria
- Paroxysmal nocturnal dyspnea – orthopnea
- Intermittent claudication
- Impotency
- CVA due to intracranial hemorrhage.

Signs
BP (To be recorded daily for 3 days):
Systolic >140 mm Hg, diastolic > 100 mm Hg
Pulse: Presence or abscence of bruits
Jugular venous distention
Peripheral edema
Eyes: Narrowing of retinal arterioles,
    Retinal hemorrhages, papilledema.
Heart and arteries: Left ventricular failure, fast rhythm, pulsus alternans.
Lungs: Rhonchi, bronchospasm
Brain: Hemiplegia
Liver: Hepatomegaly
Kidney: Uremic appearance.

Investigation
CBC – anemia
BUN – elevated
Serum creatinine – elevated
Serum electrolytes – sodium, potassium, magnesium, calcium
Serum glucose
Transaminases
Uric acid
Lipid profile – HDL cholesterol, LDL cholesterol, and triglycerides
Urinalysis : Low specific gravity, proteinuria
Ophthalmic study of retina – periodically
ECG: – Left ventricular hypertrophy
       – Q waves – significant
       – QRST interval – prolonged
Echocardiography: May show left ventricular hypertrophy
CXR (X-ray chest): Shows – cardiac enlargement
    – Coarctation of aorta
    – Ultrasonography
    – Pyelography.

Management of hypertension: Refer: The patient to the medical team.
General measures:
Lifestyle modifications:
    Behavioral changes:
    - Relief of stress, i.e. to avoid unnecessary tensions
    - Alcohol reduction/no alcohol intake

- Avoid smoking tobacco
- Moderate physical activity – at least ½ hr/day to control obesity and over weight.

Dietary intentions: Dietary measures have favorable effects on biochemical variables when compared to drug therapy:

- Avoid fried, fatty, fast food
- Increase the fibre in diet
- Moderate salt intake
- Fat restriction.

Remember DPT (Diet, Physical Activity, No Tobacco).

Drugs	Many groups of drugs available, e.g. diuretics, beta-blockers, CCB, vasodilators, angiotensin converting enzyme inhibitors (ACEI), and latest class – angiotensin II receptor blockers (ARBs), lipid lowering drugs with coexisting hyperlipidemia.
Action	Reduction of cardiac output: Diuretics and beta-blockers.

Reduction of peripheral vascular resistance:

- Other antihypertensive agents
- Alfa-blockers.

Approach
- The choice of initial antihypertensive agents is controversial. Start with small initial dose.
- Lowering of BP should be moderate initially.
- Prevention of development of postural hypotension.
- Initially use thiazide diuretics or beta-blockers, as these have shown reduction in stroke and congestive heart failure (CHF).
- Left ventricular hypertrophy (LVH) is an independent indicator of cardiovascular morbidity and mortality.

Drug combination
- Failure of initial single drug therapy to control BP is an indication for use of low dose drug combination.
- Low dose drug combination, i.e. a full dose of one drug is replaced with small doses of 2 or more drugs, in order to achieve better BP control in resistant hypertensives, and to reduce side effects, especially in patients unable to tolerate therapy with a single agent.

Combination to use
- Diuretic + beta-blocker
- Diuretic + vasodilator (CCB, ACE inhibitor, ARB)
- Diuretic + adrenergic blocker + vasodilator
- Beta-blocker + vasodilator
- ACE inhibitor + CCB.

Combination to avoid
- Two drugs from same class, e.g. beta-blocker + beta-blocker
- Centrally acting agent + beta-blocker
- Beta-blocker + diltiazem or verapamil.

Table 3.3: Selective drug therapy

Option	Age	Selective drugs	Alternative (Alt) drugs
Ist	< 50 yrs	ACEI	ARBs
	> 50 yrs	Diuretic	CCB
IInd	< 50 yrs	ACEI + CCB/or diuretic	ARBs + CCB/or diuretic
	> 50 yrs	Diuretic + ACEI	CCB + ARBs
IIIrd	< 50 yrs	ACEI + CCB + diuretic	ARBs + CCB + diuretic
	> 50 yrs	ACEI + CCB + diuretic	ARBs + CCB + diuretic
IVth	< 50 yrs	ACEI + CCB + diuretic+	ARBs + CCB + Diuretic+
	> 50 yrs	BAB/AAB/or 2nd diuretic	BAB/AAB/or 2nd diuretic

Key

ACEI: Angiotensin converting enzyme inhibitor

ARBs: Angiotensin receptor blockers.

CCB: Calcium channel blockers

AAB: Alfa-adrenergic receptor blockers

BAB: Beta-adrenergic receptor blockers

Dosage	Doses of drugs, dosing intervals, and their combinations should be evaluated for adequacy. It should be ascertained whether enough time was given for the drug to exert its maximal effect before it is declared ineffective.
Treatment	For patients not responding to sequence of drugs (Table 3.3).

Classification of Antihypertensive Drugs (as per site of action)

Diuretics	Site of action: Renal tubules
Drugs	Thiazides group:
	Chlorthiazide (diuril) 0.5–1.0 g o.d. in divided doses PO
	C/I: Electrolyte imbalance especially in patients taking digitalis
	Indication: Mild hypertension or as adjunct in severe hypertension
	Hydrochlorothiazide (esidrex) 25–50 mg o.d./b.d. PO
	Indication: Mild and severe (as adjunct) hypertension
	Loop diuretics:
	Furosemide (lasix) 20–80 mg o.d./b.d. PO
	C/I : Electrolyte imbalance (hypokalemia)
	To combat that add aldactone 25 mg t.d.s.
	Indication: Mild and severe (as adjunct) hypertension.
Beta-blockers	Site of action: Central
Drugs	Propranolol 10–120 mg b.d./or t.d.s. PO
	Indication: Mild/moderate hypertension
	C/I: CHF, diabetes, asthma
	Metoprolol 50–200 mg b.d. PO

Indication: Mild/moderate hypertension

C/I: CHF, diabetes, asthma

Atenolol 25–100 mg o.d. PO

Indication: Mild/moderate hypertension

C/I: CHF, diabetes, asthma

Phentolamine 1–5 mg IV

Indication: Pheochromocytoma

C/I: CAD.

ACE Inhibitors Drugs — Site of action: Converting enzyme (ACE inhibitors)

Enalapril 2.5–40 mg o.d. PO

Indication: Mild/severe hypertension

C/I: Renal failure, aortic stenosis, pregnancy

Captopril 6.25–50 mg t.d.s. PO

Indication: Mild/severe hypertension

C/I: Pregnancy, lactation, hypersensitivity

Other drugs — Lisinopril, perindopril, ramipril, imidapril.

Calcium Channel Blockers (CCBs): Site of action: Vascular smooth muscle

Drugs

Nifedipine 10–30 mg q.d.s. PO

Indication: Mild/moderate hypertension

C/I: Congastive heart failure, aortic stenosis

Amlodipine 5–10 mg o.d.

Indication: Mild/moderate hypertension

C/I: Pregnancy, lactation

Verapamil 40–120 mg t.d.s./q.d.s. PO

Indication: Mild/moderate hypertension

C/I: Heart failure, AV block, SA block

Diltiazem 30 mg b.d./q.d.s. PO. Max: 240 mg in divided doses

Indication: Mild/moderate hypertension

C/I: Pregnancy, sinusitis.

Vasodilator Drugs — Site of action: Vascular smooth muscle

Hydralazine hydrochloride (apresoline) 25–50 mg o.d./t.d.s.

Indication: As adjunct in moderate/severe hypertension

C/I: CAD, pregnancy, tachycardia

Diazoxide 1–3 mg/kg body wt. IV

Indication: Malignant hypertension

C/I: CHF, diabetes

Sodium nitroprusside 0.5–8 μg/kg/min IV

Indication: Malignant hypertension

C/I: CHF

Alfa blockers	Site of action: Central
Drugs	Prazosin 0.5–1 mg b.d./t.d.s Maint: 3–20 mg o.d./t.d.s.
	Indication: Mild to moderate hypertension
	C/I: CHF due to mechanical obstruction
Other drugs	Doxazosin, terazosin, phentolamine.
Adrenergic blockers	Site of action: Central/autonomic ganglia
	Clonidine 50–100 mcg t.d.s.
	Indication: Mild/moderate hypertension
	C/I: Pregnancy, lactation
	Methyldopa (aldomet) 0.5–2 g/day in divided doses
	Indication: Mild to moderate hypertension
	C/I: Hepatitis, MAO inhibitors, hypersensitivity

Specific Antihypertensive Selection (Table 3.4): of coexisting factors:

Angiotensin receptor blockers (ARBs): Site of action: Central

Drugs	Valsartan 80–320 mg/day PO
	Indication: Hypertension alone or in combination (antihypertensives)
	C/I : Hypersensitivity
	Losartan 25–100 mg/day PO
	Indication: Mild to moderate hypertension
	C/I: Hypersensitivity, pregnancy, lactation
	Candesartan 8–32 mg/day PO
	Indication: Hypertension alone or in combination (antihypertensives)
	C/I: Pregnancy, lactation, hyperkalemia

Table 3.4: Specific antihypertensive selection

Factors	Selective agents
Age < 50	ACEI or ARBs, CCB, diuretic, beta-blocker or alpha-blocker
> 50	CCB or diuretic, ACEI or ARBs, beta-blocker or alpha-blocker
Angina pectoris	Nitrates, beta-blocker, CCB, potassium channel activator
LVH	ACEI, alpha-blocker, CCB, diuretic, ARBs
CAD	Beta-blocker, CCB, ACEI
Acute MI	Nitrates, beta-blocker, ACEI, diuretic
CHF	ACEI, thiazide diuretic, ARBs, beta-blocker, alpha-blocker
CVA	Vasodilator, ACEI, CCB, beta-blocker, alpha-blocker, diuretic
Hyperlipidemia	Statins, alpha-blocker, ACEI, CCB, BBA
PVD	CCB, alpha-blocker
Diabetes mellitus	ACEI, ARBs, CCB, diuretic, alpha-blocker
Renal insufficiency	ACEI or ARBs, beta-blockers, loop diuretic, CCB
Pregnancy	ACEI, ARBs, diuretic, CCB, alpha-blocker, vasodilator
Osteoporosis	Diuretic

Acute Hypertensive Crises (Emergencies and Urgencies)

Hypertensive emergencies are those situations (DBP > 140 mm Hg) that require urgent blood pressure reduction to prevent or limit organ damage. These patients need urgent referral.

Types	CVD:
	Unstable angina
	Acute myocardial infarction
	Acute left ventricular failure
	Acute pulmonary edema
	Acute aortic dissecting aneurysm
	Cerebral:
	Acute hypertensive encephalopathy
	Cerebrovascular accident (CVA)
	Stroke/TIA
	Miscellaneous:
	Eclampsia
	Malignant hypertension
Investigations	BUN, serum creatinine and glucose, serum electrolytes
	Urinalysis
	CXR
	ECG
	CT scan.
Management	Hospitalization of the patient especially in intensive care unit (ICU)
	Elevation of head end of bed
	Monitoring of BP, neurological state, ECG, fluid balance
	Daily estimation of BUN and serum creatinine.
Drugs	Fast acting antihypertensive agents
Aim	Is to reduce DBP to 110 mm Hg within an hour and < 100 by 6 hrs.
Caution	Excessive fall of BP that may precipitate cerebral (CVA), coronary (MI) and renal ischemia should be avoided.
Drugs	Over the following 2–3 days BP should be normalized by using beta-blockers, CCB, diuretics, vasodilators or ACEI. These can be used alone or in combination:

- Beta-blocker: Atenolol 50–100 mg o.d. PO, or metoprolol 25–100 mg
- CCB: Sublingual administration of fast acting nifedipine should be avoided as degree of fall of BP may be too rapid.
- Diuretics: Furosemide 20–80 mg IV
- Vasodilators: Diazoxide (hyperstat) 300 mg IV. Is a fast acting vasodilator, without affecting (decreasing) cardiac output or renal circulation, used esp. eclampsia and malignant hypertension. Alt:
  - Hydralazine 5–20 mg IM repeat – every 2–4 hrs

> • ACEI: Enalapril 1.25 mg IV 6 hrly. Maint 2.5–40 mg PO, Alt:
> Ramipril 1.25–10 mg PO.

Maintenance	Once the BP is under control, then give drugs like diuretics or other oral antihypertensive drugs.
Renal failure	Hypertension in presence of renal failure: Failure of antihypertensive drugs is an indication for renal dialysis.

Cardiac Arrest

It is an acute medical emergency, accounting for majority of unexpected, sudden cardiac deaths (SCD).

Definition	It is defined as an abrupt cessation of cardiac pump functioning completely called asystole, or incompletely (cardiac muscle quiver very rapidly without pumping any blood) so called VF. It may be reversible by an immediate (top priority basis) management, but death may occur in its absence, due to myocardial infarction.
Etiology	Coronary artery disease (CAD) Myocardial infarction (MI) Valvular heart disorders Heart failure Shock Metabolic: Electrolyte imbalance, hypoxemia, acidosis Electrophysiological: VF, asystole, bradyarrhythmias Toxins – cardiac.
Diagnosis	Cardiac arrest is a clinical diagnosis Sudden onset of events – without any pre-warning Chest pain – acute pain of prolonged angina/MI Unconscious or collapsed patient Breathless or gasping breathing Pallor, cyanosis, cold clammy skin Pupils – dilated, pulseless, hypotension Death – sudden.
Management	Cardiac arrest is a life-threatening emergency (SCD occurs shortly within mins, if active measures not taken immediately) demanding top priority management by trained A&E staff, cardiac team, or a combination of both.

Management of collapsed unconscious person

First-aid	To be initiated immediately by a physician, nurse, paramedical staff, or trained lay persons, present at the place of attack, in order to prevent development of permanent brain damage. Time is a crucial factor.
Measures	Make the victim comfortable – lying or sitting, loosen any tight clothing • Tilt the head backwards, lift the chin, open the mouth, remove any visible foreign body from the mouth and nose.

- Mouth-to-mouth breathing
- Give a sharp blow to the breast bone (precordial)
- Call for a doctor or ambulance immediately. Avoid giving any drug, or drinks until and unless recommended by the doctor.

Management of Cardiac Arrest

Cardiac arrest is a life-threatening emergency (SCD occurs shortly within min, if active measures not taken immediately) demanding top priority management by trained A&E staff, cardiac team, or a combination of both.

Aims of treatment are

Phase I	To resuscitate (**C**ardio **P**ulmonary **R**esuscitation) the patient (Table 3.5).
Phase II	To manage the urgent precipitating conditions.
Phase III	To assess the overall situation.

Phase I	To resuscitate (**C**ardio **P**ulmonary **R**esuscitation) the patient.
Includes	• Initial response

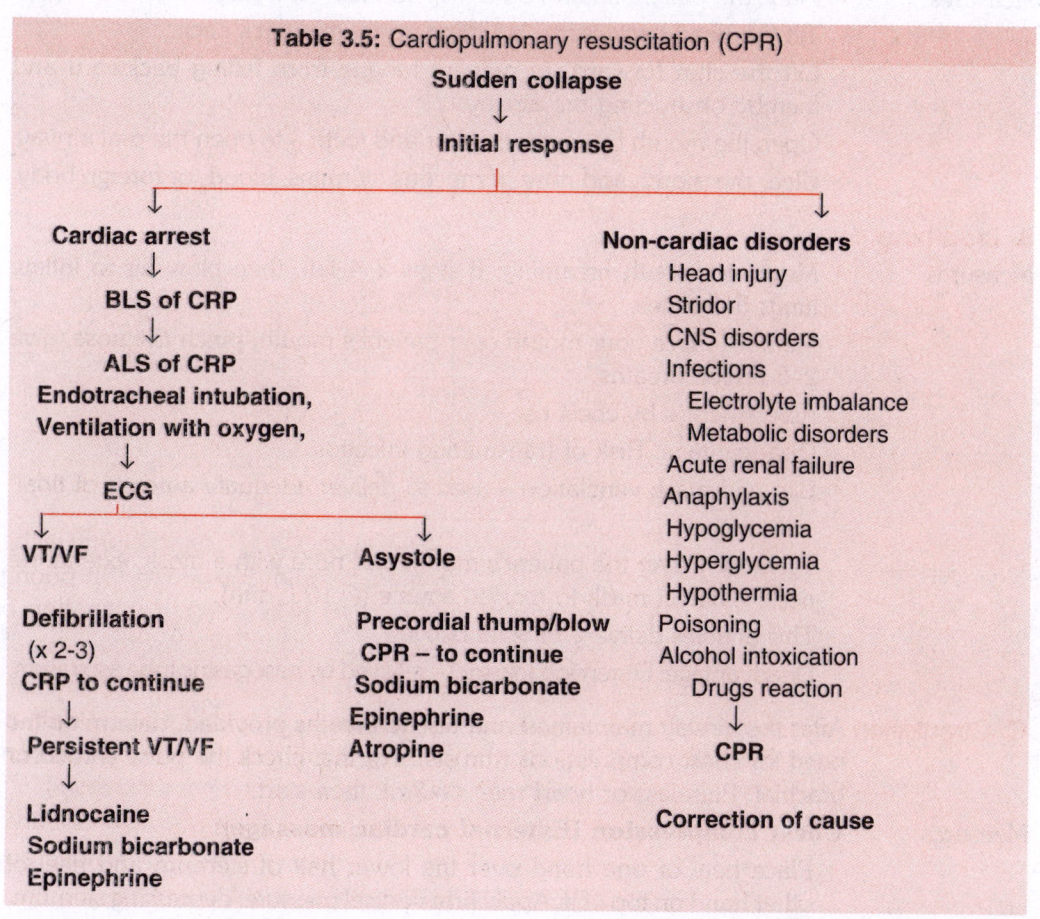

Table 3.5: Cardiopulmonary resuscitation (CPR)

Sudden collapse
↓
Initial response

Cardiac arrest
↓
BLS of CRP
↓
ALS of CRP
Endotracheal intubation,
Ventilation with oxygen,
↓
ECG

VT/VF | Asystole

Defibrillation (x 2-3)
CRP to continue
↓
Persistent VT/VF
↓
Lidnocaine
Sodium bicarbonate
Epinephrine

Precordial thump/blow
CPR – to continue
Sodium bicarbonate
Epinephrine
Atropine

Non-cardiac disorders
Head injury
Stridor
CNS disorders
Infections
Electrolyte imbalance
Metabolic disorders
Acute renal failure
Anaphylaxis
Hypoglycemia
Hyperglycemia
Hypothermia
Poisoning
Alcohol intoxication
Drugs reaction
↓
CPR

Correction of cause

- Basic life support (BLS of CPR)
- Advanced life support (ALS of CPR).

Initial response Determines whether the sudden collapse is due to cardiac arrest (by observing respiration, skin color, pulse).

Observe for any airway obstruction – stridor

Measures

Airway clearance Heimlich maneuver to remove any inhaled foreign body by:
- A precordial thump delivered firmly to the breast bone

Basic Life Support (BLS of CPR)

Follows the ABC approach, e.g. assessment followed by action, i.e. the management of airway, breathing, and circulation, in that order. This is only the initial rescue (first-aid) management. Failure to respond, then: advanced life support (ALS) – continuation of BLS.

A. Airway maintenance

Measures
- Place the patient supine on a firm surface – a trolley/hard board/bed.
- Tilt the head backwards, by lifting up the patient's neck.
- Lift the chin forward, to prevent tongue from falling backward and thereby obstructing the airway.
- Open the mouth by separating lips and teeth – to open the oral airway.
- Clear the mouth and nose of mucous, vomitus, blood, or foreign body.

B. Breathing

Measures
- Mouth to mouth breathing: If steps 2–4 fail, then blow air to inflate lungs 3–5 times.
  Method: Place your mouth over patient's mouth, pinch the nose, give 2–5 rescue breaths.
  Assessment – by chest rise
  Disadvantage: Risk of transmitting infection
- Bag and mask ventilation – used to deliver adequate amount of tidal volume
  Method: Cover the patient's mouth and nose with a mask, extend the neck, connect mask to oxygen source (@10 L/min).
  This enables delivery of 90% oxygen
  Disadvantage: Distention (gastric) – relieved by nasogastric tube aspiration.

C. Circulation
After the airway maintained and rescue breaths provided, determine the need for chest compressions (thrusts). For that check the pulse carotid or brachial. Pulseless or heart rate <60/mt, then start:

Measures
Chest compression (External cardiac massage):
- Place heel of one hand over the lower half of sternum and heel of other hand on top of it. Apply firm vertical pressure, depressing sternum,

@ of 60–90/mt. For children, use only one hand compression @ 80–100/mt.

Care: Not to injure ribs especially in a trauma case.

Monitor pulse and pupils

- Pulse – good palpable pulse is a favorable sign for compression.
- Pupils – monitor pupils size, response to light (good response – an indicator of the adequacy of the compression). Pupils that remain widely dilated, i.e. indication of cerebral hypoxia and brain damage.
- Alternate cardiac compression and pulmonary ventilation in 15:2 ratio

Reassessment   Chest compression (external cardiac massage) should always be accompanied by rescue breathing. Reassess the patient after a mt. Reappearance of spontaneous breathing and circulation—then stop the chest thrusts while ventilation to continue.

Advanced Life Support (ALS of CPR)

Aims

- To provide adequate ventilation
- To control cardiac arrhythmias
- To maintain blood pressure and cardiac output
- To reinstate organ perfusion.

Measures

- Endotracheal intubation – put endotracheal tube without any delay and attach airway to oxygen ventilator.
- Tracheostomy – may be required as an emergency measure
- Feel the pulse – carotid/femoral – present or absent.

Pulsations present

- Continue with the assisted ventilation until:
- Respiration – spontaneous respirations return.
- Pulse – palpable
- Pupils – previously dilated pupils, remain constricted.

Pulseless

- A sharp fist blow (thump) given to the midsternum area.

Still pulseless

- Defibrillation/cardioversion – to be carried out hurriedly – important criteria for the successful resuscitation. If possible, an immediate defibrillation should precede intubation and insertion of an IV line, CPR to be continued while the defibrillator is being charged.
- Monitor blood pH, electrolytes, BUN, blood for grouping and cross-matching, BSF, cardiac enzymes.
- Elevation of legs – to promote venous return
- IV fluids, vasoconstrictor drugs (use with caution), etc.

Still pulseless

Phase II   **Treatment of the urgent precipitating conditions.**

Includes   Assessment and treatment of the urgent precipitating conditions.

Aims
- To find out the underlying cause and whether it is curable or not
- To know about the nature of cardiac arrest
- To plan further necessary measures required

Monitor ECG To determine type of cardiac arrest:
- Ventricular fibrillation
- Ventricular tachycardia
- Shock (electrical activity without contraction)
- Asystole
- Sinus bradycardia.

Measures Treatment of the urgent precipitating conditions.

Ventricular Fibrillation/Tachycardia

Defibrillation DC cardioversion 200–360J. It may be necessary to use defibrillating shock to control the abnormal rhythm. Shock cycles in groups of 3. Initially 200J, 200J, 360J, with subsequent cycles at 360J.

Drugs Antiarrhythmic:
- Lignocaine 1.5 mg/kg bolus. Repeat after 2 mts for persistent VT/VF followed by IV infusion @ 2–4 mg/mt. Alt:
- Amiodarone 5–10 mg/kg bolus IV. Then 1 mg/mt IV infusion for 6 hrs and 0.6 mg/mt (next 18 hrs), Alt:
- Procainamide 500 mg IV as loading dose, followed by 2 mg/kg/hr

Persistent VF:
- Epinephrine 1 mg IV and 2–3 mg every 3–5 min during resuscitation with attempts to defibrillate between each dose.
- Sodium bicarbonate 1 mmol/kg, repeat after 2 min for persistent VT/VF
  Indication: An acidotic patient after defibrillation and intubation.

Asystole and Shock

CPR
- Continue with CPR measures for 3 min, e.g.
- Assisted respiration
- Cardiac massage
- To control hypoxemia and acidosis
- External shock – no role.
- IV fluids

Drugs
- Epinephrine 1 mg IV and 2–3 mg every 3 min by endotracheal route
- Atropine 3 mg IV should be given for asystole
- Sodium bicarbonate 1 mmol/kg, repeat every 10–15 min
- Calcium chloride 10 ml IV, repeat after 5 min as per indication.
- IV line

Sinus Bradycardia

Drugs	• Atropine 600 μg–3 mg IV bolus. Repeat if necessary
	• Isoprenaline 0.5–10 μg/min IV infusion
	• Persistent bradycardia despite atropine – may be treated with electrical pacing.
Surgery	Thoracotomy and internal cardiac massage – may be considered, if cardiac function fails to return after use of all above said measures.

Phase III	**Post-resuscitation care (follow-up measures):**
Includes	Follow up measures:

After restoration of cardiac, pulmonary, and central nervous system functions, the patient should be carefully observed, preferably in a coronary intensive care unit (CICU) for:

• Airway maintenance
• Monitor oxygenation and ventilation
• Correct hypoxia and prevent hypercapnea
• Monitor pulse oximetry to assess oxygen saturation
• Monitor ECG and CXR
• Monitor invasive hemodynamic to minimize reperfusion injury
• Maintain arterial pressures to prevent hypotensive hypoperfusion, as cerebral blood flow autoregulation is poor in the post-arrest phase
• Maintain body temperature to avoid/treat hypothermia
• Monitor U&E, calcium, magnesium
• Avoid routine use of steroids, CCB and anti-arrhythmic drugs as their role to prevent further arrhythmias is unwarranted and controversial.

Resuscitation in Trauma

MOI	• RSA
	• Fall from height.
Management	• Immobilize the cervical spine with a collar
	• Head – to be kept in neutral position
	• Airway maintenance
	• Breathing control
	• Circulation
	• IV fluids
	• Blood transfusion
	• Drugs

Refer: The patient to the orthopedic team.

Congestive Heart Failure (CHF)

Introduction	CHF remains an important public health concern, with > 22 million people worldwide suffer from CHF – a potentially debilitating disease. Despite

the treatment options for CHF, 5 years mortality remains unacceptably high at 50%.

Definition Congestive heart failure is defined as inability of the heart to maintain an output, at rest or during stress, required for the metabolic needs of the body (systolic failure) and its failure to receive blood from the body into ventricles at low pressure during diastole (diastolic failure).

Etiology
- Coronary artery disease (CAD)
- Valvular heart disease – AI/MI/TI
- Cardiomyopathy
- Congenital heart disease – left to right shunts
- Hypertension
- Upper respiratory obstruction
- Hypoglycemia
- Hypocalcemia
- Acute rheumatic fever.

Risk factors
- Myocardial infarction or ischemia
- Arrhythmias
- Dietary – excess sodium intake
- Excess fluid intake
- Drug misuse
- Alcohol abuse
- Tobacco use
- Thyrotoxicosis
- Anemia
- Pregnancy
- Physical overactivity
- Infection.

Types
- Left ventricular failure (LVF)
- Right ventricular failure (RVF)
- Both – combined left and right ventricular failure.

Diagnosis Left ventricular failure:
- Dyspnea on exertion – due to pulmonary venous engorgement and stiffness of lungs
- Orthopnea – dyspnea at rest
- Cough – due to hypertension, myocardial infarction
- Fatigue, weakness – due to reduced cardiac output
- Nocturia – due to excretion of edema fluid, and diuretic intake

Right ventricular failure:
- Anorexia
- Bloating – due to raised venous pressure
- Oliguria – present in the daytime

- Polyuria – present at nighttime
- Headache, weakness, mental aberration.

Investigation
- Complete blood count, ESR
- BUN
- Serum electrolytes
- Serum cholesterol
- Thyroid function tests – especially TSH
- ECG: Right ventricular hypertrophy – in right heart failure
  Left ventricular hypertrophy – in left heart failure
- CXR (X-ray chest): – Right atrial and ventricular enlargement in
  – Right heart failure
  – Signs of pulmonary edema
- Echocardiography: The single most useful diagnostic test in the evaluation of patients with CHF
- Coronary angiography.

Management

Aims of treatment
- To relieve from symptoms and to improve the quality of life
- To control the disease progression
- To reduce the risk of death and the need for hospitalization.

General measures
- Rest: Bed rest or sitting in a chair – reduces heart's work load and promotes sodium diuresis
- Diet: – Salt restriction to < 3 mg/day
  – Bland, low caloric-residue meal
- Smoking – cessation
- Alcohol – abstinence
- Weight reduction – daily weight measurement
- Physiotherapy: Active/passive leg exercises to prevent the development of phlebitis.

Drugs
Diuretics, ACE inhibitors, beta-blockers, digoxin, anticoagulants, angiotensin II receptor blockers, hydralazine

1. Diuretics

Indication
To inhibit renal sodium and water retention

CHF due to left ventricular systolic dysfunction, characterized by a steadily progressive state of renal sodium and water retention.

Drugs
Furosemide (a strong loop diuretic) 20–40 mg/day PO, followed by increase in dosage until urine output increased and weight reduced by 0.5–1 kg/day.

Hydrochlorothiazide (thiazide diuretic) 25–75 mg/day PO
- It decreases cardiac output, plasma and extracellular volume
  Spironolactone 25–200 mg/day PO in single or divided doses

- It causes sodium diuresis without potassium loss
- To be considered as a supplementary diuretic

Acetazolamide 0.25–0.5 g/day PO in single/divided doses
- Is a carbonic anhydrase inhibitor (inhibits HCO_3 reabsorption).

2. ACE inhibitors — To inhibit conversion of angiotensin I to angiotensin II

Indication — Heart failure due to left ventricular systolic dysfunction

Drugs
- Captopril 6.25 mg b.d., followed by doubling in dose bi-weekly
- Lisinopril 2.5 mg o.d., followed by doubling in dose bi-weekly
- Enalapril 2.5 mg b.d. followed by doubling in dose bi-weekly
- Imidapril 5 mg o.d. Max: 20 mg.

3. Beta-blockers — To prevent or reverse detrimental effects on the myocardium, by the catecholamines – released into circulation due to stimulation of sympathetic nervous system.

Indication — Heart failure due to left ventricular systolic dysfunction

Drugs
- Carvedilol 3.125 mg b.d., followed by doubling in dose b.i.w.

4. Digoxin
- To normalize the baroreceptor-mediated reflexes
- To increase cardiac output at rest and during exercise

Indication
- Heart failure due to left ventricular dysfunction, and should be used in conjunction with diuretics, an ACE inhibitors and a beta-blocker
- Heart failure with rapid atrial fibrillation

Drugs
- Digoxin 0.25–1.5 mg/day. Maint: 0.25–0.5 mg/day.

Other drugs for selective patients with systolic dysfunction:

A. Anticoagulants and antithromboembolics:

Indication — CHF with atrial fibrillation

Drugs — Warfarin 10–15 mg/day PO

Clopidogrel 75 mg/day.

B. Angiotensin II receptor blockers (ARB):

Indication — Patients intolerant to ACE inhibitor due to angioedema or cough

Drugs — Losartan 12.5–25 mg/day PO

Candesartan 16–32 mg/day PO

Indication — Patients intolerant to ACE inhibitor due to angioedema or cough.

C. Antiarrhythmic agents (class III):

Indication
- Heart failure with supraventricular tachycardia uncontrolled by digoxin or beta-blockers
- For patients with life-threatening ventricular arrhythmia who are not candidates for implantable cardiac defibrillators

Drug
- Amiodarone 300 mg IV over 1 hr via central line. Maint: 200 mg/day

D. Hydralazine 10 mg q.d.s. + Isosorbide dinitrate 10 mg t.d.s.

Indication — Patients intolerant of ACE inhibitors.

Avoid drugs that can exacerbate the syndrome of CHF and should be avoided in most patients:

- Antiarrhythmic agents – can exert important cardiodepressant and pro-arrhythmic effects. Exceptions: amiodarone and dofetilide
- Calcium channel blockers – can lead to worsening CHF and have been associated with an increased risk of CV events
- NSAID – can cause sodium retention and peripheral vasoconstriction and can enhance the toxicity of diuretics and ACE inhibitors.

Alternatives to drugs for CHF:

	• Mechanical assist devices
	• Cardiac transplantation
Limitations	• Cost
	• Infection
	• Need for chronic anticoagulation
New therapy	• Cardiac resynchronization therapy (CRT)
Actions	• To relieve symptoms
	• To improve patient's quality of life
	• To prevent re-hospitalization.

Refer: The patient to the cardiac team for management of the underlying cause.

Peripheral Vascular Disease (PVD)

Definition	As the age advances, atherosclerosis causes thickening and hardening of arterial walls, resulting in narrowing of the arteries, thus obstructing the flow of blood within it, thereby raising the morbidity and mortality.
Pathogenesis	Blockage of arteries especially smaller ones, e.g. those supplying the brain, the heart, the kidneys, arms and legs, resulting (Table 3.6) in:
Etiology	Atherosclerotic obstruction of the arteries – main cause of PVD

The blockage of arteries occurs due to:

- Narrowed artery: Due to thickening and hardening of arterial wall
- Damaged artery: Due to damage of smooth inner wall (intima)
- Blocked artery: Due to blockage by a plaque/blood clot (embolus).

Risk factors

- Age – advancing age
- Heredity
- Diet – cholesterol rich foods
- Obesity

Table 3.6: Peripheral vascular disease (pathogenesis)

Blocked artery	Target organ	Damage
Cerebral arteries	Brain	Stroke
Coronary arteries	Heart	Myocardial infarction
Renal arteries	Kidneys	Hypertension
Arm/leg arteries	Arm/leg	Gangrene

- Sedentary life – lack of exercise and stressful
- Stress
- Smoking
- Diabetes
- Hypertension.

Diagnosis
- Pain: Two types of pain, i.e.
  - Intermittent claudication – a cramp-like pain occurring commonly in the calf or foot on exercise, due to muscle ischemia, relieved with rest.
  - Rest pain – pain occurs even at rest, due to nerve ischemia so called cry of the dying nerves. Pain always worse at night, being aggravated by elevation of the limb and relieved by hanging leg over side of the bed.
- Numbness, tingling or pain in the leg, foot or toes (paresthesia)
- Leg and foot becoming cold
- Paleness of leg and foot
- Blue/red discoloration of the foot or toe (pre-gangrene)
- Dry, fragile or shiny looking skin
- Wound/ulcer – that do not heal
- Gangrene – may occur, i.e.
  - Loss of temperature
  - Loss of sensation
  - Loss of pulsation
  - Loss of function
  - Change of colour – pale, blue, black.

Investigation
- CBC
- Wassermann reaction – for syphilitic endarteritis obliterans
- Color Doppler – to measure pressure at different levels of the leg or arm
- Plain radiography for arteriosclerosis, cervical rib, gas bubbles
- Arteriography – to evaluate the condition of the arteries and extent of the blockage.

Method: Under GA inject 20 ml of 35% diodone into the artery.
Immediate skiagraphy is imperative.

Management Early diagnosis and prompt treatment done in a specialized setup, by a dedicated peripheral vascular surgeon is the essence of this day and age of superspecialization, if unnecessary amputations have to be avoided.

Refer: The patient to the vascular surgeon for management of the underlying cause.

Treatment

General measures
- Avoid cigarette smoking
- Regular exercise
- Diet – fresh fruits, vegetables, milk, fish, etc.
- Antithrombotic agents: Low molecular weight heparin and warfarin

- Reduce the risk of thrombotic occlusion to a similar extent and are also prophylactic against fatal pulmonary embolism
- Platelet inhibitors: Aspirin and oral anticoagulants are effective in the late postoperative period.

Surgical treatment:

Assessment for surgery:

- General physical examination including palpation of pulses
- Color Doppler – to measure pressure at different levels of the leg/arm A drop in pressure between two arterial segments indicates blockage in that vessel.
- Arteriography (angiography): Arteriography is the final step in the evaluation. This test uses a contrast medium that shows the arteries and extent of the blockage.

Techniques

Minimal invasive devices

- Balloon (angioplasty) catheters
- Stents
- Atherectomy

Aims   To displace the plaques, blocking the peripheral arteries

Other devices

- Thrombolytics
- Embolectomy and thrombectomy
- Thrombo-endarterectomy (disobliteration)
- Bypass surgery

Balloon Angioplasty is the most common method for opening a narrowed artery.

Method

- A deflated balloon catheter is passed over a wire through the affected vessel to the narrowed area.
- The balloon is then inflated. This flattens the plaque against the arterial wall, thereby increasing the lumen of the artery.
- Ballooning may be used alone or combined with stenting.

Disadvantage   Restenosis.

Stent Angioplasty Stent is a device, inserted to hold the vessel open. The expanded stent (resembles a piece of fence) remains in situ for long. The non-invasive nature of angioplasty is making stents especially drug coated ones – extremely popular. Drug coated stents – are small wire-mesh metal tubes, that support the affected arterial wall. The procedure is done in a catheterization lab.

Indications

- Failure of balloon catheter – restenosis
- Rescue angioplasty – done within 3 hrs of a heart attack, which is used to open a blockage while the heart attack is in progress.

Disadvantage   Cost factor.

Atherectomy Atherectomy is a method, for cutting or pulverizing plaque (soft/hard) – blocking an artery.

Thrombolytics Urokinase or streptokinase given intra-arterially through a catheter until a clot is dissolved.

Thrombectomy and Embolectomy
Indications	Organised thrombus
	Clotted blood
Method	Removal with a balloon catheter under local anesthesia.

Endarterectomy is a method, for incising the artery and removal of plaque blocking the artery.

Sites	Groin area – femoral artery
	Neck – carotid bifurcation

Bypass Surgery Is a method, for bypassing a narrowed or blocked section of an artery with a graft.

Types	Synthetic (DACRON, PTFE), or
	Venous grafts – saphenous vein from the leg – limited longivity
	Arterial grafts – conduit of choice in CABG, because of superior and event free survival.
Anticoagulants	
Heparin	Low molecular weight heparin 50 mg (5000 U) 4 hrly IV, or IV infusion 300 mg in 1.5 L normal saline in 24 hrs.
	S/E: Hemorrhage
Antidote	IV protamine sulphate (1 mL of 1% sol. Neutralizes 1000 U heparin)
Warfarin	A synthetic anticoagulant. Loading dose 30–50 mg PO
	S/E: Hemorrhage
Antidote	Phytomenadione (vitamin K) 10 mg (1 mL) PO, IM or IV. Max 40 mg o.d.
	C/I of anticoagulants: Pregnancy, peptic ulcer, hypertension, hepatic deficiency.

Deep Vein Thrombosis (DVT) syn. Phlebothrombosis
Definition	It is defined as thrombophlebitis with clot formation in a deep vein. It is an emergency (may lead to complications, e.g. pulmonary embolism – infarcts) and requires treatment on priority basis. The thrombus may commence in a venous tributary, extending into the main deep vein, where a portion may break off, causing pulmonary embolism.
Etiology	• Traumatic – major trauma
	• Surgical – postoperative
	• Physical inactivity
	• Diabetes
	• Heart disease – CHF, AMI, hypertension

	• CVA – stroke
	• Metabolic
Risk factors	• Aging
	• Obesity
	• Prolonged immobilization
	• Dyslipidemia
	• Anemia
	• Dehydration
	• IV drug use
	• Smoking
	• Pregnancy/pelvic masses
	• Shock
	• Drugs – chemotherapy, estrogens

Pathogenesis   Virchow's triad, e.g. vessel wall injury, venous stasis and state of hyper-coagulation.

Diagnosis
- Pain – calf/whole leg
- Swelling of the leg
- Discoloration
- Tenderness – calf
- Homan's sign – positive
- Pulse rate – increased
- Temperature – raised
- Respiratory symptoms/signs – suggestive of pulmonary embolism

Investigation
- Ultrasound
- Color Doppler
- MRI
- CXR

Management

Preventive
- Elevation of legs
- Elastic crepe bandage/compression stockings
- Postoperative exercises

Medical   Anticoagulants: To be continued for 8–10 days
- Oral (PO): Aspirin

         Warfarin: 1st day: 30–50 mg o.d.

                       2nd day: 10–20 mg o.d.

                       Maint.: 5–15 mg o.d.

- Parenteral:

Unfractionated heparin (UFH) 7500–10000 as initial bolus dose IV, followed by 1000 IU/hr as continuous infusion

Low molecular weight heparin (LMWH) – comparatively safe as less incidence of thrombocytopenia. Given s.c. agents:

- Enoxaparin 1.5 mg/kg o.d. or 1 mg/kg b.i.d. s.c., Alt:
- Delteparin 200 IU/kg b.i.d. s.c.

Thrombolytics: Urokinase or streptokinase given intra-arterially through a catheter until a clot is dissolved.

Dose: Streptokinase 0.75–1.5 million i.u. IV in 1 hr.
     Urokinase 50,000 i.u. in 5% dextrose/saline.

Surgical treatment

Procedures
- Femoral vein ligation, recommended in cases when anticoagulants are contraindicated.
- Thrombectomy and embolectomy: Femoral vein thrombectomy may be considered in cases not responding to conservative measures, e.g. elevation of legs, elastic crepe bandage/compression stockings, anticoagulants, fluid and electrolyte replacement, sympathetic block.

Refer: The patient to the vascular surgeon for management of the case.

Cardiac Practical Procedures

Investigations (cardiac):
1. Complete blood count (CBC)
2. ESR
3. Cholesterol total, triglycerides, HDL, LDL
4. Apoliprotein, lipoprotein
5. Creatine kinase
6. CXR (X-ray chest) – PA view
7. ECG
8. Treadmill test (exercise ECG testing)
9. Ambulatory ECG monitoring
10. Pericardiocentesis
11. Cardiac catheterization
12. Angiocardiography

New Imaging Techniques
1. Ultrasonography (US)
2. Computed tomography (CT) scan
3. Magnetic resonance imaging (MRI)
4. Nuclear medicine procedures

CXR (X-ray chest) – PA view

Shape
As a flask-shaped shadow, lying between translucent lungs, about one-third to the right and two-thirds to the left of midline. Apex of the heart– medial to midclavicular line. The right border formed by two curves, e.g. superior vena cava and arch of aorta, and the right atrium. The left border formed by four convexities, e.g. arch of aorta,

pulmonary artery, left ventricle. The right ventricle occupies main central portion in front.

Alterations in disease:

- Displacement of heart: Pleural effusion, pneumothorax, abdominal distension, obesity
- Enlarged left ventricle: Aortic incompetence, aortic stenosis, hypertension
- Enlarged left atrium: Mitral stenosis, mitral incontinence
- Enlarged aorta: Syphilitic aortitis with aneurysm, hypertension
- Pulmonary infiltration: Cor pulmonale.

ECG

Definition	A tracing or graph made by amplifying the minute electrical impulses generated in the heart. The pattern produced by these impulses, indicates whether the heart is healthy or whether it is unhealthy, and to what extent. An ECG does not affect the patient.
Technique	The instrument used is called an electrocardiograph. Electrodes connected to this apparatus are fastened over the heart and usually on both arms and a leg. They detect the tiny electric impulses produced by heart beating. The impulses are amplified by the electrocardiograph which produces a tracing on a sheet of graph paper.
Normal ECG	The waves or deflections of the electrocardiograph are designated by the letters PQRST.

P wave: Upward deflection, associated with auricular contraction, and usually best seen in lead II or chest lead VI, and are most valuable in the disorders of cardiac rhythm

QRS complex: Associated with ventricular contraction

Q wave: Downward deflection follows an upward deflection P

R wave: Upward deflection follows a downward deflection Q

S wave: Downward deflection follows a downward deflection R

T wave: Upward deflection, associated with ventricular recovery

P-R interval: From beginning of P wave to beginning of QRS complex

Electrocardiographic Abnormalities

Sinus tachycardia	ECG – normal, as the cardiac impulse arises normally
Sinus bradycardia	ECG – normal
Sinus arrhythmia	ECG – normal, apart from variation in the R-R intervals
Extrasystoles	ECG – P waves absent T wave pointing in opposite direction to QRS deflection
Paroxysmal atrial tachycardia	ECG – P waves abnormal in shape, QRS complexes normal
Atrial flutter	ECG – Auricular rate 200–400/min Auriculoventricular block of 2:1, 3:1, or 4:1
Atrial fibrillation	ECG – Auricular rate 400–600/min F (fibrillation) waves instead of P waves QRS complexes – normal, but irregularly spaced

Ventricular fibrillation	ECG – QRS complexes – grossly deformed occurring at rapid rate
Heart block	ECG – Partial heart block: PR interval > 0.22 sec
	Complete heart block: P waves and QRS complexes occur regularly but independently

Ventricular   ECG – Left: R wave – larger in leads facing left ventricle
hypertrophy   S wave – larger in leads facing right ventricle
                                      T wave – inversion
                                      ST segments – depression in lead I
                         Right: R wave – larger in leads facing right ventricle
                                      S wave – larger in leads facing left ventricle
                                      T wave – inversion
                                      ST segments – depression in leads II and III

Myocardial   ECG – Anterior: Q waves or ST segment and T wave changes or both
infarction   in lead I and chest leads facing right ventricle
                         Posterior: Q waves or ST segment and T wave changes or both
                                        in leads II and III

Ambulatory ECG Monitoring

Continuous ECG monitoring for 24 hrs, to pick up paroxysmal arrhythmias

Indications   Angina pectoris
                     Myocardial infarction

Treadmill Test (Exercise ECG Testing)

The patient undergoes a graduated, treadmill exercise test, with continuous 12 lead ECG
              and blood pressure monitoring.

Indications   Assessment of cardiac function and exercise tolerance
                     Assessment of exercise induced arrhythmias
                     Ischemic heart disease – to confirm a suspected diagnosis
                     Monitoring response to treatment

Pericardiocentesis (Pericardial Puncture)

Site   5th or 6th left intercostal space in the mammary line.
                    The mammary line is 10 cm from midline.
                    The heart apex is 9.0 cm from midline

Indication   Cardiac tamponade (life-saving measure)
                    Pericardial effusion

Method   Patient is made to sit
                    Sterile the area
                    Infiltrate with 1% procaine
                    Insert a large bore needle connected to a 3-way stopcock and a syringe,
                    into the intercostal space at the upper border of the rib, and push in the
                    direction of backwards and towards the spine.

With suction the fluid begins to flow into the syringe.

Seal the puncture site after removal of the needle.

Cardiac Catheterization

The information obtained is predominantly physiological, e.g. the flow of blood across a ventricular septal defect, or the gradient across a pulmonary stenosis.

Technique   Procedure performed in a Cath-lab.

A flexible radiopaque catheter is introduced into an antecubital or femoral vein, and manipulated within the heart and great vessels to measure pressures.

Indications   Blood samples to assess oxygen saturation

To inject radiopaque contrast medium to image the anatomy of heart

To perform angioplasty, valvuloplasty

To perform intravascular ultrasound to quantify arterial narrowing

Angiocardiography

The information obtained is predominantly anatomical. The procedure demands experience and facilities for monitoring of rhythm and other vital functions, as well as resuscitation equipment, and is an expensive procedure. The procedure should not be used solely for the purpose of diagnosis.

Technique   Taking of X-ray films while a contrast medium is injected into the heart through a catheter placed in the appropriate heart chamber, e.g. in the right ventricle just below a stenotic pulmonary valve.

Indications   Angina pectoris

Coronary artery disease

Myocardial infarction

Congenital heart disease

New Imaging Techniques

Advantages   Enhancement of diagnostic precision

Disadvantages Expensive techniques

Misuse – as a substitute for clinical workup and simple tests

Ultrasonography

Most frequently employed non-invasive imaging technique.

Technique   It consists in transducer translating reflection of sound waves from interfaces in tissues into cross-sectional images of normal and abnormal anatomy.

Indications   Cardiac ultrasonography – For congenital and acquired heart diseases (echocardiography)   – For determining effects of cardiac drugs.

Computer Tomography (CT) Scan

Technique   It consists in obtaining digitalized cross-sectional images by rapid bursts of X-rays during one revolution of both tube and detectors which are on opposite sides of patient to be scanned. It allows only limited assessment of cardiac structures.

Indications	Constrictive pericarditis
	Assessment for abnormalities of the ascending and descending aorta
	Pulmonary emboli

Magnetic Resonance Imaging (MRI)

Technique	MRI yields images reflecting magnetic differences in body tissue rather than difference in X-ray absorption or acoustic reflection. Images are obtained in the sagittal, coronal, and axial planes.
Indications	Congenital heart disease
	Assessment for intracardiac structures and great vessels

Nuclear Medicine (Radionuclide Scintography)

Nuclear medicine procedures are safe, reproducible and cost-effective.

Indication	To obtain functional information about various organ systems.
	Acute myocardial infarction
	Acute chest pain
Technique	Special imaging devices like gamma cameras and computer system give static or dynamic images. Different compounds labeled with the isotope 99 m-technetium, are utilized to evaluate various organ systems, e.g.

GIT	^{99m}Tc-sulfur colloid orphytate (oral)
Musculoskeletal	^{99m}Tc-MDP
CVS	^{99m}Tc-RBC
GUS	^{99m}Tc-DTPA
Oncology	^{99m}Tc-MDP, 201 thalidium chloride

Premedication Sedation and immobilization required.

Coronary Artery Bypass Grafting (CABG)

The number of patients who require CABG in acute MI – is limited

Indication	PTCA failure
	Tripple vessel disease
	VSD
	MR
	Cardiogenic shock from acute MI
	Left main stenosis > 50%.
Objective	Improvement in long-term survival is the main objective of CABG and has been documented in several studies

References

1. Bedell SE, et al: Survival after cardiopulmonary resuscitation in the hospital. N Engl J Med. 309:569; 1983.

2. Roberts WC, Jones AA: Standard and guidelines for cardiopulmonary resuscitation (CPR) and emergency cardiac care (ECC) JAMA. 255:290;1986

3. Silverstein MD, et al: Patients with syncope admitted to medical intensive care Units. JAMA 248: 1185;1982

4. Weissler AM. Warren JV: Syncope and shock. In: Hurst JW, et al (eds) The Heart. 4th ed. New York. McGraw-Hill. 705;1978.

5. Parrillo JE: Septic shock in humans: Clinical evaluation, pathogenesis, and therapeutic approach. In: Shoemaker WC, et al (eds) Textbook of Critical Care. 2nd ed. Philadelphia. Saunders. pp 1006–1023;1989.

6. Ingram RH Jr., Braunwald E: Pulmonary edema: Cardiogenic and noncardiogenic. In Braunwald E (ed) Heart Disease, Philadelphia, Saunders, 544;1988.

7. Parti Rohit : Syncope: Diagnosis and Management. Prime CME (10) 27–38;2009.

8. Fowler NO, et al: Cardiac tamponade: A comparison of right versus left heart compression. J Am Coll Cardiol 12:187;1988.

9. Passey R, Chopra VK: Practical Guidelines for Management of Congestive Heart Failure. Vol 5 No 3: 31–35, Family Medicine India, 2001.

10. Verma PK: Management of Heart Failure: Newer insights (Diagnostic/Prognostic/Therapeutic. Prime CME (10) 11–26;2009.

11. Constant J: The clinical diagnosis of nonanginal chest pain. The differentiation of angina from nonanginal chest pain by history. Clin Cardiol 6:11;1983.

12. Goldman L: Atypical chest pain. In: RB Taylor (ed) Difficult Diagnosis Philadelphia, Saunders, 71;1985.

13. Verheugt FWA: Acute coronary syndromes. 353 (Supple II): 1–26, Lancet;1999.

14. Mehta A, Sethi KK: Acute coronary syndromes. Vol 5 No. 3: 23–29, Family Medicine India, 2001.

15. Singh TP: Triage of acute coronary syndrome. Prime CME (10) 5–10;2009.

16. Antman EM, Rutherford JD (eds): Coronary Care Medicine: A Practical Approach. Boston, Martinus Nijhoff, 1986.

17. Ajeet B, Yadav OP: Coronary Artery Bypass Surgery: An Overview. Family Medicine India Vol 5 No 3;2001.

18. Trehan N: Developments in total arterial myocardial revascularization. Prime CME (10) 61–65;2009.

19. Sawhney JPS: Management of Dyslipidaemia: Beyond LDL-cholesterol. Prime CME (10) 39–48; 2009.

20. Goldman L, et al: A computer protocol to predict myocardial infarction in emergency department patients with chest pain. N Engl J Med 318:797;1988.

21. Mishra S, Bahl VK: Current concepts in management of acute ST-segment elevation myocardial infarction. JIMA 107(10) 680–684;2009.

22. Achari V et al: Short term mortality & complications in ST elevation myocardial infarction – the heart hospital experience. JIMA 106(10) 650–654;2008.

23. Dani SI, Patel SR: Percutaneous coronary interventions: past, present and future. JIMA 107(09) 623–626;2009.

24. Ludmer PL, Goldschlager N: Cardiac pacing in the 1980's. N Engl J Med 311:1671;1984.

25. Brugada P, Wellens HJJ (eds): Cardiac arrhythmias: Where to go from here? Mt Kisco, NY, Futura, 1987.

26. Mohan R: Management of Common Arrhythmias and Syncope. Family Medicine India Vol 5 No 3:45–50;2001.

27. Cohn PF, Braunwald E: Traumatic heart disease. In: Braunwald E (ed) Heart Disease. 3rd ed. Philadelphia, Saunders, 1988;1535.

28. Kler TS: Cardiac resynchronisation therapy. Prime CME (10) 57–60;2009.

29. Kaplan NM: Systemic hypertension: Therapy. In: Braunwald E (ed) Heart Disease, 3rd ed. Philadelphia, Saunders, 1988;862.

30. Sawhney JPS: Management of Hypertension. Diagnosis and Management. Family Medicine India Vol 5 No 3:1–6;2001.

31. Fraley EE, Feldman BH: Renal hypertension. New Engl J Med 287:550;1972.

32. Frohlich ED: Hypertension 1973: Treatment – why and how. Ann Int Med 78:717;1973.

33. Sheller JR: Asthma: Emerging concepts and potential therapies. Am J Med Sci 293:298;1987.

34. Matuschak GM, Rinaldo JE: Organ interactions in the adult respiratory distress syndrome during sepsis. Chest 94(2):400;1988.

35. Hunter D, Bomford RR: Hutchison's Clinical Methods. 14th ed Cassel, London, 1964.

36. Parkh R: Peripheral Vascular Disease: A Synopsis. Family Medicine India Vol 5 No 3:61–64;2001 .

37. Chhabra MK, Lal A, Sharma KK: Status of Lifestyle Modifications in Hypertension. JIMA 99(09) 504–508;2001.

38. Banerjee A: Coronary Artery Disease and its Problems in Management. JIMA 99(09) 474–475;2001.

39. Gupta R: Prevention of Coronary Heart Disease among Indians: focus on Primary Prevention. JIMA 98(11) 703–709;2000.

40. CHHAP: Care For Me Let Me Beat. A WHO India and GOI Biennium Project, 2004–05 41 Rains AJH, et al: Arteries and Veins. Bailey and Love's Short Practice of Surgery. 13th ed HK Lewis and Co. Ltd. 1965.

Respiratory System Emergencies and Common Disorders

- Signs and symptoms (non-specific manifestations)
- Emergencies and common disorders
  - Acute bronchitis
  - Acute bronchiectasis
  - Acute bronchial asthma
  - Acute status asthmatics
  - Acute pneumonia
  - Acute aspirated pneumonia
  - Adult respiratory distress syndrome
  - Acute adult respiratory failure
  - Acute pulmonary embolism
  - Acute tension pneumothorax
  - Acute traumatic pneumothorax
  - Acute pulmonary tuberculosis
  - COPD
  - Pleurisy
  - Lung abscess
- Respiratory practical procedures

Signs and Symptoms (Non-specific Manifestations)

1. Cough
2. Expectoration
3. Hemoptysis
4. Dyspnea
5. Chest pain
6. Cyanosis

Cough	Most common symptom of upper respiratory catarrh (URC) and lower respiratory catarrh (LRC).
Etiology	Primary: URC & LRC
	Secondary: Congestive heart failure, tuberculosis, sinusitis, otitis media, exposure to inhalation of irritating fumes
Nature	Dry or accompanied by sputum.

Expectoration (Sputum)

Etiology	Bronchitis, asthma: Mucoid expectoration
	Bacterial infection: Yellowish or greenish expectoration
	Lung abscess: Foul smelling expectoration
	Pulmonary edema: Frothy expectoration
	Bronchiectasis: Massive expectoration
	Tuberculosis: Blood in the sputum.

Hemoptysis Spitting or coughing of blood
Etiology   Bronchitis, tuberculosis, bronchiectasis, pulmonary infarction, carcinoma.

Dyspnea

Dyspnea on exertion:
Etiology   Obstruction – due to foreign body, sputum

Dyspnea at rest:
Etiology   Primary: Bronchitis, asthma, bronchiectasis, lung abscess, pneumonia
             Secondary: Congestive heart failure.

Chest Pain

Etiology   A careful history is helpful in identifying the cause of chest pain
             Primary: Pleural effusion, pneumothorax, pleurist, tuberculosis, bronchitis,
             bronchiectasis, lung abscess, pneumonia
             Secondary: Angina pectoris, myocardial infarction, congestive heart failure,
             tension pneumothorax, hemothorax.

Cyanosis High concentration of reduced hemoglobin in the blood
Etiology   Impaired diffusion from alveoli to capillaries
             Inadequate ventilation of alveoli
             Impaired perfusion/ventilation
Precipitating factors Airway obstruction
             Cold exposure.

Acute Bronchitis

Definition   It is defined as inflammation of bronchi. May be severe and life-threatening
             especially in infants and young children, due to respiratory obstruction.
Etiology   Primary: Infection – viral
                      Irritation
             Secondary: Tuberculosis, bronchiectasis, emphysema.
Diagnosis   Cough – productive, i.e. purulent type
             Breathless
             Fever
             Chest pain.
Investigation CXR – PA view
             Sputum – for culture sensitivity.
Management   Bedrest
             Smoking tobacco – prohibited
             Fluids – plenty of fluids to combat dehydration
             Steam inhalation
             Drugs: Antihistamine – to relieve bronchial inflammation

Antitussive: Codeine phosphate PO, 15–30 mg t.d.s./q.d.s.

Bronchodilator: To relieve bronchospasm

Ephedrine 25 mg PO

Antipyretic: Disprin, paracetamol

Antibiotics: To control infection:

Penicillin procaine 600,000 units IM twice daily

Penicillin G tablets 400,000 units PO, q.d.s.

Ampicillin 250–500 mg q.d.s.

Tetracycline 250–500 mg q.d.s.

Refer: The patient to the medical team for management of the underlying cause.

Acute Bronchiectasis

Definition	It is defined as dilatation of bronchi.
Etiology	Infective: Pneumonia, tuberculosis, sinusitis
	Obstructive: Foreign bodies
	Congenital: Pulmonary cyst.
Diagnosis	Cough with expectoration of purulent sputum, hemoptysis
	Fever, night sweats, loss of weight.
Investigation	Hemogram, TLC and DLC
	Sputum for culture sensitivity
	CXR – confirms diagnosis
	Bronchoscopy – reveals bronchial obstruction, bronchiectasis.
D/d	Bronchitis, tuberculosis, lung abscess
Management	Bedrest
	Isolation
	Avoid smoke, fumes, dust, smoking
	Postural drainage – elevate foot end of bed.
	Steam inhalation
	Drugs: Mucolytic agents
	Antibiotics – Broad-spectrum antibiotics (BSA)
	Surgical treatment: Pulmonary resection
	Tracheostomy.

Refer: The patient to the medical team for management of the underlying cause.

Acute Bronchial Asthma

Definition	It is defined as an inflammatory disorder of the airways associated with bronchial hypersensitivity. It may be fatal and to be treated on priority basis.
Etiology	Hypersensitivity of bronchial mucosa, in relation to non-immunological stimuli, e.g. infection, irritating inhalants, cold air, occupational hazards (industrial/mine workers), exercise, stress, etc.

Pathogenesis	Airway obstruction due to mucosal edema, excessive secretion of viscid mucus.
Diagnosis	Recurrent acute attacks of wheezing
	Cough
	Breathlessness
	Expectoration – massive, mucoid sputum
	Prolonged expiration with wheezing and musical rales
	Cyanosis
	Chest pain – pleuritic pain
	Bradycardia, arrhythmia, hypotension
	Cardiac arrest – due to prolonged hypoxia
	Exhaustion, confusion, coma.
Investigation	It is difficult to establish diagnosis on laboratory basis – as no single test It is confirmatory.
	TLC and DLC – Eosinophilia
	ABG
	CXR
	ECG
	C/S – sputum
	Culture, respiratory (isolation, identification and sensitivity)
	• BAL/bronchoscopic swabs
	Lung function tests – forced vital capacity maneuvers.
D/d	Bronchitis
	Emphysema
	Congestive heart failure.
Management	Admit patient for severe/near fatal attack
	Bed-rest – sit the patient up in bed
	Avoid smoke, fumes, dust
	Steam inhalation
	Fluids – orally or parenterally
	Smoking – prohibited
	Oxygen – especially in severe cases. Provide high flow oxygen.
Drugs	Multiple drug regimens in use – as any single drug is ineffective
	Bronchodilators:
	A. B2 agonists:
	Parenteral drugs:
	• Epinephrine is one of most potent bronchial antispasmodic agents available and is the initial drug of choice
	Dose: 0.1–0.5 mL of 1:1000 (0.1%) sol. s.c. Rept 1–2 hrly.
	Nebulized drugs:
	• Salbutamol: 100 μg/metered dose (1–2 inhalations 3–4 times/day), or

- Salmeterol 25 μg b.d. (2 inhalations/puffs), or
- Formoterol 6 μg b.d. (2 inhalations/puffs), or
- Isoproterenol 1:200 (2 inhalations) Rpt after every 30–60 mts., or
- Epinephrine 1:100 (1%) sol. oral inhalation from a hand nebulizer

B. Methylxanthines: To be instituted in case of unsatisfactory results:
- Aminophylline 0.25 g in 10–20 mL saline IV slowly, or
- Theophylline 5–10 mL t.d.s., or
- Etophylline 2–4 mL b.d./or t.d.s. IV

C. Corticosteroids: Very effective in severe cases when above said bronchodilators fail to control attacks:
- Beclomethasone 100 μg q.d.s. inhalation, or
- Hydrocortisone sodium succinate 100–200 mg IV, or
- Prednisolone 40–60 mg/day PO in divided doses, to be reduced to zero within 7–10 days
- Antibiotics – avoid routine antibiotics

ALS   For cardiac arrest (if happens to occur)
C/I   Opiates, sedatives, and tranquilizers, are to be avoided, because of respiration depression.

Refer: Patient to the medical team/ITU for requirement of ventilatory support or for failing to respond to therapy as suggested by deteriorating peak flow, hypercapnea, alarming hypoxia, drowsiness, respiratory arrest or coma.

Acute Status Asthmatics

Management   Hospitalization is mandatory
             Drugs:
- Epinephrine 0.1–0.5 mL of 1:1000 (0.1%) sol. IV, given in case of failure to respond to the drug given s.c. Rpt. 1–2 hrly
- Aminophylline 0.25 g in 10–20 mL saline IV slowly
- Hydrocortisone sod. succinate 100–200 mg IV

             Oxygen
             Endotracheal intubation – indicated in case of rising Paco$_2$
                              (ominous sign)
             IV fluids – 2–4 litres of 5% dextrose in 24 hrs, till oral intake possible
             Sedation – only after establishment of airway
             Bronchoscopy – to remove tenacious secretions.

Refer: The patient to the medical team for management of the underlying cause.

Acute Pneumonia

Definition   It is defined as acute inflammation of lung parenchyma, affecting the breathing, often fatal in young children.
Etiology   Infection:
             Bacterial: *Streptococcus pneumoniae, H. influenzae, Staph. aureus*
             Viral: Influenza.

Source	Pneumococci normally present in healthy mouth and throat.
Predisposing factors	Viral respiratory infections, exposure to cold, irritating gases/fumes, CNS depressants, heart failure.
Diagnosis	Sudden onset of shivering (chills)
	Fever – high
	Cough
	Expectoration – rust coloured sputum
	Breathlessness
	Chest pain
	Respiration – grunting type. Rate > 30/min
	Pleural friction rub may be present.
Investigation	TLC and DLC – leukocytosis
	Blood for culture sensitive test
	Sputum for smear and culture
	ABG
	CXR – show infiltration.
Management	Admit the patient
	Airway maintenance – if required, endotrachial intubation or tracheostomy
	Oxygen therapy – high flow oxygen
	Shock – if present: To be treated on top priority basis
	IV fluids and electrolytes
	Analgesics: Paracetamol, NSAID, or morphine
	Antibiotics: Penicillin G is the drug of choice, 10 million units/24 hrs
	or procaine penicillin 600,000 units 12 hrly
	or cephazolin 4 g IV
	Aspiration: Pleural fluid for smear and culture.

Refer: The patient to the medical team for management of the underlying cause.

Acute Aspirated Pneumonia

Definition	It is a severe type of pneumonia with high mortality rate.
Etiology	Aspiration of gastric materials.
Predisposing factors	Inadequate cough and/or gag reflexes
	Unconsciousness due to head injury, CVA, anesthesia, sedation
	Coma
	Postoperative
	Impaired gastric emptying, e.g. pyloric obstruction
	Alcohol
	Full stomach.
Diagnosis	Airway obstruction causing: Choking, speechlessness, dyspnea, cyanosis, cough, stridor and wheeze
	Signs and symptoms of pneumonia.

Investigation   ABG
                 CXR.
Management   Airway maintenance:
                 • Removal of airway obstruction
                 • Endotrachial intubation
                 • Ventilator with continuous oxygen therapy
                 • Bronchoscopic aspiration
                 Treatment for pneumonia.

Refer: The patient to the medical team for management of the underlying cause.

Adult Respiratory Distress Syndrome (ARDS) (syn. Shock/Pump Lung)

Definition   It is defined as a condition characterized by injury to the alveolar epithelial and endothelial barriers of the lung, interalveolar exudation and interstitial edema.

Etiology   Traumatic – RSA with shock
                 Fat embolism
                 Aspiration – gastric contents, water with near drowning
                 Inhalation – noxious gases, smoke
                 Pneumonia – bacterial/viral
                 Heart – lung perfusions.

Pathogenesis   Trauma, etc. lead to leakage from pulmonary capillary, alveolar exudation, interstitial edema, impaired perfusion ventilation, rigid lungs.

Diagnosis   Dyspnea
                 Cyanosis
                 Respiration – grunting
                 Hypotension
                 Shock.

Investigation   Blood gas estimation: Reduced Pao_2
                 Blood pH – normal or raised
                 CXR (X-ray chest) PA view shows – Patches of density
                                                 – Areas of consolidation.

Management
Preventive treatment
                 Shock: If present – top priority treatment
                 Fluid overloading – to be avoided
                 Electrolytes – salt restriction.

Specific treatment
                 Volume ventilator – Oxygen therapy to maintain Pao_2
                 Antibiotics – to control infection
                 Corticosteroids – to combat: Shock
                                              Fat embolism
                                              Aspiration pneumonia.

Refer: The patient to the medical team for management of the underlying cause.

Acute Adult Respiratory Failure

Etiology   Airway obstruction:
- Acute bronchitis
- Acute asthma
- Acute emphysema

Restrictive defects:
- Pleural effusion
- Pneumothorax
- Pneumonia
- Fibrosis – interstitial

Deformities of chest wall:
- Congenital/acquired – scoliosis, kyphosis
- Traumatic – flail chest
- Drugs – opiates overdose

ARDS/ALI.

Diagnosis   Dyspnea, headache, restlessness, dizziness, confusion, unconscious, coma.

Investigation   Blood gases: $Pao_2 < 50$ mm Hg with or without raised blood CO_2

$Paco_2 > 50$ mm Hg

Hemogram

Sputum

CXR

ECG.

Management

Airway maintenance

     Removal of airway obstruction

     Endotracheal intubation

     Ventilator with continuous oxygen therapy.

Drugs   Bronchodilators:
- Aminophylline 250–500 mg IV over 10 mts. Rpt 6 hrly
- Doxapram 0.5–1.5 mg/kg IV infusion Max 4 mg/kg
- Phenylephrine 0.5 mL in 3 mL saline, delivered by a manual aerosole
- Salmeterol 2 inhalations (50 μg) b.d. delivered by a manual aerosole
- Bambuterol 10 mg o.d. PO Max 20 mg after 1–2 wks.
- Opiates overdose: Give naloxone 200–400 μg IV bolus, followed by infusion as required

Antibiotics: To combat infection

Corticosteroids: Methyl prednisolone 30 mg/kg IV infusion Rpt 4–6 hrs.

Diuretics.

General measures: Deep breathing exercises, steam inhalation, IV access.

Refer: The patient to the medical team for management of the underlying cause.

Acute Pulmonary Embolism (APE)

Definition   It is a common cause of sudden death especially if shock occurs.

Etiology   DVT (embolism from thrombosis of deep veins of legs).

Predisposing factors

    An elderly bedridden patient

    Post-traumatic in major trauma

    Postoperative in a major surgery case

    Postpartum.

Pathogenesis   Virchow's triad: Vessel wall injury, venous stasis and hypercoagulability.

Diagnosis   Dyspnea

    Chest pain – substernal

    Cough, hemoptysis

    Syncope

    Temperature – hyperpyrexia

    Tachycardia, hypotension

    Shock.

Investigation   TLC & DLC – leukocytosis

    ESR – raised

    Serum LDH – raised

    SGOT – raised

    ABG

    CXR – pulmonary infarction, raised diaphragm, pleural effusion

    ECG

    CXR

    Pulmonary angiography.

Management:

Airway maintenance:

    Removal of airway obstruction

    Endotrachial intubation

    Ventilator with continuous oxygen therapy

    Obtain venous access

Monitor respiration, pulse, BP and urine output

Drugs   Anticoagulants:

- UFH IV 80 μ/kg as bolus followed by 18 μ/kg/hr. Infusion, Alt:
- LMWH – enoxaparin 1 mg/kg s.c. b.i.d.
- Daltaparin 120 IU/kg s.c. b.i.d.

    Thrombolytics: Streptokinase 250000 U over ½ hr

        followed by 100000 U/hr infusion for 24 hrs

    Analgesics: Diamorphine 1–2 mg s.c. or IV or

        Mepridine (pethidine) 50–100 mg IV or IM

    Antibiotics: To combat infection

Shock   If present – then treat on top priority basis.

Surgical treatment:

        Embolectomy – as a life saving measure in severe cases

        Paracentesis – removal of fluid in pleural effusion case.

Refer: The patient to the medical team for management of underlying cause.

Acute Tension Pneumothorax

Tension pneumothorax is a serious medical emergency and may be fatal, if not treated promptly.

Etiology	Unknown in majority of cases
	RSA
	Pulmonary disorder.
Pathogenesis	Tear in the visceral pleura, leads to air entry into pleural space, lung collapse, raised intrapleural pressure, cardiorespiratory disturbance.
Diagnosis	Chest pain – referred to shoulder or arm
	Dyspnea
	Cough – dry
	Movements of chest – restricted.
Investigation	CXR shows – Air in the pleural space, retracted lung.

Management

Aspiration of air

Method	Insert a large bore needle into the front of chest, into the pleural space, to relieve tension
	After relief of tension, a rubber glove drainage introduced into pleural space, other end attached to a water trap apparatus
Oxygen	Give maximal inspired oxygen to reverse hypoxia
Analgesics	Morphine 10–15 mg s.c.

Shock – if present, then treat on top priority basis.

Refer: The patient to the medical team for management of the underlying cause.

Acute Traumatic Pneumothorax

Traumatic pneumothorax is an emergency and demands priority treatment.

Etiology	Open chest wounds (sucking wounds) – due to RSA, stab injuries
	Closed chest wounds (lung puncture/laceration) due to fracture rib.
Diagnosis	Chest pain
	Dyspnea
	Movements of chest – restricted
	Hypotension.
Investigation	CXR – confirms diagnosis
	Note: Do not wait for CXR in case of airway obstruction and priority for airway management.

Management   Open chest wounds (sucking) – to be covered up with available means, e.g. bandage, shirt.

Surgery: Close the wound at earliest possible axillary.

Acute Pulmonary Tuberculosis

Definition   It is defined as an infectious disease.

Etiology   *Mycobacterium tuberculosis* – an acid-fast organism, characterized by the formation of tubercles in the lungs.

Predisposing factors

Malnutrition, diabetes, general debility, silicosis

Overcrowding

Insanitory living conditions.

Diagnosis   Cough >2/52

Hemoptysis

Fatigue, loss of weight

Symptoms due to extrapulmonary lesions: Involvement of pleura, bones and joints, GI tract, genitourinary tract, CNS (meninges) and lymph nodes.

Pediatric TB   Diagnosis of TB in children is difficult. Sputum usually cannot be obtained from them and if obtained, is often negative even on culture.

Diagnosis rests mainly on clinical history, history of contact with an infectious adult, X-ray examination and tuberculin testing.

Investigation   Sputum: For smear and culture tests:

Bacteriological examination of at least 3 samples – confirms diagnosis.

Culture is more sensitive than smear test, but is a time consuming test (4–6 weeks).

Tuberculin skin test, i.e. skin hypersensitivity to bacterial protein antigen.

Methods: Mantoux test: tuberculin injected s.c.

        Heaf test: Tuberculin injected by multiple punctures

Report: A positive reaction (induration > 10 mm) after 3/7, indicates past or current infection. But a positive test, is always not confirmatory for the presence of disease and at best can be only supportive.

A negative reaction – rules out pulmonary tuberculosis.

- Rapid culture method like: BACTEC and mycobacterial growth indicator tube (MGIT) method, continue to be costly and mostly non-available. Hence, sputum culture methods remain a limited option for majority of patients.
- Molecular biology techniques like: Polymerase chain reaction (PCR) genomic analysis, have been developed to detect the presence of drug resistance. However, these remain costly and widely non-available.

CXR: Confirms the diagnosis in majority of pulmonary tuberculosis patients.

Findings: Apical and subapical infiltrations, cavitation.

FNAC or biopsy lymph node: Histological and cultural studies – confirm diagnosis.

Management
General measures

Diet – nutritious diet

Isolation of patient

Hygiene – good

BCG vaccination – at birth to newborns, if born in an institution, and between the ages of 6 weeks and 9 months otherwise.

BCG does not protect individuals from developing adult type pulmonary TB. However, BCG prevents serious forms of TB in children.

Medication

Intermittent treatment	It has been proved by clinical trials that thrice a week (alternate day treatment) is as effective as daily treatment. However, it should be used under direct observation (DOTS), so as to ensure that the patient completes the full course of treatment and is fully cured.
Drugs	Antitubercular (AT) drugs: Primary: Isoniazid, streptomycin, PAS, ethambutol, rifampin
Isoniazid (INH)	Most effective drug, when used in combination with other (AT) drugs Dose: Adult dose: 0.60 g PO, t.i.w. Child dose: 10–15 mg/kg PO t.i.w.
Streptomycin	Less effective than isoniazid. It is not used currently, except for resistant organisms. Dose: Adult dose: 0.75–1 g (0.5 g for patients >50 yrs or <30 kg) IM, t.i.w. Child dose: 15 mg/kg IM, t.i.w. Toxicity: May cause injury to 8th cranial nerve (vertigo, deafness)

PAS (aminosalicylic acid): Less effective, but when used in combination with other (AT) drugs, it delays resistant organisms-emergence

Dose: 4–5 g PO, t.i.w.

Ethambutol	Relatively safer drug. Currently used as a substitute for PAS Dose: Adult dose: 1.20 g PO, t.i.w. Child dose: 30 mg/kg PO, t.i.w. Toxicity: Affects visual activity. To be avoided in infants and young children
Rifampin	It is one of the latest available, safe AT drug. Cost is main disadvantage Dose: Adult dose: 0.45–0.60 g PO, t.i.w. Child dose: 10–20 mg/kg PO, t.i.w.

Pyrazinamide (PZA): Less effective than abovesaid primary AT drugs.

Dose: Adult dose: 1.50 g PO, t.i.w.

Child dose: 35 mg/kg PO, t.i.w.

Toxicity: Toxic hepatitis.

Treatment Categories and Sputum Examination Schedule (Table 4.1)

Categories   There are three categories of treatment for patients suffering from tuberculosis (pulmonary or extrapulmonary).

Duration   Usually 6–8/12.

Phases
- Intensive phase (IP) of 2–4/12 and continuous phase (CP) of 4–5/12, depending upon the category of treatment.

Table 4.1: Treatment categories and sputum examination schedule

Category	TB cases	Intensive phase	Result (sputum)	Continuation phase
I	New sputum +ve, New sputum -ve, New extrapulmonary, New + HIV +ve status	2 (HRZE) t.i.w.	-ve +ve	4(HR) t.i.w. 1/4(HRZE) t.i.w.
II	Sputum +ve relapse, Sputum +ve failure, Sputum smear +ve treatment after default, Extrapulmonary relapse	3 (HRZE) t.i.w. + 2S tiw	-ve +ve	5(HRZE) t.i.w. 5(HRZE) t.i.w.
III	New sputum -ve, who are not seriously ill, Extrapulmonary, who are not seriously ill	2 (HRE) t.i.w.	-ve +ve	4(HR) tiw Refer to MO for Category II treatment

Key The number before the letters refers to number of months of treatment.
H: Isoniazid (0.60 g), R: Rifampicin (0.45 g), Z: Pyrazinamide (1.50 g), E: Ethambutol (1.20 g), S: Streptomycin (0.75 g).
Patients weighing > 60 kg receive additional 0.150 g of rifampicin.
Patients > 50 yrs of age and < 50 kg of wt., receive streptomycin 0.50 g.
Patients in categories I and II, having +ve sputum smear at the end of the initial intensive phase receive an additional month of intensive phase (IP) treatment.
Examples of seriously ill extrapulmonary TB cases are: Meningitis, disseminated TB, spinal TB with neurological complications, tuberculous pericarditis, peritonitis, bilateral or extensive pleurisy, intestinal TB and genitourinary TB.
Start afresh category II treatment for:
• Category I and Category III cases (+ve smear at 5–7/12).

Treatment categories: Phases and duration of treatment (Table 4.2)

Surgical treatment: Few patients now require surgery for pulmonary tuberculosis.

Methods: Pulmonary resection and thoracoplasty.

Pulmonary resection:

Indications
- Localized focus not responding to AT drugs for > 6 months
- Bronchial stenosis

Thoracoplasty

Indications
- Performed occasionally to reduce pleural dead space
- To close a chronic empyema space.

Refer: The severe patient to the medical and surgical teams.

Table 4.2: Treatment categories–phases and duration (doses)

Category	Duration (number of doses)		Total
	Intensive phase	Continuation phase	
I	8/52 (24 doses)	18/52 (54 doses)	26/52 (78 doses)
II	12/52 (36 doses)	22/52 (66 doses)	34/52 (102 doses)
III	8/52 (24 doses)	18/52 (54 doses)	26/52 (78 doses)

Note: In all cases of jaundice, anti-TB drugs should be stopped immediately and the patient referred for evaluation

(Source: Revised National Tuberculosis Control Programme , MOH, New Delhi)

Chronic Obstructive Pulmonary Disease (COPD)

Definition	Is defined as chronic respiratory disorder, mild to severe in intensity.
Etiology	Bacterial infection: pathogenic micro-organisms (PPMs)
Predisposing	Smoking
factors	Obesity
	Depression
Pathogenesis	PPMs in airways, causing inflammation, suppuration
Diagnosis	Age: > 35 yrs
	Breathlessness, cough, sputum, wheeze, hemoptysis
	Fever: Mild to moderate
Investigations	CBC, ESR, LFT
	Sputum analysis
	LFT: Spirometry (FEV mild <80%, moderate 30–50%, severe <30%)
	BMI
	MRC: Dyspnea score
	SaO_2: Severe COPD
	CXR
Complications	Severe COPD
	Cor pulmonale
	FEV: Rapid decline
	Infections: Recurrent
	Breathing: Dysfunctional
	Hemoptysis
Management	General measures:
	Smoking cessation
	Obesity control
	Fluids intake in plenty
	Steam inhalation
	Breathing exercises: Use of respiratory exerciser

Specific measures: Oxygen therapy

Drugs:

- Antibiotics
- Bronchodilators: Salbutamol, fenoterol, bambuterol, salmeterol,
- Mucolytic agents: To control cough
- Nebuliser therapy
- Steroids therapy: Oral or inhaler.

Refer: To Medical team for management of complicated cases.

Pleurisy

Etiology	Pulmonary tuberculosis
	Pneumonia
	Pulmonary infarction.
Diagnosis	Pain in the chest
	Dyspnea
	Fever
	Cough
	Expectoration
	Movements of chest – restricted
	Trachia – displaced, apex beat – shifted.
Investigation	CXR shows: Costophrenic angle – obliteration
	Mediastinum – shifting
	Aspiration of fluid: Fluid for smear and culture study
	Pleural biopsy: Confirms the clinical diagnosis.
Management	Thoracocentesis: Daily aspiration of fluid.

Refer: The patient to the medical team for management of the underlying cause.

Lung Abscess

Definition	It is defined as an inflammatory necrosis of lung parenchyma.
Etiology	Infection, e.g. pneumonias, bacterial septicemia.

Predisposing factors:

	Inadequate cough reflex, e.g. anesthesia,
	Bronchial obstruction
	Postoperative
	Coma
Diagnosis	Fever
	Cough
	Expectoration – foul smelling, massive sputum – brown, grey, or greenish
	Chest pain.
Investigation	Sputum for smear and culture
	CXR – A dense shadow with central radiolucency.

Management   Postural drainage

Bronchoscopic aspiration

Antibiotics

Analgesics

Expectorant.

Refer: The patient to the medical team for management of the underlying cause.

Practical Procedures

1. CXR (X-ray chest) – PA view
2. CT scan
3. MRI
4. Ultrasound
5. Bronchoscopy
6. Radioisotope imaging
7. Pleural cavity aspiration
8. Lung biopsy
9. Immunological tests
10. Pulmonary tests
11. Blood gas analysis.

CXR (X-ray Chest)

Position   Posteroanterior view

Examination   Bony cage – shape, cervical rib, crawling of ribs, scoliosis

Outline – heart and mediastinum

Costophrenic angles, diaphragm

Lung fields

Indications   Bronchitis

Bronchiectasis

Bronchial asthma

Pulmonar tuberculosis

Pulmonary fibrosis

Pulmonary embolism

Bronchogenic carcinoma

Lung abscess.

CT Scan

Aim   A series of cross-sectional images showing details of mediastinal structures and soft tissues.

Indications   Bronchiectasis

Pulmonary fibrosis

Pulmonary embolism

Bronchogenic carcinoma
Bronchitis
Bronchial asthma
Pulmonary tuberculosis
Lung abscess.

MRI

Indications   Mediastinal disorders
                  Tumors
Disadvantages Movement artifact.

Ultrasound

Indications   Examination – diaphragm movements
                  Pleural fluid presence – to differentiate from pleural thickening
                  To aid in drainage of pleural fluid.

Bronchoscopy

Indications   Bronchogenic carcinoma.

Radioisotope Imaging

Indications   Pulmonary embolism.

Pleural Cavity Aspiration

Indication   Diagnostic
                  Therapeutic, e.g. To remove pleural fluid or air
                                     To induce pneumothorax
                                     To inject antibiotics in cases of empyema.
Method   Patient sits back on the bed and leans forward.
                  Infiltrate the area with lignocaine plain 1%, down to the pleura.
                  Insert a large bore needle with a syringe, in the space along the upper
                  edge of lower rib. The site – anterior, middle, or posterior axillary line in
                  the 5th, 6th, or 7th space. Entry into the pleural cavity is indicated by
                  feeling of 'give' with suction, the fluid begins to flow into the syringe
                  Seal the skin puncture, after withdrawl of the needle.
Care   Avoid introducing air (pneumothorax).

Lung Biopsy

Indication   Tumors – to obtain samples of lung parenchyma.

Immunological Tests

Indications   Bronchial asthma – skin hypersensitivity tests
                  Tuberculosis – Mantoux and Heaf tests
                  Fungal infections – precipitating antibodies tests.

Pulmonary Tests

Spirography (Kymography)

To measure all lung volumes and capacities, except FRC (measured by an open circuit method).

Pulmonary Volumes

- *Tidal volume (TV)* is the volume of air that is breathed in or out during quite respiration (about 5 dL)
- *Inspiratory reserve volume (IRV)* is the maximal volume of air that is breathed in by forced inspiration post a normal tidal inspiration (2–3.2 L)
- *Expiratory reserve volume (ERV)* is the maximal volume of air that can be breathed out by forced expiration post a normal tidal expiration (0.7–1 L)
- *Residual volume (RV)* is the volume of air that remains in the lungs post maximal expiration (1.2 L)

Pulmonary Capacities

- *Vital capacity (VC)* is the maximal volume of air that can be breathed out from the lungs by forced expiration post a maximal inspiration. It is 4.8 L in male and 3.2 L in female. It is related to the size and physiue of the subject (2.6 L/m^2 in male and 2.1 L/m^2 in female). It is increased in swimmers and divers, and decreased in old debilitated persons and in pulmonary disorders (airway obstruction, ARDS/PARDS, emphysema, pneumothorax, pleural effusion, pulmonary edema, poliomyelitis), ascites and pregnancy. It is altered by posture (greater in upright position due to decreased pulmonary blood volume).
- *Total lung capacity (TLC)* is the volume of air that remains in the lungs post a maximal inspiration.
  Total lung capacity = Vital capacity + Residual volume (6L).
- Inspiratory capacity is the maximal volume of air that can be inspired from the resting expiratory level.
- *Functional residual capacity (FRC)* is the volume of air that remains in the lungs at the resting expiratory level.
  FRC = Residual volume + Expiratory reserve volume
  FRC is increased in emphysema and asthma due to hyperinflation of the lungs.
- *Maximum breathing capacity (MBC):* Currently maximum ventilation volume (MVV) is the maximal volume of air that can be ventilated on command during a given interval.

Blood Gas Analysis

Is the estimation of partial pressures of oxygen and carbon dioxide in the blood along with blood pH, for diagnosing respiraotory failure and acid base disturbances. Partial pressures of oxygen < 60 and of carbon dioxide > 50 mm of Hg, indicate acute respiratory failure.

References

1. Kirby WMM (editor). Modern management of respiratory diseases. M Clin North America 51:267; 1967.
2. Sheller JR. Asthma: Emerging concepts and potential therapies. Am J Med Sci 293:298;1987.
3. Goldhaber SZ (ed). Pulmonary Embolism and Deep Venous Thrombosis. Philadelphia. Saunders, 1985.
4. Pingleton SK. Complications of acute respiratory failure. Am Rev Respir Dis 137:1463;1988.
5. Lanken PN. Mechanical Ventilation in Pulmonary Diseases and Disorders, 2nd ed. AP Fishman (ed) New York, McGraw-Hill, chap. 155;1988.
6. Tobin MJ. Respiratory monitoring in the intensive care unit. Am Rev Respir Dis 138:1625;1988.
7. Arora VK. Management of tuberculosis in special situations. Current Medical Journal, 2005.
8. Swash M. Hutchison's Clinical Methods 21st Ed. Saunders, London, 2002.
9. DOTS. Revised National Tuberculosis Control Programme (RNTCP). MOH and Family Welfare, New Delhi, 2008.

Fluid and Electrolyte Emergencies and Common Disorders

Basic considerations:
- Physiology
- Normal values

Emergencies and common disorders:
- Acute water depletion
- Acute water intoxication
- Acute dehydration
- Acute overhydration
- Acute respiratory acidosis
- Acute respiratory alkalosis
- Acute metabolic acidosis
- Acute metabolic alkalosis
- Hypernatremia
- Hyponatremia
- Hyperkalemia
- Hypokalemia
- Hypercalcemia
- Hypocalcemia
- Hypermagnesemia
- Hypomagnesemia

Physiology Body fluids being distributed in two compartments (Table 5.1):
1. Intracellular fluid – bounded by cell membrane
2. Extracellular fluid – fluid outside cells. Types:
    i. Plasma of vascular system and
    ii. Interstitial (tissue) fluid – occupies extracellular tissues (spaces)
3. Transcellular fluid – separated from plasma by another epithelium, besides capillary endothelium, i.e. cerebrospinal fluid (CSF); serous fluids; synovial fluids; aqueous and vitreous humour; digestive juices of gastrointestinal tract; and urine volume and composition.

Acute Water Depletion

Etiology
- Inadequate intake due to – unconsciousness, exhaustion, esophageal obstruction, GI tract surgery – postoperatively
- Loss of water due to – hot weather, fever, vomiting, diarrhea, diabetes insipidus, diabetes mellitus, diuretics.

Diagnosis   Thirst, dry lips, flushed skin, oliguria, confusion, delirium, coma.
Investigation   Hemogram, serum electrolytes.
Management
- IV dextrose 5% or dextrose saline 2–3 L/day.
  Caution – avoid overloading
- Maintenance of intake/output charts
- Oral fluids
- Treatment of underlying cause.

Acute Water Intoxication

Etiology	• Increased intake of water due to – excessive IV fluids especially isotonic dextrose (5%), water P/R.
	• Decreased diuresis due to – insufficient renal function, CHF, cirrhosis with ascites.
Diagnosis	Headache, nausea, and incordination of movements are main features, vomiting, abdominal cramps, muscular weakness, drowsiness, coma.
Management	Restrict the water intake
	IV hypertonic saline solution – to promote shifting of ICF to ECF
	Treatment of cause.

Acute Dehydration

It is defined as decrease in the volume of both ICF and ECF, with the corresponding rise in the concentration of ICF and ECF solute.

Pathogenesis	In the blood:
	Concentration of plasma electrolyte and protein – resulting in increased plasma osmolality
	Hypovolemia – reduced renal blood flow – resulting in dysuria.
Etiology	Reduced intake of water, i.e. unconscious, esophageal obstruction
	Loss of water, i.e. hot weather, fever, vomiting, diarrhea, diabetes insipidus.
Diagnosis	Thirst, dry lips, flushed skin, oliguria, confusion, delirium, coma.
Investigation	Serum electrolytes.
Management	IV fluids – Dextrose 2.5–5.0% sol. 2–3 L/day, Alt:
	– Ringer's (lactated) sol.
	Oral fluids (ORS, i.e. oral rehydration salts)
	Treatment of underlying cause.

Acute Overhydration (syn. Dilution Syndrome)

It is defined as increase in the volume of both ICF and ECF, with the corresponding fall in the concentration of ICF and ECF solute.

Pathogenesis	In the blood:
	Water excess (overhydration) leads to increased body fluid, decreased plasma electrolyte and protein, reduced plasma osmolarity.
Etiology	Increased water intake, i.e. excessive IV fluids
	Decreased urinary excretion
	Ascites.
Diagnosis	Headache, nausea, vomiting, weakness, abdominal cramps, convulsions, coma.
Management	
Acute cases	IV hypertonic saline solution, to promote shifting of ICF fluid to ECF.

Acute Respiratory Acidosis

It is defined as a decrease in pH (increased H^+) of ECF, due to respiratory disorders.

Pathogenesis:

Hypoventilation → Elevated H_2CO_3 ↘

Elevated pCO_2 ↙

Acidosis ← Lowered pH of ECF

Etiology	Anesthesia – inadequate ventilation
	Respiratory centre depression – CNS disorders, drugs
	Lung disorders – emphysema, acute asthma, acute pneumonia
	Trauma – head injury, spinal injury.
Diagnosis	Dyspnea, breathlessness, confusion, coma.
Management	• Monitor pCO_2, Po_2, and pH of arterial blood
	• Endotracheal intubation
	• Ventilator with oxygen supply
	• IV fluids
	• Antidotes for anesthetics or drugs causing respiratory center depression
	• Bronchodilators
	• Tracheostomy may be required as an emergency measure.

Refer: The severe patient to the medical team.

Acute Respiratory Alkalosis

It is defined as an increase in pH (decreased H^+) of ECF, due to respiratory disorders.

Pathogenesis   Hyperventilation → Lowered H_2CO_3 ↘

Lowered pCO_2 ↙

Alkalosis ← Elevated pH of ECF

Etiology	Anxiety, fear
	Anesthesia – pulmonary hyperventilation
	High altitudes – hyperventilation
	Ventilator – faulty use (misuse)
	Acute asthma, acute pneumonia, pulmonary edema
	Trauma – head injury
	Drugs – salicylate poisoning.
Diagnosis	Tetany, neuromuscular irritation
	Pallor
	Hypotension
	Respiratory arrest.
Management	Anxiety: By drugs/psychotherapy
	Tetany: By rebreathing exalted air, that will increase pCO_2 and lower pH
	Respiratory arrest – treated by insufflation of CO_2.

Refer: The severe patient to the medical team.

Acute Metabolic Acidosis

It is defined as a decrease in pH (increased H^+) of ECF, due to metabolic disorders.

Pathogenesis	Metabolic disorders lead to inadequate H^+ excretion, HPO_4 retention, Na^+ K^+ Ca^{++} loss, metabolic acidosis.
Etiology	Starvation, diarrhea, ulcerative colitis, prolonged intestinal obstruction, diabetes mellitus with ketosis, renal insufficiency.
Diagnosis	Respiration – fast, noisy (hyperpnea)
	Pulse rate – increased
	Hypertension
	Urine – acidic.
Investigation	Plasma HCO_3 estimation – decreased.
Management	Removal of cause, i.e. insulin for control of diabetes
	IV fluids – Darrow's solution or saline and sodium lactate or HCO_3
	IV electrolytes replacement
	Renal insufficiency – ion exchange resins which bind K^+, reducing K^+ ion concentration, by preventing absorption of K^+ in the intestine or by hemodialysis or peritoneal hemolysis.

Refer: The severe patient to the medical team.

Acute Metabolic Alkalosis

It is defined as an increase in pH (decreased H^+) of ECF due to metabolic disorders.

Pathogenesis	Metabolic disorders lead to increased excretion of H^+, retention of HCO_3, elevation of HCO_3 in ECF, metabolic alkalosis.
Etiology	Vomiting or gastric aspiration – in pyloric stenosis
	Drugs – diuretics, corticoids.
Diagnosis	Respiration – Cheyne-Stokes respiration with periods of apnea (5–30 sec)
	Tetany – latent
	Renal insufficiency.
Management	Main aim: Replacement of potassium followed by normal saline
	Plenty of water, K^+, Na^+, Cl^-
	IV fluids (water) K^+, Na^+, Cl^-
	No lactate or HCO_3 to be given.

Hypernatremia

It is defined as increased concentration of sodium (Na) in ECF.

Etiology	Dehyderation, nephritis, cirrhosis, congestive heart failure (CHF), burns, excess of IV isotonic (0.9%) solution given.
Diagnosis	Puffiness of face, pitting edema over sacrum in severe cases, overweight
	Infants: Raised tension in the anterior fontanelle, polyuria, edema.
Investigation	Serum electrolytes.
Management	• Discontinue the saline infusion
	• Orally water or IV fluids (dextrose and water or hypotonic NaCl sol) diuretics, salt restriction, stop electrolytes.

Refer: The severe patient to the medical team.

Hyponatremia

It is defined as decreased concentration of sodium in ECF.

Etiology
- Traumatic – incld. surgical trauma
- Nausea, vomiting, diarrhea, excessive sweating in hot climate
- Intestinal obstruction, gastric aspiration
- Addison's disease, nephritis, nausea, vomiting, diarrhea,
- Nephritis
- CHF.

Diagnosis   Face drawn, sunken eyes, dry skin, tongue dry and coated, hypotension, dark coloured urine of high specific gravity.

Infants   Depressed anterior fontanelle.

Investigation   Blood – FBC, U&E, LFTs, thyroid function, osmolarity
Urine – sodium and osmolarity
ECG
CXR
Ultrasonography.

Management   Severe cases: Plasma or plasma expander
Isotonic saline solution (0.9%) IV
Less severe cases: Isotonic saline solution (0.9%) IV or Ringer's solution IV.

Refer: The severe patient to the medical team.

Hyperkalemia

It is defined as increased K^+ in ECF due to shift from ICF.

Etiology   Renal insufficiency – failure to excrete ingested potassium
Trauma – crush injury
Dehydration, burns, infection
Drugs – digitalis poisoning.

Diagnosis   Muscular weakness, paralysis, diarrhea, abdominal distention, ventricular fibrillation, cardiac arrest.

Investigation   ECG: T waves – peaked and QRS complex widened.

Management   Monitor ECG
Withhold potassium
Cation exchange resins orally or by enema
IV calcium (10 mL of 10% calcium gluconate) – as an antagonist ion
IV $NaHCO_3$
Renal failure – hemodialysis or peritoneal dialysis to remove K^+.

Refer: The severe patient to the medical (nephrology) team for emergency dialysis.

Hypokalemia

It is defined as decreased K^+ in ECF due to shift to ICF.

Etiology   Traumatic – including operative trauma
Starvation – inadequate intake of potassium

Gastroduodenal obstruction

Steatorrhea – inadequate absorption

Irritable bowl syndrome, gastroenteritis

Diabetic coma – managed by insulin

Saline solution – prolonged infusion

Burns.

Diagnosis	Patient listless, drowsiness, speech impaired, muscular weakness, paralytic ileus, incontinence of urine, gasping respirations, hypotension, cardiac arrest.
Investigation	ECG: Shows lowering/inversion of T waves and prolonged QRST interval.
Management	• Diet: Oral potassium in form of milk, meat extracts, fruit juices
	• Orally: KCl 2 g PO q.d.s,
	• Parenterally: IV potassium used with great caution, e.g. in impaired renal function with associated alkalosis: KCl 2 g in 0.5 L of 5% dextrose solution @20 drops/min. Max 3 g of potassium /24 hrly.
	• Darrow's solution – For impaired renal function without alkalosis.
	• Monitor the pulse rate during administration of potassium.

Refer: The severe patient to the medical team.

Hypercalcemia

Etiology	Hyperparathyroidism: Carcinoma breast, lungs, thyroid, kidney.
Diagnosis	Nausea, vomiting, thirst, polyuria, dehydration, anorexia, constipation, pain abdomen, muscular weakness, hangover, confusion, coma.
Investigation	Blood for FBC, U&E, LFTs, serum lipase
	Thyroid function tests
	ECG – bradycardia
	CXR – diagnostic.
Management	Removal of the cause
	Symptomatic treatment:

- Isotonic sodium chloride solution (0.9%) IV (excretion of Na^+) to be followed by excretion of Ca^{++}
- Diuretics: Furosemide may/may not be given along sodium chloride
- IV fluids along with potassium and magnesium
- Corticoids – used in case of carcinoma. Mithramycins are useful.

Refer: The severe patient to the medical team.

Hypocalcemia

Etiology	Hypoparathyroidism, renal insufficiency, rickets, malabsorption syndrome.
Diagnosis	Muscle cramps, abdominal cramps, tetany, convulsions dyspnea, polyuria, dwarfism.
Management	Removal of primary cause.
	Hypoparathyroidism – calcium with vitamin D.

Tetany:
- Hypocalcemic tetany – calcium gluconate 1–2 g IV
- Latent tetany – calcium chloride/gluconate/lactate/carbonate

Preparations and routes of administration:
- Calcium chloride (27% calcium) routes: PO or IV (10% sol)
- Calcium gluconate (9% calcium) routes: PO, IM or IV (10% sol)
- Calcium lactate (13% calcium) routes: PO
- Precipitated calcium carbonate (40% calcium) route: PO only.

Hypermagnesemia

Etiology	Renal insufficiency, excess Mg^{++} intake as a cathartic.
Diagnosis	Muscle weakness, sedation, confusion, hypotension
	Death may occur due to respiratory failure.
Investigation	ECG: Increased PR interval, broadening of QRS complex and elevated T waves.
Management	• Removal of cause – renal insufficiency
	• IV calcium gluconate/chloride – as an antagonist to Mg^{++}
	• Dialysis – may be indicated.

Refer: The severe patient to the medical team.

Hypomagnesemia

Etiology	Chronic alcoholism, starvation, diarrhea, malabsorption syndrome, prolonged GI suction, hypoparathyroidism.
Diagnosis	Hyperirritability, spasticity, cardiac arrhythmias, convulsions, death.
Management	IV fluids
	IV MgCl or $MgSO_4$ 10–40 mEq/day.

Refer: The severe patient to the medical team.

References

1. Keele Cyril A, Neil Eric: Body water and Body Fluid. Samson Wright's Applied Physiology, London, 1963.
2. Weiner M and others: Signs and symptoms of electrolyte disorders. Yale J Biol Med 43:76;1970.
3. Maxwell M, Kleeman CR (editors): Clinical Disorders of Fluid and Electrolyte Metabolism. 2nd ed. McGraw-Hill, 1972.
4. Papper S, Whang R: Hyperkalemia and Hypokalemia. Disease-A-Month. Year Book. June 1964.
5. Krupp MA: Fluid & Electrolyte Disorders. Lang Medical Publications, 1975.
6. Goodman LS and Gilman A: Water, Salts, and Ions. The Pharmacological Basis of Therapeutics, 2nd ed. Macmillan Co. 1960.

Environmental (Physical Agents) Emergencies and Common Disorders

Cold injuries:	Drowning
• Hypothermia	• Drowning and near drowning
• Chilblain	• Caisson disease
• Frostbite	• Anoxia
• Immersion foot (Trench foot)	Shock
Heat injuries:	• Electric shock
• Heat exhaustion	Irradiation
• Heat stroke	• Acute ionizing radiation
• Burns	

Hypothermia (syn. Cold Injury)

Etiology	Exposure to prolonged/extreme cold weather (wind, rain, chill)
	Unconsciousness
	Alcohol abuse
	Drug abuse – sedatives.
Pathogenesis	Cold exposure leads to – vasoconstriction, skin temp < 25°C, slowing of metabolism, increased demand for oxygen, cyanosis, tissue necrosis.
Diagnosis	Skin: cold, clammy, pale/cyanotic, urticaria
	Temp < 25°C (77°F)
	Shivering
	Hypotension, bradycardia
	Coma.
Investigation	Blood for FBC, U&E, sugar, lipase/amylase
	ECG – bradycardia, prolonged QT interval, atrial fibrillation
	CXR.

Management

Preventive measures

Keep warm, dry and moving

Active exercises of arms, legs, fingers/toes

Hot beverages – tea, coffee, etc.

Avoid alcohol, smoking.

Treatment	Warm up the body by extra-warm clothes, use of room heaters/warm AC
	Oxygen therapy
	Endotracheal intubation
	Treat the underlying cause.

Chilblain

Etiology	Exposure to prolonged/extreme cold weather (wind, rain, chill).
Pathogenesis	Cold exposure leads to–freezing with/without blistering, ulceration, hemorrhages, fibrosis.
Diagnosis	Blisters, ulcers, bleeding, fibrosis, atrophy.
Management	Rest, warmth atmosphere, hot beverages – tea, coffee, etc.
	Elevation of affected part
	Treatment of blisters, ulcers, bleeding, fibrosis.

Refer: The severe patient to the medical team.

Frostbite

Etiology	Exposure to prolonged/extreme cold weather (wind, rain, chill).
Pathogenesis	Damaged vessel walls, followed by transudation and edema (frostbitten)
	Cold exposure leads to – freezing with or without blistering/peeling (necrosis of tissues).
Diagnosis	Pain – severe burning, followed by:
	• Impaired sensations – pricking, itching, numbness
	• Stiffness
	• Blisters, followed by gangrene.
Management	Rewarming – firm steady pressure
	– immersion of part in hot water for 30 mts.
	Bed rest, wrapping in a blanket, elevation of the affected part
	Avoid trauma – friction
	Antibiotics
	Anticoagulants – heparin
	Surgery – amputation indicated in established cases.

Refer: The severe patient to the medical team.

Immersion Foot (syn. Trench Foot)

Etiology	Prolonged immersion of foot/hand in cold/muddy water.
Diagnosis	Affected foot/hand – cold, pale/cyanotic, later on turns red, hot
	Numbness followed by burning and shooting pains
	Hemorrhages
	Gangrene.
Investigation	Blood for FBC, sugar, culture
	X-ray of affected foot/hand
	CXR.

Management   Admit the patient

Protection from trauma and infection

Change the wet clothes

Bed rest

Elevate the affected part

Do not massage

Antibiotics

Surgery – amputation in advanced stages, i.e. established Gangrene.

Refer: The severe patient to the medical team.

Heat Exhaustion (syn. Heat Prostration)

Etiology   Heat exposure. Patients with cardiac, cerebral, systemic disorders, are more prone to heat exhaustion.

Pathogenesis   Heat exposure leads to water and salt depletion, resulting in collapsed peripheral circulation.

Diagnosis   Muscular weakness, muscle cramps, dizziness, headache

Skin – cold, pale, perspiration

Oliguria

Tachycardia

Hypotension

Shock.

Investigation   Hemoconcentration, electrolytes depletion.

Management   Bed rest in a cool place

Elevate feet

Massage legs

Sodium chloride 0.1% sol PO or saline IV 1–2 L

Shock: If present – then treat accordingly on top priority basis.

Refer: The severe patient to the medical team.

Heat Stroke (syn. Sunstroke)

Definition   It is a medical emergency and requires priority treatment.

Etiology   Exposure to hot weather

Affects mostly the elderly, alcoholics, weak, cardiac patients.

Pathogenesis   Sudden failure of heat-regulating system.

Diagnosis   High fever – temperature (rectal) >42°C.

Sweating – absent.

Headache, nausea, vomiting, convulsions, unconsciousness.

Skin – hot, dry, flushed.

Pulse fast, weak, and irregular.

Hypotension.

Shock.

Management
General measures

- Admit the patient in a cool place – fans/air conditioner on.
- Remove clothes
- Cool the patient by fanning or cold sponging or if possible, immerse the patient in cold water.
- Massage the limbs

Emergency treatment

- Airway maintenance – by measures include ventilator with oxygen.
- IV saline sol. 1 litre, to be given slowly.
- Antipyretics – reduce fever and also have analgesic effect.
- Aspirin 0.3–0.6 g, 4 hrly PO.
- Paracetamol 0.5 g, 3–6 times daily PO.
- Antibiotics – to control infection.
- Antishock measures – for treatment of shock (described in appropriate section, e.g. shock syndrome).
- Chlorpromazine – to control shivering and convulsions.
- Cold sponging with ice packs or ice water, with the caution – not to bring down temperature rapidly.
- Removal of the cause – eradication of the primary cause of fever should be the main aim of treatment.

Burns

Burns are due to dry heat, whereas scalds are due to moist heat.

Etiology
1. Heat: Gas flame, steam, hot water
2. Chemicals: Acids, alkalies (caustic soda)
3. Electricity
4. Radiation.

Diagnosis
Erythema with or without blisters
Discharging wounds
Shock – due to fluid loss
Infection
Scars.

Evaluation of burn injury: By considering:
1. Area of body surface involved: By Rule of Nines, i.e.

Head and neck =	9%
Arms	= 18%
Legs front	= 18%
Legs back	= 18%
Trunk front	= 18%
Trunk back	= 18%
Genitalia	= 1%

2. Depth of burn: i. Partial thickness burn

               ii. Full thickness burn.

Management

Treatment of burn shock

Due to plasma loss

      i. Plasma transfusion or plasma substitute, i.e. dextran to be given for 36–48 hrs

      ii. Blood transfusion – required in deep burns due to RBC destruction

      iii. IV fluids – Ringer's solution – to maintain plasma volume, urinary output, blood pressure

      iv. Monitor input/output fluid charts.

First aid treatment

Procedure   Toilet of burn areas and debridement of necrotic tissue:

               Toilet of burns with savlon or dettol solution

               Debridement of necrotic tissue. Puncture blebs

               Coverage with sterile dressing pads or leave the area uncovered and let it dry up by air

Severe burns   Need not be washed,

               Instead admit the patient in the A&E department and treat accordingly

Relief from pain Inj. Morphine sulphate 10–15 mg IV or IM, or

               Inj. Tramadol 100 mg IM or IV every 4–6 hrs., or

               Inj. Pentazocine 30 mg IV or 30–60 mg IM or s.c.

Antibiotics   To combat infection

               Gentamicin oint or silver sulfadiazine oint

               Inj. Tetanus toxoid IM.

Surgical treatment: Skin grafting – split skin grafting.

Refer: The severe patient to the burns specialist team.

Drowning and Near Drowning

Drowning is the third leading cause of accidental death in the USA. Children and young adults are mostly the victims, especially the males.

Risk factors   Lack of swimming training

               Avoiding to use the personal floating devices, e.g. inflated tubes

               Absence of swimming instructors

               Use of high speed boats

               Alcohol abuse while swimming or boating

               Mental disorders.

Sequence of events in drowning:

               Asphyxia – for a minute or so

               Loss of consciousness due to lack of oxygen

               Respiratory centre (initially excited) fails within another minute or so

Vasomotor centre (initially maintains vasoconstriction) fails, causing:

Peripheral vasodilatation

Hypotension

Heart beat weakens

Cardiac output ceases

Ventricular fibrillation – develops (irrecoverable)

Multiple organ failure

Death.

Pathogenesis Dry drowning: At autopsy, victims have been found without any evidence of water aspiration in the lungs. Death occurs due to asphyxia – as a result of reflex laryngospasm and airway obstruction (glottis closure)

Wet drowning: Drowning is further complicated by aspiration of water (containing solutes and solids) into the airway causing airway obstruction, asphyxia, and death.

Diagnosis Depends upon many factors include amount and type of aspirated water and speed and effectiveness of treatment

Clinically there is not any significant difference between fresh water (hypotonic) and salt (sea) water (hypertonic) drowning, as per CPR (common for both) is concerned.

S/S Fresh water drowning: Asphyxia, metabolic acidosis, hypervolemia, hemodilution, hemolysis, ventricular fibrillation

Salt water drowning; asphyxia, metabolic acidosis, pulmonary edema, hypovolemia, renal failure.

Investigation Hemogram, TLC and DLC, platelet count

Serum electrolytes

Arterial blood gas, blood pH

Urine output measurement

CXR.

Management Main aim of treatment is to correct hypoxia and acidosis as fast as possible

CPR (cardiopulmonary resuscitation) measures

Correction of circulatory changes

Correction of hemolysis

Correction of electrolyte imbalance

Corticosteroids – to control pneumonitis

Control of pulmonary edema

IV Sod bicarb ($NaHCO_3$) – to control acidosis

Antibiotics

Treatment of associated complications.

Refer: The severe patient to the medical team.

Caisson Disease (syn. Compressed Air Sickness)

It is an emergency that requires treatment on priority basis.

Etiology	Occupational disorder, prevalent in divers (who work under water, generally work in caissons – a steel chamber, filled with compressed air in which the divers are placed and sunk in deep waters) sports injury, e.g. sport of scuba.
Pathogenesis	Firstly at low depths, respiratory gases under pressure, move into blood and tissues, further diving into deeper depths, the gases in the blood and tissues, escape due to lower external pressure.
Diagnosis	Initially there may not be much discomfort except:

Nausea, vomiting

Headache, dizziness/vertigo, visual disturbances, tinnitus

Dyspnea

Bradycardia

Serious effects appear later on (during rapid decompression), e.g.

Arthralgia

Cyanosis

Bradycardia

Weakness/paralysis

Unconsciousness, coma, death.

Management

Preventive treatment: Decompression should be very gradual

First aid treatment

Airway maintenance

Oxygen supply – compressed air (recompression)

Drugs – aspirin

No sedatives/narcotics

IV fluids

Plasma transfusion.

Refer: The severe patient to the medical team.

Anoxia

Definition	Is defined as body's oxygen lack from any cause.
Etiology	• High altitudes
	• Alteration of alveolar epithelium due to poisoning with irritant gases
	• Airway obstruction (partially unventilated lungs) – asthma, bronchopneumonia, lobar pneumonia, lung collapse due to bronchial obstruction, emphysema, bronchial stenosis
	• CVS disorders – Fallot's tetralogy (arterio-venous shunt)
Pathogenesis	Inadequate pO_2 to oxygenate the hemoglobin, leading to impaired tissue oxidation

Diagnosis	Mountain sickness – nausea, vomiting, headache, depression, apathy, drowsiness or excitement, loss of self control, violent, impaired memory, impaired understanding, sensory loss, muscular weakness, fatigue
	Pulse rate > 150/min
	Hypertension
	Cyanosis
	Respiratory rate increased
Investigation	CBC
	Respiratory function tests
	Renal function tests
	CXR
Management	Symptomatic and supportive
	Hospitalisation, bed rest
	Ventilation – oxygen therapy, endotracheal intubation
	IV fluids.

Electric Shock

It is dangerous to heart as it may cause ventricular fibrillation.

Etiology	Touching a live wire, electric appliances (wet unearthed fridge/washing machine/fans/motors, etc.)
Diagnosis	Unconsciousness, or myalgia, headache, fatigue, irritation
	Skin – cold and cyanotic
	Pulseless
	Respiration – absent
	Hypotension
	Ventricular fibrillation
	Coma, death may occur.
Investigation	Hemogram, hematocrit – elevated
	Plasma volume – reduced
	Arterial blood pH
	Lumbar puncture
	ECG.

Management

Emergency care (on the spot):

Free the victim from the current by switch off the power, or severe the wire with a dry stick

CRP – if breathing is impaired (depressed/absent)

Continue CRP until spontaneous breathing and cardiac function return or beginning of rigor mortis

Specific care at hospital:

Admit the patient

Observe for – shock, cardiac disorder, hemorrhage, acidosis

               Monitor IV fluids, urine output, serum electrolytes, ECG

               Lumbar puncture (LP) – if signs of raised intracranial pressure observed

               Treatment of burns – if present.

Refer: The severe patient to the medical team.

Prognosis	Immediate death – due to ventricular fibrillation
	Late death – due to systemic infection.

Acute Ionizing Radiation

Etiology	Exposure to ionizing radiation, e.g.
	Natural sources: Radon (alpha particle)
	Cosmic rays,
	Earth's radionuclides,
	Body's radioactive elements
	Man made sources: Diagnostic X-ray
	Nuclear medicine
	Nuclear reactor accidents
	Nuclear weapon detonations
	Accidental ingestion of radionuclides.
Pathogenesis	The harmful effects of radiation depend upon degree of exposure, i.e. quantity, type of radiation and duration of exposure. Many types of injury occur following exposure to ionizing radiation, especially injury to genetic apparatus of the nucleus following structural alterations of DNA and chromosomes.
Diagnosis	Nausea, vomiting, anorexia
	Pain abdomen, diarrhea, dehydration
	Weakness, prostration
	Erythema, epidermolysis,
	Anemia, ulcerative colitis, pneumonitis
	Sterility, miscarriage, fetal death
	Bone marrow depression, leucopenia.

Management

Preventive treatment

               Avoid unnecessary exposures (diagnostic or therapeutic)

               Proper shielding from X-rays, i.e. use of lead aprons, lead goggles, lead protected screens

               Proper handling of X-ray and nuclear radiation at nuclear thermal plants equipment, by a well trained technician

Specific treatment

               No specific treatment

               Treatment depends upon extent, degree, and site of tissue injury

               Symptomatic treatment:

               Antiemetic agents: Inj. stemetil, largactil, perinorm

IV fluids and electrolytes
Blood transfusion – for anemia
Bone marrow transfusion
Antibiotics.

Refer: The severe patient to the medical team.

References

1. Chatton J Milton: Disorders due to Physical Agents. Current Medicaql Diagnosis and treatment, Lang Med Publications, Japan, 1975.
2. Orlowski JP: Drowning, near drowning, and ice water drowning (editorial) JAMA 260:390;1988.
3. Yatsu FM: Cardiopulmonary-cerebral resuscitation (editorial) N Engl J Med 314:440;1986.
4. Wallace JF: Drowning and Near-Drowning. Principles of Internal Medicine. 12th ed Vol 2:2200–02.
5. Artz CP, Moncrief JA: The Treatment of Burns. Saunders, 1969.
6. Baxter CR: Emergency treatment of burn injury. Ann Emerg Med 17:1305;1988.
7. Hunt J et al: Acute electrical burns: Current diagnostic and therapeutic approaches to management. Arch Surg 115:434;1980.
8. Mettler Jr FA, Mosely Jr RD: Medical effectes of Radiation. Orlando. Florida. Grune and Stratton. pp 1–288;1985.
9. Strauss RH, Prockop LD: Decompression sickness among scuba divers. JAMA 223:637;1973.
10. Rains AJH & Capper WM et al: Ulceration & Gangrene. Bailey & Love's Short Practice of Surgery, H.K. Lewis & Co. Ltd., London, 1965.
11. Chatterjee CC, Banerjee PK: Caisson Disease. Human Physiology, 5th ed. Books & Allied Pvt. Ltd., Calcutta, 1963.

Poisoning Emergencies

Definition
Types of poisons
Medicolegal classification of poisoning
Rules observed in a poisoning case
Poisoning emergencies:
- Acids and alkalies
- Acids
- Alkalies (corrosive)
- Alcohol (ethyl)
- Alcohol (methyl)
- Arsenic
- Barbiturates
- Mercury

- Morphia
- Phenol (carbolic acid)
- Copper sulfate (blue vitriol)
- Digitalis
- Salicylate
- Lead
- Carbon monoxide
- Animals
- Snake
- Wasp, bee sting
- Strychnine
- Chloroform

Definition

Poison is defined as a substance, that on absorption or by direct contact, causes injury to body or death. It is a difficult task to differentiate between medicine and poison. A medicine given in large dose may produce poisonous effect, whereas a poison given in smaller dose (therapeutic) may be considered as a medicine.

Types of Poisons

According to routes of administration:
1. Ingested poisons: i. Acids or alkalies (corrosives)
                       ii. Kerosene oil, petrol, paint thinner, copper sulphate
2. Inhaled poisons: Volatile acids, fumes, gases – chlorine, fluorine, vehicle exhaust gases
3. Eye contamination poisons: Acids, alkalies, fumes
4. Skin contamination poisons: Acids, alkalies, fumes, lead
5. Drugs (overdosage)
6. Snake, scorpion, insect, ant bite poisons.

Medicolegal Classification of Poisoning

Accidental (unintensional):
By mistake, e.g. swallowing of poisons – especially by young children

	By curiosity
	By spontaneous activity
	By innocence – especially children
	By habit – putting into mouth each and every objects – by children
	By negativism and imitation
	By snake bite, scorpion bite, wasp, bee sting
	By overdosage
Suicidal	(Self-killing – intensional) Opium tops the list, followed by arsenic, barbiturates, copper sulphate
Homicidal	(Murder) Arsenic tops the list, followed by aconite, opium
Stupefication	Patient behaves like a stupid.
	The aim is to rob or to rape.
	Chloral hydrate mixed with alcohol – used for stupefaction.

Rules Observed in a Poisoning Case

- Insist for presence of another medical practitioner or better send the patient to the hospital
- Inform the police and the relatives of the patient
- Preserve the vomited matter, urine, fecal matter, if any, and hand over to the police
- Do not issue death certificate and insist for a post-mortem examination.

Signs and Symptoms

- Nausea, vomiting, diarrhea
- Salivation, dryness of mouth
- Abdominal pain
- Hematemesis, melena
- Cough
- Respiration – rapid/slow
- Dyspnea
- Cyanosis, jaundice
- Palpitation
- Tachycardia/bradycardia
- Hypotension/hypertension
- Headache, drowsiness, depression
- Hallucinations, delirium, convulsions
- Coma
- Vision – blurred/colored, pupils – dilated/contracted
- Tinnitus, deafness, vertigo
- Polyuria/anuria
- Skin rash
- Anorexia, asthenia, weight loss.

Acids and Alkalies
Acids

Routes of administration	Oral intake – by mistake, or intentional
	Inhalation – of acids, fumes, gases – chlorine, fluorine
	Skin contamination (through intact or broken skin) – acids, alkalies, fumes, lead.
Pathogenesis	Corrosive effect on the skin or mucous membrane
	Circulatory collapse
	Pulmonary edema.
Diagnosis	Severe burning pain in the throat and upper GI tract
	Thirst
	Vomiting of blood
	Difficulty in breathing
	Difficulty in swallowing
	Difficulty in speaking
	Disfiguration of skin and mucous membrane in and around the mouth
	Shock.
MLD	1 ml of acid.
Management	Dilute the acid by giving orally: Milk of magnesia, aluminium hydroxide, milk, or water
	Gastric lavage: Pass gently a Ryle's tube (by nasogastric route) and lavage with milk or milk of magnesia
	Avoid bicarbonate or carbonates
	IV fluids
	Relief of pain – by analgesics/antispasmodics
	Shock – if present, to be treated on top priority basis
	Skin burns – toilet with water
	Eye burns – rinse eyes with water.

Refer: The severe patient to the medical team.

Alkalies (Corrosive) Poisoning

Common corrosive alkalies are – caustic soda, potash, ammonia.

Etiology	Accidental.
Diagnosis	Burning pain in the mouth, throat
	Nausea, vomiting, diarrhea
	Suffocation – due to inflammation of airways
	Death due to respiratory failure.
MLD	1 g.
Management	Oesophagoscopic irrigation with acetic acid, vinegar, fruit juice

Gastric lavage with gastric tubes and emetics – are contraindicated

Demulscents: Milk, white of egg, are given as buffering agents

Inj. morphine sulphate – to relieve pain

Inj. atropine sulphate – to reduce gastric motility

Airways maintenance – tracheostomy may be required.

Refer: The severe patient to the medical team.

Alcohol (Ethyl) Poisoning

Etiology	Abuse
	Dependence.
Diagnosis	CNS depressant.
Alcohol intoxication	

Nausea, vomiting, gastritis

Headache, confusion, euphoria, ataxia

Slurred speech

Impaired judgement

Sexual – aggressive behaviour (in Shakespeare's Macbeth, e.g. alcohol provokes the desire but it takes away the performance)

Coma and death.

Withdrawal syndrome

Tremors of hands, tongue, eyelids

Nausea, vomiting, headache, insomnia, hallucinations

Hypotension – orthostatic.

Delirium tremens

Disorientation, confusion, agitation hallucinations

Seizures

Death may occur due to fat embolism or cardiac arrhythmias.

MLD	300 ml.
Management	Airway maintenance

Breathing control, i.e. to control respiratory depression

Keep the patient warm up

Inj. chlorpromazine 20–50 mg IM

Gastric lavage with care to avoid pulmonary aspiration.

Drugs   Fixed schedule dosing:

Chlordiazepoxide 50–100 mg q.d.s. 1st day

                               25–50 mg q.d.s. 2nd and 3rd day

Front loading: Diazepam 20 mg orally 2 hrly until symptom free

Delirium tremens: Diazepam 10 mg IV. Repeat 5 mg every 5 mts

Abstinence: Disulfiram (anti-abuse) 250–500 mg o.d. PO.

Refer: The severe patient to the medical team.

Methyl Alcohol (Machinery Spirit) Abuse

Diagnosis	CNS depressant
	Nausea, vomiting, abdominal pain
	Headache, blindness
	Delirium, convulsions, coma
	Death may occur in severe case.
MLD	30–60 mL.
Investigation	Urine contains methanol.
Management	Gastric lavage with sodium bicarbonate solution
	IV fluids – to control metabolic acidosis
	Ethyl alcohol orally 30–40 mL – to control metabolism of methyl alcohol.

Refer: The severe patient to the medical team.

Arsenic Poisoning

Arsenic is present in pesticides (insecticides spray on fruits and vegetables) and chemicals (rat poisons).

Etiology (Medicolegal uses)	
	Accidental: May be ingested accidentally, especially by children.
	Suicidal: The drug may be taken with suicidal intention.
	Homicidal: Favourite of murderers.
Pathogenesis	Arsenic is one of most potent capillary poisons. The capillaries dilate and allow escape of plasma, resulting in marked hypotension circulatory failure, shock.
Diagnosis	Constriction of throat
	Difficulty in swallowing
	Pain abdomen
	Nausea, vomiting, diarrhea
	Muscle cramps – due to disturbed electrolytes of body fluids
	Thirst due to fluid loss
	Shock – Skin becomes cold, clammy, pale,
	Pulse – rapid and weak
	Hypotension
	Respiration – depressed
	Coma, death may occur.
MLD	100 mg.
Management	Treatment of acute poisoning:
	BAL 10% sol in oil IM 5 mg/kg 4 hrly/24 hrs
	Children dose: 2.5 mg/kg 4 hrly (6 doses)
	Induce vomiting
	Gastric lavage, milk ingestion

Shock – if present, treat it on top priority basis

Relieve pain – Inj. Morphine

IV fluids – to control fluid loss.

Refer: The severe patient to the medical team or ITU.

Barbiturates Poisoning

Pathogenesis	Barbiturates are central nervous system depressants, frequently used by physicians. The central depressant action produces calmness, sleep, inhibit convulsions, and results in basal or complete surgical anesthesia.
Etiology (medicolegal uses)	Accidental/suicidal poisoning Abuse – as sedative/hypnotic drugs.
Diagnosis	Excitement, delirium, hallucinations Depression, confusion Headache, drowsiness Respiratory depression Skin – cold, clammy, cyanotic Coma Death may occur – by ingestion of large doses of rapidly acting Barbiturates.
MLD	0.5–2.0 g.
Management	Admit the patient. Keep the patient warm. Monitor the patient's condition Airway maintenance – endotrachial intubation, ventilator, oxygen therapy Gastric lavage – to remove unabsorbed poison. Sodium sulfate 10–15 mg, may be left in the stomach, at the end of lavage, so as to hasten intestinal removal of unabsorbed poison IV fluids
Drugs	Analeptics (stimulators of respiratory centre and higher centres of CNS) Combination of picrotoxin and amphetamine
Picrotoxin	6–12 mg IV. Repeat after every 10–20 mts until some movement/twitching observed. Also given as continuous infusion @ 1–2 mg/mt Antibiotics – to prevent pulmonary infection.

Refer: The severe patient to the medical team.

Mercury Poisoning

Types	Acute and chronic mercury poisoning.

Acute Mercury Poisoning

Etiology	Oral ingestion of highly dissociated inorganic preparations. Commonly caused by mercuric chloride taken either by accident or with suicidal intent.

Pathogenesis	Mercury is a protein precipiant, affecting mucous membranes of mouth, pharynx, stomach, renal damage, distortion of electrolyte pattern of body fluids.
Diagnosis	A strong metallic taste is felt in the mouth
	Ashen grey appearance of mouth and pharynx
	Feeling of constriction and choking in the throat
	Burning sensation, extending from mouth down to stomach
	Severe abdominal pain
	Thirst
	Nausea, vomiting, diarrhea
	Anuria
	Muscle cramps
	Shock, death – mainly due to renal failure.
MLD	70 mg.
Management	Admit the patient
	Give milk with whites of beaten eggs – as precipitant, followed by gastric lavage
	Sodium formaldehyde sulfoxylate – as local antidote
	BAL (dimercaprol) IM – to inactivate already absorbed mercury
	$NaSO_4$ 30 g in water – as cathartic
	Treat oliguria, anuria accordingly
	Hemodialysis – to flush out mercury speedily.

Chronic Mercury Poisoning

Etiology	Exposure to mercury for longer period, i.e. industries utilizing mercury.
Diagnosis	Stomatitis
	Colitis
	Anorexia
	Peripheral neuritis
	Anemia
	Renal damage
	Depression, insomnia, hallucinations.
Management	Treatment is symptomatic
	Removal of patient from mercury contact
	Improvement of nutritional condition
	BAL IM.

Refer: The patient to the medical team.

Morphia Poisoning

Types	Acute and chronic morphine poisoning.

Acute Morphine Poisoning

Etiology	Suicidal: Opium is drug of choice in suicide, as the death is painless
	Accidental – overdosage.

Routes of administration

1. Poultice containing large amounts of opium
2. Local application to a wound
3. Inj. of morphine
4. As enema
5. Per vaginal.

Pathogenesis	Morphine exerts narcotic action, manifested by analgesia, sleep, and respiration depression.
Diagnosis	Nausea, vomiting
	Headache, depression, asleep or stuporous
	Respiratory depression
	Pulse – fast and weak
	Pinpoint pupils
	Convulsions
	Shock
	Coma, death – due to respiratory failure.
MLD	65 mg.
Management	Admit the patient
	Airway maintenance
	Ventilator with oxygen
	Respiratory stimulation – caffeine and sodium benzoate, aminophylline, nikethamide
	Ephedrine and amphetamine – respiratory stimulants and antinarcotics
	Naloxone 0.8–2 mg IV or IM. Rept at 2–3 mts intervals if necessary
	Nalorphine hydrochloride 5–10 mg IV. Repeat 10–15 mts
	Total dose not to exceed 40 mg
	The effects on respiration and circulation are dramatic
	Gastric lavage – if poison taken orally
	Sodium sulfate 30 mg in water – as cathartic
	IV fluids and electrolytes – to control dehydration and acidosis
	Plasma – to combat shock.

Refer: The severe patient to the medical team.

Chronic Morphine Poisoning (Opium Addiction)

Etiology	Habitual smoking, IV (addicts – for euphoria, thrill).
Diagnosis	Addict – shabbily dressed, cunning, malicious, degenerate criminal (due to disturbed financial, nutritional, social position).

Withdrawal Symptoms

Expresses craving and need for the drug

Feeling of sickness, apprehensive, irritable

Indulgence in criminal activities – theft, violence – to obtain drug

Deep sleep (yen) followed by

Restlessness, miserable, sweating, tremor

Muscular weakness, depression

Nausea, vomiting, colic

Hypertension

Headache, delirium

Death – may occur due to cardiovascular failure.

Management	Combined medical, nursing, and psychiatric treatments are essential
	Admit the patient
	Detailed physical and laboratory examinations
	Withdrawal – may be abrupt, rapid, or slow
	Substitution of methadone for morphine and subsequent withdrawal of methadone
	Psychological and sociological rehabilitation of patient required after withdrawal symptoms disappear
	Personality and environmental adjustments required to remove the root cause of death.

Phenol (Carbolic Acid) Poisoning

Etiology	Accidental, rarely homicidal – due to strong colour and smell.
Route of administration: Oral.	
Pathogenesis	Acts as a corrosive agent locally and remotely acts as a narcotic poison affecting CNS and CVS.
Diagnosis	Local action on skin – burning sensation, tingling, and numbness
	PO – burning sensation in the mouth, throat, and stomach, thirst
	Nausea, vomiting, pain abdomen, muscle cramps
	Oliguria
	Respiratory and circulatory failure
	Coma.
MLD	2 g
Management	Give milk, water orally
	Gastric lavage
	Activated charcoal left in the stomach after gastric lavage
	Drugs: Inj. Atropine sulfate – to reduce the motility of stomach
	Inj. Morphine – to relieve pain
	IV saline drip with noradrenaline – to elevate blood pressure
	Asphyxia – endotracheal intubation attached to ventilator with oxygen
	Burns – toilet of wound with soap and water, followed by application of olive oil.

Refer: The severe patient to the medical team.

Copper Sulfate (Blue Vitriol) Poisoning

Copper sulfate is a metallic irritant.

Etiology	Suicidal – as easily available without permit
	Homicidal – unsuitable for homicidal poisoning, due to its deep blue colour and a disagreeable metallic taste
	Accidental – may occur in young children, mistakenly sucking it as a lozenge.
Diagnosis	Symptoms appear within 15–20 mts after poison is consumed
	Strong metallic taste, thirst, salivation
	Sensation of constriction in the throat, headache
	Burning pain in the stomach
	Nausea, vomiting – bluish/greenish vomitus, diarrhea
	Jaundice – due to fatty degeneration of liver
	Oliguria
	Convulsions, paralysis, coma
	Death – may occur within 1–3 days, earlier in children.
MLD	1 oz.
Management	Demulcents -- egg albumin given as an antidote
	Gastric lavage – with potassium ferrocyanide, that forms insoluble cupric ferrocyanide, which is washed out by water
	IV saline, or dextrose solution, to control dehydration
	Inj. Morphine – to relieve pain
	BAL IM may be given.

Refer: The severe patient to the medical team.

Digitalis Poisoning

Etiology	It is due to continued ingestion of the drug in amounts greater than are destroyed or eliminated.
MLD	Unknown.
Diagnosis	Nausea, vomiting, diarrhea, anorexia, headache, fatigue, malaise, drowsiness, are the earliest features of digitalis poisoning
	Skin rashes, blurred vision
	Pulse – irregular, slow
	Hypotension
	Ventricular fibrillation
	Shock.
MLD	Unknown.
Management	Give milk, water, activated charcoal, followed by gastric lavage or emesis
	Do not use any stimulant drug – may induce ventricular fibrillation
	Sodium bicarbonate – to correct acidosis
	Calcium gluconate – to correct hyperkalemia
	Atropine 1–2 mg IV – to correct bradycardia/AV block

Lidocaine or beta-blocker – to correct VT
Digibind (digoxin antibody) – to correct arrhythmias and hyperkalemia
IV Dextrose 5% – add KCl 2 g, to be monitored by ECG
Ventricular fibrillation – use defibrillator along with other measures.

Refer: The severe patient to the medical team.

Acute Salicylate Poisoning

Etiology	Accidental – overdosage (in the treatment of acute rheumatic fever) Suicidal.
MLD	10–30 g of sodium salicylate – may cause death in adults Lethal dose of methyl salicylate – considerably < sodium salicylate Children: 4 ml of methyl salicylate may be fatal.
Diagnosis	Headache, dizziness, tinnitus, impaired hearing, dimness of vision Nausea, vomiting, diarrhea, thirst Cold, clammy skin, sweating Epistaxis, bleeding from gums, retinal hemorrhage, hematuria Confusion, drowsiness, delirium, coma Death – may occur due to respiratory or circulatory failure.
Management	Admit the patient, warmth Withdrawal of salicylate medication Gastric lavage – with warm saline Demulscents – milk, egg Stimulants IV fluids and electrolytes.

Refer: The severe patient to the medical team.

Lead Poisoning

Lead is a slow acting, but powerful poison.

Etiology	Lead poisoning is mostly chronic because of slow absorption

1. Exposure in industry: Lead is inhaled in dusts or fumes, i.e. workers exposed to lead mining, smelting, and refining,
2. Printers, painters – also prone to lead poisoning
3. Household poisoning: Contaminated drinking water with lead in piping supply.

Diagnosis	Patient is moody, excited in early stages Skin – face is ashen in colour, lips – pale Blue line (Burtonian line) – seen on the margin of gums Metallic taste, thirst Nausea, vomiting, anorexia, constipation Abdominal colic Headache, dizziness, irritability, insomnia

	Muscle fatigue
	Hypotension.
Investigation	Urine – scanty, positive for lead, trace of albumin
	TLC and DLC: Increase in reticulocytes.
MLD	Uncertain.
Management	Admit the patient
	Gastric lavage magnesium sulfate or sodium sulfate, followed by water
	Lead colic – IV calcium gluconate 10 ml of 20% sol or
	IV calcium chloride 5 ml of 10% sol
	If not relieved of colic, then give Inj. atropine
	If pain not relieved, then give morphine or methadone
	Cathartic – to eliminate unabsorbed lead from the bowl
	Barbiturates – to control excitement, convulsions
	Purgatives – 1 oz magnesium sulfate for relief of constipation.

Carbon Monoxide Poisoning

Etiology	Accidental: Use of gas or coal burning heaters in an unvented room resulting in deaths.
	Suicidal: Exhaust fumes inhalation for commiting suicide
Pathogenesis	$CO + Hb$ = Carboxyhemoglobin – causing tissue anoxia.
Diagnosis	Nausea, vomiting, headache, giddiness, faintness, unconsciousness, cyanosis, death.
Management	Shift the patient to fresh air immediately
	Airway maintenance – use ventilator and supply oxygen (100%)
	Tracheostomy – may be required sometimes
	IV Dextrose 50 ml of 50% sol – to combat cerebral edema
	Maintain BP and body temp.

Refer: The severe patient to the medical team.

Animals Poisoning
Snake Bite (Ophitoxemia—Ophidia means snake or serpent)

Poisonous (venomous) snakes: Sea snakes, viper, krait or karet, cobra.

Poison	The venom of poisonous snakes is either neurotoxic or hemotoxic.
Etiology	Accidental, suicidal, homicidal – seldom.
Pathogenesis	Neurotoxin results in respiratory paralysis while hemotoxin causes hemorrhage due to hemolysis and damage to blood vessels lining.
Diagnosis	Pain: Burning pain at the site of bite
	Nausea, vomiting, thirst, perspiration
	Swelling, redness
	Local tenderness
	Collapse
	Shock

Death (immediately from shock or within ½ hr to 30 hrs) due to:
- Fright causing neurogenic (mental) shock, or
- Paralysis of medullary respiratory center, or
- Failure of vasomotor center, cardiac failure, or
- Intravascular thrombosis especially of pulmonary arteries.

Management   Immobilization of the part

Apply tourniquet – to be released for few mts. after every 1 hr, to avoid onset of gangrene

Incision and suction – removes 10% venom, if performed during first ½ hr

IV antiserum (antivenom) – after testing sensitivity

Shift the patient immediately to the hospital for admission and for the definitive treatment

IV fluids

Blood transfusion

Corticosteroids – given with caution, and not to be given if the patient getting antiserum

Analgesics/sedatives.

Refer: The patient to the medical team.

Wasp, Bee, Sting Poisoning

Etiology   Accidental

Diagnosis   Pain, swelling, itching

Management   Cold sponging

Rubbing/massage with any iron object

Analgesics, antihistaminics

Inj. Epinephrine hydrochloride 1:1000 solution 0.2–0.5 ml IM or s.c. followed by diphenhydramine hydrochloride 5–20 mg IV

Shock – if present, then treat accordingly.

Refer: The patient to the medical team.

Strychnine Poisoning

Strychnine poisoning is not rare.

Etiology   Accidental poisoning is common in children due to consumption of sugar coated cathartic pills containing strychnine.

Suicidal poisoning – rare now as CNS depressants being favored now.

Pathogenesis   Strychnine is a spinal poison, affecting the anterior horn cells.

Diagnosis   Symptoms are mainly of CNS stimulation

Bitter taste, dryness of tongue, feeling of choking in the throat

Stiffness of face and neck, followed by muscle twitchings

Hyperextension of the body (opisthotonos)

Arms and legs – rigidly extended, fists – clenched

Jaw – trismus

Face – risus sardonicus

Respiratory arrest – due to diaphragm involvement

Convulsive seizures

Death – due to medullary paralysis.

MLD	Adults: ½ gr. Young children: 1/60 gr.
Management	Aims of treatment:
	1. To prevent convulsions
	2. To protect medulla from anoxia and stimulation
Drugs	Barbiturates: Depress the hyperexcitability of spinal cord and also block impulses entering spinal cord from higher centers.
	Pentobarbital sodium IV 0.3–0.7 g, given to combat convulsions and keep patient asleep, with great care not to depress the respiration
	Emetics: Inj. Apomorphine hydrochloride 1/10–1/5 gr.
	Gastric lavage with potassium permanganate 1:1000 sol.

Refer: The severe patient to the medical team.

Chloroform Poisoning

It is a volatile liquid with strong aromatic smell.

Etiology	Accidental.
Diagnosis	Burning pain in the mouth, throat, and stomach
	Nausea, vomiting
	Skin – cold and clammy
	Face – cyanosed
	Pupils – dilated
	Respiration – slow
	Pulse – rapid, feeble, irregular
	Hypotension
	Death – may occur due to respiratory or cardiac failure.
MLD	4–6 hrs. Fatal period: 4–6 hrs.
Management	Gastric lavage – with water
	Demulscents
	Inj. Atropine sulfate, nikethamide, adrenaline
	Warm up the body with blankets
	Airway maintenance – ventilate the patient with oxygen.

Refer: The severe patient to the medical team.

References

1. Goodman LS, Gilman A (ed):General principles of toxicology. The Pharmacological Basis of Therapeutics, 4th ed. Macmillan, New York.
2. An Experienced Teacher: Notes on Medical Jurisprudence and Toxicology Current Publishers, Calcutta, 1965.

3. Dreisbach Robert H, Krupp Marcus A, Chatton Milton J (editors): Poisons. Lange Medical Publications, Japan.
4. Reid HA: Jhekaston RDG: The management of snakebite. Bull WHO 63:885–95;1983.
5. Russell FE: Snake venom poisoning. Philadelphia: JB Lippincot Co. 291–300;1980.
6. Saitz R, O'Malley S: Pharmacotherapies for alcohol abuse. Med Clin North Am 81:881–907;1997.
7. Schorling JB, Buchsbaum DG: Screening for alcohol and drug abuse. Med Clin North Am 81:845–65;1997.
8. Basu D, Singh J: Drug and alcohol abuse: General physician's perspective. JIMA 103:88–98;2005.
9. Goel SP: Common poisonings and their management in children CMJ India 11:7–14.
10. Ghai OP, Piyush G: Poisonings and accidents. Essential Pediatrics 640–41;2004.
11. Steentoft A: Fatal digitalis poisoning. Acta Pharmacol 32:353;1973.
12. Wyatt JP, Illingworth RN, Robertson CE, Clancy MJ, Munro PT: Poisoning. Oxford Handbook of Accident and Emergency Medicine 174–202;2005.

Blood (Hematology) Emergencies and Common Disorders

Signs and symptoms (non-specific manifestations)

Emergencies and common disorders:

Blood disorders:

- Blood coagulation
- Bleeding disorders
- Fibrinogenopenia
- Hemophilia
- Vitamin K deficiency
- Vitamin K antagonists
- Phenindone (dindivan)
- Diagnosis of coagulation disorders

Anemias:

- Iron deficiency anemia

- Pernicious anemia
- Aplastic anemia
- Hemolytic anemia

Hemoglobin disorders:

- Thalassemia – minor and major

Leukemias:

- Acute leukemia
- Chronic myelocytic leukemia

Multiple myeloma

Hodgkin's disease

Agranulocytosis

Signs and Symptoms (Non-specific Manifestations)

1. Headache
2. Dyspnea
3. Giddiness
4. Palpitation
5. Asthenia
6. Edema feet
7. Hemorrhage
8. Anemia
9. Jaundice
10. Melena.

Blood Coagulation

Physiology   The essential blood coagulation reaction is – conversion of soluble fibrinogen into insoluble fibrin protein, by an enzyme thrombin. Fibrinogen exists freely in circulating blood, while thrombin does not. When blood is shed, thrombin is formed from inactive circulating precursor prothrombin (formed in liver under influence of vitamin K – which is synthesized by intestinal bacteria especially *B. coli.*) under influence of Ca⁺⁺ and thromboplastin – derived from damaged tissues, disintegrated platelets, and plasma (Table 8.1).

Blood Clotting Factors—Synonyms

Factor I: Fibrinogen
Factor II: Prothrombin
Factor III: Thromboplastin (tissue)
Factor IV: Calcium
Factor V: Proacclerin – labile factor, AC globulin
Factor VII: Proconvertin – stable factor
Factor VIII: Antihemophilic factor (AHF), antihemophilic globulin (AHG)
Factor IX: Christmas factor.

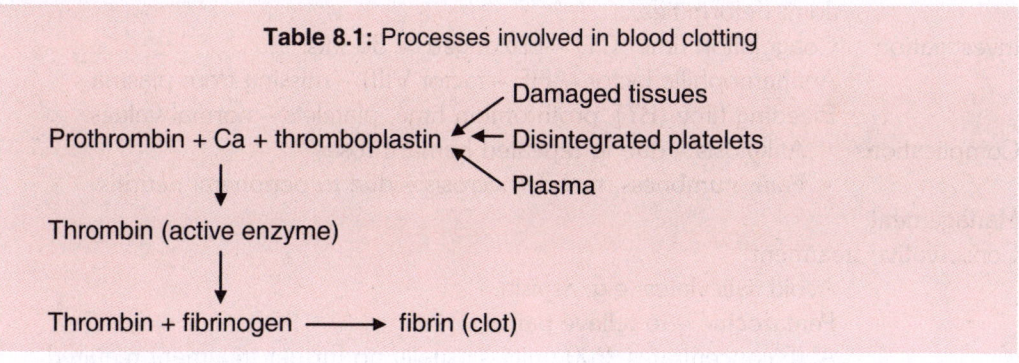

Table 8.1: Processes involved in blood clotting

Prothrombin + Ca + thromboplastin ← Damaged tissues
← Disintegrated platelets
← Plasma

Thrombin (active enzyme)

Thrombin + fibrinogen ⟶ fibrin (clot)

Bleeding Disorders

Etiology
• Due to defects in coagulation, i.e.
• Lack of fibrinogen (fibrinogenopenia)
• Lack of factor VIII (hemophilia)
• Deficient prothrombin – due to lack/absence of vitamin K
• Deficient factor V, factor VII, or factor IX
• Increased platelet destruction, due to defective capillary contractility (purpura).

Fibrinogenopenia A rare congenital defect with bleeding tendencies
Occurs during pregnancy – associated with premature separation of placenta.

Etiology   Multiple embolism of small tissue fragments.
Pathogenesis   Multiple embolism of tissue fragments (rich in thromboplastin) resulting in clot formation, depletion of plasma fibrinogen, failure in clot formation, hemorrhages.
Diagnosis   Severe bleeding per vaginum.
Investigation   Blood clotting time–defective.

Management   IV fibrinogen sol.
               Blood transfusion.
Refer: The severe patient to the obstetric team.

Hemophilia   It is an inherited bleeding disorder, transmitted by females to males who manifest signs of the disease, while the females themselves show no sign/symptoms of the disease.
Etiology   Lack of factor VIII, resulting in deficiency of plasma thromboplastin factor.
Diagnosis   History of bleeding in a male
                  Prolonged bleeding even after minor trauma
                  GI tract bleedings
                  Hematuria
                  Hematomas formation
                  Pain
                  Joint deformities.
Investigation   Coagulation time (CT) – prolonged > 30 mts
                  Antihemophilic factor (AHF – factor VIII) – missing from plasma
                  Bleeding time (BT), prothrombin time, platelets – normal values.
Complications   • Ankylosis – due to repeated hemarthroses
                  • Pain, numbness, muscle necrosis – due to peripheral neuritis.
Management
Conservative treatment
                  Avoid salicylates, e.g. aspirin.
                  Pentazocine – to relieve pain
                  AHF concentrates 200 units – usually no further treatment required
                  Plasma 15–20 ml/kg during 1–2 hrs. Repeat 12 hrly
                  Factor IX – proplax 10 units/kg.
Surgical treatment
                  Aspiration of joint
                  Rest to the joint.
Refer: The patient to the orthopedic team.

Purpura   Hemorrhagic disorder due to increased platelet destruction, as a result of defective capillary contractility.
Etiology   Primary – idiopathic: Mostly seen in children.
                  Occasionally congenital or hereditary
                  Secondary – symptomatic: Allergic or infective, e.g. endocarditis, typhus
                  Drugs, e.g. quinine, quinidine, thiazides, aminosalicylic acid, ergot, bismuth
Diagnosis   Petechial hemorrhages – subcutaneous, mucous membranes, epistaxis, bleeding gums, vaginal bleeding, GI tract bleeding, hematuria.
Investigation   • Platelet count decreased
                  • Bleeding time prolonged
                  • Clotting time normal.

Management
Preventive treatment

Avoid – trauma, sports injury, elective surgery, tooth extraction, unnecessary drugs

Specific treatment

Drugs   Corticosteroids indicated in severe purpura.

Prednisolone 10–20 mg q.d.s. PO

Surgical treatment: Splenectomy

Indications: Purpura of > 1 year duration

Severe purpura.

Refer: The severe patient to the medical team.

Vitamin K deficiency Vitamin K is indispensable for the synthesis of prothrombin by liver.

Etiology   Obstructive jaundice: Stone, tumour.

Pathogenesis   Biliary obstruction leads to absence of bile in the intestine, absence of bile salts in the intestine, prevention of vitamin K absorption from intestine, decreased factor VII and prothrombin, prolonged prothrombin time, prolonged clotting time, hemorrhages.

Diagnosis   Itching, pale skin, pale conjunctiva, diarrhea, hepatitis

Hemorrhages, death may occur due to uncontrolled bleeding.

Management   Orally – bile salts and vitamin K

Inj. vitamin K IM.

Refer: The severe patient to the medical team.

Vitamin K Antagonists

Dicoumarol   Acts as an anti-vitamin K, by replacing vitamin K in the liver, prevents vitamin K from synthesizing prothrombin, resulting in reduced plasma prothrombin, factor VII activity decreases, blood clotting is depressed.

Uses   As an anticoagulant in phlebitis, coronary thrombosis, given orally

Dose   Adult: 100–200 mg initially. Repeat 12.5–50.0 mg every 1–4 days determined by results

Phenindone (Dindevan)   It is an anticoagulant. Depresses factor VII.

Action – quick

Duration – short

Uses   Severe hepatic or renal dysfunction

Hemorrhagic disorders

Dose   Adult: 200 mg PO Maint: 100 mg/day

Children: Not recommended

Warfarin   It is vitamin K antagonist (reduces action of vitamin K dependent clotting factors in the liver)

Uses   Thromboembolic disorders
Dose   Adult: 10 mg o.d. PO
               Children: Not recommended.

Diagnosis of Coagulation Disorders

History of bleeding:
               Inquire about onset of bleeding, i.e. old or recent onset
               Inquire about number of episodes
Circumstances of bleeding: Inquire about trauma, minor surgery, e.g. tooth extraction or
               tonsillectomy
Duration   Inquire about duration of bleeding episode
Family history Inquire about family history of bleeding
Character of bleeding   Inquire about type/character of bleeding, e.g.
   • Purpuric spots: Suggest capillary or platelet defect
   • Hematomas, hemarthroses, large ecchymoses – hemophilia
   • Postoperative, postpartum severe hemorrhages: Suggest fibrinogen
     deficiency.

Anemias   Anemia is a blood disorder characterized by low red blood corpuscles
               (RBC) or low hemoglobin (Hb). It is usually not a disease, but a symptom
               of a disease.
Normal values RBC count = Adult male: 5–6.5 (5.5) million/cu mm
               Adult female: 4–5.5 million/cu mm
               Hb = Adult male: 14–16 (15.6) g/dL
                   Adult female: 12–16 (13.7) g/dL
                   (Measured by Sahli's hemoglobinometer)
Laboratory classification of anemias:
1. Cell volume (MCV): Macrocytic, normocytic, microcytic
2. Hemoglobin concentration (MCHC): Normochromic or hypochromic, e.g. pernicious
   anemia – is a macrocytic anemia
   Iron deficiency anemia – is a normocytic or microcytic hypochromic anemia

Clinical classification of Anemias

1. Iron deficiency anemia
2. Pernicious anemia
3. Hemolytic anemia
4. Aplastic anemia.

Iron Deficiency Anemia

Definition   It is a normocytic or microcytic hypochromic anemia. It is the most
               common type of anemia, mostly found in women.
Etiology   Diet – lacking proteins, vitamins

Age: Common in infants and young children

Women – in the active reproductive life

Pregnancy – due to increase in plasma volume

Hemorrhage (blood loss):

- External hemorrhage: Trauma
- Internal hemorrhage: Menorrhagia, GI tract bleeding.

Infection – especially in infants, e.g. PUO, bronchitis

Diagnosis	Pallor, dizziness, difficult breathing, anorexia, fatigue, palpitation.
Investigation	Hb – low
	RBC – normocytic or microcytic, hypochromic
	WBC – normal
	Platelets – normal or increased.
Management	
Iron therapy	Oral or parenteral
Oral	Ferrous sulfate 0.2 g t.d.s. after meals or
	Ferrous gluconate 0.3 g t.d.s. after meals
	Oral iron to be given for 3 months (till Hb values return to normal)
Parenteral	Indications:

- Intolerance to oral iron
- GI tract disorders
- Severe continued hemorrhage

Dose	250 mg for each g of Hb – below normal
	Imferon (iron dextran) 50 mg (1 ml) deep IM. Maint. 100–250 mg o.d. or EOD. A test dose of (0.5 ml) should preferably be given first, to avoid unusual reaction blood transfusion.

Refer: The severe patient to the medical team.

Pernicious Anemia

Definition	It is a macrocytic anemia. The RBCs fail to develop normally, although large number of immature cells are present in the bone marrow.
Etiology	Due to lack of intrinsic factor with a consequent failure in the absorption of vitamin B_{12} which regulates the maturation of nucleated red cells in the bone marrow.
Diagnosis	Pallor, sick, irritable, jaundice, dyspnea, palpitation, anorexia, glossitis, indigestion, diarrhea, numbness, tingling of legs and arms, fatigue.
Investigation	RBC count < 1 million/cu mm
	PCV 95–160 μm^3 (average 87 μm^3)
	MCHC 35% (normal) Hb conc./cell – reduced
	MCH 50 μg (normal 30)
	Platelets reduced
	Serum bilirubin elevated
	Bone marrow aspiration study: Megaloblastic bone marrow.

Management	Vitamin B$_{12}$ 100 μg IM 1–3 times/week until normal, then 100 μg/month
	May need vitamin B$_{12}$ injections throughout life.
Prognosis	Untreated pernicious anemia is fatal.

Hemolytic Anemia

Definition	It is defined as anemia due to increased red cell destruction coupled with increased erythropoiesis.
Etiology	RBC damage due to:

- Bacterial toxins poisoning – by direct action

Incompatible blood transfusion reactions:
- Appearance of abnormal hemolysins in the blood, which may hemolyse compatible blood cells and even patient's own red cells
- Chemicals poisoning – by direct action, e.g. ether, chloroform, benzene
- Snake venoms poisoning – by direct action, e.g. viper venom
- Drugs, e.g. quinine, sulphonamides, phenacetin, nitrites, chlorates.
- Osmotic disturbances, e.g. addition of distilled water or hypotonic saline solution, increases the cell volume – causing hemolysis
- Hypersplenism.

Diagnosis	Pallor, jaundice, anemia, malaise, fatigue, splenomegaly.
Investigation	Hematocrit – reticulocytosis
	Hemogram – Hemoglobin level increased
	Indirect bilirubin and urobilinogen – level increased
	Coombs' test +ve
	Bone marrow study – marked erythroid hyperplasia.
Complications	Acute hemolytic anemia, shock, abdominal pain, purpura.
Management	Removal of underlying cause.
Medical treatment	
	Prednisolone 10–20 mg 4 times o.d. PO, until normal Hb values achieved.
Surgical treatment	
	Splenectomy – likely to be of value.

Refer: The severe patient to the medical team.

Acute Hemolytic Anemia

Etiology	• As a complication of hemolytic anemia
	• Drugs: Penicillin, sulphonamide, methyldopa
	• Bacterial infections: Streptococcal hemolytic septicemia, *E. coli* infections, *Clostridium welchii* infections
	• Thrombocytopenic purpura
	• Neoplastic: Hodgkin's disease, chronic lymphatic leukemia
Diagnosis	Fever, sudden onset with chills, nausea, vomiting, pain abdomen, backache, pallor, jaundice, splenomegaly, red or black urine.

Investigation   MCV – normocytic

Hb conc – normochromic

Urine – hemoglobinuria

Bone marrow – hyperplastic.

Complications   Shock, acute renal failure.

Management   It is a medical emergency and requires priority treatment,

Medical treatment

Hospitalize the patient

Removal of cause

Discontinue all medicines

IV fluids

Blood transfusion – to combat shock or anoxia

Packed red cells – prefered over whole blood

Prednisolone – given if response to above measures fail/poor

Dose: 10–20 mg q.d.s. PO, given until Hb value is normal and serum and urine are clear of hemolytic products.

Surgical treatment: Splenectomy rarely indicated.

Refer: The severe patient to the medical team.

Aplastic Anemia

Definition   It is a normocytic or macrocytic normochromic anemia, results from marked reduction in precursor cells, colony forming progenitors of mature granulocyte, megakaryocytes, erythroid cells, and stem cells, due to destruction/damage of bone marrow.

Etiology   Unknown

May occur at any age

May occur as a toxic reaction to:

Chemicals: Cosmetics, hair dyes, insecticides, X-ray radiations, etc.

Diagnosis   Pallor, fatigue, progressive weakness, petechiae, GI tract bleeding, hematuria, tachycardia, headache.

Investigation   RBC count < 1 million/cu mm

Cells – macrocytic

WBC count < 2000/cu mm

Platelets count < 3000/cu mm

Serum bilirubin < normal

Bone marrow aspiration – fatty bone marrow.

Management   It is a medical emergency, that requires priority treatment.

Medical treatment

Hospitalize the patient

Removal of cause

Discontinue all medicines

Androgens therapy:
- Testosterone enanthate 250 mg IM every 2/52
- Nandrolone decanoate 25–100 mg IM weekly

Blood transfusion: Packed red cells/whole blood for platelet depletion

Antibiotics – to control infections.

Surgical treatment:

Splenectomy – in case of failure of above said treatment

Bone marrow transplantation

Stem cell therapy (SCT).

Prognosis
Poor (fatal period – few months)

Hemorrhage and infection are causes of death.

Refer: The severe patient to the medical team.

Hemoglobin Disorders
Sickle Cell Anemia

Definition
It is a recessive hereditary disorder, confined to blacks (African and American) and aboriginal tribes in India. The abnormal Hb is transmitted as dominant trait.

Pathogenesis
The RBCs become deformed into irregular, pointed shapes (sickles), which do not slip easily through capillaries, arterioles and venules, and thus the circulation is impaired, causing anoxia, infarction of tissues, e.g. liver, spleen, muscles and bones.

Diagnosis
A black patient

Anemia, jaundice, fever, myalgia, malaise, fatigue, pain abdomen

Headache, convulsions, paralysis.

Investigation
Hemogram

Serum LDH – elevated

Screening tests (peripheral blood smear):
- Sodium metabisulfite test: 1 drop of patient's blood + 1 drop of reagent (mixed on a slide) results in sickening of RBC within few mts (deoxygenated RBC become distorted as Hb becomes insoluble).
- Sickledex solubility test: 0.02 ml of blood + 2 ml of reagent (sodium dithionate as reducing agent + saponin and phosphate buffer as precipitating agents) results in SHb producing a cloudy tube (normally a clear tube).

Management
Monitoring of crisis (under observation)

Oxygen therapy

Analgesics

IV fluids

Blood transfusion

Antibiotics

Newer treatment modalities:
- Fetal Hb production stimulators: Hydroxyurea, butyrates
- HbS solubility increasing agents: Urea, cyanate, phenylalanine
- Red cells HbS concentration reducing agents: DDAVP
- Bone marrow transplantation (BMT).

Prognosis   Majority of patients die during childhood due to cerebral hemorrhage, shock, or uremia.

Refer: The severe patient to the medical team.

Thalassemia

Definition   It is defined as a heterogenous group of hereditary disorders, characterized by absence or reduced hemoglobin synthesis, resulting in a microcytic hypochromic anemia of varying degree. RBCs are not fully filled up with Hb.

Types   Thalassemia minor and major.

Pathogenesis   Reduced synthesis of one of the globin chains of RNA. In beta thalassemia, beta chains are abnormal while alpha chains are normal, while in alpha thalassemia, it is reverse. The unbalanced synthesis causes precipitation of normal chains, causing premature destruction (hemolysis) of RBC, in the bone marrow.

Thalassemia minor is heterozygous (adult/fetal Hb – 90/10%) form of disorder.

Thalassemia major is homozygous (adult/fetal Hb – 10–30/70–90%) form of disorder.

Thalassemia Minor
Thalassemia minor occurs, when a person inherits only one thalassemia gene, having minimal ill effect on beta chains synthesis.

Diagnosis   Common in Chinese
Pain abdomen
Anemia
Splenomegaly.

Investigation   RBC > 6 million/cu mm
MCV (50–70 μm^3)
MCHC – reduced
Target cells and stippled cells – common
Bone marrow – increased number of nucleated RBC
Hemosiderin – present.

Management   No treatment required.
Patients have normal lifespan.

Thalassemia Major
Thalassemia major occurs, when a person inherits 2 thalassemia genes, one from each parent. The double genes cause severe anemia, that requires regular blood transfusion throughout life.

Diagnosis	Anemia – paleness, fussiness, weakness and slow growth
	Abdomen bulges – due to hepatomegaly, splenomegaly.
Investigation	RBC – hypochromic, microcytic red cells with erythroblasts
	Target cells – seen
	Fetal Hb – elevated
	X-ray – skull and long bones: Medullary portion – increased
	Cortex – thinning.
Management	Regular blood transfusion after every 1 month
	Surgical treatment:
	• Splenectomy – indicated if secondary hemolytic anemia develops
	• Bone marrow transplantation
	• Stem cells replacement

Refer: The severe patient to the medical team.

Leukemias	The leukemias are a group of disorders in which one or other of the types of white cells undergo malignant change. The bone marrow becomes diffusely infiltrated with primitive cells (myelocytic, lymphocytic, or monocytic) and the corresponding primitive forms appear in the peripheral blood.

Acute Leukemia

Definition	It is a disorder of the blood forming tissue, characterized by an abnormally large number of WBCs in the blood, bone marrow and other blood forming tissues.
Etiology	Unknown
	Age – may involve any age group – mainly during first 5 yrs.
	Race – no bar
Types	Acute and chronic and lymphatic and myelocytic.
Diagnosis	Fever, pallor, anorexia, petechiae, weakness, malaise, anemia
	Myalgia and arthralgia
	Lymph nodes – enlarged, splenomegaly, hepatomegaly.
Investigation	Hemogram – anemia
	TLC – leukocytosis
	Platelet count < 100,000/cu mm
	Blood smear – immature and abnormal cells seen
	Auer bodies in the cytoplasma of myeloblasts
	Bone marrow (BM) – proliferation of myeloblasts/lymphoblasts
	Philadelphia chromosome +ve
	X-rays bones – marked osteoporosis, periosteal elevation, osteolytic lesions.
D/d	Acute myeloblastic leukemia – presence of cytoplasmic granules
	Acute lymphatic leukemia – absence of cytoplasmic granules
Complications	GI tract hemorrhage, cerebral hemorrhage (ICH), systemic infection.

Management

Treatment of acute lymphatic leukemia

Aim
- To destroy each and every leukemic cell in the body, to prevent relapse due to multiplication of residual cells.
- To kill all leukemic cells by multiple drug therapy, that attacks the leukemic cells in different phases of mitotic cycle.

Drugs
Vinca alkaloids:
- Vincristine adult: 1.4–2 mg/sq m IV weekly for 4/52
  children: 1.5–2 mg/sq m
- + Prednisone 40 mg/sq m
- Others: Vinblastin, vinorelbine

Antimetabolites:
- Methotrexate (inhibits DNA, RNA, and protein synthesis)
  Dose: 2.5–3.3 mg/sq m + Prednisolone 60 mg/sq m IV b.i.w.
- Mercaptopurine 2.5 mg/kg o.d. PO b.i.w.

Management of relapses:
- Vincristine and prednisone as above for 4–7/7.

Treatment of acute myeloblastic leukemia

Aim
- To prolong remission as permanent cure is not currently possible.
- To kill all leukemic cells by multiple drug therapy, that attacks the leukemic cells in different phases of mitotic cycle.

Drugs
Alkylating agents:
- Busulfan (Myleran) – is drug of choice
  Dose: 0.6 mg/kg/day PO till TLC comes down to 10000/cu mm
  Drug may be discontinued/given intermittently
- Melphalan (alkeran) 10 mg/day PO for 1/52
- Cytarabine 100–200 /sq m b.i.d. in 2 divided doses for 4–6/7 plus
- Thioguanine (antimetabolite)
  Dose: 2.5 mg/kg o.d. PO in 2 divided doses for 4/7. Rept. every 2/52
- Cyclophosphamide – an alkylating agent
  Dose: 2–3 mg/kg/day PO

Vinca alkaloids:
- Vincristine adult: 1.4–2 mg/sq m IV weekly for 4/52
  children: 1.5–2 mg/sq m
- + Prednisone 40 mg/sq m

Radiotherapy
Total body irradiation/local therapy
- Radiophosphorus (32P) 1–2.5 mCi (millicurie) IV. Rept every 2/52 till TLC < 10,000/cu mm
  Check up – every 6/52.

Treatment of complications

> Fever – antibiotics
>
> Haemorrhage – platelet concentrates given to raise platelet count – at least to 60,000/cu mm
>
> Hyperuricemia – Allopurinol 100 mg, 3–4 times daily given to combat high uric acid
>
> IV fluids.

Refer: The patient to the oncology and medical team.

Prognosis

Acute lymphatic leukemia:	Using the above approach, survival for many yrs. In 15–25% of all patients
Acute myeloblastic leukemia:	Up to 50% of patients will achieve remissions on above two regimens.

Chronic Myelocytic Leukemia

Definition	It is a disorder of the blood forming tissue, characterized by proliferation of immature leukemic cells.
Etiology	Unknown Generally considered to be neoplastic – inevitably fatal May involve any age group – mainly adults.
Diagnosis	Mostly diagnosed accidentally Pallor, fever, malaise, anorexia, petechiae Weakness, anemia Pain – bone and joint Splenomegaly.
Investigation	Hemogram – normochromic, normocytic anemia TLC – leukocytosis (> 500,000/cu mm) Platelet count > 1,000,000/cu mm Blood smear – immature and abnormal cells (nonfilamented neutrophils, myelocytes and metamyelocytes) seen. Blast cells – 5% Auer bodies in the cytoplasm of myeloblasts Bone marrow (BM) – massive proliferative myeloblasts Philadelphia chromosome +ve X-rays bones – Marked osteoporosis, periosteal elevation, osteolytic lesions.
Management	Usually a disease of adults.

General measures: Palliation of symptoms and correction of anemia

Chemotherapy

Drugs

- Busulfan (myleran) – an alkylating agent, is drug of choice
  Dose: 2–6 mg o.d. PO, till TLC comes down to 10000/cu mm
  Drug may be discontinued or given intermittently
- Alkeran 10 mg o.d. PO, for 1/52

- Cytarabine 2–3 mg/kg o.d. IV in two divided doses for 4 days plus
- Thioguanine 2.5 mg/kg o.d. PO, in two divided doses for 4 days repeat every 2/52
- Cyclophosphamide – an alkylating agent
  Dose: 2–3 mg/kg/day PO
- Vincristine 2 mg IV o.d. PO, for blastic crises. Used in combination with prednisone 200 mg o.d. PO. Rpt. every 2 wks until bone marrow clears
- Mercaptopurine 2.5 mg/kg/day PO. Maint: half dose
- Hydroxyuria 20–30 mg/kg/day PO
- Interferon alpha-2a 3–9 million i.u. s.c./or IM
- Imatinib 600 mg o.d. PO.

Radiotherapy   Total body irradiation or local therapy
Radiophosphorus (^{32}p) 1–2.5 mCi (millicurie) IV. Rept every 2/52 till TLC < 10,000/cu mm
Check up – every 6/52.

Stem cell therapy (SCT) – highly effective, but expensive procedure.

Refer: The patient to the oncology and medical teams.

Multiple Myeloma (Plasma Cell Myeloma)

Definition   Multiple malignant, endosteal tumors (proliferation of plasma cells) resulting in marked bone destruction.

Etiology   Unknown.

Risk factors
- Radiation exposure – nuclear industry workers
- Insecticides exposure – farmers, horticulturists
- Virus exposure – herpes virus

Diagnosis   Age – usually appears in 6th and 7th decades of life and is rare in < 40 yrs.
Race – seen in all races.
Sex – twice common in males
Site – skull, spine, sternum, ribs, femur, tibia
Severe bone pain – aggravated by motion
Bones are involved in 90% of patients, pathological fractures
Fever, thirst, nausea, headache
Anemia, fatigue, loss of weight.

Investigation   Hemogram – anemia: Normocytic, normochromic type
Rouleau formation – marked
ESR – raised
TLC and platelet count – normal
Serum alkaline phosphatase – elevated
Serum globulin – elevated
Urine – Bence Jones proteinuria – present in 40% of patients
X-ray skull – show typical punched out areas

	MRI – highly accurate in detecting an early epidural involvement
	Bone marrow (aspiration) biopsy – shows plasma cells.
D/d	Skeletal metastasis – from breast, thyroid, prostate, kidney
	Hyperparathyroidism
	Amyloidosis – always associated with plasma cell neoplasia.
	Abnormal gamma globulin products, especially those of Bence Jones type, are directly involved in these tissue (amyloid) infiltrates.
Management	No effective treatment known and the disease is always fatal
Aims	• Relief from pain and reduction of tumor masses
	• Ambulation of patient to combat negative calcium balance
	• Prevention of exposure to trauma to avoid occurrence of the pathological fractures

Treatment

General measures

Blood transfusion – to combat anemia

Analgesics – for control of pain

Chemotherapy

Drugs   Alkylating agents:
- Melphalan (alkeran) – most effective agent available.
  Dose: 10 mg o.d. PO, for 7/7 + prednisone 100 mg o.d.
  Maintenance dose: 10 mg o.d. every 4/52
- Cyclophosphamides 50 mg/kg IV for 7/7
- Vincristine: Adult: 1.4 2 mg/sq m IV weekly for 4/52
                    Children: 1.5–2 mg/sq m
  + Prednisone 40 mg/sq m

Radiotherapy • For control of pain and for reducing tumor mass.

Surgery   • Decompression with radiotherapy – for cord compression
              • Stem cell (bone marrow) transplantation (SCT) – for selective patients.

Prognosis   Average survival time after diagnosis is 2 years. Occasionally a patient may live for many years in apparent remission.

Refer: The patient to the oncology and medical teams.

Hodgkin's Disease

Definition   It is a malignant tumor of hematopoietic origion. It is characterized by abnormal proliferation, in one or several lymph nodes, of lymphocytes, histiocytes, eosinophils, and Reed-Sternberg giant cells.

Etiology   Unknown.

Diagnosis   Age – usually appears in young adults

              Race – seen in all races.

              Sex – twice common in males

              Severe bone pain – aggravated by motion

	Lymphadenopathy – regional lymph nodes (commonly cervical nodes) enlarged, non-tender, elastic and rubbery to feel
	Fever – Pel-Ebstein type, fatigue, pruritis
	Pressure symptoms – edema, engorged neck veins, cyanosis
	Fatigue, anemia, loss of weight, pruritis
	Hepatosplenomegaly.
Investigation	TLC and DLC – lymphocytopenia, occasionally eosinophilia,
	CXR
	X-ray bone (regional) – shows rarefaction
	Ultrasound – abdomen
	Lymph node biopsy
	Bone marrow biopsy
	Liver function tests.

Staging	O	Undetectable
	I	Single lymph node affected
	II	2 or > 2 lymph nodes affected
	III	Both sides of diaphragm affected but involvement of regional lymph nodes, splenomegaly
	IV	Involvement of – bone marrow, lung parenchyma, pleura, GI tract, hepatomegaly, CNS, renal.

Management	
Radiotherapy	It is treatment of choice for stages I, II, and III.
Chemotherapy	For stages III, or IV
	Combination chemotherapy: It is treatment of choice
Drugs	• Cyclophosphamide—2-3 mg/kg IV o.d. for 6 days followed by 50–100 mg PO o.d. in divided doses.
	• Vinblastin: Adult: 1.4 mg/sq.m/wk. IV. Max: 11.1 mg/sq.m
	Children: 2 mg/sq m/wk. IV. Max: 7.5 mg/sq m
	• Vincristine 1.4 mg/sq m/wk IV +
	Prednisone 40 mg/sq m o.d. PO for 2/52
	• Chlorambucil – 0.1–0.2 mg/kg PO o.d. in divided doses.

Refer: The patient to the oncology and medical team.

Agranulocytosis

Etiology	Exact cause unknown.
Risk factors	Drugs and chemicals, e.g. antithyroids, sulphonamides, aminopyrine, thiazines.
Diagnosis	Fever, chills, sore throat, mouth and throat ulcers, lymphadenopathy.
Investigation	TLC and DLC – lekcopenia (depleted granulocytes, lymphocytes and monocytes), ESR – raised
	Bone marrow (BMB) biopsy – hypoplastic.
Management	Admission and isolation of the patient

IV fluids

Discontinue the suspected drugs or chemical agents

Antibiotics – to control infection

Corticosteroids – to control toxemia.

Refer: The severe patient to the medical team.

References

1. Keele CA, Neil E (editors): The Blood. Samson Wright's Applied Physiology, 10th ed., London, 1961.
2. Wintrobe MM, et al: Clinical Hematology, 7th ed. Lea and Febiger, 1974.
3. Krupp MA, Chatton MJ: Current Medical Diagnosis and Treatmant, Maruzen Asian Ed., Bombay, 1975.
4. George E: Multiple Myeloma: Recognitin and Management, Family Medicine India, Vol. 4 No.2, 22–28;2000.
5. Charnley J: Diseases of Bones. Bailey and Loves Short Practice of Surgery, 13th ed. H.K.Lewis and Co. Ltd. London, 1965.
6. Goodman LS, Gilman A: The Pharmacological Basis of Therapeutics, 2nd ed. The Macmillan Co. New York, 1960.
7. Arora V: Drug Update, Vol. 7 Issue 2;2010.
8. Gulhati CM: MIMS, Vol. 28 No 9;2008.
9. Mishra L: Drug Today, Vol. 1 and 2, Issue 7–9;2008.

Gastrointestinal Tract and Liver Emergencies and Common Disorders

Signs and symptoms (non-specific manifestations)
Emergencies and common disorders:
- Acute abdomen
- Candidiasis (syn. Moniliasis, Thrush)
- Acute gastritis
- Acute corrosive esophagitis and gastritis
- Gastro-esophageal reflux disease (GERD/GORD) syn. Heartburn
- *Helicobacter pylori* (*H. pylori*) infection
- Postgastrectomy syndrome (dumping syndrome)
- Crohn's disease syn. Regional (enteritis, ileitis, enterocolitis)
- Acute ulcerative colitis
- Acute peptic ulcer
- Hemorrhoids (piles)
- Acute anal fissure (fissure-in-ano)
- Acute anorectal abscess
- Acute fistula-in-ano
- Liver disorders
- Jaundice
- Hepatic coma (syn. liver insufficiency)
- Porta-systemic encephalopathy syndrome
- Hepatitis
- Pylephlebitis

Liver abscesses
- Amebic liver abscess
- Pyogenic liver abscess

Signs and Symptoms (Non-specific Manifestations)

1. Nausea and vomiting
2. Constipation
3. Diarrhea
4. Flatulence
5. Irritable bowel syndrome
6. Gastrointestinal bleeding
7. Acute abdomen (pain abdomen)

Nausea and Vomiting

Definition   Nausea is defined as feeling of sickness, discomfort or uneasiness in the stomach, which is normally relieved by vomiting. It may occur singly or concurrently.

Vomiting (emesis) occurs as a result of muscular contractions (retching) that expel the ingested food or any other matter in the stomach, normally following nausea.

Etiology	Faulty dietary habits – overeating, or eating fatty, spicy or too hot foods, foods infected by bacteria, eating gellfish or rotten pork.
	Irritation of GI tract, e.g. cholecystitis
	Inflammation of GI tract, e.g. appendicitis
	Obstruction in GI tract, e.g. small intestinal obstruction
	Poisons, e.g. exogenous and endogenous toxins
	Drugs, e.g. digitalis, morphine, aspirin, antibiotics, sulphonamides
	Miscellaneous, e.g. sea sickness, morning sickness of pregnancy, sight of blood or violence, smell of rotten meat/fish

Management

Acute cases   Admit the patient

IV fluids

Nothing by mouth till symptoms persist

Drugs:

- Prochlorperazine (stemetil)
  Dose: Adult: 5–10 mg b.d. or t.d.s. PO or 12.5 mg IM
            Children: 10 kg body wt. 0.25 mg/kg PO
- Promethazine (avomine)
  Dose: Adult 25 mg b.i.d./t.d.s. PO or 25 mg IM, children 12.5 mg IM
- Metoclopramide HCl (perinorm, reglan)
  Dose: Adult 10 mg t.d.s. PO, children 0.5–1 mg/kg PO
- Trifluopromazine HCl (Siquil) 20–50 mg o.d. PO or 1–3 mg IV or 5–10 mg IV
- Chlorpromazine HCl 25–50 mg IM. Rept – every 4–6 hrs or
                 10–50 mg PO rept every 4–6 hrs

Specific treatment: Removal of underlying cause.

Constipation

Definition	Decrease in frequency of bowel movements (2 or fewer/week) and difficulty in expressing (straining) of hard and dry stools	
Etiology	Functional	Diet – reduced intake of dietary fibre
		Age – elderly
		Sedentary life – little or no exercise
		Immobilization – bed ridden, e.g. postoperatively
		Anxiety
	Organic, e.g.	Intestinal obstruction
		Irritable bowel syndrome
		Anorectal stenosis, stricture
		Anal fissure, hemorrhoids
		Anorectal/perineal abscesses
		Neoplastic–carcinoma colorectal
		Endocrinal – hypothyroidism

	Pregnancy
	Neuromuscular – cerebral palsy, spinal cord lesions
	Drugs – opium, morphine.
Investigation	Barium enema
	Endoscopy – lower GI tract.
Management	
General treatment	

Reassure the patient, e.g. a daily bowel movement is not essential to health, and the patient should be helped to develop normal bowel habits.

Adequate fluids – to assist passage of intestinal contents

Adequate residue diets (whole wheat flour, fruit and vegetables)

Adequate physical exercise – helpful

Drugs:

- Milk of magnesia (cremaffin) 10–15 ml; children 5 ml
- Liq. paraffin (agarol) 10 ml; children 5 ml
- Bisacodyl (dulcolax) 1–2 tab PO at bedtime or
- As suppository P/R (1 inserted rectally)

Specific treatment: Treatment of the cause.

Acute Diarrhea

Definition	It is defined as diarrhea of infectious origin that begins acutely. Infection is associated with high morbidity and mortality especially in malnourished children and elderly patients.
Etiology	Infections:

- Rotavirus, Norwalk virus
- Bacterial, e.g. *Escherichia coli*, *Shigella*, *Salmonella*
- Protozoal, e.g. *Entamoeba histolytica*, giardiasis, *Vibrio cholerae*

Miscellaneous:

- Psychogenic, e.g. nervous diarrhea
- Neurologic, e.g. tabes dorsalis, diabetic
- Metabolic, e.g. hyperthyroidism
- Food allergy
- Malabsorption
- Malnutrition.

Investigation	Stools: Microscopical examination and bacterial cultures for parasites and inflammatory cells
	Proctoscopy: Indicated in dysentery cases and in those showing no improvement within a week
	Serum electrolytes: To determine replacement therapy.
Management	Admit the patient

IV fluids and electrolytes – especially in infants and elderly

Oral rehydration therapy (ORT) – oral rehydration salts (ORS)

Antidiarrheal drugs:

- Loperamide HCl 4 mg PO. Rept 2 mg after each motion
- Nalidixic acid 1 g q.d.s. PO for 7 days; children 2.5–10 ml t.d.s.
- Furazolidine 100 mg q.d.s. PO; children ½ to 1 tspf. q.d.s.
- Metronidazole 400 mg t.d.s. PO for 7 days
- Colistin sulph. susp. 5–15 mg/kg/day in divided doses

Specific treatment: Removal of the cause.

Flatulence

Definition | It is defined as an uncomfortable collection of air/wind in the stomach or the intestines, and the discomfort is relieved by expulsion of gas (flatus) from the mouth or the anus.

Etiology | Functional

Organic disorders of the digestive system

Management

Aim | To minimize public embarrassment by following means:

- Good hygiene and eating habits
- Diet: Nutritious. Avoid milk and milk products
- Specific treatment: Removal of the cause

Irritable Bowel Syndrome

Definition | It is one of the most frequent gastrointestinal disorders.

Etiology | Functional

Organic disorders of GI tract.

Diagnosis | Diarrhea, constipation

Feeling of incomplete evacuation

Pain abdomen.

Management | General treatment:

Diet: Avoid fried, spicy, fast foods, alcohol, coffee

Drugs: Gastrointestinal sedatives:

- Dicyclomine HCl 10–20 mg t.d.s. PO; children (2–12 yrs) 10 mg t.d.s.
- Chlordiazepoxide 10–20 mg o.d. PO; children: Not recommended
- Ranitidine 150 mg b.i.d. PO for 4–8/52
- Clidinium brom. 2.5 mg t.d.s. before meals and at bedtime
- Specific treatment: Removal of the underlying cause.

Gastrointestinal Bleeding

Definition | Hematemesis is defined as the vomiting of blood, whereas melena as the bleeding per rectum, rendering stools black and cherry. It is a common serious emergency and requires priority treatment.

Source	Upper GI tract 90%
	Large intestine 9%
	Small intestine 1%.

Etiology

Upper gastrointestinal bleeding:

Peptic ulcer of the duodenum, stomach, oesophagus

Esophageal varices

Mallory-Weiss syndrome (esophagogastric mucosal tear)

Gastritis

Alcohol abuse

Blood dyscrasias – purpura, hemophilia, pernicious anemia

Carcinoma stomach

Lower gastrointestinal bleeding:

Hemorrhoids

Anal fissure

Traumatic – forcing of foreign bodies into rectum (torture)

Diverticula colon

Carcinoma colon

Diagnosis	History of weakness or fainting
	Hematemesis
	Melena
	Pain abdomen.
Investigation	Hemogram, hematocrit, platelet count, BT and CT

- Liver function tests, e.g.
  - Serum bilirubin
  - Serum proteins
  - Alkaline phosphatase
  - Prothrombine concentration
- Plain X-ray abdomen
- Ultrasound abdomen and pelvis
- Endoscopy – very helpful in diagnosis
- Angiography – in case endoscopy fails to locate the site of bleeding
- Proctoscopy
- Sigmoidoscopy
- CT scan

Management

General treatment

Admit the patient

Monitor fluid intake, urine output

Insert a nasogastric Ryle's tube, a Foley's catheter

Recording of BP, pulse, respiration every ½ to 1hr

IV fluids – Ringer's or dextrose saline

Plasma transfusion or plasma expanders, e.g. Hemaccel – while blood transfusion is prepared

Blood transfusion – for treatment of shock

Diet: Liquid diet followed by bland diet

Drugs: Antacids, e.g. Alum. Hydrox. Gel 200–400 mg q.d.s. PO
            Mag. trisilicate 0.5–1.0 g o.d. PO

Endoscopic hemostatic procedures:
- Sclerotherapy (injection therapy) for bleeding varices:
  Sclerosants: Polidocanol, ethanolamine, alcohol, hypertonic saline
- Thermal therapy: Cautery or laser electrocoagulation
- Hemostatic clip or band ligation

Specific treatment: Treatment of the underlying cause.

Refer: The severe patient to the medical and surgical team.

Acute Abdomen (Pain Abdomen)

Described in appropriate section of general surgery emergencies.

Aphthous Ulcer (Syndrome Canker Sore, Ulcerative Stomatitis)

Definition	Is a shallow mucosal ulcer or multiple ulcerations on an inflamed oral mucosa.
Etiology	Unknown.
Predisposing factors	Infective: Viral
	Inflammatory: IBS, Behçet's syndrome, infectious mononucleosis, PUO
	Agents: Physical, chemical or microbial
	Alcohol abuse, e.g. drinking too much alcohol
	Allergic, e.g. certain food items, e.g. nuts, chocolates, citrus fruits
	Stress.
Pathogenesis	Ulcer covered with a pseudomembrane.
Diagnosis	Burning pain
	Ulcer/s
Investigation	CBC, ESR
	Blood sugar
Management	
General measures	
	Bland mouth rinses
	Analgesics, sedatives
	Antibiotics
	Corticosteroids
	Local: Hydrocortisone ointments

Refer: The patient to the medical team.

Candidiasis (Syndrome Moniliasis, Thrush)

Definition	Is a fungal infection of the mouth.
Etiology	Fungal infection – *Candida albicans*.
Predisposing factors	Acute fever
	Debilitating
	Antibiotics abuse
	IBS
	Alcohol abuse, e.g. drinking too much alcohol
Pathogenesis	Lesions covered with curd-like patches in the mouth
Diagnosis	Pain
	Fever, malaise, lethargy
	Lymphadenopathy
Investigation	CBC, ESR
	Culture of lesions scraps.

Management

General measures: Symptomatic and supportive.

Diet: Nutritious with vitamin supplements

Bed rest

Mouth rinses

Specific treatment

Drugs :

• Antifungals:

Nystatin – 0.5 million units tds

Gention violet 1% sol. locally tds

Miconazole nitrate crème – locally tds

Clotrimazole crème – locally tds.

Refer: The patient to the medical and surgical team.

Acute Gastritis

Definition	It is defined as inflammation of the stomach, and is one of the most common disturbances of the stomach.
Etiology	Faulty dietary habits, e.g. eating spicy food, drinking too much coffee
	Alcohol abuse, e.g. drinking too much alcohol
	Drugs/chemical irritants, e.g. salicylates, NSAIDs, alkalies, acids
	Infective, e.g. bacterial and viral
	Allergic, e.g. certain food items
Diagnosis	Anorexia – may be the only presenting symptom
	Fullness – epigastric,
	Nausea and vomiting, diarrhea
	Flatulence, epigastric heaviness, pain abdomen
	Fever, chills, headache, malaise, muscle cramps.

Investigation TLC and DLC – leukocytosis or leukopenia

Endoscopy – helpful in D/d.

Management

General treatment

Nothing by mouth until acute symptoms have subsided, then give liquid, followed by a soft diet.

Drugs Gastrointestinal sedatives and antispasmodics:

- Oxyphenonium bromide. 5–10 mg q.d.s. PO; children 2.5 mg b.i.d.
- Cimetidine 400 mg b.i.d. or t.d.s. PO for 4–8/52
- Famotidine 40 mg PO at bedtime for 4–8/52; children: not advised
- Ranitidine HCl 150 mg b.i.d. PO for 4–8/52; children: not advised
- Hyoscine butylbromide (buscopan) 20 mg q.d.s. PO
- Metoclopramide HCl (perinorm, reglan) 5–10 mg t.d.s. PO
  Suspension 5 mg/5 ml; children 2.5 mg b.d.

Acute Corrosive Esophagitis and Gastritis

Etiology Ingestion of corrosive and irritant substances:

Corrosive substances:

- Acids, e.g. mineral, sulphuric, nitric, hydrochloric
- Alkalies, e.g. caustic soda, potash, ammonia

Irritant substances:

- Oxalic acid, carbolic acid, salicylic acid;
- Mercury, arsenic, copper sulfate, lead, phosphorus

Diagnosis Corrosion of lips, tongue, mouth, pharynx

Pain – severe burning, cramping in the epigastrium

Nausea, vomiting, diarrhea, thirst, dysphasia

Local tenderness – positive over the epigastrium

Shock.

Investigation TLC and DLC: Leukocytosis

Urine: Proteinuria

Analysis of aspirated gastric fluid

Endoscopy – to determine tissue damage

Management Admit the patient

Insert nasogastric Ryle's tube – gastric suction

IV fluids and electrolytes

Gastrointestinal sedatives and antispasmodics:

- Oxyphenonium bromide 5–10 mg q.d.s. PO; children 2.5 mg b.i.d.
- Cimetidine 400 mg b.i.d. or t.d.s. PO for 4–8/52
- Famotidine 40 mg PO at bedtime for 4–8/52; children: Not advised
- Ranitidine HCl 150 mg b.i.d. PO for 4–8/52; children: Not advised
- Hyoscine butylbromide (buscopan) 20 mg q.d.s. PO

- Metoclopramide HCl (perinorm, reglan) 5–10 mg t.d.s. PO Suspension 5 mg/5 ml; children 2.5 mg b.d.

Antacids and sedatives:

- Alum. hydrox. tab/gel PO

Antidote – specific antidote to be administered immediately

Surgical treatment: Emergency laparotomy – to resect the damaged tissues.

Refer: The severe patient to the medical and surgical team.

Gastro-Esophageal Reflux Disease (GERD/GORD) syn. Heartburn

Definition	Is a disagreeable substernal burning pain, resulting from an irritating stimulus of the distal esophagus.
Etiology	Reflux of acid-peptic gastric contents (peptic esophagitis).
Predisposing factors	Alcohol abuse, e.g. drinking too much alcohol
	Allergic, e.g. certain food items
	Pregnancy – high incidence, disappears after delivery
Pathogenesis	Gastric acid causing esophageal erosion
Diagnosis	Burning substernal pain
	Nausea
	Vomiting
	Lethargy
Investigation	CBC, ESR
	Esophagoscopy – in recurrent cases
	CXR
	Plain X-ray abdomen
	Ultrasound abdomen

Management

General measures:

Elevate end of the bed

Maintaining an erect posture post eating

Maintain fluid and electolyte balance

Nothing by mouth until acute symptoms have subsided

IV dextrose infusion

IV potassium supplementation

Diet: Small dry meals

Specific treatment:

Drugs:

- Anticholinergics: Inhibit parasympathetic innervations, thereby reduce secretion and motility of the stomach (dicyclomine, propantheline, atropine, belladonna alkaloids, hyoscine)
- Histamine H-2 Receptor Inhibitors: Reduce gastric acid output, thereby healing peptic ulcers and relief in reflux esophagitis

- Reflux suppressants: Forms a raft that floats on the stomach contents, buoyed by CO_2, providing a mechanical barrier to reflux (antacids or carbenoxolones)
- *Protone pump inhibitors:* Inhibit gastric acid by blocking hydrogen-potassium adenosine triphosphatase enzyme system (proton pump) in gastric parietal cells (omeprazole, pantoprazole, iansoprazole)
- Prokinetic agents: Increase the tone of the lower esophageal sphincter (cisapride). Banned in many countries such as USA, UK, India etc. due to reported deaths from arrhythmias.

Surgery: For treating gastro-esophageal reflux in patients with extra-esophageal manifestations, i.e. asthma.

Refer: The patient to the medical and surgical team.

Helicobacter Pylori (H. Pylori) Infection

Definition	Is defined as an infection with *H. pylori*, an important cause of morbidity related to the upper GI tract, especially stomach and duodenum, common amongst children of underprivileged communities – a current realization. It is associated with duodenal ulcers (95%) and gastric ulcers (70%), thereby eradication of *H. pylori* is an essential part of the management of these disorders.
Etiology	Bacterial infection: *Helicobacter pylori* (*H. pylori*).
Pathogenesis	Erosions of gastri and duodenal walls, ulceration.
Diagnosis	Nausea, vomiting
	Pain abdomen: Epigastric
	Vertigo, headache
	Fever
	Hypertension or hypotension
	Palpitations
Investigation	CBC, ESR, blood sugar, blood cholesterol profile, LFT, RFT,
	ECG
	X-ray chest
	Plain X-ray abdomen
	Ultrasound abdomen
	ENT check up: For vertigo
	Neurology check up: To rule out any neurological deficit
	MRI and CT angioscan of brain
Management	Medical treatment:
	Combination regimens for eradication of *H. pylori*
	First line (one week) triple therapy regimens:
	Antibiotic: Amoxycillin 1 g bid and Clarithromycin 0.5 g bid PO
	Penicillin hypersensitivity:
	Metronidazole 0.4 g bid PO + Clarithromycin 0.25 g bid PO

Acid suppressants: Proton pump inhibitor:
- Omeprazole 20 mg bid PO, or
- Pantoprazole 40 mg bid PO, or
- Rabeprazole 20 mg bid PO

Second line (one week) quadruple therapy regimens:

Antibiotic: Oxytetracycline 0.5 g qid PO, plus

Metronidazole 0.4 g tid PO

Acid suppressants: Proton pump inhibitor:
- Omeprazole 20 mg bid PO, or
- Pantoprazole 40 mg bid PO, or
- Rabeprazole 20 mg bid PO

Cytoprotectant: Tri-potassium dicitratobismuthate 0.12 g qid PO.

Refer: The patient to the medical team.

Postgastrectomy Syndrome (Dumping Syndrome)

Definition	Is a syndrome that occurs after gastrectomy.
Etiology	Gastrectomy.
Predisposing factors	Provoked by soluble, hypertonic carbohydrates. Sympathetic vasomotor responses
Pathogenesis	Rapid flow of fluid into small intestine, increased plasma kinins, increased peripheral blood flow, modest drop in plasma volume, increased hematocrit, decreased serum.
Diagnosis	Nausea, vomiting, or diarrhea
	Sweating, warmth
	Epigastric fullness and grumbling
	Abdominal cramps
	Pallor, weakness
	Syncope.
Investigation	CBC, ESR
	Blood sugar – lowered
	ECG – changes noticed
D/d	Reactive hypoglycemia – occurs much later after the meal and relieved by ingestion of food.

Management

General measures:

Diet: Frequent, small, feedings high in protein, fat and low carbohydrate

Fluid to be taken between meals and not with meals

Specific treatment:

Drugs:
- Sedatives and anticolinergics.

Refer: The patient to the medical and surgical team.

Crohn's Disease Syndrome Regional (Enteritis, Ileitis, Enterocolitis)

Definition	Is defined as a chronic, recurrent inflammatory disease affecting any part of GI tract. It involves young adults, running an intermittent clinical course with mild to severe disability and frequent complications.
Etiology	Unknown.
Pathogenesis	Whole thickness of the intestinal wall involved, with normal areas (skip lesions) between affected ones. Marked submucosal thickening with lymphedema, lymphoid hyperplasia and granulomas, overlying mucosa ulcerated
Diagnosis	Onset – insidious
	Age – common in young adults
	Nausea, vomiting, diarrhea
	Fever – low grade, chills, anorexia, malaise, loss of weight
	Abdominal pain (RLQ) – cramping, swelling, tenderness
Investigation	CBC – anemia (macrocytic)
	Stools – for occult blood and cultures
	Barium meal study – rose thorn ulcers and strictures
	Sigmoidoscopy
	Biopsy – selective.
D/d	Acute appendicitis, ulcerative colitis, amebic colitis, tuberculosis
Risk factor	Carcinoma intestine (small and large).
Management	General measures:
	Diet : High calorie, high protein, high vitamin, plenty of fluids orally
	Avoid raw fruits and vegetables
	Drugs:
	• Acute exacerbations: Corticosteroids (systemic & parenteral)
	• Maintaining remission: Azathioprine
	• Controlling diarrhea: Codeine phosphate.
	• MMR vaccine – without much evidence.
Surgery	Non-curative although desired in most cases.

Refer: The patient to the medical and surgical team.

Acute Ulcerative Colitis

Definition	Is defined as recurrent inflammatory disease of the large intestine.
Etiology	Unknown.
Pathogenesis	Multiple, irregular ulceration of colon (esp. recto-sigmoid), thickened wall with scarring and polypoid structures.
Diagnosis	Diarrhea: Bloody and mucoid
	Fever, malaise, weight loss
	Abdominal pain, distention, tenderness
	Anemia.

Investigation	CBC – hypochromic microcytic anemia due to blood loss
	TLC and DLC–polymorphonuclear leukocytosis
	ESR – elevated, platelets increased
	C-Reactive protein
	Stools – blood, mucous and pus
	– cultures
	Electrolytes balance – disturbed
	LFT
	Barium meal study – may show regional to generalized irritability, pseudopolyps, narrowed lumen
	Colonoscopy and sigmoidoscopy – may show ulceration and polypoids
	Biopsy.
D/d	Dysentery – amebic or bacillary
	Lymphogranuloma venereum – history and Frei test
	Crohn's disease
	Intestinal diverticulitis
	Intestinal neoplasm
Management	General measures:
	Bed rest
	Diet – nutritious, supplemented with vitamins
	– avoid milk and milk products
	Acute case:
	Hospitalisation of patient
	IV fluids, nothing by mouth
	Corticosteroids
Surgery	Total colectomy with ileostomy – in refractory disease, neoplasm, massive hemorrhage

Refer: The patient to the medical and surgical team.

Acute Peptic Ulcer

Definition	It is an acute ulceration of a part of the GI tract.
Types	Duodenal and gastric.
Etiology	Hyperacidity, hypersecretion of hydrochloric acid
	Decreased tissue resistance – alcohol abuse
	Drugs, e.g. corticosteroids, salicylates, NSAIDs
	Severe burns
	Hemorrhagic disorders
	Food poisoning
	Bacteremia.
Diagnosis	Pain abdomen in the epigastrium.
	• Pain – gnawing, cramp-like, or heartburn type
	• Pain may radiate to back or shoulder

	Hematemesis
	Local tenderness over epigastrium.
Investigation	Anemia – hypochromic
	Stools – occult blood
	Gastric analysis – shows acid > 5 mEq/hr
	Plane X-ray abdomen – may show an ulcer crater
	Endoscopy – a valuable adjunct in diagnosis of duodenal ulcer.

Management

Conservative treatment

Admit the patient

Diet: Nutritious diet, regular meals. Begin with liquid diet and hourly antacids, followed by a bland diet and later on a regular diet.

Do not give milk as 'therapy'

Avoid coffee, tea, cola, beverages, spicy foods, alcohol

Drugs   Antiulcer and antisecretory:

- Antacids: Alum hydrox. tab. 600 mg t.d.s. PO suspension: Gel 5–10 ml t.d.s. PO after meals
- Cimetidine 400 mg b.i.d. or t.d.s. PO for 4–8/52
- Famotidine 40 mg PO at bedtime for 4–8/52; children: Not advised
- Ranitidine HCl 150 mg b.i.d. PO for 4–8/52; children: Not advised
- Hyoscine butylbromide (buscopan) 20 mg q.d.s. PO
- Metoclopramide HCl (perinorm, reglan) 5–10 mg t.d.s. PO
  Suspension 5 mg/5 ml; children 2.5 mg b.d.

Anticholinergics (antispasmodics and intestinal motility):

- Propantheline 15 mg t.d.s. before meals and 30 mg PO bedtime
- Dicyclomine 10–20 mg t.d.s.
- Others: Atropine, ambutonium, hyoscine, clidinium, belladonna alkaloid

Proton pump inhibitors: Inhibit gastric acid by blocking proton pump (Hydrogen – potassium adenosine triphosphatase enzyme system):

- Omeprazole 20 mg o.d. PO for 8/52
- Others: Lansoprazole, esomeprazole, pantoprazole

IV fluids and electrolytes

Blood transfusion – for hematemesis.

Surgical treatment: Emergency laparotomy – indicated in acute perforation for surgical closure.

Refer: The severe patient to the medical and surgical team.

Hemorrhoids (syndrome Piles)

Definition	Hemorrhoids are varices of anorectal veins, originating in the venous hemorrhoidal plexus, formed by radicles of superior, middle, and inferior hemorrhoidal veins.
Types	External or internal to the dentate margin (pectinate line). External covered by skin, while the internal clothed by mucous membrane.

Etiology   Hereditary
                    Constipation – straining factor
                    Overpurgation
                    Diarrhea, dysentery, colitis.

Precipitating factors:
                    Constipation, straining at stool, prolonged sitting – to pass stool
                    Anal abscess
                    Fissure in ano.

Diagnosis   Bleeding per rectum
                    Prolapse on defecation
                    Mucoid discharge per rectum
                    Pruritus, pain
                    P/R examination
                    Proctoscopy.

Management

Conservative treatment
                    Diet: Low-roughage diet
                    Improving bowl habits
                    Sitz baths
                    Analgesics – to control pain
                    Antibiotics – to combat infection

Injection therapy   Indicated in 1st degree hemorrhoids. It is effective, but with much recurrence rate.

Surgery treatment   **Refer** the severe patient to the medical and surgical team.

Surgery   Hemorrhoidectomy.

Indications   3rd degree hemorrhoids and failure of the conservative measures

Acute Anal Fissure (syndrome Fissure-in-Ano)

Definition   It is defined as an elongated ulcer in the long axis of the anal canal, extending upwards from the anal margin into the rectum.

Site   Midline posteriorly–common, and midline anteriorly.

Etiology   Unknown
                    May be due to pressure exerted by the passage of hard stools, over the posterior wall at level of anorectal junction (anatomical curvature).

Diagnosis   Age – common in younger and middle age
                    Sex – more common in women
                    Pain – sharp, agonizing, aggravated on defecation
                    Stools – blood stained
                    Discharge per rectum
                    A sentinel skin tag can be seen.

Management

Conservative treatment

> Analgesics
>
> Lignocain ointment – introduced by patient himself daily
>
> Dilatation of anal canal, by passing a gloved finger lubricated with lignocain ointment. This is followed by passing of anal dilators.

Surgical treatment **Refer** the severe patient to the surgical team for surgery.

Surgery   Division of transverse fibres of internal sphincter

                   Excision of sentinel pile.

Acute Anorectal Abscess

Etiology   Traumatic – penetration of rectum by a foreign body (torture)

                   Infective – infected anal gland, blood-borne infection

Types   Perianal, ischiorectal, pelvirectal, submucous, depending upon site

Diagnosis   Pain – aggravated on defecation, difficulty in sitting and walking.

Management

Conservative treatment

> Analgesics
>
> Antibiotics

Surgical treatment: **Refer** the patient to the surgical team for surgery.

Surgery   Incision drainage under general anesthesia.

Acute Fistula-in-Ano

Definition   It is defined as a track, lined by granulation tissue which opens deeply in the anal canal or rectum and superficially on the skin around the anus.

Types   High level and low level, depending upon its internal opening is above or below the pectinate line.

Etiology   Anorectal abscess

                   Tuberculosis – multiple fistulae

Diagnosis   Discharge per rectum – sero-purulent type

                   Itching

                   Pain.

Investigation   Rectal examination: Internal opening felt as a nodule

                   Proctoscopy: Reveals an internal opening of the fistula

                   CXR (X-ray chest): To rule out tuberculosis.

Management

Conservative treatment

> Analgesics
>
> Antibiotics

Surgical treatment: **Refer** the severe patient to the surgical team for surgery.

Surgery   Incision or excision of the fistula.

Liver Disorders

Functions
- Storage organ: Glycogen, fats, proteins, vitamins A and B_{12}
- Synthesis: Plasma proteins, fibrinogen, prothrombin, heparin (mast cells)
- Secretion: Bile
- Formation and destruction: RBCs
- Detoxication and protection:
  - Metabolism: Carbohydrates, fats and proteins
  - Excretion: In bile: Bile pigments, cholesterol, bacteria, toxins, heavy metals, bacteria, toxins.
  - Heat regulation

Table 9.1 Liver function tests (LFT)

Test	Method	Units	Normal range
Bubin direct	Photometry	mg/dL	0–0.20
Bilirubin total	Photometry	mg/dL	0.30–1.20
Bilirubin indirect	Calculated	mg/dL	0–0.9
Alkaline phosphatase	Photometry	U/l	M: 53–128 F: 42–98
SGOT	Photometry	U/l	M: 0–37 F: 0–31
SGPT	Photometry	U/l	M: 13–40 F:10–28
Protein total	Photometry	g/dL	6.6–8.3
Albumin	Photometry	g/dL	3.5–5.2
Globulin	Photometry	g/dL	2.30–3.50
Albumin/globulin ratio	Calculated	Ratio	0.9–2.0

Urine
Bilirubin
Urobilinogen
Stercobilinogen

Jaundice

Definition
Is defined as a yellow color of the skin, conjunctive and other tissues, caused by the presence of an excess of bilirubin in the plasma and tissue fluids.

Etiology
Infective or toxic damage to the liver cells (hepatocellular jaundice)
Obstructive: Bile ducts obstruction (obstructive jaundice)
Hemolytic: Excessive breakdown of RBCs (hemolytic jaundice)

Predisposing factors
Infections: Viral hepatitis, infectious mononucleosis, spirochetal

Drugs
Chemical irritants – salicylates, NSAIDs, acids, alkalies, chlorpromazine, methyl testosterone, antibiotics – ampicillin, amoxicillin, doxycycline, isoniazid, BSA
Alcohol abuse, e.g. drinking too much alcohol
Allergic, e.g. certain food items

Diagnosis
Anorexia – may be the only presenting symptom
Nausea and vomiting, diarrhea

Flatulence, URQ heaviness

Pain abdomen

Fever, chills, headache, malaise, muscle cramps

Hepatomegaly, ascitis, fetor hepaticus, pruritus.

Investigation CBC – leukocytosis or leukopaenia, ESR – raised

LFT – Table 9.2 (Sample: Serum; Method: Photometry and calculated)

CT scan: Diagnostic in detecting SOL of liver (abscess, tumors, cysts)

Liver biopsy (percutaneous): Diagnostic in diffuse hepatic disorder

Management Symptomatic and supportive

Refer: The severe patient to the medical and surgical team.

Hepatic Coma (syn. Liver insufficiency)

Definition Is an acute emergency that demands priority attention and treatment.

Etiology Toxemia

Cirrhosis – hemorrhage into GI tract

Predisposing Infections: Viral hepatitis, infectious mononucleosis, spirochetal

factors

Drugs Chemical irritants – salicylates, NSAIDs, acids, alkalies, narcotics
chlorpromazine, methyl testosterone, antibiotics – ampicillin, amoxicillin,
doxycycline, isoniazid, BSA

Alcohol abuse, e.g. drinking too much alcohol

Allergic, e.g. certain food items

Pathogenesis Transportation of toxic substances to various parts of the body due to
failure of detoxicating functions of the liver.

Table 9.2 Liver function tests

Tests	Normal values	Units	Hepatocellular jaundice	Obstructive jaundice
Bilirubin – Direct	0–0.20	mg/dL	Increased	Increased
Bilirubin – Total	0.30–1.20	mg/dL	Increased	Increased
Bilirubin – Indirect	0–0.9	mg/dL	Increased	Increased
Alkaline Phosphatase	M: 53–128 F:42–98	U/l	Increased	Increased
SGOT	M: 0–37 F:0–31	U/l	Increased	Unchanged
SGPT	M: 13–40 F:10–28	U/l	Increased	Unchanged
Protein – Total	6.6–8.3	g/dL	Unchanged	Unchanged
Serum Albumin	3.5–5.2	g/dL	Decreased	Unchanged
Serum Globulin	2.30–3.50	g/dL	Unchanged	Unchanged
Albumin/globulin ratio	0.9–2.0	Ratio	Unchanged	Unchanged
Prothrombine time (Response to vit. K)	40–100% (15% increase)	24 hrs.	Prolonged	Prolonged
Cholesterol Total	100–250	mg/dL	Decreased	Increased
Urine : Bilirubin			Increased	Decreased
Urine : Urobilinogen			Increased	Decreased
Stool : Urobilinogen			Increased	Decreased

Diagnosis	Fetor hepatis
	Lethargy
	Jaundice
	Disorientation
	Convulsions
	Death
Investigation	CBC – leukocytosis or leukopaenia, ESR – raised
	Serum electrolytes estimation
	LFT – Table 9.1 (Sample: Serum; Method: Photometry and Calculated)
	CT scan: Diagnostic in detecting SOL of liver (abscess, tumors, cysts)
	Liver biopsy (percutaneous): Diagnostic in diffuse hepatic disorder

Management

General treatment

Maintain fluid and electrolyte balance

Nothing by mouth until acute symptoms have subsided

IV dextrose infusion

IV potassium supplementation

High carbohydrate diet

Specific treatment

Hemodialysis – to remove toxic substances from blood

Renal transplant

Refer: The patient to the medical and surgical team.

Porta-Systemic Encephalopathy Syndrome

Definition	Is an acute emergency that demands priority attention and treatment.
Etiology	Cirrhosis – hemorrhage into GI tract
Predisposing	Diet: High protein
	Hemorrhage: Upper GI tract
Pathogenesis	Porta-systemic venous shunt passage of protein (breakdown) end products include ammonia, from GI tract into systemic circulation transportation of toxic substances to various parts of the body due to failure of detoxicating functions of the liver.
Diagnosis	Disorientation and a flapping tremor of outstretched hands
	Rigidity – cogwheel rigidity of the limbs
	Convulsions
	Coma, death may occur.
Investigation	CBC – leukocytosis or leukopaenia, ESR – raised
	Serum electrolytes estimation
	LFT – Table 9.1 (Sample: Serum; Method: Photometry and Calculated)
	CT scan: Diagnostic in detecting SOL of liver (abscess, tumors, cysts)
	Liver biopsy (percutaneous): Diagnostic in diffuse hepatic disorder

Management

General treatment

        Maintain fluid and electrolyte balance

        Nothing by mouth until acute symptoms have subsided

        IV dextrose infusion

        IV potassium supplementation

        High carbohydrate diet

Specific treatment

        Hemodialysis – to remove toxic substances from blood

        Surgery: Sub-total colectomy

        Tracheostomy – for prolonged unconsciousness

Refer: The patient to the medical and surgical team.

Hepatitis

Definition	Is defined as inflammation of liver.
Types	Infectious : Viral hepatitis–A, B, C, D and E
	Fulminating
	Alcoholic

Viral Hepatitis

Etiology	Viral infection : A, C, D and E by RNA virus and B by a DNA virus.
Hepatitis A	Described in Section 13 of Pediatric Emergencies and Common Disorders
Hepatitis B	Described in Section 13 of Pediatric Emergencies and Common Disorders
Hepatitis C	Described in Section 18 of Emerging and Re-emerging Acute Infections
Hepatitis D	Described in Section 18 of Emerging and Re-emerging Acute Infections

Fulminating Hepatitis

Etiology	Is an acute inflammation of liver, which may take a rapidly progressive course terminating in less than 2/52.
Pathogenesis	Extensive necrosis of liver leading to acute atrophic liver
Diagnosis	Nausea, vomiting, diarrhea
	Fever, rigor, malaise, loss of weight
	Pain abdomen in RUQ
	Jaundice – may be absent or minimal
	Coma
Investigation	LFT – show extreme hepatocellular damage.
Management	Corticosteroids – inconsistently effective
	Exchange transfusions.

Refer: The severe patient to the medical team.

Pylephlebitis (syn. Portal Pyemia)

Definition	Is an acute emergency that demands priority attention and treatment.
Etiology	• A suppurative disease in any drainage part of the portal system
	• A complication of appendicitis or diverticulitis
Pathogenesis	Thrombophlebitis of a vein draining infected lesion – spreading infection into liver – liver abscess.
Diagnosis	Fever, chills, malaise
	Nausea, vomiting, diarrhea
	Hepatomegaly, tenderness, rigidity
	Ascites, jaundice
Investigation	CBC – leukocytosis or leukopaenia, ESR – raised
	Serum electrolytes estimation
	LFT – Table 9.1 (Sample: Serum Method: Photometry and Calculated)
	Blood culture
	CT scan: Diagnostic in detecting SOL of liver (abscess, tumors, cysts)
	Liver biopsy (Percutaneous): Diagnostic in diffuse hepatic disorder

Management
General treatment

Maintain fluid and electrolyte balance

Nothing by mouth until acute symptoms have subsided

IV dextrose infusion

Blood transfusion

Antibiotics: BSA – tetracyclines

Specific treatment

Surgery: Laparotomy – to drain the abscess.

Refer: The patient to the medical and surgical team.

Liver Abscesses

Amebic Liver Abscess

Etiology	Is one of terminations of amebic hepatitis – a complication of amebic dysentery.
Predisposing factors	Alcohol abuse
Pathogenesis	Pathogen: *Entamoeba histolytica*
	Entamoeba histolytica from a focal lesion in colonic wall enters liver via portal vein, causing localized liquefaction necrosis, an abscess formed, liver enlarges, abscess encapsulated (remain dormant), or burst into right lung, peritoneal cavity, pleural cavity.
Complication	Bacterial infection
Diagnosis	Fever, chills, malaise
	Nausea, vomiting, diarrhea
	Pain abdomen RUQ, referred to right shoulder
	Hepatomegaly, tenderness, rigidity.

Investigation   CBC – leukocytosis or leukopaenia, ESR – raised

Serum electrolytes estimation

LFT – Table 9.1 (Sample : Serum   Method : Photometry & Calculated)

Stools: For *Entamoeba histolytica*

Chest X-ray

Plain X-ray abdomen

CT scan: Diagnostic in detecting SOL of liver (abscess, tumors, cysts)

Liver biopsy (percutaneous): Diagnostic in diffuse hepatic disorder

Management

General treatment

Maintain fluid and electrolyte balance

Nothing by mouth until acute symptoms have subsided

IV dextrose infusion

Blood transfusion

Antibiotics: Chloroquine 0.6 g od po for 2/7 followed by 0.3 g od 2/52

BSA – tetracycline 0.25 g qds

Emetine

Specific treatment

Surgery:

• Aspiration of the abscess

• Incision drainage of the abscess.

Refer: The patient to the medical and surgical team.

Pyogenic Liver Abscess

Definition   Single or multiple pyogenic abscesses form in the liver without any obvious cause.

Etiology   Mostly the cause is apparent, or may be ascertained:

Traumatic: Direct invasion from penetrating wound, empyema, subdiaphragmatic abscess, infectious process

By portal vein: Appendicular abscess, diverticulitis, ulcerative colitis, typhoid, actinomycosis of right iliac fossa

By bile ducts: Cholelithiasis (impacted), stricture bile duct

By hepatic artery: Pyemia, septicemia

By umbilicus: Umbilical vein of newborn, para-umbilical veins

Pathogenesis   Liver destruction proportionate to size of abscess, hepatomegaly

Diagnosis   Fever – steady or swinging, rigors occur occasionally.

Pain abdomen – localized to right hypochondrium or epigastrum, referred occasionally to right shoulder

Local tenderness – RUA, rigidity in acute cases

Nausea, vomiting, malaise, loss of weight

Hepatomegaly

Investigation   CBC – polymorphonuclear leukocytosis, ESR raised
Stools examination – for amebae
CXR – diaphragm elevated (right-side abscess)
Scanning liver – intra-hepatic disorders
D/d   Amebic abscess.
Management
General treatment

Maintain fluid and electrolyte balance
Nothing by mouth until acute symptoms have subsided
IV dextrose infusion
Blood transfusion
Antibiotics: Chloroquine 0.6 g od po for 2/7 followed by 0.3 g od 2/52
BSA – tetracycline 0.25 g qds.

Specific treatment

Surgery
* Aspiration of the abscess
* Incision drainage of the abscess–in case of failure to aspirate abscess.

Refer: The patient to the medical and surgical team.

Acute Intestinal Obstruction
Described in appropriate section of General Surgery Emergencies

Acute Appendicitis
Described in appropriate section of General Surgery Emergencies

Acute Cholecystitis
Described in appropriate section of General Surgery Emergencies

Acute Pancreatitis
Described in appropriate section of General Surgery Emergencies

Acute Peritonitis
Described in appropriate section of General Surgery Emergencies

Acute Diverticulitis
Described in appropriate section of General Surgery Emergencies

Acute Salpingitis
Described in appropriate section of General Surgery Emergencies

Acute Intussusception
Described in appropriate section of General Surgery Emergencies

Acute Renal Colic

Described in appropriate section of General Surgery Emergencies

Anal Abscess

Described in appropriate section of General Surgery Emergencies

Viral Hepatitis

Described in appropriate section of Pediatric Emergencies.

References

1. Midwinter A: Vomiting in pregnancy. Practitioner 206:743;1971.
2. Loening Baucke V: Chronic constipation in children. Gastroenterology 105:1557–64;1993.
3. Reynolds JC, et al: Chronic severe constipation. Gastroenterology 92:41;1987.
4. DrummB, et al: Peptic ulcer in children. Paediatrics 82:410–14;1968.
5. Steer ML, Silen W: Diagnostic procedures in gastrointestinal haemorrhage. N Engl J Med 309–646;1983.
6. Blacklow NR, Cukor GC: Viral gastroenteritis. N Engl J Med 304:397;1981.
7. Drossman DA et al: Psychosocial factors in the irritable bowel syndrome. Gastroenterology 95:701; 1988.
8. Goulston KJ: Clinical diagnosis of the irritable colon syndrome. MJ Australia 1:1122;1972.
9. Krejs GY, Fordtran JS: Diarrhoea in Gastrointestinal Disease. MH Sleisenger, JS Fordran (eds). Philadelphia, Saunders, chap 16;1983.
10. Levitt MD: Intestinal gas production. J Am Dietet A 60:487;1972.
11. Allen R, et al: Corrosive injuries of the stomach. Arch Surg 100:409;1970.
12. Harding Rains AJ et al (eds) Bailey and Love's Short Practice of Surgery. 13th ed, 1965.
13. Parks AG: Haemorrhoidectomy. Advances Surg 5:1;1971.
14. Jackman RJ: Anorectal fistulas: Current concepts. Dis Colon Rectum 11: 247;1968.
15. Alexander RM, Manheim SD: Anal fissures in infants and children. Am J Dis Child 96:29;1958.
16. Puri R: Hemostatic Clip in Gastrointestinal Bleeding. Family Medicine India. Vol.6 – No. 1. IMA College of General Practitioners, 2002.
17. Carbone JV et el: Gastrointestinal Tract and Liver. Current Medical Diagnosis and Treatment. Maruzen Asian ed., Tokyo,1975.
18. Das K: Clinical Methods in Surgery. 6th ed., Calcutta, 1962.

Endocrine and Metabolic Emergencies

Symptoms and signs (non-specific manifestations)
Emergencies:
- Diabetic coma
- Acute hypoglycemia
- Diabetic ketoacidosis

- Thyroid storm
- Myxedema coma
- Acute adrenal insufficiency
- Acute renal failure

Symptoms and Signs (common presenting complaints)

Obesity – in Cushing's syndrome
Growth – delayed (dwarfing) – in hypothyroidism or
  – excessive (gigantism) – pituitary or hypothalamic disorders
Weakness/wasting – especially in diabetes mellitus, thyrotoxicosis
Skin – abnormal pigmentation, e.g. hyperpigmentation/vitiligo
Hirsutism – one of chief presenting complaints of women
Appetite – anorexia – in Addison's disease or
  overeating – in thyrotoxicosis
Polyuria and polydipsia – in diabetes mellitus/or diabetes insipidus
Gynecomastia – in thyrotoxicosis, adrenal tumors, estrogen therapy
Precocious puberty – in hypothyroidism
Cryptorchidism – in hypogonadism
Mental retardation – in hyperthyroidism, Addison's disease
Tetany – in hypoparathyroidism

Diabetic Coma

Definition | It is a life-threatening emergency, characterized by absolute insulin deficiency.
Etiology | Diabetes related causes:

- Hypoglycemia – due to overdoses of hypoglycemic drugs
- Hyperglycemia – due to absolute insulin deficiency
- Lactic acidosis – due to accumulation of poisonous acetoacetic acid

Non-diabetes related causes:

- Traumatic – head injury, CVA, hemorrhagic shock
- Infective – CNS infections

- CVS disorders – MI, hypertension
- Renal failure
- Metabolic – intracranial tumors
- Alcohol abuse
- Drug toxicity.

Diagnosis   Nausea, vomiting, constipation
Headache, pain abdomen
Breathing – deep and sighing (air hunger). Breath – acetonic smell
Palpitation, sweating, tachycardia, anxiety, malaise
Loss of consciousness – due to dehydration and acidosis
Coma.

Investigation   Diabetes profile – CBC, glucose (fasting + PP), glycosylated HBa1C,
Total/HDL/LDL cholesterol, triglycerides, microalbumin, creatinine, uric acid
BUN
HCO_3
Urinalysis – glucose, microalbuminuria, acetone, magnesium
X-ray skull, CT scan of brain
EEG
Angiography
Lumbar puncture.

Management   It is a life-threatening emergency and top priority should be given to maintain life and an emergency treatment to be started immediately

Emergency treatment

- Admit the patient
- Airway maintenance
- Artificial ventilation
- Oxygen therapy
- Treatment of shock – if present
- Catheterize the patient
- IV fluids and electrolytes:
  - When blood sugar >500 mg/dL, give IV normal saline 0.45 sol @ 1 L/hr. Add $NaHCO_3$, 44 mEq/50 ml ampule to saline sol
  - When blood sugar falls to <250 mg/dL, give 5% glucose solution with insulin therapy (glucose prevents hypoglycemia and cerebral edema) Repeat every 2–4 hrs, till ketonuria cleared.
  - IV mannitol 0.5–1 g/kg @ 60 drops/mt, to reduce raised ICP
  - IV corticosteroids, to control brain edema
- Gastric intubation (Ryle's tube) and gastric lavage with the sodium bicarbonate solution.
- No sedation

- Monitor plasma glucose, serum electrolytes, sodium bicarbonate, urine glucose and ketones, input/output chart
- Insulin therapy: Regular (short acting) insulin initially IV or s.c.
  Dose: IV 50–100 IU and s.c. 50–100 IU, every 2–3 hrs.
  Doses depend upon responses of hyperglycemia and ketoacidemia $KHPO_4$, 40 mEq/hr: to combat potassium loss due to polyuria and vomiting >200 mEq. However, serum potassium is usually normal or high during first few hrs
- Antibiotics – to control infection
- Treatment of any associated complication, e.g.
- Acute hypoglycemia
- Acute cerebral edema
- Acute renal failure.

Refer: The severe patient to the medical team.

Prognosis Poor in elderly patients and in patients getting delayed treatment
Death may occur due to complications, e.g.
- Acute myocardial infarction
- Acute renal failure
- Acute cerebral edema.

Acute Hypoglycemia

Definition It is one of the most commonly encountered acute complications of diabetes.

Etiology Overdosage of insulin or oral hypoglycemic agents – attempted or homicidal suicide
Meal – fasting, missed, delayed or inadequate
Strenuous physical exercises, e.g. cycling, swimming, running especially after taking insulin
Pituitary insufficiency
Alcohol misuse
Drugs – salicylates, MAO inhibitors, NSAIDs, methotrexate, clofibrate prootentiate the action of hypoglycemic drugs
Hepatic failure.

Pathogenesis
- Accumulation of acetoacetic acid
- Acidemia
- Renal failure – circulatory failure

Diagnosis Headache, nausea, vomiting, constipation, pain abdomen, hunger, fatigue, cold sweat, trembling of hands
Breathing – deep and sighing (air hunger)
Palpitation, confusion, abnormal behavior, loss of consciousness
Convulsions, coma, death – may occur.

Investigation CBC
Serum C-peptide

Glucose – fasting + PP
Glycosylated HBA 1c
Cholesterol – Total/HDL/LDL
Triglycerides
Microalbumin
Serum electrolytes – Na, K, Cl
Creatinine
Uric acid
Urinalysis.

Management

Emergency measures

Hypoglycemia associated with unconsciousness or stupor (glucose < 2.2 mmol/L) should be treated on an emergency basis:

- Glucagon 0.5–1 mg (0.5-1 I.U.) IV, IM, or s.c.
  If the patient does not respond within 10–15 mts, the dose may be repeated or IV glucose – 25–50 ml of 50% of glucose solution over a period of 2–3 mts should be administered. Medical attention is required. When consciousness has been regained, oral carbohydrates should be ingested.

Prophylactic measures

- Diabetics should be advised to carry a diabetic patient identity card about themselves indicating their clinical history for the use of other in case of emergency, and they should carry some sugar or a few biscuits with them.
- Do not delay, skip, or reduce the food intake
- Take a snack containing carbohydrate, before exercise
- Avoid exercise during peak time period of insulin action
- Avoid alcohol
- Avoid sulphonylureas, if having hepatic or renal insufficiency.

Refer: The severe patient to the medical team.

Diabetic Ketoacidosis (DKA)

Etiology   Hyperglycemia.

Diagnosis   Polyuria, polydipsia, visual blurring, lethargy, weight loss, nausea, vomiting, deep breathing (Kussmaul's respiration)
Breath – fruity odor of acetone
Hypotension, tachycardia – due to dehydration and salt loss
Stupor, coma.

Investigation   Complete blood count
Diabetes profile – glucose (fasting + PP), glycosylated HBa1C, Total/HDL/LDL cholesterol, triglycerides,
Microalbumin, creatinine,

Uric acid

BUN

Serum electrolytes – Na, K, Cl, HCO_3

Urinalysis – glucose, microalbuminuria, acetone, magnesium

ECG

X-ray skull, brain scan.

Management

Emergency treatment

Monitor laboratory values in relation to therapeutic maneuvers

Catheterize (indwelling) the patient

Recording of fluid intake/output. Recording of medications

Gastric intubation and lavage with sodium bicarbonate solution

No sedation

Insulin therapy: Regular (short acting) insulin initially

IV 50–100 IU and s.c. 50–100 IU, every 2–3 hrs

$KHPO_4$, 40 mEq/hr

Antibiotics

IV normal saline 0.45% sol @ 1 L/hr

Add $NaHCO_3$, 44 mEq/50 ml

When blood glucose falls to < 250 mg/dL, then glucose 5% given and insulin therapy repeated every 2–4 hrs until ketonemia cleared.

Refer: The severe patient to the medical team.

Thyroid Storm It is a life-threatening form of thyrotoxicosis.

Etiology
Iodine refractoriness

Thyroidectomy

Stress

Adrenocortical insufficiency.

Diagnosis
Nausea, vomiting, diarrhea, dehydration, anorexia, fever, dyspnea, exophthalmos, stare, tremor, tachycardia, atrial fibrillation, CNS irritability and delirium, even death may occur.

Investigation
CBC, ESR

Thyroid panel – T3, T4, TsH

Serum electrolytes

Serum cholesterol

ECG: Tachycardia, P and T wave changes, atrial fibrillation

X-ray: Barium meal study

Ultrasound scanning

Bones densitometry – demineralization.

Management

Emergency measures

Admit the patient

Airway maintenance

Artificial ventilation, oxygen therapy

Iodine: Sodium iodide 1–2 g IV. Repeat 12 hrly

Antithyroid drugs (inhibit synthesis of thyroxine and tri-iodothyronine):

- Carbimazole 15–40 mg o.d. PO in divided doses
  C/I: Airway (tracheal) obstruction
- Propylthiouracil 600–900 mg o.d. PO Max: 1200 mg/day
  C/I: Pregnancy, lactation
- Sodium iodide 1–2 g IV. Rept. Every 12 hrs.
- Corticosteroids

Treatment of complications

General measures

Cold sponging

Sedatives.

Refer: The severe patient to the endocrinologist.

Myxedema Coma It is a life-threatening medical emergency with a high mortality rate.

Etiology		
Primary	Autoimmune	: Thyroiditis
	Iatrogenic	: Iodine treatment, thyroidectomy, irradiation of neck
	Drugs	: Iodine excess, lithium, antithyroid drugs, INF-alpha
	Iodine deficiency	
	Infiltrative	: Amyloidosis, sarcoidosis
Transient	Withdrawal of thyroxine in patients with intact thyroid	
Secondary	Hypopituitarism : Trauma, pituitary adenoma	
	TSH deficiency	
	Adrenals – hypofunctioning.	
Risk factors	Sepsis	
	Exposure to cold	
	Hypoventilation – causing hypoxia and hypercapnia	
	Pneumonia	
	CHF	
	CVA	
	Hypoglycemia	
	Hyponatremia.	
Diagnosis	Almost always occurs in the elderly	
	Level of consciousness – reduced	
	Seizures – sometimes	
	Hypothermia	
	Hypoxia and hypercapnia.	
Investigation	Complete blood count, ESR	
	Thyroid stimulating hormone (TSH)	

Thyroid peroxidase antibodies

Creatine phosphokinase

Total cholesterol, HDL, LDL, triglycerides

Serum electrolytes

ECG

Ultrasound scanning

Bones densitometry – demineralization.

Management   It is a life-threatening emergency, if treatment is withheld too long.

Emergency measures

Admit the patient

Airway maintenance

Artificial ventilation

Oxygen therapy

Drugs   Thyroid hormones:
- Sodium thyroxine IV bolus of 500 μg serves as loading dose Repeat 50–100 μg/day or
- Hydrocortisone 50 mg 6 hrly
- Antibiotics.

Refer: The severe patient to the medical (endocrinologist) team.

Acute Adrenal Insufficiency

It is an acute medical emergency and should be treated on priority basis.

Etiology   Traumatic – RSA, direct violence, hemorrhage

Infective – severe viral and bacterial especially meningococcal infection

Adrenalectomy

Sudden withdrawal of adrenocortical hormone, in patients receiving hormonal therapy

Stress, fasting

Pituitary gland disorders

Metabolic – carcinoma

Diagnosis   Nausea, vomiting, diarrhea, dehydration, headache, lethargy, confusion, high fever, pain abdomen, hypotension coma.

Investigation   CBC, TLC and DLC, blood glucose, serum sodium, potassium, BUN, blood culture, ECG.

Management

Emergency treatment

Admit the patient

Airway maintenance

Artificial ventilation

Oxygen therapy

IV fluids

Plasma transfusion

Hydrocortisone phosphate or succinate 100 mg IV. Rept. IV infusion of 50–100 mg every 6 hrly

Antibiotics

No sedatives.

Refer: The severe patient to the medical team.

Acute Renal Failure

It is an acute emergency and should be treated on priority basis.

Definition	It is defined as a series of syndromes (uremias) with abrupt impairment of renal functions, e.g. failure to excrete nitrogenous waste products, acidemia, raised serum potassium, and cellular dehydration.	
Etiology	Prerenal	Traumatic – RSA, crush injury, direct violence
		Hemorrhage
		Shock – traumatic, surgical, MI
		CHF
		Spinal anesthesia
		Burns
		Dehydration – vomiting, diarrhea, excessive sweating
	Intrinsic renal	Shock – hypotension >2 hrs.
		Acute pyelonephritis
		Infections – Gram-negative bacterial
		Drugs – nephrotoxic
		Toxins – arsenics, mercury, carbon tetrachloride
		Hemolysis – due to incompatible blood transfusion
		Abortion
	Postrenal	Calculus
		Acute glomerulonephritis.

Risk factors   Age > 65 yrs
Family history of renal diseases
Diabetics
Autoimmune diseases
Systemic infections
UTI
Urinary tract obstruction
Drugs – NSAID.

Diagnosis

Oliguric phase   Nausea, vomiting, anorexia, lethargy, dehydration, oliguria or anuria, hematuria, proteinuria, hypertension, shock

Diuretic phase   Urine volume – increases in increments of few mL to 100 mL/day, until 300–500 mL/day excreted (renal function returns slowly to normal)
Electrolytes – heavy loss of sodium and potassium

Obstructive phase (postrenal)

Renal colic, oliguria or anuria, headache, drowsiness,

Kidney – tendered and may be palpable.

Investigation   CBCt

Serum electrolytes – sodium, potassium and chloride

Serum creatinine, creatinine clearance

GFR < 60 mL/min/1.73 m²

BUN, uric acid

Urinalysis – sediment, proteinuria, albuminuria

CXR, ultrasonography.

Management

Emergency treatment

Catheterize the patient

Fluid and electrolytes:

- IV 5% dextrose with little or no potassium
- IV mannitol

Caution   **No electrolytes to be given until diuresis recommences.**

Management of life-threatening complications

Shock – if present, then treat accordingly as top priority

CHF – if present, then treat accordingly

Hemorrhage – blood transfusion

Hypertension – to be lowered gradually by:

- Nitroprusside IV infusion or
- Labetalol IV infusion
- Frusemide IV

Hyponatremia (due to fluid overloading) – treated by:

- Fluid restriction and hypertonic saline infusion

Hyperkalemia causing sudden death due to cardiac toxicity treated by:

- Calcium gluconate IV over period of 10 mts or
- Sodium bicarbonate sol. IV infusion over a period of 15 mts

Metabolic acidosis – treated by sodium bicarbonate

- Persistence of acidosis – needs dialysis

Mercury or arsenic poisoning – treated by antidote BAL

Infection – treated by antibiotics

Convulsions – if present, then give P/R paraldehyde or barbiturates:

- Pento/amobarbital sodium or chlorpromazine

Uremia – treated by dialysis, may be indicated in severe oliguric phase

Dialysis   To remove uremic toxins (endogenous and exogenous), transfiltration, and to maintain fluid, electrolyte and acid-base balance

Indications   CHF, pulmonary edema, severe acidosis, severe hyperkalemia, neurological disorders

Types   Hemodialysis and peritoneal (preferred in children).

Renal transplant

Indications   Best option for renal failure especially for dialysis patients.

General measures
                 Bed-rest
                 Diet – protein free, mineral free, strictly-limited fluid regimen
                 Glucose – IV or PO to combat ketosis
                 Monitor daily fluid input and output
                 Smoking – abstinence (stop)
                 Obesity – to be controlled.

Surgery   Removal of renal calculus (stone)

Indication   Post-renal anuria (calculus anuria).

Refer: The severe patient to the medical team.

References

1. Alberti K, et al: Small doses of intramuscular insulin in the treatment of diabetic "coma." Lancet 2:515;1973.
2. Swerdloff R: Atypical diabetic coma. California Med 119:29, Oct 1973.
3. Shah SN: Hypoglycaemia: Prevention, consequences and management. JIMA 100:166;2002.
4. Magnus Novo Nordisk Services: Management of Hypoglycaemia. Banglore.
5. Felig P: Diabetic ketoacidosis. New England J Med 290:1360;1974.
6. Ashkar FS, et al: Thyroid storm treatment with blood exchange and plasmapheresis. JAMA 214:1275; 1970.
7. Becker Ce: Coma in myxedema. California Med 110:61;1969.
8. Jain PK: Myxedema coma. Current Medical Journal of India 10:17;2005.
9. Frawley TF: Treatment of adrenal insufficiency states including Addison's disease. Mod Treat 3:1328; 1966.
10. Flamenbaum W: Pathophysiology of acute renal failure. Arch Int Med 131:911;1973.
11. Merrill JP: Kidney disease: Acute renal failure. Advances Int Med 10:127;1960.
12. Rains AJH, Capper WM: Anuria. Bailey & Love's Short Practice of Surgery, H.K..Lewis & Co. Ltd. London, 1108;1965.

Nervous System Emergencies

- Stupor and coma
- Syncope (fainting)
- Stroke (cerebrovascular accident)
- Seizures (epilepsy)

- Status epilepticus
- Parkinsonism (paralysis agitans)
- Narcolepsy
- Tension headache

Stupor and Coma

Definition	Stupor is defined as partial to almost complete loss of consciousness, whereas coma is defined as complete loss of consciousness (for a long time) from which the patient cannot be aroused, even by the most painful stimuli.
Etiology	Intra- or extracranial
Intracranial	Traumatic – head injuries
	Cerebrovascular accidents (CVA)
	Raised intracranial pressure (ICP) CNS infections
	Convulsive disorders (disturbed brain electrical activity) – epilepsy
	Reduced cerebral blood flow
	Neoplastic: Intracranial tumors
Extracranial	Traumatic: RSA, e.g. multiple injuries
Endocrinal	Diabetic ketoacidosis, hypoglycemia, uremia, hepatic coma, hypercapnia, hypercalcemia, hypothyroidism
	Cardiovascular: MI, hypotension, hemorrhage, shock
	Renal failure encephalopathy
	Osmolarity disorders: Hyponatremia
	Drugs misuse: Barbiturates, narcotics, tranquilizers
	Alcohol abuse
	Toxins: Endogenous toxins
	Physical agents exposure, e.g. hypo/hyperthermia, burns, electric shock Poisons, e.g. snake bite.
Diagnosis	Case history: Interrogate patient, his relatives, friends, to find out cause
	Physical examination: Signs of underlying cause.
Investigation	CBC, BUN, blood sugar

Serum electrolytes

Urine analysis

ECG

X-ray skull

CT scan of brain

MRI

Ultrasonography of abdomen

EEG

Angiography – cerebral

Lumbar puncture – CSF examination.

Level of consciousness – recorded by:

- Using Glasgow Coma Scale (GCS), i.e. by observing three types of responses – eye opening, verbal and motor responses to the commands of speech and pain. Maximum score is 15. Any reduction in the score is an indication of a loss in the unconscious level (Table 11.1). Alt:
- Using AVPU system, i.e. alert, responds or unresponsive to the commands of vocal and painful stimuli.

Management   Coma is a life-threatening emergency and top priority should be to maintain life until a precise diagnosis made and an appropriate treatment can be started.

Emergency treatment

Maintenance of airway

Artificial ventilation, oxygen therapy

Treatment of shock – if present

Catheterize the patient

IV access is established

Table 11.1 : Glasgow Coma Scale (GCS)		
Response to commands		*Score*
Eye opening	Spontaneously	4
	To speech	3
	To pain	2
	None	1
Verbal	Oriented	5
	Confused	4
	Inappropriate	3
	Incomprehensible	2
	None	1
Motor	Obeys commands	6
	Localises pain	5
	Withdraws (pain)	4
	Flexion (pain)	3
	Extension (pain)	2
	None	1

IV dextrose for hypoglycemia

IV naloxone for narcotic overdose

IV heparin for basilar thrombosis

IV sucrose 50–100 mL given slowly over 20 mts. for raised ICP or

IV urea 30% sterile sol in 10% invert sugar 1 g/kg @ 60 drops/mt

Indication – to reduce raised intracranial pressure (ICP)

IV corticosteroids – to control brain edema.

Refer: The patient to the neurosurgeon for management of the underlying cause.

Syncope (syn. Fainting)

Definition	Syncope is defined as a sudden transient loss of consciousness with associated loss of postural tone, whereas faintness is defined as impending loss of consciousness (presyncope), with lack of muscular strength.
Etiology	Reduced cerebral blood supply (transient interruption) – due to:

A. Vasovagal (vasodepressor) and neutrally mediated: Mid/post acts, e.g. sneezing, coughing, swallowing, defecation, micturition.

B. Sympathectomy – due to antihypertensives use

C. Orthostatic: Hypovolemia, diabetic ketoacidosis, alcohol, infection, drugs – antihypertensives, opiates, nitrates, and elderly patients

D. Carotid sinus syncope

E. Hypovolemia – GI tract hemorrhage

F. Cardiovascular disorders causing reduced cardiac output:
- Obstructive: Pulmonary stenosis, pulmonary embolism, pulmonary hypertension, aortic stenosis, mitral stenosis
- Myocardial: Acute myocardial infarction
- Pericardial: Cardiac tamponade
- Arrhythmic:
  - Bradyarrhythmias: AV block – 2nd and 3rd degree, Stokes-Adams syndrome, sinus bradycardia, carotid sinus, glossopharyngial neuralgia
  - Tachyarrhythmias: Supraventricular tachycardia, ventricular tachycardia and ventricular fibrillation

G. Cerebrovascular disorders, e.g. CVA, cerebral ischemia, anemia

H. Emotional disorders, e.g. anxiety, stress, fear, hysteria, sad news

I. Unexplained syncope – 50% of patients.

Pathogenesis	Impairment of brain metabolism due to hypotension with transient reduction of cerebral blood flow.
Diagnosis S/S	History taking and thorough physical examination – crucial to diagnosis. Nausea, yawning, anxious appearance, restlessness, palpitation, perspiration, face – pale, cold, moist, blurring of vision, epigastric distress, muscular weakness, hypotension, sudden loss of consciousness.
Investigation	CBC – to confirm anemia Serum electrolytes – to confirm disorders causing arrhythmias

ECG (12-lead) – to confirm CAD, MI, AV blocks

CXR – to confirm cardiomegaly, valvular heart disease

TMT – to confirm CAD

Holter monitor (24 hr.) – to confirm arrhythmia

Head-up tilt test – to confirm unexplained neurocardiogenic syncope

MRI, CT scan and EEG – to rule out any neurological cause.

Management

Preventive treatment

Aims	To prevent recurrences
	To prevent injuries due to fall
	To reduce risk of mortality
Measures	Tilt training

Emergency treatment

Position: Place the patient in the recumbent position (permits with head lower than rest of body, and the head turned to the side

Any tight clothing – to be loosened

Splash – water on the face

Subnormal temperature – to be covered with a blanket

Inhalation of aromatic spirits of ammonia

Treatment of underlying cause:

- Priority should be given to management of serious causes, e.g. MI, cardiac arrhythmias, and hemorrhage. Treatment of these inducing syncope is discussed in Chapter of Cardiovascular Disorders.
- Vasovagal syncope – to avoid emotional excitement
- Vasomotor: Ephedrine and phenobarbital
- Neurocardiogenic: β-blockers, fluorocortisone acetate, midodrine
- Aftercare: Observe the patient carefully – to save an elderly from fall.

Refer: The patient to the medical/neurological team.

Stroke (Cerebrovascular Accident)

Definition	It is defined as a focal neurological disorder due to a pathologic process (coronary hemorrhage/block). In majority of cases, the onset is abrupt with rapid evolution.
Etiology	Thrombosis
	Embolism
	Hemorrhage
	Hypertension
	Syncope.
Risk factors	Ageing
	High fat content in the blood, obesity
	Sedentary life – lifestyle changes
	Diabetes mellitus

	Smoking
	Alcohol abuse
Diagnosis	Sudden onset of signs and symptoms
	Hyperesthesia, impaired speech, headache, neck rigidity, fever, vomiting, momentary visual impairment, transient weakness of a limb, convulsions, coma.
Investigation	Lumbar puncture – CSF: Pressure raised, blood due to hemorrhage
	ECG – to rule out MI
	X-ray skull – may show aneurysm with calcification
	EEG – impaired
	Carotid angiography – to rule out aneurysm and carotid obstruction

Management

Preventive treatment: Prior to stroke/transient ischemic accident (TIA):

Antiplatelet treatment – routine use (prolonged) beneficial

Aspirin – safe and cheap, but less effective than anticoagulants

Dose: 75 mg/day or

Aspirin 75 mg/day + dipyridamole (safe and more effective but costly)

Anticoagulants: Reduce risk of stroke, but with risk of hemorrhage

Alternative to anticoagulants (contraindicated): Aspirin

Cholesterol reduction: For CHD patients

• Statins – may be beneficial to patients with history of CHD

Hypertension – to be controlled.

Emergency treatment

Admit the patient

Bedrest

Agitated – sedatives/tranquilizers

IV fluids

Catheterization – for nonvoiding

Lumbar puncture – with care in case of hemorrhage

Anticoagulation – for cerebral thrombosis.

Surgery	Carotid endarterectomy – beneficial in carotid stenosis
	Percutaneous transluminal angioplasty – role inadequate.

Refer: The patient to the neurosurgeon for management of the underlying cause.

Seizures (Epilepsy)

Definition	A brain seizure or convulsion is characterized by an abrupt onset of transient alterations in the cortical electrical discharge, manifested clinically by a change in level of consciousness or by a motor, sensory, psychic, or autonomic symptom.
Etiology	Organic brain disease
	Head injury
	Cerebrovascular accidents (CVA)

Brain infections
Hypoglycemia
Hypocalcemia
Uremia
Intoxications.

Types Partial or focal seizures:
- Simple partial seizure
- Complex partial (psychomotor) seizures
- Secondary generalized seizures

Primary generalized seizures:
- Grand mal (tonic-clonic) seizures
- Petit mal (Absence) seizures
- Febrile seizures
- Myoclonic seizure
- Atonic seizure

Status epilepticus (recurrent seizures with/without intervals).

Diagnosis Partial or focal seizures:

A. Simple partial seizure:
   Consciousness: Fully preserved during seizure
   Seizure: May be motor, sensory, autonomic or psychic in type
   Motor activity: Twitching of one part of the body
   Sensory symptoms: Paresthesia, vertigo, hallucinations
   Autonomic and psychic symptoms: Fear, anger, hallucinations
   Jacksonian seizures: Clonic convulsions in thumb/greater toe, mouth's
   corner, and may soon involve the whole side (generalized)
   EEG: Regular spike discharges with intervening irregular discharges

B. Complex partial (psychomotor) seizures:
   Consciousness – impaired, symptomology is complex
   Aura: Unusual sensation (smell of burning rubber, wood), abrupt
   emotional stress, illusions, hallucination
   Motor activity disturbances: Automatisms
   Amnesia: For events taking place during seizure
   EEG: Unilateral/bilateral spikes, sharp/slow waves discharges

C. Secondary generalized partial seizures:
   Consciousness: Loss of consciousness
   Motor activity: Convulsive
   Aura: Twitching, eye deviation, aphasia
   EEG: Shows presence of a postictal focal neurological deficit

Primary generalized seizures:

A. Grand mal (tonic-clonic seizure):
   Consciousness: Sudden loss of consciousness

Aura: A typical aura may herald a major seizure, e.g. spasm of a limb, turning of head and eyes, numbness, due to an irritating focus in the opposite prefrontal region.

Tonic phase: Contraction of respiratory muscles, followed by:

- Clonic convulsions of whole body
- Fall to the ground and emit a cry
- Frothing at the mouth
- Tongue bitting, bruises
- Loss of bladder and bowel control
- Pupils dilated, deep reflexes absent
- Dyspnea and cyanosis

EEG: Tonic phase: Shows low voltage fast activity

Clonic phase: Shows bursts of sharpe waves with slow waves during pauses

B. Petit mal (absence seizures):

Consciousness: Sudden, brief losses of consciousness, without loss of postural control. Seizures last for few seconds. Consciousness returns as suddenly as it was lost.

Motor activity: Without any convulsive motor activity

EEG: Shows brief 3-Hz spike and wave discharges

C. Febrile seizures:

Age – infancy and early childhood

S/S – convulsive movements with fever

EEG: Shows spasms and hypsarrhythmia

D. Myoclonic seizure:

Consciousness: Fully preserved during seizure

Motor activity: Convulsive movement – sudden and brief, involve part/whole body

EEG: Shows polyspike and wave discharges or sharp and slow waves

E. Atonic seizure:

Consciousness – briefly impaired and without any postictal confusion

Motor activity: Postural muscle tone – sudden and brief

EEG: Shows polyspikes and slow waves

Status epilepticus: Prolonged/repetitive seizures without a period of recovery between attacks – may occur with all forms of seizures, frequently of serious import. Comatosed patients apt to become exhausted, hyperthermic and may die.

EEG: Shows polyspike and wave discharges or sharp and slow waves.

Investigation	EEG
	Skull X-rays
	CSF analysis
	Blood glucose and calcium
	Brain scan.

Management	Aim of treatment is complete suppression of symptoms
	Avoid alcohol consumption
	Avoid hazardous occupations and driving
	Treat emotional factors
	Anticonvulsant measures
Drugs	Aims: To prevent seizures by maintaining an effective plasma concentration of anti-epileptic drugs
	Start with low dose and then increase gradually until control of seizures
	Abrupt withdrawal of antiepileptic should be avoided
Agents	Barbiturates:

Barbiturates:
- Phenobarbitone 30–120 mg o.d. PO in divided doses
  Indications: All types of seizures
- Others: Methyl-phenobarbitone

Benzodiazepines:
- Clonazepam 1–1.5 mg o.d. PO Maint: 4–8 mg/day
  Indications: All types of seizures, status epilepticus
  Ist drug of choice: Myoclonic seizure
- Carbamazepine 100–200 mg o.d. PO Max: 400 mg b.d./t.d.s.
  Indications: All types of seizures
  Ist drug of choice: Grand mal (tonic clonic) and partial (focal) seizures
  Others: Oxcarbazepine

Hydantoins:
- Phenytoin 150–300 mg o.d. Max: 300 mg
  Indication: Grand mal (tonic clonic) and partial (focal) seizures
  Ist drug of choice: Grand mal (tonic clonic) and partial (focal) seizures
- Diphenylhydantoin sod. (dilantin) 0.3–0.6 g:
  Indications: Grand mal/petit mal
- Others: Methoin
- Sodium valproate 600 mg o.d. PO Max: 2.5 g/day
  Indications: All types of seizures
Ist drug of choice: Myoclonic and petit mal seizures
- Other drugs:
  Acetazolamide (diamox) 1–3 g: Grand mal/petit mal
  Chlordiazepoxide (librium) 15–60 mg: All types of seizures
  Diazepam (valium) 8–30 mg: All types of seizures.

Status Epilepticus

It is a life-threatening disorder and requires priority treatment
Maintenance of airway, ventilation, oxygenation
Maintenance of temperature
IV dextrose

Drugs	Lorazepam 2–3 mg o.d in divided doses PO or IV Max: 10 mg
	Ist drug of choice
	Other drugs: Diazepam, clonazepam, followed by:
	Phenytoin. If not controlled, then give:
	Phenobarbitone 1 mg/kg/mt IV. If does not respond, then give:
	Paraldehyde 1–2 ml diluted in saline IV slowly + sodium pentothal.
Surgery	Corpus callosotomy – for tonic or atonic seizures
	Resection of parts of cortex, e.g. temporal lobe.

Parkinsonism (syn. Parkinson's Disease, Paralysis Agitans)

Definition	Defined as a chronic, slowly progressive disorder, characterized by involuntary tremors, rigidity and akinesia.
Pathogenesis	Degeneration of dopaminergic neurons in the nigro-striatal pathway, resulting in dopamine deficiency.
Etiology	Idiopathic – exact cause unknown in majority of cases
	Traumatic – head injury
	Inflammatory – complication of encephalitis, neurosyphilis
	Degenerative:

- Progressive supranuclear palsy
- Multiple system atrophy
- Cortical based ganglionic degeneration
- Diffuse Lewy body disease
- Parkinson dementia ALS complex
- Huntington's disease
- Wilson's disease

	Vascular – arteriosclerosis
	Poisoning – carbon monoxide, mercury, alcohol
	Drugs: Dopamine receptor blocking agents (antipsychotic), reserpine, methyldopa, lithium
	Metabolic: Parathyroid disorders
	Neoplastic: Brain tumor.
Diagnosis	Age – common in 50–60s. But may occur in youngsters also
	Speech – impairment
	Involuntary tremors – pill rolling movements of hands – max. at rest.
	As the disease advances, muscular tremors may affect the whole body
	Facial expression – fixed (mask-like) with eyes fixed and unblinking
	Rigidity of limb muscles (lead pipe) – upon passive motion
	Gait – slow, shuffling, festinating.

Management
General measures

Reassurance and psychologic support
Alcohol – moderate use to relax tension

Physiotherapy: Massage, stretching of muscles, active exercises

Medical treatment: Mainly symptomatic

Indications	Rigidity, spasms and akinesia (weakness)
Drugs	• Levodopa – drug of choice. It is a precursor of dopamine

  Dose: 250 mg t.d.s. PO; Max dose 4–8 gm
  S/E: Nausea, vomiting, anorexia, hypotension, cardiac and CNS disturbances, involuntary movements
  C/I: Psychosis, narrow angle glaucoma, pregnancy
• Amantadine: 100 mg o.d. PO. for 1st week. Max dose 100 mg b.d.
  S/E: Nausea, vomiting, dizziness, confusion, constipation, hypotension
  C/I: Convulsions, gastric ulceration, renal disease

Antimuscarinics (anticholinergics):
• Procyclidine: 2.5 mg t.d.s. PO; Max dose 30 mg o.d.
  S/E: Nausea, vomiting, headache
• Orphenadrine: 50 mg t.d.s. PO, increasing to four times daily
  S/E: Nausea, vomiting, confusion, agitation, insomnia
  C/I: Narrow angle glaucoma, prostatic enlargement
• Diphenhydramine
  Dose: 50 mg t.d.s.
  C/I: Drowsiness

Others	• Dopamine antagonists: Phenothiazines, metoclopramide and domperidone
	• Ergot derivatives: Bromocriptine, cabergoline and lisuride
	• Antimuscarinics (anticholinergics): Benzhexol, benztropine

Oculogyric crisis

Drug	Biperiden, cycrimine
	Dose: 1.25–5 mg t.d.s.

Surgical treatment: **Refer** the patient to surgical team for surgery

Indication: Selective cases – severe motor fluctuations and dyskinesia

Types of surgery

Methods	• Pallidotomy (globus pallidus) and thalamotomy (thalamus): A small area of brain is permanently destroyed by heating or freezing.
	• Deep brain stimulation (DBS) surgery – with probes: The same areas of the brain are temporarily made hypoactive by very high frequency stimulation, by electrodes placed in those areas connected to a pacemaker stimulator placed surgically under skin and subcutaneous tissue under the collar bone.

Narcolepsy

Definition	Defined as a clinical syndrome of unknown etiology characterized by excessive episodes of uncontrollable daytime sleep.
Etiology	Unknown
Risk factors	Brain (hypothalamus) damage – due to head injury, infection, or tumor
	Emotional (laughing, crying, overexcited)

Diagnosis	Recurrent daytime sleepiness
	Cataplexy – transient loss of muscle tone
	Sleep paralysis – inability to move between sleep and arousal
	Nocturnal awakenings
	Hypnagogic (hallucinations – visual, auditory, sensory) at onset of sleep
	Behavior – absent minded
	Sex – more in males.
Investigation	CSF examination – very low levels of hypocretin.
Management	

Scheduling of nocturnal sleep

> Instructions to patient – to maintain a scheduled bedtime/arising time. He/she may indulge in brief activities, e.g. reading, watching TV, eating, etc. followed by an attempt to sleep.

Scheduling of daytime sleep

> Naps – short and longer are advised. These are refreshing ones and are scheduled mostly during post-lunch hour and post-work (upon returning home).

Counseling	Narcolepsy patients do require special assistance/conseling at school, at working place.
Caution	Narcolepsy patients are at greater risk for motor vehicle accidents due to falling sleep at the wheel. They should be cautioned to avoid long drives and stop driving upon feeling sleepy. Cataplexy patients may better avoid driving till fully cured.
Drugs	Stimulants (antidepressants):

- Amphetamines (may cause mood and growth impairment):
  - Dextroamphetamine 5–10 mg t.d.s. Children: Not recommended
  - Methylphenidate 10–20 mg t.d.s. Children: Not recommended

Modafinil – non-amphetamine wake promoting agent

Dose: 100–400 mg/day in divided doses. Children: Not recommended

TCADs: Alleviate/eliminate cataplexy's symptoms

- Amitriptyline 10–25 mg t.d.s. PO. Max: 200 mg/day
- Imipramine 25–50 mg t.d.s. PO. Max: 200 mg/day

SSRIs: More tolerable than TCADs but comparatively less effective

- Fluoxetine 20–60 mg/day PO in divided doses
- Sertraline 50 mg/day PO

SNRIs (5-HT): Chemically unrelated to other SSRIs

- Venlafaxine 75 mg/day PO.

Tension Headache

Definition	Is the commonest of all types of headaches.
Etiology	Muscle spasm or contraction caused by disorders of the muscles of the forehead, scalp, occiput, or adjoining structures.

Predisposing factors	Traumatic: Head injury
	Inflammatory: Cervical spondylitis, cervical arthritis
	Infective: Otitis media, sinusitis, toothache, gingivitis, tonsillitis, PMS
	CVS: Hypertensive
	Metabolic: SOL
	Endocrinal: Diabetic ketoacidosis
	GI tract: Gastritis, abdominal distention
	Eyes: Eyestrain – prolonged use of eyes
	Emotional: Anxiety, anger, excitement, irritation
	Alcohol abuse
	Smoking
	Drugs abuse
	Postural: Stooping, straining, sexual intercourse
	Exertion: Overexertion, strenuous exercises, fatigue.
Pathogenesis	• Distention, traction, dilatation of intra/extracranial arteries
	• Traction, displacement of intracranial venous sinuses
	• Traction, compression of cranial and spinal nerves
	• Meningeal irritation
	• Raised ICP
	• Spasm – cranial and cervical muscles
Diagnosis	*Headache*
	• *Character:* Mostly dull, aching, occasionally burning or singing, or feeling of tightness, bursting or pressure
	• *Degree of incapacity:* Severe migraine attack incapacitate day's work, awakens from sleep during night or disturbs sleep
	• *Site:* Usually occipital and supraorbital, or variable in case of headache due to extracranial causes, many a times localization uninformative or misleading
	• *Duration:* Single, brief, momentary, or in migraine sets in morning/or daytime, peaks in an hour or so, lasts for hrs, in case of brain tumor may occur at any time – day/night, lasts for min to hrs. with increasing frequency.
	Nausea, vomiting
	LOC: Disturbed.
Investigation	CBC, ESR, blood sugar
	X-ray skull
	ECG
	EEG
D/d	Traumatic: Head injury
	Inflammatory: Cervical spondylitis, cervical arthritis

Infective: Otitis media, sinusitis, toothache, gingivitis, tonsillitis, PMS

CVS: Hypertensive

Metabolic: SOL

Endocrinal: Diabetes mellitus

GI tract: Gastritis, abdominal distention

Eyes: Eyestrain – prolonged use of eyes

Emotional: Anxiety, anger, stress, excitement, irritation

Alcohol abuse

Smoking

Drugs abuse

Postural: Stooping, straining, sexual intercourse

Exertion: Overexertion, strenuous exercises.

Management   General measures: Rest, relaxation, freedom from stress

Physiotherapy: Heating pads, warm bath, traction for cervical spondylitis

Drugs: Analgesics, muscle relaxants, barbiturates, tranquilizers.

References

1. Day SC, et al: Evaluation and outcome of emergency room patients with transient loss of consciousness. Am J Med 73:15;1982.
2. Kapoor WN, et al Diagnostic and prognostic implications of recurrencesin patients with syncope. Am J. Med 83:700;1987.
3. Silverstein MD, et al: Patients with syncope admitted to medical intensive care units. Jama 248: 1185;1982.
4. Sutherland JM, Eadie MJ: The Epilepsies, 3d ed. Edinburgh, Churchill Livingstone, 1980.
5. Weissler AM, Warren JV: Syncope and shock. In The Heart. 4th ed. JW Hurst, et al (eds) New York. McGraw-Hill, 1978, p 705.
6. Plum F, Posner J: The diagnosis of Stupor and coma. Davis, 1966. TD: The differential diagnosis of coma. New Engl J Med 290:1062;1974.
7. Browne TR, Poskanzer DC: Treatment of strokes. (2 parts) New Engl J Med 281:594,650;1969.
8. Martin WE and Others: Pakinson's disease. Neurology 23:783;1973.
9. Black JE, Brooks SN: Narcolepsy: Evolution and Management. CNS News, 200510.
10. Sandhu PS: Managing pediatric epilepsies and epilepsy syndromes. Current Medical Journal of India. 31–36: Vol XI No.6;2005.

Psychiatric Emergencies and Disorders

Psychiatric disorders:
- Classification

Psychiatric assessment (diagnosis):
- History (interrogation)
- Medical examination

Management
- Medical treatment
- Drugs
- Convulsive therapies (electroconvulsive therapy)
- Surgical treatment (leucotomy)
- Hospitalization of a psychiatric patient
- Psychological treatment

Neuroses:
- Anxiety neurosis
- Phobic neurosis
- Acute hysterical neurosis
- Anorexia nervosa
- Obsessive neurosis
- Acute depression
- Suicide
- Acute mania

Psychosis:
- Acute schizophrenia

Organic:
- Dementia
- Autism

Sexual and allied problems:
- Impotence (erectile dysfunction)
- Sterility
- Frigidity
- Sexual perversions

Menstrual disorders

Alcoholism and drug addiction:
- Alcoholism (syn. alcohol abuse)
- Acute alcoholism (intoxication)
- Chronic alcoholism
- Withdrawal symptoms
- Delirium tremens

Drug abuse
- Narcotics abuse, barbiturates abuse

Psychiatric Emergencies/Disorders

Definition   Defined as abnormal psychological states, in which the patients 'behavior or experiences are qualitatively or quantitatively beyond the range of socially accepted behavior and experience. During the last three decades, the psychiatric disorders have changed remarkably in quality, severity, and frequency.

Classification   Common psychiatric emergencies/disorders (Table 12.1).

Etiology   • Situational aberration: Adjustment reactions aberration
                    • Child: Rejection (unwanted child, illegitimate child, stepchild, handicapped child) accompanied by failure to attend to normal needs

of child, unfavorable comparisons, admission to child's disliking school, unnecessary scolding, overprotection
- Parents: Misinterpreted behavior, mismatched expectations, parenting style, coping mechanism
- Environment: Stress, support.

Table 12.1: Common psychiatric emergencies/disorders	
Disorder	*States (behavior/experiences)*
Transient situational	Adjustment reactions of infancy to late life, e.g. development maladjustments, transient feeding problems, disobedience, lying, stealing
Behavioral	Abnormal behavior, e.g. hyperkinetic reaction, runaway reaction, withdrawing reaction, overanxious reaction, group delinquent reaction
	Attention held easily or fleeting
	Disinterest in the surroundings
	Consciousness – conscious or confused
	Intelligence – intelligent or dull
Neurosis	Anxiety states, hysterical – conversion and dissociation, phobic neurosis, obsessive neurosis, reactive depression
Psychosis	Schizophrenia, manic depressive, paranoid, autism, catatonic – excited
Special symptoms	Speech disorders, sleep disorders, feeding disorders, learning disorders, enuresis, Tic, encopresis
Organic	Disordered functioning of personality, due to an organic diffuse involvement of the brain – infective (meningitis, encephalitis, syphilis) vitamin B complex deficiency, hypoxia, diabetic, myxedema, pregnancy depression, hyperemesis gravidarum, head injury, CVA, degenerative diseases (Alzheimer's disease, senile dementia, Huntington's chorea), alcoholic – intoxication,hallucinosis, delirium tremens, brain tumors
Personality	Antisocial, hysterical,paranoid, schyzotypal, schizoid, obsessive-compulsive
Sexual deviation	Homosexuality, pedophilia, fetishism, exhibitionism, sadism, etc.
Alcoholism	Addiction, excessive drinking – episodic and habitual
Drug abuse	Opium, pethidine, barbiturates, cocain, hashish, marijuana, halucinogens, psychostimulants
Social mal-adjustment	Marital discord, dejected love affair, occupational discord
Mental retardation	Mild, moderate, severe

Psychiatric assessment (diagnosis)

Diagnosis   Psychiatric diagnosis is based upon the history (interrogation) and examination.

History (interrogation) – should include:

Psychiatric (Mental) History

- Inquire from the patient – if he is co-operative, intelligent, fully alert
- Inquire from the parents – in case of a young child.
- Inquire from the relatives/friends – in case of patients suffering from any psychiatric or neurological disorders

Complaints	As per patient's point of view, e.g.

- Problems of bad habits
- Anxiety – source known or unknown
- Orientation – in time, space, and person
- Habit: Nail bitting, thumb sucking, enuresis
- Dietary: Food refusal, overeating, vomiting, anorexia
- Sleep: Insomnia, narcolepsy, cataplexy, nightmares, sleep walking
- Personality: Anger, fears, jealousy, shyness
- Antisocial: Lying, steating, cruelty, gangsters, terrorists
- Speech: Stammering, stuttering
- Sexual: Masturbation, hypersexuality, homosexuality, incest

Present illness	Date and factors responsible for onset of symptoms
	Aggravating and relieving factors
	Additional symptoms
Past illness	Illnesses, incapacity, hospitalization, disability, stress, fear, anger, medication
Family history	Disturbance in family, e.g. death in the family, separation of relatives, property disputes, illnesses, parents' divorce
Personal history	Anxiety, fear, stress, truancy, failure in examinations, illnesses, job dissatisfaction, unemployment, alcohol abuse, drug abuse, relationship to others.
Sexual history	Contacts with opposite sex, perverted sex, masturbation.

Psychiatric (Mental) Examination

The mental condition of the patient is assessed by:

- Observing his/her appearance and behavior
- Response to questions

Appearance and behavior:

Observe the patient's appearance and behavior while lying in bed, e.g. whether patient is disturbed, agitated, or feared.

Appearance	Neat and clean or unkempt
Behavior	Attention held easily or fleeting
	Showing any interest/disinterest in the surroundings
	Consciousness – conscious or confused
	Intelligence – intelligent or dull

Response to questions:

Reaction to inquirer – friendly or discourteous

Conversation – slower or faster.

Medical Examination

Should include complete physical examination, i.e. as for any other case and necessary investigations (Section 1: Case taking).

Investigations

Psychological evaluation: To assess intelligence, personality, feelings, differentiate psychic problems from organic ones.

Assessment   Objective: To assess qualitative evaluation versus standard norms

- Intelligence tests – to assess IQ:
  - Minnesota multiphasic personality inventory (MMPI) – to assess depression, hysterical, schizophrenic status
  - Aptitude and interest tests – to assess the environmental changes benefits
  - Subjective – to assess the conscious and unconscious attitudes judged from patient's responses
- Sentence completion – to assess the patient's skill
- Thematic appreciation – to assess the personal conflicts.

Neurologic evaluation

- EEG – useful in epilepsy, localization of cerebral tumors and other expanding intracranial lesions
- X-ray skull
- MRI
- CT scan
- Cerebral angiography – useful in localization of cerebral tumors and vascular lesions.

Management
- Medical treatment
- Psychological treatment
- Behavioral treatment.

Medical Treatment
Drugs
I. Sedatives, Tranquilizers, and Hypnotics:

A. Benzodiazepins:

Action: Sedative, hypnotic, tranquiliser, muscle relaxant

Indication: Anxiety with or without insomnia, alcohol withdrawal

C/I: Psychosis, phobia, glaucoma, respiratory depression

S/E: Drowsiness, confusion, vertigo, skin rashes, nausea

Drugs: Chlordiazepoxide   5–10 mg t.d.s. PO Max 50 mg

      Alprazolam   0.25–5 mg b.d.s./or t.d.s. PO

      Diazepam   5–30 mg o.d. in divided doses children 1–5 mg PO

      Lorazepam   2–3 mg/day in divided doses PO

      Nitrazepam   5–10 mg at bed time PO.

B. Barbiturates:

Action: CNS depression, mild sedation to anesthesia

Indications: Anxiety tension states (anxiety, mania, convulsions)

C/I: Hepatic and renal impairment, alcohol

S/E: Nausea, vomiting, diarrhea, pain abdomen, fatigue, tremor, polydipsia, ployuria, confusion, dizziness, rashes

Drugs: Phenobarbitone

Adult: 15–30 mg o.d. PO. Max 210 mg in divided doses

Children: 1–2 mg/kg body wt.

> Chlordiazepoxide and phenobarbital (long acting) along with chloral hydrate (short acting) provide a safe dosage schedule.

C. Phenothiazines:

Action: Antipsychotic and anxiolytic

Indication: Schizophrenia and anxiety tension conditions

C/I: Blood dyscrasias, hepatic malfunction, brain damage, coma, circulatory collapse

Side effects: Drowsiness, postural hypotension, arrhythmias, skin rash

Drugs: Chlorpromazine (largactil)

> Adult dose: 10–25 mg t.d.s. PO
>
> Children: > 5 yrs. Age – 1/3rd to ½ of adult dose
>
>   < 5 yrs. Age – 0.5 mg/kg body weight
>
> Alprazolam (alprax) 0.25–0.5 mg b.d.s. or t.d.s. PO
>
> Propranolol (betaspan, inderal) 80 mg o.d. Max 240 mg PO
>
> Trifluoperazine (trinicalm) 5–15 mg o.d. PO and 10 mg IM.

D. Butyrophenone:

Action: Sedative and tranquilising

Indication: Anxiety, psychoses, acute mania, acute schizophrenia

C/I: CNS depression, coma

S/E: Nausea, vomiting, drowsiness, skin reactions

Drugs: Haloperidol 2–3 mg/day PO.

II. Antidepressants:

A. Tricyclic Antidepressants (TCA)

Action: Antidepressant

Indications: Depression, mood disorders, e.g. guilt, helplessness, inferior complex, insomnia

C/I: Glaucoma, heart block, hepatic impairment

S/E: Nausea, vomiting, diarrhea, dryness of mouth, constipation, anorexia, weight loss, headache, agitation, phobia, enuresis, sexual dysfunction, glaucoma, postural hypotension, cardiac arrhythmias, coma, death

Drugs: Imipramine 25–75 mg t.d.s. PO. Max: 200 mg in divided doses

> Amitryptyline 10–25 mg t.d.s. PO. Max: 150 mg o.d.
>
> Lithium 600 mg o.d. PO Max
>
> Mirtazapine 15–45 mg o.d. PO.

B. Selective Serotonin Reuptake Inhibitors (SSRIs)

Action: Antidepressant

Indications: Depression, mood disorders, e.g. guilt, helplessness, inferior complex, insomnia

C/I: Glaucoma, heart block, hepatic impairment

S/E: Nausea, vomiting, diarrhea, dryness of mouth, constipation, anorexia, weight loss, headache, agitation, phobia, enuresis, sexual dysfunction, glaucoma, postural hypotension, cardiac arrhythmias, coma, death

Drugs: Fluoxetine HCl   20–80 mg o.d. PO

Sertraline HCl   50–200 mg o.d.day PO

Paroxetine HCl   20–50 mg o.d. PO

Fluvoxamine HCl 50–200 mg o.d. PO.

Convulsive Therapies: Electroconvulsive Therapy (ECT)

Mode of action Unknown.

Indications   Severely depressed patients, especially if they are suicidal.

It is administered 2–3 times a week and as per rules 6–12 sittings are required.

Premedication   Antiarrhythmic: Inj. atropine – to combat cardiac arrhythmias

Sedative and muscle relaxant: Barbiturate to combat violent effects of the fit.

Method   A seizure is produced by passing an electric current through the head (bitemporarily or unilaterally).

S/E   Confusion – some degree

Memory – becomes temporarily poor especially in elderly patients

Intellegence – some difficulty with intellectual tasks

Mania – rarely a patient becomes maniac during ECT

Fractures – may occur though very rare.

C/I   MI

CHF

Past history of subarachnoid hemorrhage.

Leukotomy

Leukotomy   In this procedure, the fibers connecting the frontal lobe to the thalamus are severed.

Indications   Chronic depressions not responding to adequate treatment within three years.

Complication   Frontal lobe syndrome development – causing loss of drive and disinhibition, which are likely to hinder the patient's return to work.

Hospitalization of a Psychiatric Patient

Admission   Acute cases: Admit to a psychiatric ward – full/part time.

Part time stay in the hospital, i.e. staying during the day, and going home at night or stays the night in the hospital while attending to work during day, or stay only for a few hrs/day.

Shelter homes: Provide homely atmosphere, e.g. foster homes for the children and cares for disabled and elderly patient.

Indications
- Unable to look after himself/herself
- Harmful to himself or others
- For diagnostic and observation purposes
- For special treatment, e.g. ECT, leukotomy, medical trials.

Disadvantages
- Demoralization, e.g. no self-confidence
- Stigma of being a psychiatric patient
- Cost factor, i.e. expensive treatment
- Segregation of psychiatric patient from other patients.

Solution (alternative)
- Period of hospitalization to be shortened
- Acceptable treatment
- Lessening of stigmatization
- Selective staff for psychiatric patient.

Psychological Treatment

Aim
These patients to be given the understanding of their abnormal behavior and helped (counseled) to recognize and to avoid stressful situations. There is hardly any evidence about group counseling being more effective than superficial psychotherapy.

Types of Counseling

1. Individual counseling: Means counseling provided by a psychotherapist (health professional) to a single patient, depending primarily on verbal talks to alleviate psychological complaints, encourage more adaptive behavior patterns and promote emotionally meaningful personal knowledge.

Short-term (Crisis) Counseling: Daily to weekly basis for a couple of weeks.

Indication
Stress.

Aims
Preventive and therapeutic – relief of symptoms and learning.

Mid-term (Eclectic) Counseling: Weekly basis for a couple of months.

Indication
Stress.

Aims
To support and encourage the defence mechanisms – the patient needs medications, frequently used in conjunction with the psychotherapy arrangements for family contacts to be made whenever necessary.

Long-term (Analytic) Counseling: Daily for a couple of years.

Indication
Unresolved conflicts.

Aims
To assist the patient in resolving his transference feelings and reach self-understanding.

2. Group Counseling: Means counseling provided by a psychotherapist to two or more patients utilizing verbal and non-verbal procedures to change complaints, especially those arising from maladaptive personal behavior styles.

Individuals Counseling: Means counseling amongst unrelated individuals, who can learn about their behavior by getting feedback from others, watching similar behavior in others, and thereby practicing new style of behavior.

Indication   Difficulty in establishing and maintaining relationships.

Couples counseling: Means counseling amongst two or more couples.

Indication   To recognize own's behavior by watching other's behavior.

Families counseling: Means counseling amongst two or more families, to interact with each other to examine and modify personal and family interaction styles which are thought to be the cause of complaints amongst members of the family.

Indication   To relieve complaints

               To help family members learn new methods to deal with stress.

Behavioral Treatment: Means educating the patient to acceptable behavior and his training with patience and understanding. The counseling involves co-ordination amongst patients/parents (in case of child), teachers and psychologist, in order to bring about change.

Aims   To forget about those destructive/unproductive types of behavior, resulting from faulty learning.

Methods   Imitation: Learning by imitation.

               Indication: Patients with low self-esteem.

               Rewarding/encouraging: Maintenance of behavior by eliciting rewards.

               Indication: The child learns soon that good behavior is rewarded.

               Aversion: To ward off/dislike/hate.

               Indication: Enuresis, alcoholism, homosexuality.

Neuroses

Definition   Defined as an emotional or mental disorder accompanied by obsessional (excessive anger, anxiety, jealousy, or a phobia – unreasoned fear or hatred) behavior, without any logic/reason.

Types   Anxiety neurosis

               Phobic neurosis

               Hysterical neurosis

               Anorexia nervosa

               Obsessive neurosis.

Anxiety Neurosis

Definition   Defined as a feeling of being worried about an event that may happen or may have happened and keep on thinking about it all the time. What may be trivial for one person may be overwhelming to another who is vulnerable in a certain way.

Etiology   Response to a threatening life situation, e.g. maladjusted attempt to resolve internal conflicts, i.e. unresolved, childhood problems, e.g. insecurity, dependency, hostility, need for affection, intimacy, depression, disturbed occupational, social or domestic environment.

Diagnosis	Anxiety, fear, tension, restlessness, palpitations, tremor of hands, breathlessness, dryness of the mouth, headache, dizziness, depression, perspiration, diarrhea, indigestion, fatigue, muscle cramps, hypertension, tachycardia, memory – disturbance, polyuria, sleep disturbances.
Management	
Psychologic	It is treatment of choice.
	Reality or transactional analysis – for personal relationship conflicts
	Individual group therapy – for family conflicts
Behavioral	Desensitization, by exposing the patient to the situation. Compulsions are treated by saturating the patient with anxiety/fear producing situation
Social	Family counseling
Drugs	Anxiolytics: Sedatives and tranquilizers:
	Benzodiazepins:
	Action: Anxiolytic, hypnosedative, muscle relaxant
	Indication: Anxiety disorders, tension states, muscle spasm

- Chlordiazepoxide: 5–10 mg t.d.s. PO Max 50 mg
- Alprazolam: 0.25–5 mg b.d.s./or t.d.s. PO
- Diazepam: 5–30 mg o.d. in divided doses. Children 1–5 mg PO
- Lorazepam: 2–3 mg/day in divided doses PO
- Nitrazepam: 5–10 mg at bedtime PO.

Beta-blockers:
- Propranolol: 40 mg t.d.s. Max: 80–160 mg/day

Other drugs: Oxprenolol, metoprolol.

Refer: The patient to the psychiatric team.

Phobic Neurosis

Definition	Defined as a strong unreasonable condition in which patient is usually anxious, but also have an abnormal fear of something (claustrophobia).
Etiology	Fear, apprehension, guilt.
Diagnosis	Anxiety
	Abnormal fear (claustrophobia):

- Fears of animals – fear of snake, dog, cat, lion, etc.
- Obsessive fears – fear of being infected, fear of school
- Hysterical fears – fear of being alone in house, fear of traveling alone.

Management	
Psychological	Supportive psychotherapy to help the patient find specific alternatives to harmful ways of dealing with his/her problems.
Behavioral	Best treated by family doctor preferably with the aid of a relative.
	Fear provoking situation is presented to the patient in small doses.
	Reassurance – to an upset patient.
Medical	
Drugs	Anxiolytics: Sedatives and tranquilizers:

- Chlordiazepoxide: 5–10 mg t.d.s. PO Max 50 mg

- Oxazepam: 10–15 mg t.d.s./or q.d.s.
- Haloperidol 2–3 mg o.d. PO.

Refer: The patient to the psychiatric team.

Acute Hysterical Neurosis

Etiology	It is a conditioning in which the patient suddenly feels very nervous, anxious, excited and is unable to control his/her emotions.
	Hysteria is not the same as malingering (consciously feigns illness) as the hysteric is unaware of the motivation of the symptom.
Diagnosis	Patient has a tendency to be indifferent to the queries and relates manifestation in a detached manner.
	Psychological conflict – being partly solved by the adoption of physical symptoms, without any organic base.
	Conversion symptoms:

- Physical: Thyrotoxicosis, hypoglycemia
- Psychological: Amnesia, pseudodementia, anxiety, abnormal behavior – difficulties with others, depression.

Management
Psychotherapy– Individual group therapy is helpful
Situational readjustment
Social measures
Avoid attacking conversion symptom

Medical   Anxiolytics: Sedatives and tranquilizers:

- Chlordiazepoxide: 5–10 mg t.d.s. PO Max 50 mg
- Diazepam 5–10 mg o.d. PO
- Oxazepam: 10–15 mg t.d.s./or q.d.s.
- Haloperidol 2–3 mg o.d. PO.

Refer: The patient to the psychiatric team.

Anorexia Nervosa

Definition	Defined as a mental disorder in which young women stop eating as they believe themselves fat and want to loose weight to be thin.
Etiology	Age – common in younger persons
	Dieting – for anxiety over weight gain
	Exercise – excessive
	Vomiting – self induced
	Abuse – of laxatives, appetite suppressants, diuretics
	Depression.
Diagnosis	Failure to eat – sometimes eat well, but in secret make themselves vomit
	Vomiting
	Depression – fear of gaining weight
	Hypotension
	Loss of weight, starvation to death.

Investigation   To check for hypoglycemia and hypokalemia
Management
Psychological: Psychological (encouraged) and physical (forced) measures are required
                  to prevent these patients from deliberately starving themselves to death
Medical   Admit the patient: For hypotension or hypokalemia
Drugs   Sedatives and tranquilisers:
                  • Chlordiazepoxide: 5–10 mg t.d.s. PO Max 50 mg
                  • Diazepam 5–10 mg o.d. PO
                  • Oxazepam: 10–15 mg t.d.s./or q.d.s.
                  • Haloperidol 2–3 mg o.d. PO.
                  Treatment of complications – metabolic, cardiac.
Refer: The patient to the psychiatric team.

Obsessive Neurosis

Definition   Defined as an extreme unhealthy interest in something or worry too much
                  about something, or repeat particular actions again and again (compulsion
                  to action from which patient cannot free himself/herself, although he/she
                  realizes that it is senseless, or at least that it is persisting and dominating
                  without cause.
Etiology   Anxiety, fear, tension, unhealthy interest, worry, compulsion.
Diagnosis   Obsessions: Constantly recurring thoughts, e.g. fear of hitting someone
                  Compulsions: Repetitive actions, e.g. need to re-check the things they
                  have already done, rituals of locking door and so on. Patient is forced to
                  do something against his will.
                  Depression.
Management
Psychological: Regular visits for discussion and reassurance
Medical   Admit the patient (serious condition): To be kept fully occupied
Drugs   Anxiolytics: Sedatives and tranquilizers:
                  • Chlordiazepoxide: 5–10 mg t.d.s. PO Max 50 mg
                  • Oxazepam: 10–15 mg t.d.s./or q.d.s.
                  • Haloperidol 2–3 mg PO.
                  Antidepressive drugs:
                  • Imipramine 75–300 mg o.d. PO.
Surgery   Leukotomy – indicated, if conservative treatment fails.
Refer: The patient to the psychiatric team.

Acute Depression

Definition   It is defined as a feeling of sadness, that makes one feels extremely unhappy
                  about a hopeless future, so that he/she cannot live a normal life.
Etiology   Primary depression due to endogenous events:
                  • Restlessness, feelings of guilt, loneliness and hopelessness, anorexia,
                    loss of weight and insomnia

Secondary depression due to:
- Organic brain syndromes, schizophrenia, drug reactions

Reactive depression due to exogenous events:
- Stress, anger, guilt, loss of a person, job or status, ignoring someone or something.

Diagnosis	According to diagnostic and statistical manual of psychiatric disorders (DSM), diagnosis of a major depressive disorder requires presence of at least 5 out of following 13 signs/symptoms present for 2/52:

- Presence of depressed/irritable mood nearly every day for most of the days – mild sadness to deep gloom
- Markedly diminished interest or pleasure in activities enjoyed earlier
- Anorexia
- Insomnia – loss of sleep or decreased/increased sleep
- Psychomotor agitation or retardation
- Lethargy – fatigue/loss of energy – getting easily fatigued
- Feelings of worthlessness, hopelessness or inappropriate guilt
- Lack of satisfaction
- Loss of libido
- Impaired concentration – loss of concentration or indecisiveness
- Loss of weight
- Recurrent thinking about contemplating suicide or death
- Reluctance to speak.

Management
Acute phase

Triage	Assess whether the patient can be managed as OPD patient or will require hospitalization
Treatment	Hospitalization – mandatory in case of expressed/assessed suicidal risk
	Work continuation – work will be therapeutic in mild depression
Drugs	Antidepressant drugs – indicated only in moderate to severe depression

- Choice of drug depends on age, sex, comorbid medical and psychiatric illness, symptoms, doctor's choice, and experience with drugs
- Patient's preference of drug and prior response to a given drug
- Onset of action, side effects, and cost decide the choice of drug for each particular case

Drugs: Antidepressants:

Selective serotonin reuptake inhibitors (SSRIs):
- Fluoxetine HCl 20–60 mg o.d. PO
- Sertraline HCl 50–200 mg o.d. PO
- Paroxetine HCl 20–50 mg o.d. PO
- Fluvoxamine maleate 50–300 mg o.d. PO Max 300 mg o.d.

Tricyclic antidepressants (TCAD):
- Imipramine (tofranil) 75–100 mg o.d. PO
- Desipramine (norpramin) 50–150 mg o.d.PO
- Amitryptyline (sarotena) 10–25 mg t.d.s. PO Max 150 mg o.d.

Serotonin noradrenaline reuptake inhibitors (SNRIs):
- Venlafaxine 25–150 mg o.d. in divided doses Max 375 mg
- Mirtazapine 15–45 mg o.d. PO Max 60 mg o.d.
- Lithium 300 mg t.d.s. PO along with major tranquilizer
- Haloperidol 10 mg o.d. PO and for emergency control 10–30 mg IM

Maintenance	6/12 from time of complete remission of symptoms, as chances of relapse are high during first 6/12 following remission of symptoms.

Convulsive therapies: Electroconvulsive therapy (ECT)

Mode of action: Unknown

Indications: Severely depressed patients, especially if they are suicidal

It is administered b.i.w. or t.i.w. and as per rules 6–12 sittings are required.

Refer: The patient to the psychiatrist for further treatment.

Suicide

Definition	A possible danger in depression and the psychiatrist should make a careful assessment of this risk, e.g. a broken home in childhood, a depressed parent with fears of harming his/her child. It is a psychiatric emergency and should be admitted to the hospital immediately.
Etiology	An intentional or voluntary determination to end one's life
	Willingness to die initiates within the person
	Presence of a known or hidden reason forces one to end one's life
	Alternatives, other choices/options – being not considered prior suicide.
Risk factors	Age: Suicide rates increase with age
	Sex: Male – more prone to commit suicide
	Marital status: Single, never married, divorcee or widowed
	Occupation: Unemployed
	Psychiatric patients
	Past history of suicidal attempt
	Scizophrenia
	Alcohol dependence
	Family: Unresponsive, isolated.
Diagnosis	Past history of suicidal attempt/attempts
	Suicidal thoughts, intent, plans
	Depression.
Management	
Preventive treatment	
	Identifying the problem in its various dimensions
	Understanding risk factors
	Developing interventions

Management of immediate crisis:

> Admit the patient
>
> Calm down the patient
>
> Reduce the immediate risk of suicide
>
> Enhance hope and confidence
>
> Improve effectiveness in tackling problems
>
> Family/friends support
>
> Arrange follow-up for patients at high suicide risk irrespective of whether they have a mental disorder; negative life events often precede suicide whether or not patients have a mental disorder.

Refer: The patient to the psychiatric team for:

> Treatment of specific psychiatric disorder
>
> Treatment of depression
>
> Treatment of schizophrenia
>
> Treatment of alcohol dependence.

Acute Mania

Definition
: It is defined as a very strong feeling for something/someone, and for that he behaves in a stupid or dangerous way. There may be brief periods of depression lasting for only few seconds. These patients are overactive, overtalkative and overcheerful. They start many projects but never manage to complete them.

Etiology
: Unknown

: Excitement, stress, depression, surgery or infection – aggravate mania.

Diagnosis
: Common in young adults

: Attacks are often recurrent, and last for a few weeks or a few months

: Flight of ideas – based on chance association include similar sounds

: Irritability, irresponsibility

: Elevated mood – marked cheerfulness to wild hilary, hallucinations

: Depression – very short period

: Exhaustion

: Intercurrent infection.

Investigation
: CBC

: Serum electrolytes

: Renal function tests.

Management
: Admit the patient

Drugs
: • Lithium is the drug of choice for the treatment of acute mania

: Dose: 300 mg t.d.s. PO along with major tranquilizer

: Monitor serum lithium level weekly at 0.8 mmol/L

: Discontinue lithium, if response not satisfactory within 2/52.

In view of neurotoxicity, lithium usually not reintroduced.
- Haloperidol 10 mg o.d. PO and for emergency control 10–30 mg IM
- Carbamazepine – started as a mood elevator after stopping lithium
Dose: 200 mg/day Max: 400 mg b.d./or t.d.s.

Refer: The patient to the psychiatric team.

Acute Schizophrenia

Definition	It is a serious mental disorder characterized by abnormal thinking, disturbed emotions, and disruption of communication links with others, unbased on real happenings around.
Etiology	Unknown.
Diagnosis	Agitation, unhappiness, frustration, disappointment, emotional imbalance:

- Thought disorder: Normal steady progress of thought may be interrupted and the train of thought then starts again on a new track.
- Formal thought disorder: Patient is able to form concepts and make generalizations but includes too much and his thought is illogical. Thus unusual combinations of ideas occur.
- Perceptual disorders: Presence of hallucinations (voices, visual, pain, touch, pressure and sexual sensations), which are perceptions without a relevant object in the external world.
- Emotional disorders: Depression, anxiety, elation, bewilderness. There is change of emotional expression.
- Motor and behavioral disorders: Experience of passivity in which the patient has the experience that his/her thoughts, actions or emotions are not his own, but they are forced upon him/her by some external power.

Management	
Medical	The acute phase is a medical emergency with high risk of morbidity and mortality, if left untreated.
Aims	Treatment should be realistic and oriented toward specific living problems Admit the patient
Drugs	Antipsychotics: Ist generation antipsychotics
Action	Alleviate agitation and psychotic symptoms
Benefits	Prompt management of the acute psychosis
S/E	Extrapyramidal side effects (EPS) – acute dystonia, sedation. Akathisia

A. Benzodiazepins:

Drugs: Anxiolytics: Sedatives and tranquilizers:
- Chlordiazepoxide: 5–10 mg t.d.s. PO Max 50 mg
- Oxazepam: 10–15 mg t.d.s./q.d.s. PO
- Diazepam 10–30 mg o.d. PO
- Lorazepam 2–3 mg o.d. IM
- Alprazolam 0.25–0.5 mg t.d.s. PO

B. Phenothiazines:

Action: Alleviate agitation and aggressiveness

Drugs: Chlorpromazine 10–25 mg t.d.s. PO or 25–50 mg IM

C. Butyrophenons:

Action: Alleviate agitation

Drugs: Haloperidol 5–10 mg o.d. PO

Emergency control 10 mg IM. Rpt every 4 hrs. until patient calms down

D. Tranquilizers

Action: Sedation – very effective:

- In controlling troublesome hallucinatory voices,
- In dumping down the drive behind persecutory delusions,
- In diminishing the severity of formal thought disorder and
- In allaying excitement.

Drugs: Phenobarbitone 30–120 mg/day in divided doses

Action: Sedation

2nd generation antipsychotics :

Action: Alleviate agitation and psychotic symptoms

Benefit: Use of these agents along with benzodiazepine – may show better efficacy and safety, than the 1st generation agents

S/E: EPS – fewer incidences

Drugs: Clozapine 12.5 mg o.d./b.d. Continue to increase by 50–100 mg o.d. over 2–3 wks. Max 900 mg/day in divided doses

Olanzapine 5–20 o.d. PO

Aripiprazole 10–15 mg o.d. PO Max 30 mg o.d.

Risperidone 2–6 mg o.d. PO Max 16 mg o.d.

Ziprasidone 40–160 mg o.d. PO

Trifluoperidol 0.5 mg o.d. PO Max: 8 mg o.d.

Shock therapy (ECT): Indicated where medical treatment fails.

Refer: The patient to the psychiatrist for further treatment.

Senile Dementia

Definition It is defined as a disorder affecting the brain and memory, and gradually the patient loses the ability to think and behave normally. It is the progressive dementing illness in which the histological findings are the same as those in Alzheimer's disease.

Etiology Traumatic – head injury

Infective

Metabolic

Vascular

Degenerative

Neoplastic – cerebral tumors.

Diagnosis	Age – disease of elderly, e.g. usually begins over the age of 70
	Sex – females > in males
	Intellectual ability – markedly declined
	Amnesia – memory loss
	Delusions – depressive/manic mood
	Depression – transient
	Anxiety, irritability
	Hallucinations
	Epileptic fits
	Death – due to infection or general vegetative decay.
Investigation	CBC
	Blood sugar
	Blood cholesterol
	Urine analysis
	X-ray skull
	EEG.
Management	Admit the patient
	No specific treatment
	Drugs: Phenothizines – initially small doses, increase slowly
	Treatment of the cause.

Refer: The patient to the psychiatric team.

Autism

Definition	A severe mental disorder that affects children and prevents them from communicating with other persons.
Etiology	Unknown.
Hypothesis	Neurological – injury to reticular formation of brainstem (intrauterine)
	Psychological – parental maltreatment of the child
	Genetic – common twins (inidentical and fraternal)
	Organic – neurological dysfunctions.
Diagnosis	Emotional deprivation
	Failure to develop normal relationship with others
	Failure to react to a situation
	Response to stimuli – unusual
	Speech – poorly developed/not developed at all.
Management	No drug to treat autism till date
	Try to contact and communicate with the child
	Provide a favorable atmosphere
	Physiotherapy:
	• Occupational therapy
	• Speech therapy.
Prognosis	Reserved
	Only few children grow up to lead self-supporting lives.

Alzheimer's Disease

Described in section of geriatric emergencies.

Sexual and Allied Problems

Impotence (Erectile Dysfunction): It is a major quality of life issue for an increasing healthy ageing population.

Definition	Impotence is defined as complete inability to perform sexual act to premature ejaculation, whereas erectile dysfunction (ED) is defined as inability to achieve or maintain an erection adequate for sexual satisfaction.
Prevalence	Common in men >40 years of age. Prevalence and severity increases with age.
Etiology	Psychological: Anxiety, shame, fear or failure
	Marital disharmony
	Organic disorders: Diabetes mellitus, endocrinal disorders, spinal cord disorders, disseminated sclerosis, hypertension, alcohol and drug abuse, malformations and deformities of penis and testis, e.g. absence of penis, hypospadias, absence of testicles, undescended testis
	Drugs: Antihypertensive, antidepressants, phenothizines.
Diagnosis	Erection – Primary ED: Never had an erection
	Secondary ED: Moderate or incomplete erection
	Ejaculation - premature
	Libido – lack of sexual drive
	Sexual satisfaction – decreased or absent.
Investigation	Blood sugar, urine analysis.
Management	Psychological treatment – reassurance and a sexual moratorium for 4/52.
	Premature ejaculation is less a disorder than a matter of the patient not having learned techniques to delay ejaculation
	Drugs:
	• Sildenafil 50 mg PO taken an hr. prior to sexual activity
	• Tadalafil 10–20 mg PO taken an hr. prior to sexual activity
	Treatment of the cause.

Medicolegal aspect: **Divorce** can be claimed/granted legally on the basis of impotence.

Sterility	Incapacity on the part of the male to impregnate and on the part of the female to conceive. Sterility and impotency may be present in the same person or may exist separately in male and female.
	Sterility mainly referred to females, while impotence to males.
Etiology	Psychological: Anxiety, fear, hysterical fits
	Malformation of genitalia: Absence of vagina, uterus, ovaries
	Diseases: Vaginitis, cervicitis, salpingitis, leukorrhea.
Management	Psychological treatment: Reassurance and a sexual moratorium.
	Treatment of the cause.

Frigidity	The early stages of intercourse are pleasurable, but the woman does not achieve an orgasm.
Etiology	In women is due to – Fears, marital disharmony, poor sexual technique, e.g. lack of arousal or clitoral stimulation by her partner. Dyspareunia Vaginismus.
Management	Psychological treatment: The couple should receive instructions in coital technique with a view to breaking down any prudery and inhibitions about sexual behavior which may be present. Treatment of the cause.

Refer: The patient to the psychiatric team.

Sexual Perversions

Definition	Perversions comprise deviations in the aim of sexual satisfaction, or in the selection of a sexual partner, that are considered as unnatural and unacceptable. As long as activities in sexual foreplay are intended as a prelude to vaginal intercourse, they cannot be presumed as perversions.
Etiology	Family discords Parental attitudes – behavioral problems, e.g. dominance, rejection, unrealistic expectations, overcriticism, discrimination, unfavorable comparison, etc. Early sex experience Environmental factors – school/college, prison Experience (+ve/–ve) – with same or opposite sex.

Types of Perversions

Homosexual	Sexually attracted to a person of the same sex. When a partner of the same sex is preferred (Gay – a man sexually attracted to other man; Lesbian – a woman sexually attracted to other woman). Homosexuality is relatively common these days, and social and legal attitudes toward homosexuality have markedly changed recently. But in general male homosexual's threat to boys, is not greater than male heterosexual's to girls.
Bisexuals	Sexually attracted to both male and female. Those having relationships with either sex, and frequently are homosexuals who have been denying his/her homosexual preference. Bisexuality often ends by establishing a sexual preference.
Trans-sexualism	Someone who wants to be or look like a person of the opposite sex. An attempt to deny and reverse the biological sex and to achieve an opposite sex identification. The trans-sexual male attempts to assume interests, dress, behavior of opposite sex.
Pedophilia	When a child is chosen/preferred as the sexual outlet.
Gerontophilia	When an elderly partner is chosen/preferred

Incestuous	Relationship between close relatives, e.g. between father and daughter, mother and son, brother and sister, due to marital discords or family problems and modern cultural influences.
Bestiality	Sexual intercourse with an animal – due to deprivation of other outlets and psychological disorders.
Necrophilia	Sexual intercourse with a dead body
Voyeurism	Sexual gratification by looking at a nude body or a sexual act
Extragenital intercourse	Anal or oral sex
Exibitionism	Sexual gratification by exposure of one's body or genitals to the opposite sex, e.g. indecent exposure versus striptease.
Transvestism	Someone who enjoys dressing like a person of the opposite sex. Sexual gratification (masturbation, orgasm) by wearing clothes, make up, of opposite sex
Sadomasochism	Sexual gratification by inflicting or experiencing pain. Death may occur in extreme acts.
Diagnosis	Sexual drive: Increased/decreased Sexual satisfaction: Deviations, e.g. decreased/absent Variations: In the choice of sexual partner, objects and practices.

Management

Medical

Drugs	Anxiolytics: Sedatives and tranquilizers:

- Chlordiazepoxide: 5–10 mg t.d.s. PO Max 50 mg
- Oxazepam: 10–15 mg t.d.s./q.d.s. PO
- Diazepam 10–30 mg o.d. PO
- Lorazepam 2–3 mg o.d. IM
- Alprazolam 0.25–0.5 mg t.d.s. PO

Treatment of underlying cause:
- Alcohol abuse, drugs abuse, impotency, frigidity, libido alteration, diabetes mellitus, neurological disorders.

Psychologic counseling

As long as activities in sexual foreplay are intended as a prelude to vaginal intercourse, they cannot be presumed as perversions.

Perversions are often multiple and resistant to the psychotherapy. If they are isolated perversions in a reasonably stable person, they may respond to behavior or aversion therapy. Psychological treatment is successful, provided the patient is co-operative, often not in majority of cases. It is often successful in exhibitionism, fetishism, voyeurism.

Pedophilia: Difficult to treat. The simplest way to prevent the subject from giving way to his perverse desires to seduce children is for him to take large doses of estrogen for the rest of his life. This will remove all sexual drive, both perverse and normal, which is not an excessive price to pay for liberty.

Homosexual: Individual/couple counseling, helpful

Marital conflicts: Couple counseling is treatment of choice

Behavioral counseling:

Usually disappointing in homosexuality

Voyeurism or fetishism: Modeling and role playing may be helpful

Frigidity: Couple therapy is treatment of choice – instructions regarding sexual activities (Masters and Johnson, and Kamasutra)

Aims   To alleviate anxiety due to past failures

Social counseling:

Homosexual: Family counseling is helpful.

Social conditions inhibiting sex (lack of privacy, work schedule, e.g. different shifts for both working partners, joint families)

Menstrual (Described in details in the chapter of obstetrics and gynecology)

Etiology   Psychological factors:

Amenorrhea   Due to psychological factors or a radical change in the mode of life, depressive illness.

Menorrhagia   Due to psychological stress, depressive illness

Dysmenorrhea   Due to neurotic traits (disorder of neurotic women).

Management   Reassurance to patient – patients to be firmly assured that they do not suffer from any serious physical or mental disorder.

Premenstrual tension syndrome:

May be severe in neurotic unstable patients.

Patient becomes anxious, depressed, irritable, emotionally labile, suspicious and sensitive.

Management   Reassurance to patient: Patients to be firmly assured that they do not suffer from any serious physical or mental disorder.

Drugs   Oral diuretics daily, starting few days before the psychological symptoms usually occur and to continue until the onset of menstruation.

If fails – then ethisterone 10 mg orally daily for the last 14 days of the menstrual cycle.

Alcoholism (syn. Alcohol Abuse)

Definition   An alcohol addict may be defined as one who has lost control over his drinking and has a compulsion to keep on drinking with resultant deterioration of emotional, social and work activities.

Etiology   Any social or cultural factor which leads to the rapid excessive consumption of alcohol will tend to cause alcohol addiction.

Reasonably stable persons who are exposed to an alcoholic environment may become addicted.

Some tense anxious individuals may begin drinking to allay anxiety and depression and then become addicts.

Psychological individuals may drink heavily as part of their generally disorganized behavior and finally become addicted to alcohol.

Diagnosis	Blackout – temporary loss of memory
	Loss of tolerance to alcohol
	Tremors
	Obsessive drinking – secret drinking
	Craving for alcohol – for that he will lie, steal, or cheat to get it.

Management
General measures

Admit to hospital – to dry him out

Diet – adequate

Vitamin B complex IV – to avert delirium tremens

Drugs	Chlorpromazine – for relief of withdrawal symptoms
	Prochlorperazine – for relaxation, sleep, nausea and vomiting
Aversion therapy	Disulfiram: Prevents breakdown of acetaldehyde, formed during metabolism of alcohol in the body.
	Dose: 1st day 0.75 g, 2nd day 0.5 g, 3rd day and 0.25 g subsequently.
	Sensitization: To alcohol develops after 2–3 hrs. Due to acetaldehyde poisoning (nausea, vomiting, dyspnea flushing of face, tachycardia.
	• Apomorphine: Patient is allowed to drink as much as he likes
Antidote	Apomorphine 2–8 mg is then given s.c. for 3/7, following that, the patient will vomit even at sight or smell of alcohol
	This helps him to stop drinking.
Psychotherapy	Patient is encouraged to find something to fill the gap.

Acute Alcoholism (Intoxication)

Alcohol intoxication is time limited, reversible and the onset depends on tolerance, amount ingested and absorbed.

Diagnosis	History of alcohol abuse
	Euphoria, disinhibition, mild co-ordination problems
	Confusion, impaired consciousness – may progress to anesthesia
	Mood lability, impaired judgment, sexual or aggressive impulses
	Speech – slurred
	Nystagmus, ataxia,
	Pupils – normal or dilated
	Respiration – slow and noisy
	Tachycardia
	Skin – cold and clamy, hypothermia
	Stupor, coma, death.
Investigation	GGT, MCV, and CDT markers levels: To detect excessive use of alcohol.
	Alcohol screening tests (Table 12.2)
	Alcohol use disorder identification test (AUDIT): Consists of 10 questions. A score of 8 or more is positive.

CAGE questionnaire: Consists of four questions. A score of 4 or more is positive. One positive test is suggestive of underlying disorders

Michigan alcohol screening test (MAST): Consists of 25 questions. A score of 5 or more is taken as positive.

Table 12.2: Alcohol screening tests

Test	Questions	Score	Interpretation
AUDIT	10	8 or >	+ve
CAGE	4	2 or >	+ve
MAST	25	5 or >	+ve

Management   Admit the patient

Dry him/her out – abstinence from alcohol

Patient should be kept warm

Artificial respiration with oxygen or CO_2 with oxygen – to control respiration depression.

Gastric lavage – with care to prevent pulmonary aspiration of the return flow

Analeptics – to hasten emergence from acute alcohol intoxication

Caffeine – as an antagonist to alcohol.

Given P/R or IM along with sodium benzoate (0.5 g)

Ephedrine or other stimulants, e.g. amphetamine

Hypertonic glucose sol IV to treat cerebral edema

Combined glucose and insulin therapy – have promising results

Careful nursing care – to prevent trauma and hypostatic pulmonary complications

When a person takes too many drinks: Symptoms depend on the amount of alcohol in the system, e.g. staggering gait, drowsiness, stupor, alcoholic blackout, coma, death.

Refer: The patient to the medical team for further treatment.

Chronic Alcoholism

Definition   Social drinking, leads to problem drinking, physical dependence (addiction), personality changes

Diagnosis   Loss of appetite, vitamin deficiency

Delirium tremens, convulsions, dementia, death.

Refer: The patient to the medical team for further treatment.

Withdrawal Symptoms

Anxiety, delirium tremens, e.g. confusion, tremor, visual hallucinations, seizures.

Management   Admit the patient – if the condition warrants

Sedative – as a substitute to overcome anxiety and depression

	Drugs: Diazepam 20 mg PO every 2 hrs till symptomless
	Psychotherapy – is the basic treatment. Group therapy – helpful
Drugs	Heavy doses of vitamin B complex given IV to avert delirium tremens.
	Chlorpromazine (largactil) and prochlorperazine (stemetil) are both very useful in the relief of alcohol withdrawal symptoms
	Chlordiazepoxide 50 mg q.d.s. Maint 25–50 mg every 1–2 hr.

Refer: The patient to the medical team for further treatment.

Delirium Tremens

	Defined as a syndrome commonly seen in chronic alcoholism and confined to heavy drinkers.
Etiology	Unknown – may occur without an apparent cause
	Traumatic: Head injury – subdural hemorrhage
	Infective
	Withdrawal of alcohol
	Metabolic disorders.
Diagnosis	Tremor – violent tremor affecting the mouth, hands, and the upper part of trunk
	Delirium
	Hallucinations – visual, auditory
	Disorientation, confusion, agitation
	Restlessness – marked
	Vomiting, dehydration, malnutrition
	Insomnia – complete
	Amnesia or dementia
	Seizures, coma, death.
Management	Admit the patient
Psychotherapy	To provide encouragement and reassurance.
Medical	Vitamin B complex IV – rapidly control the delirium.
	Chlordiazepoxide 100 mg IM
	Haloperidol 10 mg IM. Rpt every 4 hrs until patient calms down
	Chlorpromazine 10–25 mg t.d.s.

Refer: The patient to the medical team for further treatment.

Drug Abuse The drug addict is one who is psychologically or physically dependent on a drug. He intends to increase the dose, develops some tolerance of its toxic effect and has an overwhelming need to continue taking it. In certain cases, physical dependence and marked tolerance are the outstanding features, while in others the dependence appears to be more psychological than physical.

Triad of drug addiction:

- Psychological craving or dependence in procurement of the drug

- Physical dependence with withdrawal symptoms on stopping of drug
- Tolerance – need to increase the dose to obtain desired effects.

Addictive drugs • Narcotics:

Drugs: Morphine and opium alkaloids, e.g. morphine, codein, heroin

- Sedatives and hypnotics:

Drugs: Barbiturates, alcohol, bromide, paraldehyde, chloral hydrate

- Stimulants:

Drugs: Cocaine, amphetamines.

Diagnosis Gait – defective

Tremors

Headache, heaviness (clouding) of head, visual disturbances

Nausea, vomiting, diarrhea.

Investigation To induce withdrawal symptoms – by:

- Withdrawal of the drug
- Inj. morphine antagonist.

Management Admit the patient in acute cases

Abstinence from drugs

Sedatives – as substitute for alcohol to combat anxiety

Individual, group, and family counseling.

Narcotics Abuse

Narcotic causes relief from pain, stupor, sleep

Drugs Morphine and opium alkaloids, e.g. codein, heroin, pethidine

S/E Addiction or dependence – if repeatedly used and ultimately results into tolerance.

Pneumonia, infection, peripheral neuritis.

Diagnosis Confusion, stupor, euphoria, aggressive behavior

Speech – slurred, impaired

Miosis/mydriosis

Drowsiness, sleep, coma, death.

Withdrawal S/S Restlessness, irritability, dysphoria, bodyaches, anxiety, perspiration, lacrimation, flushes, nausea, vomiting, tachycardia, hypertension

Management

1. Overdosage Admit the patient

Give an antagonist, e.g.

- Naloxone 0.4 mg IV. Repeat after 10 mts.
- Clonidine 0.1–0.3 mg PO 3–4 times

IV fluids

Monitor the patient carefully

2. Withdrawal symptoms

> Admit the patient
>
> Naloxone as antagonist
>
> Methadone 10 mg PO or IM
>
> Psychotherapy, individual therapy, may be of some help.

Refer: The patient to a drug dependency clinic and his own GP, for seeking help to stop his habit.

Barbiturates Abuse

Affect both behavior and physiology. Addictions are observed with, e.g. phenobarbitone and chlordiazepoxide

Diagnosis	Drowsiness, loss of memory, sleep
	Impaired speech
	Respiratory depression
	Hypotension
	Nausea, vomiting, abdominal cramps, anorexia
	Tremors, seizures, hallucinations, depression, coma
MLD	10 mg/dL for long-acting barbiturates
	3 mg /dL for short-acting barbiturates.
Management	Admit the patient
	Drugs: As these drugs are cross-dependent, anyone of them may be used for treatment of detoxification.

• Phenobarbitone 200 mg PO. Repeat 4 hrly

> Family counseling.

Refer: The patient to a drug dependency clinic and his own GP, for seeking help to stop his habit.

Reference

1. Freedman AM, Kaplan HI: Comprehensive Textbook of Psychiatry. Williams and Wilkins, 2009.

2. Solomon P, Patch VD (editors): Handbook of Psychiatry, Lange, 2008.

3. A Short Guide to Mental Illness. May and Baker Pvt Ltd., Bombay, 1967.

4. An Experienced Teacher: Notes on Medical Jurisprudence and Toxicology Current Publishers Calcutta, 1965.

5. Vahia VN, Shah AB, Shah AA: Management of depression in primary care. JIMA 103:68–70;2005.

6. American Psychiatric Association – Diagnostic and Statistical Manual of Mental Disorders. 4th ed, Text Revision. Washington DC: American Psychiatric Association, 2000.

7. Trivedi JK, Srivastava RK, Tandon R: Suicide risk: Management. JIMA 103:78–84;2005.

8. Mann JJ: A current perspective of suicide and attempted suicide. Ann Int Med 136: 302–11;2002.

9. WHO–Report on Suicide Prevention: Emerging from Darkness. WHO, 2001.

10. Basu D, Singh J: Drug and Alcohol Abuse. JIMA 103:88–98;2005.

11. Schorling JB, Buchsbaum DG: Screening for alcohol and drug abuse. Med Clin North Am 81:845–65;1997.

12. Kissen B: Medical management of alcoholic patient. In: Kissen B, Begleiter H, (eds). Treatment and Rehabilitation of the Chronic Alcoholic. New York: Plenum Publishing Co, 1997.

13. Franklin CA: Modi's Medical Jurisprudence and Toxicology. 21st ed. Bombay: NM Tripathy Pvt Ltd, 531–3;1993.

Pediatric Emergencies and Common Disorders

Immunization schedule
- For pregnant woman and for children

Normal values
- Normal height and weight
- Normal teething progress
- Temperature
- Pulse
- Respiration

Drug dosage
- Children's drug dosage
- Calculation of child's dosage
- Normal laboratory values

Pediatric critical care
- Pediatric intensive care unit (PICU)
- Assessment of a seriously ill child
- Monitoring
- Pulse oximetry
- Pediatric cardiopulmonary resuscitation (PCPR)
- Pediatric basic life support (PBLS)
- Pediatric advanced life support (PALS)
- Adjuncts for airway and ventilation
- Resuscitation in trauma

Sudden infant death syndrome (SIDS) syn. Cot death

Congenital heart diseases
- Pulmonary stenosis
- Coarctation of aorta, aortic stenosis
- Atrial septal defect (ASD)
- Ventricular septal defect (VSD)
- Patent ductus arteriosus (PDA)
- Fallot's Tetralogy (FT)
- Pulmonary stenosis with reverse interarterial shunt
- Tricuspid atresia (TA)

- **Eisenmenger's syndrome (ES) (syn. pulmonary hypertension)**

Pediatric fevers
- Pyrexia of unknown origin (PUO)/fever of unknown origin (FUO)

Pediatric infections
- Viral infections
  - Chickenpox (varicella-zoster)
  - Pediatric acquired immune deficiency syndrome (PAIDS)
  - Chickenpox (varicella-zoster)
  - Measles (rubeola)
  - Mumps
  - German measles (rubella)
  - Acute encephalitis
  - Poliomyelitis
  - Viral hepatitis
    - Hepatitis A
    - Hepatitis B
    - Hepatitis C
  - Rabies (hydrophobia)
  - Dengue fever
- Bacterial infections:
  - Acute influenza (HiB disease)
  - Acute meningitis
  - Diphtheria
  - Pertusis (whooping cough)
  - Tetanus
  - Typhoid fever
  - Acute osteomyelitis
  - Acute septic arthritis
  - Tuberculosis in childhood
  - Acute pneumonias
  - Acute bronchitis

- Acute bronchiolitis
- Bronchiectasis
- Pleurisy
- Pleural effusion
- Empyema
- Lung abscess
- Protozoal infections

Acute (severe) malaria

Acute respiratory distress syndrome (ARDS)

Pediatric practical procedures:

- Injection (parenteral therapy)
  - Subcutaneous injection
  - Intradermal injection
  - Intramuscular
  - Intravenous (venous access)
  - Venipuncture
  - Intravenous infusion
  - Intravenous cannulation
  - Arterial puncture
  - Intraosseous infusion
  - Intraperitoneal infusion
- Bone marrow aspiration

- Bone marrow trephine biopsy
- Lumbar puncture
- Pericardiocentesis
- Liver biopsy
- Renal biopsy
- Fine needle aspiration study (FNAS)
- Gastric lavage
- Manual removal of foreign body from airway
  - Removal in an infant
  - Removal in a child older than 1 yr
  - Maneuver in conscious child
  - Maneuver in unconscious child
- Assisted ventilation
  - Types of ventilation
    - Manual ventilation
    - Bag and mask ventilation
    - Continuous positive airway pressure (CPAP)
    - Mechanical ventilation

New imaging techniques:

- Ultrasonography, CT scan, and MRI
- Nuclear medicine (radionuclide scintigraphy)

Immunization Schedule (Tables 13.1 and 13.2)

Table 13.1: Immunization schedule for pregnant woman	
Early in pregnancy	Tetanus toxoid (TT-1) injection
One month after TT– 1	TT–2 or booster (injection)

Table 13.2: Immunization schedule for children		
Age	Vaccine	Dose
Birth	BCG	Single dose
6/52	Oral polio	1st dose
	Tripple antigen (DPT)	
	(Diphtheria, Pertussis, Tetanus)	1st dose
	HiB vaccine (Hemophilus B)	1st dose
	Hepatitis B	1st dose
10/52	Oral polio	2nd dose
	Tripple antigen (DPT)	2nd dose
	HiB vaccine (Hemophilus B)	2nd dose
	Hepatitis B	2nd dose
14/52	Oral polio	3rd dose
	Tripple antigen	3rd dose

Contd...

Contd...

	HiB vaccine (Hemophilus B)	3rd dose
18/52	Oral polio	4th dose
24/52	Oral polio	5th dose
30/52	Hepatitis B	3rd dose
36/52	Measles	Single dose
12/12	Chickenpox vaccine	Single dose
	Hepatitis A	1st dose
Age	*Vaccine*	*Dose*
15/12	Measles, mumps, rubella (MMR)	Single dose
16–18/12	Oral polio	1st booster
	Tripple antigen (DPT)	1st booster
	HiB vaccine	Booster dose
	Hepatitis A	2nd dose
2 yrs	Typhoid vaccine	1st dose
5 yrs	Oral polio	2nd booster
	Tripple antigen (DPT)	2nd booster
	Typhoid vaccine	Repeat every 3 yrs
	Hepatitis B	Booster dose
10 yrs	Tetanus toxoid (TT)	Booster dose
16 yrs	Tetanus toxoid (TT)	Booster dose
		(Repeat in case of injury)

Caution:
1. Immunization is effective only when regular and complete dose is given
2. Avoid immunization if the child is ill. Although mild cough, cold, fever, diarrhea, are not contraindications for immunization
3. Information before immunization is to be provided about allergies, convulsions and drug reactions
4. Vaccines retain their potency and efficacy, if stored at requisite temperatures
5. Disposal syringes and needles of standard quality are to be used.

Normal Values (Tables 13.3 to 13.7)
Weight and Height: Up to the age of one year.

Table 13.3: Normal weight and height

Age	Weight in kg	Weight in lb	Height in cm	Height in in.
At birth	3.5–4.0	7.5–9.0	53	21
At 4/52	4.3–4.7	9.5–10.5	56	22
At 12/52	5.5–5.9	12–13	62	24
At 24/52	7.6–7.8	16.5–17	69	27
At 36/52	8.4–8.6	18.5–19	70	28
At 1/12	9.5–9.9	25.0–26	85	34

Teething

Table 13.4: Normal teething progress		
Teeth	*Upper*	*Lower*
Central incisors	6–8/12	5–7/12
Lateral incisors	8–11/12	7–10/12
Cuspids	16–20/12	16–20/12
First molars	10–16/12	10–16/12
Second molars	20–30/12	20–30/12

Respiration: Counted by watching the movements of the abdomen

Table 13.5: Respiration	
Age	*Rate per minute*
Newborn infants	40
2nd year	35
5th year	25
15 year	20
Ratio of respiration: Pulse	1:4

Pulse

Table 13.6: Pulse	
Age	*Rate per minute*
Newborn infants	140
Ist year	130
2nd year	115
3rd year	105
5th year	100
8th year	95
12th	80

After that gradually slows down to normal adult rate. During sleep, the pulse rate falls about 10–15 beats

Temperature

Table 13.7: Temperature

In young children, the temperature should be taken by placing the thermometer in

1. Rectum – a rectal thermometer to be used
2. Axilla
3. Groin

The rectal temperature is normally higher than the mouth or axillary temperature

Temperature conversion table: 9 Centigrade = 5 Fahrenheit – 160

Centigrade to Fahrenheit = Centigrade × 9/5 + 32 = F

Fahrenheit to Centigrade = Fahrenheit – 32 × 5/9 = C

Table 13.8: Normal hematology and blood chemistry values

Hematology	At birth	Child	Adult	Unit
Hemoglobin	16–18	15–16	14–16	g/dL
RBC count	3–7	1–2 or <	0.5–2	%
Eosinophil count	2–3	4–6	up to 6	%
Platelet count	0.2	0.15–2	0.15–0.5	m/cmm
ESR	15	10–15	0–10	mm/1st hr.
Bleeding time (BT)	1–3	2–5	2–7	min.
Clotting time (CT)	3–10	3–11	3–11	min.
Prothrombin time	10–15	12–20	12–25	sec.
Blood Chemistry				
Cholesterol	50–100	100–200	150–250	mg%
Glucose	60–100	70–120	80–159	mg/dL
Proteins total	4.5–7.0	6.4–7.5	5–7.0	g/dL
Albumin	2.5–5.0	3.7–5.0	4–5.5	g/dL

Children's (Drug) Dosage

Calculation of child's dosage: By one of following calculating rules/factors:

Body weight: The average dose of a drug is calculated on basis of dose of an adult male weighing 70 kg (155 lb).

Clark's rule:
$$\frac{\text{Weight in pounds} \times \text{Adult dose}}{150} = \text{Child's dose}$$

Age

Young's rule:
$$\frac{\text{Age in years} \times \text{Adult dose}}{\text{Age} + 12} = \text{Child's dose}$$

Bastedo's rule:
$$\frac{\text{Age in years} + 3 \times \text{Adult dose}}{30} = \text{Child's dose}$$

Cowling's rule:
$$\frac{\text{Age of child at next birthday} \times \text{Adult dose}}{24} = \text{Child's dose}$$

Sir Lauder Brunton:
$$\frac{\text{Age of child at next birthday} \times \text{Adult dose}}{25} = \text{Child's dose}$$

Scale of doses: Based on:

Body weight   : mg or g/kg of body weight
Body surface area : mg or g/sq.m. of body surface area
Age   : fraction of adult's dose (Table 13.9)

Table 13.9: Scale (age) of doses, the adult dose being represented as 1

Age (yrs)	Dose	Age (yrs)	Dose
< 1	1/12	< 7	1/6
< 2	1/8	< 12	1/2
< 3	1/6	< 18	2/3
<4	1/4	> 18	1

Pediatric Emergencies
Pediatric Critical Care
Pediatric Intensive Care Unit (PICU)

Pediatric intensive care unit (PICU) has got a vital role to play in improving the child survival. The aim is to provide special care of each disordered system to re-establish normal functioning and to prevent multiple system disorder. In the tertiary care hospitals especially with surgical units, 10–20% of total pediatric beds to be earmarked for PICU. The PICU team should include, dedicated physicians and nurses well trained in intensive care and well versed with resuscitation. Care of a child in PICU requires regular assessment and monitoring. Recording of all the monitoring on a pre-designed chart. The decision making in the PICU should proceed in the evaluation, intervention, re-evaluation. Attention should be paid to diet, sedation and analgesia, and control of infection. Also mandatory to communicate with the parents/attendants regularly and apprise them of child's condition.

Indications for pediatric intensive care:

A. Cardiopulmonary emergencies
- Shock
- Cardiac arrest
- Pulmonary edema
- Cardiac tamponade
- Arrhythmias
- Congestive heart failure
- Hypertensives crises (emergencies and urgencies)
- Respiratory failure – impending or established
- Pediatric respiratory distress syndrome
- Status asthmatics
- Artificial ventilation
- Cyanosis and hypoxia
- Acute pneumonia

B. Nervous system emergencies
- Coma
- Acute meningitis
- Status epilepticus
- Viral encephalitis
- Cerebral malaria

C. Endocrinal and metabolic emergencies
- Diabetic ketoacidosis
- Acute renal failure
- Impaired electrolytes – sodium, potassium, calcium, BUN

D. Emergency procedures
- Peritoneal dialysis
- Exchange transfusion

E. Miscellaneous

> Transfusion reactions
> Poisoning
> Gastrointestinal hemorrhage
> Acute abdomen
> Acute diarrhea
> Hepatic failure
> Electrical injuries.

Facilities to be Available in PICU

> Beds
> Resuscitation equipment
> Monitoring equipment for cardiopulmonary functions
> Ventilator with oxygen supply
> IV fluids and emergency medicines
> Support of well-equipped laboratory for:
> - Hemogram profile
> - BUN
> - Electrolytes estimation
> - Glucose estimation
> X-ray unit
> Ultrasonography
> ECG.

Assessment of a Seriously Ill Child

It is mandatory to recognize a sick child at the earliest, in order to improve chances of survival of seriously ill children, based on interrogation (history) and examination, e.g. proper case taking – including interrogation of child and parents, and examination. To begin with, ABC's are quickly assessed, e.g. airway patency, breathing, and circulation. Any abnormality in these requires life support /resuscitation on top priority basis. Followed up by recording of pulse rate, respiratory rate, temperature, examination of different systems, necessary investigations, and interventions performed.

Monitoring of Critically Ill Children Monitoring of critically ill children is an essential part of management.

Aims
1. Helpful in diagnosis and management by intermittent or continuous measurement of main physiological indices
2. Monitoring the important changes in the child's condition
3. Evaluation of criteria that would help in assessment of treatment and prognosis.

Monitoring Respiration, pulse, blood pressure, temperature, blood, urine, and monitoring of hepatic, renal, and hematologic parameters.

Respiratory Monitoring

Definition   Monitoring of rate and rhythm of respiration.

Pulse Oximetry

Definition   A non-invasive method of measuring oxygen (%) saturation of Hb

Technique   Based on Beer-Lambert law and ratio of oxyhemoglobin to the sum of total hemoglobin (reduced hemoglobin and oxyhemoglobin)

Estimation   By measuring absorption at wavelengths of 660 nm (red) and 940 nm (infrared).

Pulse (Hemodynamic) Monitoring

Definition   Monitoring of rate and rhythm of pulse

Technique   Pressure applied with thumb over forehead – resulting in blanching. Return of color, on pressure removal.

Estimation   By assessment of capillary filling time.

Blood Pressure Monitoring

Definition   Monitoring of blood pressure by:
- Manual sphygmomanometer or
- Invasive methods – by placing a catheter in an artery and thereby recording of BP
- Non-invasive methods – by Doppler manometers (continuous or intervals monitoring).

Urine Monitoring

Monitoring   of urine output.

of hepatic, renal, and hematologic parameters.

Pediatric Cardiopulmonary Resuscitation (PCPR)

Aims   i. To maintain organ viability during cardiac arrest

ii. To assist in return of spontaneous circulation.

Components   1. Pediatric basic life support (PBLS)

2. Pediatric advance life support (PALS).

Pediatric Basic Life Support (PBLS)

PBLS (backbone of effective resuscitation) is a cardiopulmonary resuscitation (CPR) protocol mandatory in cases of cardiopulmonary arrest, till advanced life support is instituted

PBLS   Follows the ABC approach. Assessment followed by action, e.g. management of airway, breathing, and circulation, in that order. This is only the initial rescue (first-aid) management. Failure to respond, then PALS (pediatric advanced life support).

Measures of PBLS: Place the child supine, on a hard surface. Extend the neck.
1. Airway maintenance: Clear the airway – from any obstruction, e.g. foreign body, saliva, vomitus.
2. Breathing:
   i. Spontaneous breathing – airway maintenance
   ii. No spontaneous breathing – rescue breathing must be provided and airway to be kept patent concurrently
   A. Mouth-to-mouth breathing – to be provided for as long as necessary
   Method: Place your mouth over child's mouth (+nose in infant)
   > Pinch the nose
   > Give 2–5 rescue breaths
   > Assessment – by chest rise
   Disadvantage: Risk of transmitting infection
   B. Bag and mask ventilation – to deliver adequate amount of tidal volume
   Method: Cover the child's mouth and nose with a mask
   > Extend the neck
   > Connect mask to oxygen source (@10 L/min)
   > This enables delivery of 90% oxygen
   Disadvantage: Distention (gastric) – relieved by nasogastric tube aspiration
3. Circulation: After the airway maintained and rescue breaths provided then determine the need for chest compressions (thrusts).
   > For that check the pulse – carotid (children) or brachial (infant)
   > If pulseless or heart rate <60/mt, then start chest compressions:
   > Place the heel of the hand over lower part of sternum
   > Press down firmly, so as to depress the sternum by 1–1.5 cm
   > Repeat very fast @ 90–120/mt

   Pulse   Good palpable pulse is a favorable sign for compression
   Pupils   Monitor pupils size, response to light (good response – an indicator of the adequacy of the massage)
4. Reassessment: External cardiac massage should always be accompanied by rescue breathing. Reassess the child after a mt.
   Reappearance of spontaneous breathing – stop the chest compression, while ventilation to continue, till return of adequate spontaneous breathing.

Pediatric Advanced Life Support (PALS)
PALS   Refers to assessment and support of pulmonary and circulatory function in the intervals before, during and after an arrest.
Components   • PBLS
              • Establishing and maintaining oxygenation, ventilation, and perfusion
              • Diagnosis and management of arrhythmias clinically and by ECG monitoring
              • Establishing and maintaining venous access – ideally central vein lines

- Diagnosis and treatment of reversible causes of arrest, e.g. hypoxia, hypothermia, hypovolemia, tamponade, tension pneumothorax
- Top priority treatment of cardiac and respiratory arrest
- Management of trauma, shock, respiratory failure, and other pre-arrest disorders.

Adjuncts for Airway and Ventilation

1. Oxygen therapy

Indications	Seriously ill children
	Respiratory insufficiency
	Shock
	Trauma
	After CPR to overtide ventilation perfusion mismatch
Method	Administration: By face masks, nasal cannula, pharyngeal/laryngeal mask, tracheal tubes with ventilation

2. Endotracheal intubation

Most effective and reliable method of ventilation

Objectives	Ensures airway patency, reduces dead space,
	Provides protection from gastric distention and aspiration,
	Allows tracheal suctioning and positive end-expiratory pressure
Indications	Airway obstruction
	Fatigue – due to exhaustive breathing
	Apnea – due to inadequate CNS control of ventilation
	CPR – for prolonged duration
Tube size	Depends on child's age, i.e.

Diameter (in mm): <1 yr 3.5–4.0

$$>1 \text{ yr} = \text{Age in yrs}/4 + 4$$

Length (in cm) : From angle of mouth

$$>2 \text{ yrs Age in years}/2 + 12$$

After intubation: Assess position of tube by ensuring symmetrical chest rise

3. Vascular access

Intravenous access: Accessible vein: Femoral, internal, and external jugular

Objectives	Provide more secure access to circulation
	Permit administration of drugs, e.g. vasopressors, calcium, sodium bicarbonate

4. Intraosseous access

Indications	Failure of vascular access to administer fluids, drugs, blood products
Sites	Proximal tibial bone marrow, distal femur, iliac spine

5. Fluid therapy

Objective	Early restoration of the circulating blood volume – to prevent – shock or cardiac arrest

| Fluids | Ringer's lactate or normal saline |
| | Blood transfusion – for hemorrhagic shock |

6. Drug therapy

Drug	Epinephrine IV/IO 0.01 mg/kg (0.1 mL of 1:10,000 sol)
Indication	Cardiac arrest – pulseless
	Bradycardia

| Drug | Lidocain 1 mg/kg IV/IO followed by infusion 20 µg/kg/mt IV/IO/ET |
| Indication | VF/VT |

| Drug | Amiodarone 5 mg/kg IV/IO |
| Indication | Pulseless VF/VT |

| Drug | Atropine 0.02 mg/kg |
| Indication | Bradyarrhythmias |

| Drug | Sodium bicarbonate 1 mEq/kg IV/IO slowly |
| Indication | Metabolic acidosis |

| Drug | Calcium gluconate 1 mL/kg IV/IO slowly |
| Indication | Hypocalcemia |

| Drug | Naloxone 0.1 mg/kg IV/IO/ET |
| Indication | Opioid intoxication |

7. Defibrillation: Defibrillation is the asynchronous depolarization of myocardium

Indication	Ventricular fibrillation (VF)
	Ventricular tachycardia (VT)
Method	One small paddle is placed over right side of upper chest and second paddle over the apex of heart (left of nipple)
Dose	2 Joules/kg If unsuccessful, a double dose is repeated
	Failure of 3 attempts – then repeat defibrillation after giving Epinephrine and CPR for 30–60 sec
	Failure of 4th attempt – give Amiodarone 5 mg/kg bolus Lidocain 1 mg/kg or Epinephrine – high dose followed by Defibrillation 4 J/kg within 30 sec

Simultaneous correction of hypoxia, acidosis and hypothermia is mandatory to improve outcome of defibrillation

| Prognosis | Depends on the etiological factor(s) |
| | However, increasing number of infants and children can be successfully resuscitated, if external cardiac massage is begun immediately on detection. |

Shock   **Described in appropriate section III of General Symptoms.**

Sudden Infant Death Syndrome (SIDS) syn. Cot Death

Definition	Sudden death in infancy with unknown cause.
Etiology	Unknown.
Risk factors	Airway obstruction
	Viral infection
	Winter season
	Smoking – passive (parental smoking)
	Drug abuse – by pregnant mothers
	Prone sleeping.
Prevention	Sleep – supine position
	Avoid passive smoking
	Avoid overheating.
Management	Until and unless signs of postmortem (rigidity/staining) appear, continue resuscitation measures
	Urgent call to consultants A&E and pediatrics
	Immediately following death, prepare yourself, and in presence of a senior staff nurse, inform the parents about the death in a dignified manner, and inform about the measures, e.g. postmortem.
	Involve a religious leader and a social worker to help the parents
	Inform the parents about police visiting them later that day
	Inform the GP to arrange for a home visit.

Congenital Heart Diseases

Definition	Is the commonest cause of congestive heart failure in infants, whereas in older children are the rheumatic fever and rheumatic heart disease.
	Congenital heart disease patients relatively have better myocardium (Keith)
Classification	*Without Shunt:*
	Right-sided: Pulmonary stenosis
	Left-sided: Aortic stenosis, coarctation of aorta
	With Shunt:
	Acyanotic:
	Atrial septal defect (ASD)
	Ventricular septal defect (VSD)
	Patent ductus arteriosus (PDA)
	Cyanotic:
	Fallot's Tetralogy (FT)
	Pulmonary stenosis with reverse interarterial shunt
	Tricuspid atresia (TA)
	Eisenmenger's syndrome (ES)
Pathogenesis	Stenosis of a valve/or vessel: Ventricular hypertrophy, heart failure.
	Shunt (left to right): Blood shunting from left atrium/or ventricle to the

right atrium/or ventricle, increased workload of right ventricle, increased pulmonary blood flow over systemic flow, exaggerated on exercise, causing pulmonary hypertension, shunt reversal (right to left).

Shunt (right to left): Blood shunting from right atrium/or ventricle into left atrium/or ventricle, aorta, bypassing pulmonary circulation, arterial unsaturation, low pulmonary blood flow.

Complications	Polycythemia, cerebral thrombosis, brain abscess, bacterial endocarditis
Diagnosis	• Stenosis: Manifestations of heart failure.
	• Shunt (left to right): Dyspnea on exertion, fatigue, pulmonary hypertension, hemoptysis
	• Shunt (right to left): Dyspnea on exertion, fatigue, cyanosis, clubbing, polycythemia, syncope, cerebral thrombosis.

Cardiac signs:
• Precordial bulge, substernal thrust, apical heave, thrills, bruits.
Murmurs: Functional (innocent) or structural (congenital)

Investigation	*CXR:* Cardiac size and shape, pulmonary vascularity, edema, skeletal anomalies
	ECG (13-lead): To assess anatomical and hemodynamic changes :
	P waves: Tall, spiked from right atrial hypertrophy (pulmonary stenosis), widened from left atrial hypertrophy (VSD, MS)
	ST segment: Depression and T wave inversion (LVH)
	QT interval: Prolonged (ventricular arrhythmias)
	Echocardiography (M-mode): To study anatomy and functioning of valves and septa.
	Doppler echocardiography: To study abnormalities of blood flow (shunts).
	MRI: Diagnostic and therapeutic values in congenital heart disease.
	Angiography: To identify and quantify shunts.
	Cardiac catheterization: Diagnostic value.
	Interventional catheterization: Therapeutic value (pulmonary stenosis, aortic stenosis, ASD, PDA).
D/d	Cyanosis with clubbing: Congenital pulmonary AV fistula, cor-pulmonale
	Cyanosis without clubbing: Peripheral venous stasis due to low cardiac output.

Pulmonary Stenosis

Definition	That to maintain the cardiac output in the presence of pulmonary stenosis, the right ventricular pressure has to rise considerably, above the level of systemic pressure in severe cases.
Etiology	Unknown
Pathogenesis	Increased resistance to outflow due to pulmonary stenosis, raises the right ventricular pressure, thereby limiting the pulmonary blood flow

Diagnosis	Mild stenosis (right ventricular – pulmonary artery gradient < 50 mm Hg)

* Asymptomatic

Moderate/severe stenosis (gradients > 80 mm Hg) causes:
* Dyspnea on exertion, fainting, chest pain
* Right ventricular failure: Edema, increased dyspnea, fatigue
* Palpable right ventricular heave
* Thrill: Left 2nd and 3rd ICS parasternally
* Murmur: 3rd and 4th ICS

Investigations	ECG: Peaked P waves, right axis or right ventricular hypertrophy

CXR and fluoroscopy: Mild to moderate cardiac enlargement, pulmonary artery dilated, pulmonary vascularity – normal/or diminished.

Angiography: Delineates anatomy of the lesion

Cardiac-catheterization: To estimate the gradient across pulmonary valve

Management: Surgical correction of the lesion.

Refer: The patient to the medical/pediatric team.

Coarctation of Aorta, Aortic Stenosis

Definition	Is defined as localized stricture of the aortic arch, at or near the insertion of ligamentum arteriosum (distal to the origin of left subclavian artery). To maintain the renal circulation, arterial pressure proximal to coarctation increases considerably, causing elongation of the ascending aorta, resulting in substernal arterial pulsation (diagnostic).
Etiology	Unknown
Hemodynamics	Arterial pressure proximal to coarctation increases considerably, causing elongation of the ascending aorta, resulting in substernal arterial pulsation (diagnostic).
	Cardinal feature of aortic valve stenosis is a systolic gradient across the aortic valve (systolic pressure difference between left ventricle and aorta). Narrowing of valvular area increases the gradient, the increased left ventricular systolic pressure leads to left ventricular hypertrophy, and low cardiac output. Left atrial pressure increases on exertion, leading to left ventricular failure and low cardiac output.
Complications	Triad of syncope on exertion, left ventricular failure, and angina pectoris
Diagnosis	Dyspnea on exertion, fatigue, palpitation, giddiness, weakness, syncope
	Pulsations: Arterial visible in the neck and suprasternal notch, femoral pulsations weak or absent as compared with brachial pulse. Collateral arteries visible or palpable in the ICS and along scapular borders.
	Chest: Localized heaving PMI, left of MCl
	Pulse: Small amplitude, sloping upstroke (plateau pulse), or tidal wave higher than percussion wave (anacrotic pulse)
	Respiratory rate: Normal in the absence of pulmonary congestion
	Left ventricular failure: Features present in acute, severe cases

Apical impulse: Less forceful, to left of MCL

Thrill: Systolic thrill over aortic area

ACD increased to left and down

Heart sounds: A2 normal or delayed and weak 3rd heart sound, atrial fibrillation.

Murmur: Systolic, ejection murmurs at the base

BP: Normal or systolic normal with high diastoiic

Investigations ECG: Left ventricular hypertrophy.

CXR: Scalloping of ribs due to enlarged collateral ICS arteries, left ventricular hypertrophy.

Angiography: Aortic, coronary and left ventricle – to evaluate degree of valvular regurgitation and valvular and coronary stenosis

Cath-lab: Right and left heart catheterization – to evaluate degree of valvular regurgitation and valvular and coronary stenosis

Echocardiography – to demonstrate impaired or absent valve motion

D/d Supravalvular obstruction

Management Medical treatment:

- Sedation
- Propranolol

Surgical treatment:

Indications: Progressive left ventricular failure, syncope from cerebral ischemia, angina pectoris due to low cardiac output of aortic stenosis.

Surgery:

- Myotomy and resection (limited) of hypertrophied muscle.
- Reconstruction: Valve replacement: prosthetic or homograft valve – procedure of choice in severe congenital stenosis.

Refer: The patient to the medical/pediatric team.

Atrial Septal Defect (ASD)

Definition Is defined as persistence of mid-septal, ostium secundum (most common) and/or low-septal ostium primum (rare), involving endocardial cushion.

Pathogenesis Blood flows through the defect, from left atrium into right (twice the systemic blood flow) atrium, increased right ventricular output and pulmonary blood flow.

Diagnosis Mild to moderate shunts: Asymptomatic.

Large shunts: Dyspnea on exertion, cardiac failure

Pulsations: Right ventricular visible and palpable

Pulse: Normal

Murmur: Loud systolic ejection murmur in 2nd and 3rd ICS parasternally. A functional tricuspid apical or xiphoid mid-diastolic murmur often present.

Heart sound: 2nd widely split, uninfluenced by respiration.

Investigations ECG: Incomplete or complete right bundle branch block, left superior axis deviation.

CXR: Enlarged right atrium and ventricle, large pulsating pulmonary arteries, increased pulmonary vascularity.

Cardiac catheterization: Reveals physiological information – to measure volume of shunted blood, intra-cardiac and pulmonary pressures, and pulmonary vascular resistance.

Angiocardiography: Reveals precise anatomical information.   :

Management Mild to moderate shunts: No surgical treatment required.

Large shunts: Surgery indicated.

Refer: The patient to the medical/pediatric team.

Ventricular Septal Defect (VSD)

Definition Is defined as a lesion characterized by persistent opening in the upper interventricular septum due to failure of fusion with the aortic septum, resulting in shunting of blood from high pressured left ventricle into low pressured right ventricle.

Pathogenesis Blood flows through the defect, from high pressured left ventricle into low pressured right ventricle, pressures equalize in the ventricles in large ventricular septal defects, shunt depending on relative pulmonary and systemic vascular resistance, causing right and left ventricular strains.

Diagnosis S/S: Depend upon size of the lesion and presence/or absence of raised pulmonary vascular resistance:

Mild to moderate shunt: Asymptomatic.

Large shunts: Dyspnea on exertion, cardiac failure

Pulsations: Right ventricular heave palpable

Pulse: Normal

Murmur: Loud systolic ejection murmur in left 3rd and 4th ICS parasternally.

A mid-diastolic flow murmur often present.

Heart sound: An apical 3rd heart sound often present.

Investigations ECG: Normal/or right, left, or bi-ventricular hypertrophy as per size of lesion and pulmonary vascular resistance.

CXR: Enlarged right and left ventricles, left atrium, and pulmonary arteries, and increased pulmonary vascularity.

Cardiac catheterization: Reveals physiological information – to measure volume of shunted blood, intra-cardiac and pulmonary pressures, and pulmonary vascular resistance.

Angiocardiography: Reveals precise anatomical information.

Management Mild to moderate shunts: No surgical treatment required.

Large shunts: Surgery (closure of lesion) indicated.

C/I: Pulmonary vascular resistance > one-third of systemic vascular resistance.

Refer: The patient to the medical/pediatric team.

Patent Ductus Arteriosus (PDA)

Definition	Is defined as ductus arteriosus failure to close and persisting as a shunt connecting left pulmonary artery and aorta, near origin of left subclavian artery.
Pathogenesis	Blood flows through the lesion, from left aorta into pulmonary artery, in systole and diastole, increased workload of left ventricle. In right to left or bi-directional shunt, obstructive pulmonary vessels, cause pulmonary hypertension.
Diagnosis	Mild to moderate shunts: Asymptomatic.
	Large shunts: Dyspnea on exertion, cardiac failure
	Pulsations: Right ventricular visible and palpable
	Pulse pressure: Wide
	Murmur: Continuous, rough machinery murmur in left 1st and 2nd ICS Parasternally
	Heart sound: 2nd widely split, uninfluenced by respiration.
Investigations	ECG: Normal/or left ventricular failure.
	CXR: Enlarged left atrium and ventricle, prominent pulmonary artery, aorta, and left atrium.
	Cardiac catheterization: Left-to-right shunt.
	Angiocardiography: Reveals precise anatomical information. :
Management	Mild to moderate shunts: No surgical treatment required.
	Large shunts: Surgery (division and closure) indicated in children and adults.

Refer: The patient to the medical/pediatric team.

Fallot's Tetralogy (FT)

Definition	Is defined as a syndrome consisting of pulmonary stenosis, VSD, right ventricular enlargement, and overriding aorta, i.e. aorta arising astride VSD, causing blood entering it both from right and left ventricles.
Pathogenesis	Pulmonary stenosis and a large VSD cause equalization of pressure in both ventricles, right ventricular blood entering partly into pulmonary trunk (artery) through pulmonary stenosis, and partly through VSD, into aorta, admixture of de-oxygenated blood with left ventricular's oxygenated blood, causing cyanosis and clubbing of fingers
Diagnosis	Dyspnea: Relieved by squatting, fatigue, syncope
	Cyanosis and clubbing of fingers
	Heave: Right ventricular
	Murmur: Harsh, systolic, left-parasternal
	Heart sound: Loud 2nd sound
Investigations	ECG: Prominent P-waves
	CXR: Boot-shaped heart (concave pulmonary artery segment) :
	Cardiac catheterization: Establish diagnosis
	Angiocardiography: Reveals precise anatomical information.

Management	Surgical: Using extracorporeal circulation.
	Blalock type shunt oxygen therapy – for severe cyanosis.
	Propranolol: For syncope.

Refer: The patient to the medical/pediatric team.

Pulmonary Stenosis with Reverse Interarterial Shunt

Definition	Is defined as pulmonary stenosis with atrial septal lesion, causing reversed interarterial shunt (venous blood passing from right atrium into left atrium through atrial septal lesion).
Pathogenesis	Elevated right ventricular pressure causes right ventricular hypertrophy and decreased distensibility, venous blood passing from right atrium into left atrium through atrial septal lesion, resulting in arterial unsaturation, causing cyanosis.
Diagnosis	Dyspnea on exertion, fatigue
	Cyanosis, clubbing of fingers, polycythemia
	Pulsation: Right pulmonary artery pulsation and heave
	Murmur: Long, harsh, pulmonic systolic, thrill
Investigations	ECG: Prominent P-waves, right ventricular hypertrophy
	CXR: Heart enlargement, dilated pulmonary artery, decreased pulmonary vascularity.
	Cardiac catheterization: Establish diagnosis
	Angiocardiography: Reveals precise anatomical information.
Management	Surgical: Correction of pulmonary stenosis and ASD.
	Blalock type shunt oxygen therapy – for severe cyanosis.

Refer: The patient to the medical/pediatric team.

Tricuspid Atresia (TA)

Definition	It is defined as narrowing of tricuspid valve, that may occur as an isolated defect, with pulmonary artery narrowing, along with ASD, or with VSD or patent ductus arteriosus.
Hemodynamics	Blood from right atrium shunting into left atrium, reaches lungs, via VSD into right ventricle, or shunting from aorta into pulmonary circulation through patent ductus (rudimentary right ventricle and pulmonary artery).
Complications	Hepatomegaly, cardiac cirrhosis, right heart failure.
Diagnosis	Hepatomegaly, ascitis, edema, jaundice
	Pulse pressure: Wide, resting pulse rate increased to maintain cardiac output
	Respiratory rate: Normal in the absence of pulmonary congestion
	Giant alpha wave in jugular pulse with sinus rhythm
	Thrill: Mid-diastolic thrill between left sternal border and PMI
	Heart sounds: M1 often loud
	Murmur: Loudest over 3rd–5th ICS, transmitted to apex
	BP: Normal.

Investigations	ECG: Left axis deviation or left ventricular hypertrophy wave (water-hammer, collapsing, or Corrigan pulse) deviation or left ventricular hypertrophy
	CXR: Showing enlarged left atrium and left ventricle
	Cardiac catheterization: Diagnostic
	Angiography: Diagnostic.
Management	Surgical treatment: Blalock (anastomosis of subclavian and pulmonary arteries) – procedure of choice.
Prognosis	Poor–hardly reach adulthood.

Refer: The patient to the medical/pediatric team.

Eisenmenger's Syndrome (ES) (syn. Pulmonary Hypertension)

Definition	Is defined as a syndrome of many congenital cardiac lesions, whereby the status of the pulmonary vascular bed is often the principal determinant of the clinical manifestations, course, and the feasibility of surgery. There occurs a large communication between the systemic and pulmonary circulation at the aorto-pulmonary, ventricular, or atrial levels, with predominantly right-to-left shunts, due to high resistance and obstructive pulmonary hypertension.
Etiology	Unknown: Majority of cases, may be present from birth.
Predisposing factors	Accompaniment of many congenital cardiac lesions – right ventricular hypertrophy.
Pathogenesis	Obstructive/obliterative structural changes: In pulmonary vascular bed increased pulmonary blood flow and/or increased resistance, increased pulmonary arterial blood pressure, elevated pulmonary venous pressure, right ventricular hypertrophy, variable shunt reversal – blood moves from left to right and vice versa.
Diagnosis	Dyspnea: On exertion – moderate to severe
	Cyanosis
	Clubbing
	Polycythemia
	Pulsations: Pulmonary artery and right ventricular
	Murmur: Systolic, along the left sternal border
	Thrill: Pulmonic systolic ejection.
Investigations	CBC, ESR
	ECG: P waves – peaked, right ventricular hypertrophy
	CXR
	Fluoroscopy: Pulsating pulmonary arteries with reduced vascularity
	Angio-cardiography, cardiac catheterization – to establish shunt site.
Management	No specific treatment proved effective for obstructive pulmonary vascular disorder.

Refer: The patient to the medical/pediatric team.

Pediatric Fevers

Definition   Fever is defined as raised body temperature, e.g.

Rectal temperature: > 38°C (100.4°F)

Normally rectal temperature is 0.5°C (1°F) > than oral temp.

Prolonged, raising of rectal temperature > 41°C (106°F) may cause brain damage.

Rectal temperature > 43°C (109°F) may cause death.

Etiology   Pyrexia/fever of unknown origin (PUO/FUO)

Infections: Viral, rickettsial, bacterial, protozoal, fungal

Inflammation

Trauma

Head/spinal cord injuries

Heat stroke, dehydration

Drug/pyrogen reactions, serum sickness, anaphylactic shock, chemical poisoning.

Diagnosis   Fever

Signs and symptoms of underlying cause.

Investigation   Extensive laboratory studies:

- TLC and DLC
- Peripheral blood smear examination – for malaria and filarial
- Serological tests – for typhoid, toxoplasmosis, amebiasis
- Microscopic examination of blood, urine, sputum, throat, stool
- Cultures of blood, urine, sputum, throat, CSF, gastric/lymph node aspirate,
- CXR (X-ray chest), ultrasonography, CT scan, MRI, may be required for diagnosis.

Management   Removal of the underlying cause of fever

General measures:

- Oral or IV fluids – to combat loss of fluid from perspiration, etc.
- Hydrotherapy (to reduce fever) cold sponges, alcohol sponges, ice bags
- Antipyretic and analgesics – to reduce fever
- Aspirin 10–20 mg/kg/dose PO. Rept 4 hrly
- Acetaminophen (paracetamol) 15 mg/kg/dose PO. Rept 4 hrly.

Refer: The child to the pediatric team.

Pyrexia of Unknown Origin (PUO)/Fever of Unknown Origin (FUO)

Definition   It is defined as prolonged undiagnosed fever of unknown origin, with temperature above 38.5°C (101°F) on many occasions for > 3/52 duration.

Etiology   Infective – obscure abscess in liver/kidney/brain/bone/peritoneum/dental

Endocrinological and metabolic – diabetese, thyrotoxicosis

Autoimmune disorders – rheumatoid arthritis, SLE, polyarteritis

Neurogenic

Neoplastic – leukemia, Hodgkin's disease, lymphoma

Travel – to remote areas with epidemiology of disease

Miscellaneous – drug induced fever, sarcoidosis.

Diagnosis   History

Examination.

Investigation   TLC and DLC

Peripheral blood smear examination – for malaria and filarial

Serological tests – for typhoid, leishmaniasis, amebiasis

Cultures – blood/urine/sputum/throat/CSF/liver aspirate

PCR – to diagnose an infective agent

Seroimmunological tests – to diagnose an antibody

X-ray chest (CXR)

Biopsy – lymph node/tissue

Ultrasonography

CT scan

MRI.

Management

General measures

Admit the child

Cool and airy atmosphere

Hydrotherapy – ice cold water sponging

Fluids – oral or IV saline/dextrose

Drugs   Paracetamol 15 mg/kg. Rpt after every 4 hrs.

References

1. Strader DB et al: Diagnosis, management and treatment of hepatitis C. Hepatology, Vol. 39, No. 4, 2004
2. Alter MJ: Prevention of spread of hepatitis C. Hepatology, Vol. 36(suppl 1): 593–598;2002
3. Rewari BB, Sukarma T: Emergencies in HIV medicine. JIMA, Vol. 107: 317–322;2009

Pediatric Infections
Viral Infections
Pediatric Acquired Immune Deficiency Syndrome (PAIDS)

Definition   It is called 20th century plague, with fatal outcome.

Etiology   Human immunodeficiency virus (HIV 1) of retrovirus group.

Risk factors   Mothers indulging in prostitution

Hetrosexual mothers with bisexual husbands, addicted mothers

Blood transfusion without testing for HIV

Obesity and its accompaniment

Non-alcoholic fatty liver disease

Hepatitis B & C.

Diagnosis   Incubation period (time period from exposure to virus to the development of disease)

	3 months to 5 yrs
	Fever
	Night sweats
	Loss of weight
	Diarrhea
	Gastrointestinal bleeding
	Rashes
	Pneumonia.
Investigation	TLC and DLC – lymphopenia < 2000/cmm
	Platelet count – thrombocytopenia
	Raised levels of mmunoglobulins – IgA, IgG, IgM
	ELISA test
	Culture of virus
	T cell growth factors.
Management	
Prevention	Counseling of mothers (with AIDS) to change the lifestyle
	Screening of blood donors
Specific	No specific treatment either for HIV infection or the resulting immunodeficiency.
	At present, available therapy can neither eradicates the virus nor provides any definitive cure.
	Early diagnosis and control of infections by aggressive use of antibiotics may prolong the life of suffering child.
	Antiretroviral therapy: Many combinations of drugs are in use for therapy.
	Drugs: Interferon, ribavirin, suramin, zidovudine
	Chose the simplest regimen possible, reducing the dose frequency and no. of pills
	Chose the drugs with less no. of side effects
	Monitor response by HIV copy no. and CD4 lymphocyte count.

Refer: The child to the pediatric team.

Chickenpox (Varicella-zoster) Infection

Definition	It is an acute viral and highly contagious disease of childhood, and may prove fatal. A single attack confers permanent immunity.
Etiology	Varicella-zoster virus.
Transmission	Direct or indirect contact – person to person
	Air-borne infection – uncommon.
Diagnosis	Incubation period: 14–16 days
	Prodromal symptoms – minimal, e.g.
	Low grade fever, chills, malaise
	Headache, backache
	Rash – appears on first day, has a characteristic centripetal distribution

Lesions– pass through stages rapidly, e.g. macule, papule, vesicle, pustule and crust

Site: Lesions appear mainly over trunk, back, shoulders, face, limbs

The condition generally improves within a week's time

The disease is more severe in adults.

Complications	URC, otitis media, encephalitis, persistent diarrhea, hepatitis.
Investigation	TLC and DLC – leukopenia
	Serological tests – ELISA and complement fixation test.
Management	No specific treatment is available. Treatment is mainly symptomatic and supportive.

General measures

Quarantine (home/ward isolation) the child – till crusts disappear

Bed-rest – till afebrile

Personal hygiene to be optimized

Antipyretics – acetaminophen 15 mg/kg/dose PO

Antihistaminics – to combat itching

Local application of calamine lotion

Antibiotics – to combat secondary infections

Acyclovir (zovirax) to reduce number of skin lesions and drug of choice

Dose: 20 mg/kg/dose q.d.s. 5 days

Treatment of complications:

Secondary infections, pneumonia – treated by antibiotics

Encephalitis – treated symptomatically.

Prophylaxis	Active immunization: A live attenuated chickenpox (varilrix) vaccine given within 3 days of exposure
	Passive immunization: Vericella-zoster immunoglobulin (VZIG)
	125 units/10 kg s.c. within 4 days of exposure

Refer: The child to the pediatric team.

Measles (Rubeola)

Definition	It is the most common and most infectious viral infections of childhood. A single attack confers permanent immunity.
Etiology	Measles virus (RNA virus of paramyxovirus group).
Transmission	Direct or indirect contact
	Droplet infection.
Diagnosis	Incubation period: 10–18 days
	Fever, cough, running of nose, sneezing, redness of eyes
	Koplik spots – appear on 2nd or 3rd day, on the inner side of cheek, opposite 2nd molar, these may be single or multiple, bluish or grayish
	Rash – appears on 4th day, erythematous and blanches on pressure
	Site – rash appears on face, behind ears, neck, trunk, limbs
	Fever and rash normally last for a week.

Complications URC, otitis media, bronchitis, pneumonia, encephalitis.
Investigation TLC and DLC – leukopenia
Serological tests – ELISA for detecting measles antibody.
Management No specific treatment is available. Treatment is mainly symptomatic and supportive.
General measures

Isolate the child – till crusts disappear
Bed rest – till afebrile
Personal hygiene to be optimized
Antipyretics – acetaminophen 15 mg/kg/dose PO
Antihistaminics – to combat itching
Local application of calamine lotion
Antibiotics – to combat secondary infections
Acyclovir (zovirax) to reduce number of skin lesions
Dose: 20 mg/kg/dose q.d.s. for 5 days.

Treatment of complications:

Secondary infections, pneumonia – treated by antibiotics
Encephalitis – treated symptomatically.

Prophylaxis Active immunization: Live attenuated measles vaccine 1000 TCID-50 s.c.
Refer: The child to the pediatric team.

Mumps

Definition It is a viral infection of the salivary glands. A single attack confers permanent immunity.
Etiology RNA virus of paramyxoviridae group.
Transmission Direct contact
Air-borne droplets.
Diagnosis Incubation period: 2–3 weeks
Fever
Headache, pain near ear
Nausea, malaise
Loss of appetite
Difficulty in chewing
Swelling behind angle of jaw.
Investigation TLC and DLC – leukopenia
Culture of throat washings, spinal fluid, urine
Serological tests – ELISA, complement fixation test.
Complications Orchitis, epididymitis, pancreatitis, encephalitis.
Management Treatment is mainly symptomatic
General measures

Analgesics – paracetamol or aspirin

Fomentation

Bed-rest, support

Steroids – to combat pain and swelling.

Treatment of complications

Encephalitis – management of cerebral edema, airway, vital functions

Secondary infections – treated by antibiotics

Orchitis – scrotal support, corticosteroids,

Pancreatitis – symptomatic relief.

Prophylaxis   Isolation of the child

Active immunization: Live attenuated mumps vaccine 1000 TCID 50 s.c.

May be given at age of 15–18 months.

Refer: The child to the pediatric team.

German Measles (Rubella)

Definition   It is a less contagious viral infection, commonly seen in older children and adults. A single attack confers permanent immunity.

Etiology   Myxovirus.

Transmission   Direct contact

Droplet infection

Diagnosis   Incubation period: 14–21 days

Fever/chills

Cough, sneeze, running nose

Malaise

Rash (small red spots) – appear on 5th day over face, trunk, limbs

Koplik's spots – inside cheeks

Lymphadenopathy – cervical.

Complications   Mental and growth retardation, otitis media, pancreatitis, deafness, dental malformations, pneumonia, encephalitis.

Investigation   TLC and DLC – leukopenia

Serological tests: ELISA, complement fixation test.

Management   No specific treatment is available. Treatment is mainly symptomatic and supportive.

Preventive   Quarantine – home or hospital.

General   Bed-rest

Measures   Diet – liquid/semiliquid

Antipyretics and analgesics – paracetamol or ibuprofen

Antibiotics – to control/prevent infections.

Treatment of complications

Secondary infections, pneumonia – treated by antibiotics

Encephalitis – treated symptomatically

Pancreatitis – symptomatic relief.

Prophylaxis   Isolation of the child

Active immunization: Live attenuated mumps vaccine 1000 TCID 50 s.c.
         May be given at age of 15–18/12.

Refer: The child to the pediatric team.

Acute Encephalitis

Definition	It is an acute inflammation of the brain.
Etiology	Viruses: Arboviruses, herpes simplex, rabies virus, mumps virus, poliovirus, enteroviruses.
Risk factors	Post-exanthematous disorders of childhood, e.g. varicella, measles, rubella
	Post-vaccination – smallpox, triple, rabies
	Reactive – drugs, chemicals, poisons, bacterial toxins.
Diagnosis	Fever, malaise, URC, nausea, vomiting, stupor, coma, convulsions, paralysis.
Investigation	CBC
	TLC and DLC – lymphocytic leukocytosis
	Lumbar puncture – CSF pressure and protein content increased
	Blood culture – for virus
	Serological tests.
Complications	Pneumonia, UTI, parkinsonism, epilepsy.

Management

Preventive	Active immunization against infectious disorders during childhood.
General	Airway maintenance
measures	Oxygen therapy
	Nasogastric tube feeding
	IV fluids.

Treatment of complications

     IV mannitol – to reduce intracranial pressure

     Control of convulsions – by use of anticonvulsants, e.g. phenobarbitone, phenytoin or carbamazepine

     Control of infection – by use of antibiotics.

Poliomyelitis

Definition	It is an acute infectious viral disease, prevalent worldwide, especially in the communities with poor vaccination status.
Etiology	Enterovirus (an RNA virus).
Transmission	Oropharyngeal route.
Diagnosis	Incubation period: 7–14 days
	Fever
	Sore throat, bodyaches
	Nausea, vomiting, anorexia
	Flaccid paralysis of lower motor neuron type (involvement of anterior horn cells) lower limbs affected more than upper limbs

Sensations – intact

Bladder involvement – of short duration

Bowel involvement – of long duration.

Complications	UTI, pneumonia, pulmonary edema, skeletal deformities.
Investigation	Isolation of virus from stools and throat swab.
Management	No specific treatment. Treatment is primarily symptomatic and supportive

Bed-rest

Relief of pain – by application of warm packs to muscles and analgesic

Physiotherapy – to combat deformities and for building up muscle tone
good nursing care

Diet – nutritious, balanced

Suction – to clear secretions

Tracheostomy – may be required

Assisted respiration with mechanical ventilator.

Treatment of complications

Bulbar poliomyelitis – requires: ICU, airway maintenance, ventilation, endotrachial intubation, tracheostomy, oxygen therapy

Secondary infections, pneumonia – treated by antibiotics

Pulmonary edema – treated symptomatically

Skeletal deformities – treated by active exercises, braces/splints.

Prophylaxis	Active immunization with polio vaccine

Types of vaccine: Salk vaccine (killed) injectable
Sabin vaccine (live) oral polio drops.

Viral Hepatitis

Types	Five types of viral hepatitis: A, B, C, D, E.
Etiology	A, C, D, and E are caused by an RNA virus

B caused by a DNA virus.

Hepatitis A

Transmission	Direct contact: Fecal–oral route

Contaminated food and water.

Diagnosis	Incubation period: 3–5/52

Fever, malaise

Nausea, vomiting, anorexia, pain abdomen

Urine – dark colored

Jaundice – may appear

Liver – enlarged and tendered

Spleen – palpable.

Investigation	ALT, AST, alkaline phosphatase, are elevated.
Management	No specific treatment.

General measures

        Bed-rest

        Diet: Nutritious diet, rich in carbohydrates and proteins and fat restriction.

Prophylaxis   Active immunization: Human normal immunoglobulin 1 mL IM

Hepatitis B

Etiology	DNA virus.
Transmission	Contaminated blood transfusion
	Cotaminated hypodermic needles – for multipurpose use
	Shaving razors – shared by different persons
	Sexual contact – with infected partner
	Infected mother – to fetus especially in last (3rd) trimester or during delivery.
Diagnosis	Incubation period: 6/52–6/12
	Clinical picture is same as that of hepatitis A.
	Rash, urticaria, arthralgia, weakness, purpura
	Confusion, restlessness, tremors.
Investigation	TLC and DLC – lymphocytosis
	SGPT and alkaline phosphatase – elevated.
Management	No specific treatment.

General measures

        Bed-rest with early ambulation

        Diet – rich in carbohydrates, avoid proteins

        IV dextrose 10%

        Blood transfusion – may not be beneficial

        Drugs: Interferon 5–10 million units/sq m IM t.i.w. for 4–6/12

            Lamivudine – limited use in children.

Treatment of complications:

        Secondary infections, pneumonia – treated by antibiotics

        Encephalitis – treated symptomatically.

Prophylaxis   Active immunization: By hepatitis B vaccine 1 mL IM (into deltoid)

        Children 0.5 mL IM (into thigh)

        Repeat: 2nd dose after 1 month and 3rd dose after 6/12.

Hepatitis C : Described in section 18 of Emerging and Reimerging Emergency.

Hepatitis E : Described in section 18 of Emerging and Reimerging Emergency.

Rabies   : Described in section 18 of Emerging and Reimerging Emergency.

Bacterial Infections
Acute Influenza (HIB Disease)

Etiology	*Haemophilus influenzae* – a gram-negative coccobacillus, present in the nasopharynx of non-immunized persons.
Transmission	Direct contact
	Droplet infection

Diagnosis	Incubation period – variable
	Signs/symptoms depend upon involved system, e.g.
	Septicemia
	Cellulitis, suppurative arthritis
	Pneumonia
	Menigitis
	Pericarditis
Investigation	Smears for culture sensitivity test
	Serological test – slide agglutination with type specific antisera
Management	Antibiotic cephalosporins, e.g. cefotaxime and ceftriaxone – parenterally or chloramphenicol and ampicillin may be given.
Prevention	HIB vaccine

Refer: The child to the pediatric team.

Acute Meningitis

Definition	It is an inflammation of the brain due to infection of the pia–arachnoid mater and CSF.
Etiology	Bacterial infections (purulent type):

- *Haemophilus influenzae*
- *Streptococcus pneumoniae*
- *Neisseria meningitidis*
- *Staphylococcus aureus*

Viral infections (aseptic type):

- Mumps virus
- Enteroviruses
- Poliovirus

Granulomatous meningitis:
- *Mycobacterium tuberculosis*

Meningovascular meningitis:
- *Treponema pallidum* (syphilis).

Predisposing Factors	Age – common in children
	URC
	Pneumonia
	Head injury
	Metabolic – Hodgkin's disease, multiple myeloma.
Diagnosis	Fever, headache, nausea, vomiting, malaise, sore throat, cough, diarrhea
	Rash – patechial
	Neck and back stiffness
	Kernig and Brudzinski signs – positive.
Investigations	TLC and DLC – leukocytosis
	CSF – Pressure : raised

Cells : >1000/mL
Proteins : >45/dL
Glucose : <40 mg/dL
CSF culture +ve
Blood culture +ve
CXR – may show an area of pneumonitis or abscess
X-ray skull and sinus – may show # skull or sinusitis
CT scan – to confirm sinusitis or brain abscess.

Complications Cranial nerve palsies, deafness, epileptic fits, shock, coma.

Management

General Monitor – vital signs
measures IV isotonic electrolyte sol. – to achieve volume expansion.

Treatment of complications

IV isoproterenol – to control shock
IV corticosteroids – to boost action of isoproterenol
IV heparin 50 U/kg – to control intravascular clotting
IV mannitol 2 g/kg or urea 0.5 g/kg – to control cerebral edema

Specific Antimicrobials:
measures Penicillin G
Adults: 18–24 mU IV o.d. in divided doses
Children: 400,000 U/kg o.d. in divided doses
Ampicillin
Adults: 12–18 g IV o.d. in divided doses
Children: 400 mg/kg o.d.
Chloramphenicol
Adults: 4–6 g IV o.d. in divided doses
Cephalosporins (3rd generation – cefotaxime, ceftriaxone)
Adults: 2 g IV o.d. undivided doses
Children: 200 mg/kg o.d. in divided doses

Prophylaxis HIB vaccine.

Diphtheria

Definition It is an acute bacterial disease.
Etiology *Corynebacterium diphtheriae* – a gram-positive rod.
Transmission Droplet infection.
Diagnosis Incubation period: 2–6 days
Sore throat, difficulty in swallowing
Nasal discharge
Fever, malaise
Tonsils – covered with a grayish-white membrane.
Investigation Smear examination

Culture test

Fluorescent antibody technique.

Management Antitoxin: Antidiphtheritic serum (ADS) 20–100 thousand units IM or IV

Antibiotics: Penicillin, erythromycin, rifampicin or clindamycin for 2/52

Prophylaxis Active immunization with DPT or DT.

Refer: The child to the pediatric team.

Pertussis (Whooping Cough)

Etiology *Bordetella pertussis* – a gram-negative bacillus.

Transmission Droplet infection

Direct contact.

Diagnosis Incubation period: 6–14 days

Fever, rhinitis, sneezing

Cough – paroxysmal, i.e. bouts of cough with inspiratory whoop

Anxiety

Vomiting.

Investigation TLC and DLC – lymphocytosis

ESR – low

CXR (X-ray chest) – shows infiltration, atelectasis, or emphysema

Smear for culture test

ELISA – to detect IgM, IgG, IgA – directed towards pertussis toxin.

Management

General measures

Isolation of patient

Cough syrups

Sedatives

Oxygen therapy

Maintenance of fluids and dietary intake

Antibiotics:

- Erythromycin is drug of choice. Dose: 50 mg/kg/day for 2/52, or
- Cotrimoxazole, ampicillin, amoxicillin, or
- Chloramphenicol for 5–7 days

Corticoids – in severe cases.

Prophylaxis Active immunization with DPT.

Refer: The child to the pediatric team.

Tetanus

Etiology *Clostridium tetani* – gram-positive bacillus, present in soil, dust, feces of animals and humans.

Transmission Contaminated wound

Contaminated umbilical cord – cutting of cord with septic knife/scissors.

Pathology	Bacilli after entering circulation, get attached to the motor endplate in the muscles and motor nuclei of nervous system, muscle spasms, respiratory or circulatory paralysis.
Diagnosis	Incubation period: 3–14 days, shorter the period, worst prognosis
	Pain, muscle spasms, cramps
	Difficulty in swallowing
	Irritability, restlessness, convulsions
	Death.
Management	Antitoxin (ATS)IM or IV Children 0.1 million international units (IU)
	Newborns 30000–50000 IU
	Active immunization: Toxoid 0.5–1.0 ml, followed by booster doses after every 3/52
	Antibiotics – Penicillin is drug of choice
	Human tetanus immunoglobulin (HTIG) 500–3000 IU given IM stat
	Intrathecal HTIG – of value.
General measures	Isolation of patient in a dark, quite room
	Good nursing care
	Maintenance of fuid and dietary intake
	Antispasmodics –· to control muscle spasms, e.g. diazepam, phenobarbital, paraldehyde, magnesium sulfate
	Oxygen therapy
	Tracheostomy –may be required.
Prophylaxis	Active immunization with tetanus toxoid.

Refer: The child to the pediatric team.

Typhoid/Paratyphoid Fever

Definition	Serious infectious disease.
Etiology	Bacterial infection, e.g.
	Salmonella typhoid – typhoid fever
	Salmonella paratyphoid – paratyphoid fever.
Transmission	Source: Unhygienically prepared or undercooked food, contaminated milk, water, foods, and over-ripened fruits, vegetables
	Route: Fecal–oral – by ingestion of food contaminated by urine and feces of patients suffering from typhoid and of carriers (harbouring germs in their GI tract, gallbladder, or bone marrow).
Epidemiology	Endemic in tropical countries – due to poor hygiene/sanitation.
	Incubation period: 14 days.
Diagnosis	Fever – temperature continues to rise – often to 41°C (105°F)
	Chills and sweating
	Headache, vomiting
	Constipation or diarrhea

Skin rash (red spots) – appears on 6th day of fever

Splenomegaly.

Complications	Intestinal hemorrhage – due to perforation of the ulcerated area of intestine, peritonitis, shock, death.
Investigations	CBC
	Hb and ESR
	Blood culture – isolation and identification
	Widal test.
Management	
Prevention	Do's:

- Maintain a high standard of personal hygiene – wash hands before and after meals
- Drink only bottled or boiled water
- Eat only thoroughly cooked food that is served hot

Don't:

- Avoid raw/undercooked seafood
- Avoid uncovered food served by street hawkers/unhygienic food joints
- Avoid tap water, ice-cubes, ice-creams, cut fruits

Specific	Antibiotics: Chloramphenicol 1 g PO – until fever disappears, or ampicillin 100 mg/kg/day PO
	Antipyretics
	IV dextrose sol.
	Treatment of complications
Prophylaxis	Typhoid vaccination:
	Active immunization: 0.5 mL s.c. or IM. Repeat after 1/12

- Oral vaccine 3 capsules taken over 5 days (days 1, 3, 5)

Acute Osteomyelitis (Acute Pyogenic Infection of Bone/Acute Osteitis)

Etiology	Bacterial infection, e.g. *Staphylococcus, Streptococcus, Pneumococcus, Meningococcus, Gonococcus, Haemophilus influenzae*, gram-negative bacilli.
Transmission	Direct: Compound fractures
	Indirect: Hematogenous – through bloodstream.
Diagnosis	Age – common in children
	Bone – tibia, femur, humerus are commonly affected
	Site – bone ends (metaphysis)
	Onset – sudden
	Pain – severe
	Fever with chills
	Swelling

	Skin – hot, red Local tenderness – over the bone Swelling of joint – absent initially, may present later on Movements – free initially, and later on may be painful and restricted.
Investigation	Hemogram TLC and DLC – leukocytosis ESR – raised Blood culture X-ray: Normal in early cases. Later on there occurs rarefaction of the metaphysis, and subperiosteal bone formation.

Complications

General	Toxemia, septicemia, pyemia
Local	Septic arthritis Fracture – pathological Deformity/shortening.

Management

General measures

      Bed-rest

      Immobilization – by splint, traction

      Elevation of the part

Specific	Antibiotics

  • Penicillin, ampicillin or tetracycline, given IM or IV soon after taking blood for culture sensitivity.

  • Rational drug therapy is based upon drug sensitivity tests

      Aspiration of abscess – for culture sensitivity

      Analgesics

      IV fluids

      Blood transfusion.

Surgery

Indications	Abscess formation – causing persistent pain, local tenderness and fever
Procedures	• Incision and drainage of subperiosteal abscess • Decompression of the medullary canal by drilling/fenestration.

Refer: The child to the orthopedic team.

Acute Septic Arthritis

Etiology	Bacterial infection, e.g. *Staphylococcus*, *Streptococcus*, *Pneumococcus*, *Meningococcus*, *Gonococcus*, *Haemophilus influenzae*, gram-negative bacilli.
Diagnosis	Onset – sudden Pain – severe Fever with chills Swelling of joint

	Skin – hot, red
	Local tenderness
	Movements – painful and restricted.
Investigation	Hemogram
	TLC and DLC – leukocytosis
	ESR – raised
	Blood culture
	Synovial fluid analysis: Leukocytosis
	Smear and culture study of causative organism
	X-ray: Normal in early cases, but later on shows demineralization, bony erosion, narrowing of joint space, osteomyelitis.

Management

General measures

 Bed-rest

 Immobilization of joint by splint, traction

 Elevation of the part

 Warm fomentation

 Antibiotics

 Analgesics

 Fluids – PO or IV

Surgical measures

 Aspiration of joint

 Incision and drainage.

Refer: The patient to the orthopedic team.

Tuberculosis in Childhood

Tuberculosis is prevalent worldwide with nearly 0.17 million children dying of it every year. It is a major health problem in economically poor countries of Asia, Africa and South America.

Incidence	Children: 5–15% of all tubercular cases.
Etiology	*Mycobacterium tuberculosis.*
Transmission	Tuberculous patient – discharging tubercle bacilli in sputum or nasopharyngeal secretions
	– direct contact.
Diagnosis	Cough for 3/52 or more
	Fever – evening rise of temperature
	Night cramps
	Sweating
	Loss of weight
Investigation	CBC
	ESR

Tuberculin test:
- Mantoux test: 0.1 ml of diluted tuberculin is injected ID on the anterior surface of forearm. A wheal is raised.
  Report: After 48–72 hrs. Induration > 10 mm – infection and should be treated. A negative test does not rule out tuberculosis.
- Multiple puncture test: Sputum smears (3) or laryngeal swab for acid-fast bacilli (AFB)
- Serological test: TB ELISA – not for diagnosis of childhood TB
  PCR: Sensitivity and specificity of PCR for CSF and pleural fluid high
  CXR (X-ray chest) PA view – may be positive or negative.

Management	
General measures	
	Isolation – to pollution free atmosphere
	Diet – nutritious diet
	Nursing care.
Drugs	Antitubercular drugs: Short course chemotherapy is accepted by:
	WHO, American Academy of Pediatrics and IUATLD. It is treatment of choice these days.
	Isoniazid 10–15 mg/kg
	Rifampicin 10 mg/kg
	Pyrazinamide 35 mg/kg
	Streptomycin 15 mg/kg
	Ethambutol 30 mg/kg

The standard short course chemotherapy regimen consists of two phases:
Intensive phase: Aims: To eliminate bacterial load
                               To prevent emergence of drug resistant strains.

Pneumonia

Definition	It is defined as inflammation of lung parenchyma, caused by infection.
Etiology	Infection – bacterial or viral
	Bacterial: *Pneumococcus, Streptococcus, H. influenzae*
	Viral: Influenza, measles, chickenpox
	Mycoplasma: Pneumoniae
	Fungal: Coccidomycosis
	Rickettsial: Typhus
	Miscellaneous: Drowning, foreign body.
Diagnosis	Sudden onset
	High fever, chills
	Cough with rust colored sputum
	Vomiting, diarrhea
	Chest pain.
Investigation	TLC and DLC – leukocytosis

Sputum – for Gram's stain and culture

Blood culture

CXR (X-ray chest) – shows infiltration, lobar consolidation.

Management	
Emergency measures	Airway maintenance – by endotracheal intubation
	Oxygen therapy
	Shock – if present, should be treated as a top priority
	Pulmonary edema – treat accordingly
	Fluids, cough syrups, antipyretics
	Antibiotics:

- Penicillin G is drug of choice for *Pneumococcus*
- Cloxacillin + ampicillin/gentamicin for *Staphylococcus*
- Ampicillin or penicillin + chloramphenicol for *H.influenzae*
- Penicillin + kanamycin or gentamicin for *Klebsiella*.

Refer: The child to the pediatric team.

Acute Bronchitis: Described in appropriate section of Respiratory Disorders

Acute Bronchiolitis: Described in appropriate section of Respiratory Disorders

Bronchiectasis: Described in appropriate section of Respiratory Disorders

Pleurisy: Described in appropriate section of Respiratory Disorders

Pleural Effusion: Described in appropriate section of Respiratory Disorders

Empyema: Described in appropriate section of Respiratory Disorders

Lung Abscess: Described in appropriate section of Respiratory Disorders

Acute (severe) Malaria: Described in section of Emerging and Re-imerging Infections

Acute Respiratory Distress Syndrome (ARDS): Described in appropriate section of Respiratory Disorders.

Practical Procedures

Subcutaneous injection (sc): Only non-irritating drugs can be given

Sites	Outer surface of upper arm
	Anterior surface of forearm
Indication	Vaccination – measles, MMR
	Drugs – insulin, atropine, etc.
	Hormones
Method	Hold the child to prevent movement of arm
	Clean the skin with spirit or an antiseptic sol
	Pinch up skin
	Insert a subcutaneous needle into skin at an angle of 60°
	Care not to enter a blood vessel – check by drawing plunger
	Inject the drug and then withdraw
Care	Do not rub the site.

Routes of administration of Drugs/Fluids/Blood/Vaccines (Table 13.10)

Table 13.10: Routes of administration of drugs/fluids/vaccines

Routes	Sites	Indications	Adv.	Disadv.
Subcutaneous	Upperarm Forearm	Vaccination, drugs, hormones	Slow absorption	Infection, sloughing
Intradermal (ID)	Upperarm Forearm	Vaccination, Tuberculin (Mantoux) test	Slow absorption	Infection, sloughing
Intramuscular	Thigh, arm, buttocks	Aqueous sol., oily sol., irritating substances	Safe, even absorption	Infection, abscess
Intravenous (IV)/ venous access	Umbilicus, scalp, arm, thigh, neck	Blood sampling, IV drugs, fluids, blood transfusion, monitoring BUN, BP	Rapid absorption	Allergic reactions
Umbilical vein	Umbilicus			
Scalp vein	Temporal			
Antecubital	Elbow			
Femoral	Thigh			
External jugular	Neck			
Internal jugular	Neck			
Intravenous infusion	Wrist hand/foot	Fluids, blood transfusion, drugs in aqueous sol.	Emergency measure	Allergic reactions
Venesection	Leg, wrist	Failure to establish IV approach	Emergency measure	Allergic reactions
Arterial puncture	Wrist	BUN analysis Monitoring of BP	Emergency measure	Arterial damage
Intraosseous infusion	Tibia, femur	Failure to establish IV approach	Emergency measure	Infection cellulitis
Intraperitoneal infusion	Abdomen	Failure to establish IV approach	Emergency measure	Bladder injury
Bone marrow aspiration	Iliac crest	Histopathological examination	Diagnostic	Infection
Bone marrow trephine	Iliac crest	Histopathological examination	Diagnostic	Infection

Intradermal (ID) Injection

Sites   Outer surface of upper arm
               Anterior surface of forearm
Indication   Vaccination – BCG, tuberculin (Mantoux) test
Method   Hold the nervous patient/child to prevent movement of arm
               Clean the skin with spirit or an antiseptic sol
               Stretch the skin
               Insert the needle into skin – only needle tip to enter skin
               Inject the vaccine, etc.
Care   Do not rub the site.

Intramuscular (IM)

Sites   Infants/younger children: Anterolateral surface of mid-thigh
               Older children (5–11): Upper and outer quadrant of buttocks (gluteal)
               Adolescents (12–16): Mid-deltoid
Indications   Drugs – aqueous sol., oily sol.,
               Alternative to s.c. – irritating substances which cannot be given s.c.
               Disadvantage: Infection – abscess formation, pain

Intravenous (IV), syn. Venous Access

Sites   Neonatal (newborn): Umbilical vein
               Infants/younger children: Scalp vein
               Older children: Dorsum of hand/foot
               Adolescents: Wrist, dorsum of hand/foot, antecubitus
Indications   Emergencies
               Certain irritating and hypertonic solutions
               General anesthesia
Disadvantages Unfavorable reactions
               No retreat after the drug is injected
               Scarring of veins due to repeated IV injections
Caution   Unless specifically indicated, drugs should never be given IV.

Methods
Umbilical Vein

Indication   Exchange transfusion in newborn infants
               IV infusion
               Monitoring blood gas and blood pressure
Method   Sterilization of cord area
               Cutting the cord close to base of stump
               Three blood vessels (pair of arteries and a vein) visible
               Insert the catheter into vein gently
               Blood flows into catheter. Connect catheter to the infusion set
               After withdrawal of catheter, the tip of catheter is sent for culture.

Scalp Vein

Advantages   Easy to insert
               Minimal trauma
               Steadiness and stability
               Constant in location
               Preservation of veins for future needs
Method   Hold the head of child
               Shave and prepare the selected area

Fix the vein by stretching skin taut with fingers

Insert the needle at an angle of 30°

Blood flows into scalp vein

Connect scalp vein set to the drip set.

Antecubital   Commonly used in older children.

Method   Arm is firmly gripped above the elbow, and by holding the arm fully extended and supinated, clean the skin with a spirit swab. A scalp vein needle is introduced into an antecubital vein. A 2–3 way stopcock is attached to the catheter end. The stop cock is removed, when blood sample is to be taken.

Femoral   Seldom used because of danger of gangrene of toes

Method   Holding leg fully abducted at hip and knee flexed to 90°

Palpate femoral artery below inguinal ligament

Femoral vein entered by introducing needle just medial to artery

After obtaining blood, needle withdrawn gently

Apply firm, steady pressure for 2–3 min.

External Jugular

Method   Turn head to one side and keep it at lower level than the body.

Vein – stretched, becomes visible, crossing sternomastoid.

Puncture the vein and draw blood.

Withdraw needle and apply pressure for 2–3 min.

Disadvantage   Hematoma formation

Internal Jugular (Central venous catheterization)

Method   Insert needle at midway down the posterior border of sternomastoid, directing towards suprasternal notch. After obtaining blood, the catheter is introduced over a guide wire and advanced into the vessel. The needle withdrawn gently. Apply firm, steady pressure for 2–3 min.

Disadvantage   Hematoma formation, injury to lungs

Intravenous Infusion (IV Infusion)

Sites   Neonatal (newborn): Umbilical vein

Infants/younger children: Scalp vein

Older children/adults: Antecubital, wrist veins, back of hand, leg

Wrist Veins, Dorsum of Hand/Foot

Method   Arm is firmly gripped above the wrist/ankle, clean the skin with a spirit swab. Introduce the cannula riding a metal needle, into the vein.

Withdraw the needle, leaving cannula in the vein. Cannula can be retained in the vein for 2–3 days.

Venesection

Indications	Failure to establish IV approach (unavailable peripheral vein).
C/I	Fracture, osteomyelitis, osteoporosis, cellulitis.
Sites	Leg: Anterior to the medial malleolus.
Method	Under local anesthesia, a transverse skin incision given across the vein. Two silk sutures looped around proximal and distal to the venesection site. The distal suture is tied firmly, to prevent venous return.
	A sharp cut made in the wall of the vein, and the catheter is introduced up, blood starts flowing, IV set attached to the catheter end, the silk loops tied up. Suturing of skin wound, and dressing.

Arterial Puncture

Indications	BUN analysis
	Monitoring of blood pressure
Sites	Radial, brachial, femoral, tibial, dorsalis pedis and temporal arteries.
Method	Sterile the area
	Local anesthesia given
	Insert a heparinized syringe, blood flows into syringe
	After collecting blood, withdraw needle, apply pressure for 2–3 min.

Intraosseous Infusion

Indication	Failure to establish IV approach
Advantages	It is a safe, rapidly achieved and reliable alternative to IV route, for the infusion of isotonic, sodium chloride solution, plasma, whole blood.
C/I	Fracture, osteomyelitis, osteoporosis, cellulitis
Sites	Proximal tibia – anteromedial surface 2 cm (1") below tubercle, Alt: Distal tibia and distal femur
Method	Sterile the area
	Local anesthesia given
	A bone marrow needle or spinal needle, introduced into marrow
	Remove stilet and flush the needle with saline solution
	Blood flows into syringe. Connect the needle to IV set.

Intraperitoneal Infusion

Indication	Failure to establish IV approach
Advantage	Seldom employed clinically but is a common laboratory procedure.
	Peritoneal cavity offers a large absorbing surface, for fluids and blood.
Disadvantage	Danger of infection and adhesions
Method	Sterile the area
	Insert needle at junction of upper one-third and lower two-thirds between umbilicus and pubic symphysis.
	Connect needle to IV set, void the bladder during procedure.

Bone Marrow Aspiration

Indications	As an alternative to IV, e.g. circulatory collapse, edema, burns, restless patient.
	Infusion of isotonic sodium chloride solution, plasma, whole blood.
	Non-irritant drugs.
C/I	Osteomyelitis
	Bacteremia
Sites	Children > 2 yrs: Iliac crest – anterior superior iliac crest
	Children < 2 yrs: Tibia – anteromedial aspect of proximal part
Method	Sterile the area
	Local anesthesia given
	Insert the trocar and cannula through skin, periosteum, cortex, into bone marrow. Remove trocar.
	Aspirate marrow by suction with a syringe attached firmly to the cannula.
	After aspiration, replace trocar, and then withdraw the needle.

Bone Marrow Trephine

Indication	Histopathological examination
C/I	Osteomyelitis, bacteremia
Sites	Iliac crest
Method	Sterile the area.
	Local anesthesia given.
	Skin incision given.
	Stylet of Tamshidi-Swain trephine is locked and the handle introduced into the incision, till it touches the iliac crest. The needle is driven into bone with clockwise and anticlockwise movements, till feeling of "Give".
	Stylet is removed, and the needle rotated to break the specimen.
	Needle withdrawn and specimen removed from needle with a probe.
	Aspirate specimen smeared on glass slides before being placed into a fixative, for histopathological study.

Lumbar Puncture

Indication	Diagnostic and therapeutic.
C/I	Papilledema – may cause herniation of medullary cone (fatal)
	Lumbar spine disorders
	Skin infections
Site	L4–L5 intervertebral space
Method	• Hold the child in sitting/lateral recumbent position, with neck flexed to the chest and knees flexed to abdomen
	• Sterile the area (3rd–4th intervertebral space)
	• Local anesthesia (lignocaine plain 1%) given

- Introduce a lumbar puncture needle with stylet in position, through skin, between spines, through ligamentum flavum
- Withdraw the stylet
- Collect the CSF
- Replace the stylet and then withdraw the needle
- Seal the puncture site with tinc. benzoin co.

Fine Needle Aspiration Study (FNAS)

Indication   Diagnostic, e.g. histopathological study of a tumor or a lymph node
                  Therapeutic – determining course of management
C/I   Bleeding disorder
Method   • Sterile the area
                  • Local anesthesia (lignocain plain 1%) given
                  • Insert the needle perpendicular to skin
                  • Pull the plunger to apply negative pressure
                  • Remove the needle, and aspirated specimen smeared on glass slides before being placed into a fixative, for histopathological study.

Pericardiocentesis

Indication   Cardiac tamponade (life saving measure)
                  Pericardial effusion (diagnostic measure).
Site   Inferolateral of xiphoid sternum (5th left intercostal space).
Method   • Sterile the area
                  • Local anesthesia (lignocaine plain 1% infiltration) given
                  • Needle – 16/18/20 gauge for infant/older child
                  • Insert the needle (attached to a 50 ml syringe) into left 5th space, just inferior and left to xiphoid sternum, directing the needle towards tip of patient's left scapula.
                  • Aspirate the fluid, after entering the pericardial space
                  • Withdraw the needle. Seal the puncture site.
Aftercare   Monitor the patient and ECG for at least 6 hrs.

Gastric Lavage

Indication   Diagnostic – tuberculosis and carcinoma of stomach
                  Therapeutic – Poisoning
                             – Hemorrhage – upper GI tract.
Method   • Place the child supine with head overextended
                  • Open the mouth, and put in mouth gag
                  • Advance the lubricated Ryle's tube, through mouth/nose, into throat, continue advancing tube as per mark on tube (1 transverse line at 40 cm, i.e. teeth – cardiac orifice distance, and 3 transverse lines at 57 cm i.e. teeth – pylorus distance).

- Confirm the presence of tube in the stomach – by pushing air through the tube, while auscultating over stomach.
- Suction out the gastric contents.
- Fix the tube firmly on the face with adhesive tape

Caution   Not to enter tube into trachea

Liver Biopsy

Indication   Diagnostic, e.g. hepatits, cirrhosis, tuberculosis
C/I   Bleeding disorder
Caution   Prothrombin time – must be within normal range
Site   Right 10th intercostals space – midaxillary line
Method
- Sterile the area
- Local anesthesia (lignocaine plain 1%) given
- Lie down the child supine with hands behind the head
- Introduce the liver biopsy needle (Tru,-Cut needle) with stylet, through the 9th or 10th intercostal space, pushed further into liver
- Withdraw the stylet, advance the inner and outer needles into liver
- Withdraw the whole needle assembly
- Seal the skin wound with tinc. benzoin co
- Remove the tissue from the gutter of needle and put into formalin.

Renal Biopsy

Indication   Diagnostic, e.g. hematuria, nephrotic syndrome, renal failure.
C/I   Bleeding disorder
             Polycystic kidney
             Hypertension
             Hydronephrosis
Site   2 cm inferior and medial to the tip of 12th rib (inferior border)
Method
- Sterile the area
- Local anesthesia (lignocaine plain 1%) given
- Insert a 20–21 needle parallel to spine, into kidney
- Entry into kidney is confirmed by movement of needle with the respiration, remove the needle
- Introduce a biopsy (Tru-Cut) needle with stylet into kidney
- Remove the stylet
- Cutting of kidney tissue by rotating the biopsy needle
- Remove the biopsy needle
- Seal the puncture site
- Removed tissue is put into formalin.

Foreign Body Removal (Manual) from Airway

Diagnosis — Cough, stridor, gagging, cyanosis, wheezing,
Respiratory distress.

Management

Caution — Avoid removal of the foreign body by finger sweep, as it may further push back the foreign body into airway.

Method — Separate techniques are used for removal of a foreign body in infants and older children.

Removal in an Infant

Method — Back blows chest thrusts
- Hold the infant face down on your forearm.
- Support the head of child by holding the jaw, and keeping the head lower than trunk, deliver 4–5 hand's blows between infant's shoulder blades.
- Turn around the infant to supine position while firmly supporting head and neck. Exert 4–5 quick chest thrusts in a similar manner used for the chest compressions.
- Repeat the whole process until the foreign body is expelled out.

Removal in a Child > 1 year

Method — Heimlich maneuver (subdiaphragmatic abdominal thrusts)

Age — > 1 year

Aim — To increase the intrathoracic pressure and create an artificial cough, that forces the foreign body out of the airway

C/I — Infants – because of the danger of liver injury.

Maneuver in Conscious Child

Method —
- Stand behind the child and encircle him/her by putting both arms directly under his/her axillae. Place one fist against the child's abdomen in midline, slightly above umbilicus and well below the xiphoid.
- By holding this fist with other hand, exert quick upward thrusts, taking care not to press the xiphoid or lower rib cage.

Maneuver in Unconscious Child

Method —
- Position of the child: Supine position.
- Kneel at child's feet. Place one hand on child's abdomen in the midline, just above the naval, much below the rib cage. Press the 2nd hand on top of the 1st.
- Deliver quick upward thrust into the abdomen.
- Press down firmly, so as to depress the sternum by 1–1.5 cm

Assisted Ventilation

Definition   It is defined as life-sustaining mechanical provision of respiratory gas exchange, in order to maintain gaseous concentration and pH of blood at an optimal level in the event of respiratory failure.

Indications   Congenital – malformations
Traumatic – birth trauma, head injury, meconium aspiration
Inflammatory – epiglottitis, bronchiolitis
Infective – diphtheria, croup, bronchopneumonia
Cardiovascular – cardiac arrest, shock, CHF
Neurologic – acute polio, CNS infections, HIE, apneic attacks.

Ventilator

It is defined as a mechanical device for providing artificial pulmonary ventilation.

Types   Manual ventilator (hand operated), or
Mechanical ventilator – may be automatic to control and monitor pulmonary flow of air.

Types of ventilation

1. Intermittent positive pressure: Pulmonary ventilation is provided by administrating oxygen for inflation of the lungs under positive pressure.
2. Continuous positive pressure: Pulmonary ventilation is provided by administrating oxygen or inflation of the lungs under continuous positive pressure, that is never allowed to return to zero.

Manual Ventilation

A. Bag and mask ventilation: This life-saving procedure, performed by a self-inflating Ambu bag, that is capable of delivering 90% oxygen, if a corrugated tube is attached to the bag.
Indication: Asphyxiated/apneic neonate.

B. Continuous positive airway pressure (CPAP): Provides a continuous supply of humidified oxygen – air mixture. Patient exhales against a water column kept at a level to maintain the required pressure resistance. May be administered by a facemask/nasal prongs/nasopharyngeal catheter/endotracheal tube.
Indications: RDS (HMD), inflammatory disorders, atelectasis.

Mechanical Ventilation

Principles   Maintenance of normal gas exchange depends on oxygenation and ventilation.
Oxygenation   To administer oxygen at higher pressures (hyperbaric oxyzgen therapy)
Ventilation   To maintain the gas exchange pulmonary function.
Indications
• Acute respiratory failure due to polio, Guillain-Barre syndrome, tetanus poisoning.
• Failure of 100% oxygen or CPAP to revert apnea/respiratory failure.
Method   Mechanical ventilation needs intubation of the trachea.
Types
• Conventional ventilators

Monitoring
- Oscillator or high frequency jet ventilators.
- Admit acutely ill patients needing mechanical ventilation, to ICU
- Continuous ECG monitoring
- Vital signs, serum electrolytes, fluid balance and urine output
- Mental and neurological status – ventilator parameters and tracheal cuff pressures
- Arterial pH, pCO_2 and PO_2 – to assess alveolar ventilation and arterial ventilation by clinical and investigative measures is vital
- Adequate ventilation: Patient shows pink color, adequate air entry and chest expansion, absence of chest retraction, prompt capillary filling in < 2 sec, BP – normal. Pulse oximetry – 90–95% oxygen saturation. Blood gas – PAO_2 60–90 mm Hg, $PaCO_2$ 40–45 mm Hg, pH 7.3–7.45.

Weaning from Ventilator

Indications
- Hemodynamics status – stable
- Neurological status (level of consciousness) – stable
- Fractional inspired oxygen FiO_2 – reduced
- Underlying disease and complications – improved

New Imaging Techniques

- Ultrasonography (US)
- Computed tomography (CT) scan
- Magnetic resonance imaging (MRI)
- Nuclear medicine procedures

Advantages   Enhancement of diagnostic precision

Disadvantages   Expensive techniques

Misuse – as a substitute for clinical workup and simple tests.

Ultrasonography

Most frequently employed non-invasive imaging technique in childhood.

Technique   The transducer translates the reflection of sound waves from interfaces in tissues into cross-sectional images of normal and abnormal anatomy.

Indications   Neuro-ultrasonography: For hydrocephalus, intracranial disorders, intracranial hemorrhage, tumors

Cervical ultrasonography: For cervical adenitis

Cardiac ultrasonography: For congenital and acquired heart diseases, (echocardiography) for determining effects of cardiac drugs

Abdominal ultrasonography: For pyloric stenosis, intussusception, appendicitis, cholelithiasis, etc.

Skeletal ultrasonography: For congenital dislocation of hip

Prenatal ultrasonography: For evaluation of fetus growth

Misuse: For sex determination.

Computed Tomography (CT) Scan

Technique	It consists in obtaining digitalized cross-sectional images by rapid bursts of X-rays during one revolution of both tube and detectors which are on opposite sides of child to be scanned. It can distinguish among structures.
Indications	Evaluation of trauma – head and neck injuries, hydrocephalus
	Planning reconstructive craniofacial surgery
	Detecting – bronchiectasis, pulmonary metastases.

Magnetic Resonance Imaging (MRI)

Technique	MRI yields images reflecting magnetic differences in body tissue rather than difference in X-ray absorption or acoustic reflection.
	Images are obtained in the sagittal, coronal, and axial planes
Indications	Displaying brain tumors and demyelinating diseases
	Spinal cord and canal imaging – procedure of choice
	Congenital heart disease
	Tumors of skeletal tissues, liver, pelvis, mediastinum
	Epiphyseal injuries.

Nuclear Medicine (Radionuclide Scintigraphy)

Nuclear medicine procedures are safe, reproducible and cost-effective.

Indication	To obtain functional information about various organ systems.
Technique	Special imaging devices like gamma cameras and computer system give static or dynamic images. Different compounds labeled with the isotope 99 m-technetium (^{99m}Tc), are utilized to evaluate various organ systems, e.g.
	GIT: ^{99m}Tc-sulfur colloid orphytate (oral).
	Musculoskeletal: ^{99m}Tc-MDP
	CVS: ^{99m}Tc-RBC
	GUS: ^{99m}Tc-DTPA
	Oncology: ^{99m}Tc-MDP, 201 thalidium chloride
	Premedication: Sedation and immobilization required.

References

1. Petersdorf R. Fever of unknown origion. An old friend revisited. Arch Intern Med 152:21;1992.
2. Baun S, Litman N: Mumps virus.In: Mandell GL, Bennett JE, Dolin R; (eds). Infectious Diseases. Fourth edition. New York: Churchill Livingstone 1496–1501;1995.
3. Pawlotsky JM. Use and interpretation of virological tests for hepatitis C. Hepatology 36 (suppl 1): S65–S73;2002.
4. Thomas DL. Hepatitis C and human immunodeficiency virus infection. Hepatology 36 (suppl 1): S201–S209;2002.
5. Dubey AP. Hepatitis B immunization in children. Acad Today 3:43–4;1998.
6. Lemon SM, Thomas DL: Vaccines to prevent viral hepatitis. N Engl J Med 336:196–204;1997.

7. Rigau Perez JG, Clark GG, Gubler DJ, et al. Dengue and dengue hemorrhagic fever. The Lancet 352:971–7;1998.

8. Diphtheria, Pertusis and tetanus. Recommendation for vaccine use and other preventive measures. MMWR 40:RR-10;1991.

9. Wesley AG, Pather M: Tetanus in children: An 11-year review. Ann Trop Pediatr 7:32;1987.

10. Hunter D, Bomford RR (editors): Hutchison's Clinical Methods, 14th ed. Cassel, London, 1964.

11. Gill D, O' Brien N: Pediatric Clinical Examination. London : Churchill Livingstone. 1988.

12. Mandell GL, Bennett JE, Dolin R. Principles and Practice of Infectious Diseases. New York: Churchill Livingstone; 1995.

13. Gupte S: The Short Text Book of Pediatrics, 10th ed. Jaypee Bros. New Delhi.

14. Tuberculosis in Children. Guidelines for diagnosis, prevention and treatment (A statement of the Scientific Committees of the IUATLD. Edited by Hershifield E.) Bulletin of International Union against Tuberculosis and Lung diseases. 66:61–7, 1991. WHO. Stop TB at source. WHO report on TB epidemic. Geneva 1995.

15. Brooks MH, Kiel FW, Sheeby TW, Barry JG: Acute pulmonary edema in falciparum malaria. A clinicopathological correlation. N Engl J Med 279:732–7;1968.

16. Looareesuwan S, Wilairatana P: Guideline in management of severe malaria. JIMA 10:628–31; 2000.

17. Warrel DA: Cerebral malaria: clinical features, pathophysiology and treatment. Ann Trop Med Parasitol 91:875–84;1997.

18. Ghai OP, Gupta P, Paul VK: Ghai Essential Pediatrics, 6th ed.

19. Dengue Hemorrhagic Fever: Diagnosis, Treatment, Prevention and Control. 2nd ed. World Health Organization. Geneva 1997.

20. Rigau Perez JG, Clark GG, Gubler DJ, et al. Dengue and dengue hemorrhagic fever. The Lancet 352:971–7;1998.

21. Goetting MG: Progress in Pediatric CPR. Em Med Clin North Am 13:291–320;1995.

22. Brown K, Bocock J: Update in pediatric resuscitation. Emerg Med Clin North Am. 20:1–26;2002.

23. Guidelines 2000 for cardiopulmonary resuscitation and emergency. Cardiovascular care. Pediatric basic life support. Circulation 102:253–90;2000.

24. Henretig FM, King C: Practical Emergency Procedures. Hong Kong: Williams and Wilkins, 1997.

25. Guidelines 2000 for cardiopulmonary resuscitation and emergency cardiovascular care. Pediatric advanced life support. Circulation 102:291–342;2000.

26. Tiwari UC, Singh S, Singh H, Rajput R Meena. Pulmonary Manifestations in Malaria. Jima 10:612–14, 200.

27. Tobias JD: Shock in children: the first 60 mts. Pediatr Ann 25:330–38;1996.

28. Graeffe R: Practical Pediatric Procedures. New York Hobel, 1997.

29. Singhi SC: Intraosseous infusion. Indian Pediatr 29:253;1992.

30. Katariya S: Pediatric imaging today. In: Gupte S (ed). Recent Advances in Pediatrics. Vol 8. New Delhi: Jaypee Brothers, 1998.

Geriatric Emergencies and Common Disorders

Geriatric illnesses	Frozen shoulder (periarthritis of shoulder)
Alzheimer's disease (dementia)	Osteoarthritis (degenerative joint diseases)
Parkinson's disease (syn. paralysis agitans)	Ischemic heart disease
Recurrent fall (falls in elderly)	Hypertension in elderly
Osteoporosis	Chronic pulmonary disease

Geriatric Illnesses

Increase in life expectancy, worldwide, over the last two decades, because of control of communicable diseases, better healthcare and health awareness, and improved economic scenario, has increased the ageing population above 60 years. The huge burden of ageing population has become the prey of several geriatric illnesses:

1. Neurological disorders, e.g.
   Alzheimer's disease (dementia)
   Parkinson's disease
   Falls in elderly
   Stroke
2. Inflammatory disorders, e.g.
   Osteoporosis
   Frozen shoulder
   Osteoarthritis
   Rheumatoid arthritis
   Cervical and lumbar spondylosis
   Tuberculosis
   Syphilitic
3. Cardiovascular disorders
   Ischemic heart disease
   Hypertension in elderly
4. Pulmonary diseases, e.g.
   Acute bronchitis
   Acute pneumonia
   Acute asthma

             Acute pulmonary edema

             Lung abscess

5. Traumatic disorders, e.g.

             Fracture: Neck of femur

                      Spine

                      Colles'

             Dislocation, sprain

6. Neoplastic disorders

             Carcinoma: Lungs

                      Breast

                      Prostate

                      Thyroid

                      Kidneys

                      GI tract

                      Genitourinary tract

7. Miscellaneous disorders

- Osteosclerosis, deafness, cataract, blindness,
- Diabetic retinopathy

Note: Most of these disorders described in appropriate sections of Respiratory, Orthopedic and Neoplastic (Oncology) Disorders.

Alzheimer's Disease (Dementia)

Definition	It is a clinical syndrome characterized by acquired loss of cognitive and emotional abilities (loss of memory and cognitive functioning) that impairs with daily living activities, and as the illness progresses, it results in various behavioral and psychiatric symptoms. It is an elderly disease and that prevalence increases exponentially with age. More specifically the prevalence doubles with every five years increase in age.
Etiology	Traumatic – head injury
	Infective – cerebral infection, tuberculosis, syphilis
	Vascular – arteriosclerosis of cerebral arteries
	Malnutrition – deficiency of vitamin B_{12} and folic acid, cholinergic
	Alcohol abuse
	Endocrinal disorders – diabetes mellitus, estrogen depletion
	Emotional – stress, anxiety
	Toxic – amyloid, glutamate
	Metabolic disorders – brain tumors
Risk factors	Senility, female sex, less education, family history of dementia, Down syndrome, stroke, hypertension, heart disease, hyperlipidemia, thyroid disorders, hydrocephalus
Protective factors	Antioxidants, e.g. vitamin E, C, turmeric.

	Estrogen supplements
	Anti-inflammatory drugs, e.g. NSAIDs
	Education and social status, e.g. higher education and healthy status
Diagnosis	Age > 60 years
	Loss of memory and cognitive functioning
	Impaired daily living activities
	Behavioral and psychiatric disturbances
	Family history of dementia
	Malnourishment
Investigation	Complete hemogram, ESR
	Serological tests for syphilis:

Serological tests for syphilis:
- Complement fixation (Wassermann)
- Flocculation (VDRL)

Serum proteins, serum cholesterol, serum electrolytes
BUN, blood glucose
CSF examination.

Management A person suffering from Alzheimer's disease (AD)/dementia needs medical care. Family members are counseled by psychologist. They are explained about the diagnosis, its implication and how to handle the patient.

Treatment of the cause:

Results from recent therapeutic trials in AD are both encouraging and discouraging. Etiologic hypotheses and drugs currently available or under study for Alzheimer's disease are:

Cholinestrase inhibitors

Drugs Donepezil 5–10 mg o.d.
S/E: Nausea, vomiting, diarrhea, muscle cramps

Galantamine 8–24 mg o.d.
S/E: Anorexia, weight loss

Rivastigmine 3–12 mg o.d.
S/E: Nausea, vomiting, diarrhea

N-methyl-D-aspartate (NMDA) receptor antagonist

Drugs Memantine 5–10 mg o.d.
S/E: Nausea, vomiting, diarrhea

Anti-inflammatory drugs (NSAIDs): Results are not encouraging

Drugs Celecoxib 100–200 mg o.d. PO
S/E: GI tract, liver, renal toxicity

Diclofenac 75 mg o.d./bid IM followed by 60 mg b.i.d. PO

Estrogen replacement therapy (ERT): Results are not encouraging

Drugs Conjugated estrogens, raloxifene 1.25 mg o.d.
S/E: Deep venous thrombosis

Antioxidants:

Drugs   Vitamin E 1000 IU b.i.d. PO

Near future therapies

Amyloid inhibitor agents

Drugs   Vaccination with amyloid beta-42, amyloid beta, gamma-secretase Inhibitors, may dramatically improve AD therapy, but not available currently for general clinical use.

Note: The medical and surgical treatments have remarkably upgraded the management of AD, but so far the results are dismal.

Refer: The patient to geriatric, psychiatric and medical teams.

Parkinson's Disease (syn. Paralysis Agitans)

Described in appropriate section of Nervous System Emergencies.

Recurrent Fall (Falls in Elderly)

Definition   Falls are a major health problem amongst the elderly, and the rate increases with the advancing age, resulting in fractures and contributory factor in admissions in the hospitals/nursing homes.

Risk factors   *Neurological:* Cerebral, cerebellar and spinal cord disorders affecting balance, e.g. Parkinson's disease, AD, peripheral neuropathy

Musculoskeletal: Muscular weakness of lower limbs, PIVD, sciatica, arthritis, deformed lower limbs

Visual disorders: Cataracts, glaucoma, retinal degeneration

Hearing defects: Vertigo, deafness

Psychological: Cognitive impairment or depression postural hypotension

CVS: Arrhythmias, IHD

Environmental – defective street lights, uneven/broken roads, slippery pathways.

Assessment   Medical

Mental status

Visual acuity, perimetry, audiometry

Sensory – vibration and proprioception testing

Muscle power

Blood pressure

Environmental

Management

Preventive treatment

Health promotion and falls prevention:
* Ensuring safety around the home, e.g. proper environment
* Regular check up/counseling by family/attached doctor
* Regular vision and hearing check up
* Regular exercise

Medication review

Avoidance of psychotropic medications in the first instance. Need for long-term support when reducing psychotropic medications.

Exercise

An exercise regime at home, better under the guidance of an expert physiotherapist/yoga teacher, reduces the risk of falls in elderly at home. Safety is prime consideration in determining an aged person's ability to participate in a home exercise regime especially where balance exercises are performed.

Home modifications

- Adequate lighting in the home
- Walkways and corridors – to be kept clear and well lit
- Repair and replace carpets with worn areas, holes, shreds
- Tables and benches – do not have sharp edges
- Doors – open easily
- Clear away garden tools from the walkways and keep paths well swept and non-slippery

Injury minimization

- Calcium and vitamin D: For reducing incidence of fractures in elderly due to osteoporosis
- Use of a walking aid: Stick, umbrella or crutches
- Avoid use of worn or slipping and poorly fitting shoes, high/narrow heels.

Osteoporosis

Osteoporosis is a worldwide phenomenon, being considered now as a common geriatric disorder. No race or sex has been spared.

Definition

It is defined as a progressive systemic disease characterized by reduced bone mass and deteriorating bone tissue (matrix), thereby resulting in increased bone fragility and subsequently a fracture may occur with a minor injury, when the bone loss > 30%.

Etiology

Primary   Unknown

Secondary   Traumatic: Prolongaed immobilization

Inflammatory: Rheumatoid arthritis, tuberculous, syphilitic

Endocrinal: Lack of androgens – senile osteoporosis

Lack of estrogens: Post-menopausal osteoporosis

Hypopituitarism: Hypogonadism

Hyperthyroidism: Thyrotoxicosis

Hyperparathyroidism

Excessive ACTH or corticosteroids – Cushing's syndrome

Diabetes mellitus

Pregnancy

Metabolic   Calcium deficiency

Neoplastic	Multiple myeloma.
Risk factors	Age: > 60 yrs.
	Sex: F: M ratio 6:2
	Race: Asian
	Built: Thin
	Menopause: Early
	Alcohol abuse: Excess intake
	Smoking: Cigarettes
	Diet: Poor diet
	Life style: Sedentary
	Activity: Lack of physical activity (exercise)
	Drugs: Heparin and corticosteroids – prolonged use.
Diagnosis	Asymptomatic to severe backache
	May be found accidently on X-ray examination for a fracture
	Fracture: Occurrence of a fracture is the most common finding, e.g.
	Sites: Fracture neck of femur
	Fracture vertebral body (crush)
	Colles' fracture
	Pain: Low backache – localized or radiating
	Deformity
	Height: Loss of height.
Investigation	Serum calcium, phosphate and alkaline phosphatase – are normal.
	X-ray shows: Areas of demineralization of spine, pelvis, limbs
	Fracture: Compression fracture of vertebral body
	Fracture neck of femur
	Colles' fracture

Bone densitometry (BMD) measurement: May be an important test in early diagnosis of bone mineral loss.

Technique: Ultrasound (US) of the os calcis

Other sites: Lumbar spine, neck of femur and distal end of radius

The BMD measurement is recorded as a T score:

(Patient's BMD compared to BMD of a healthy young adult)

And a Z score:

(Patient's BMD compared to BMD of same sex and age person)

Interpretation: Depending on the T score the patient's fracture risk can be calculated and treated accordingly (Table 14.1).

CT scan	Quantitative CT scan
MRI	Quantitative MRI
DEXA	(Dual Energy X-ray absorptiometry) – is a valuable test
Disadvantage	It is an expensive procedure
Bone Biopsy	Rarely done – being an invasive and time consuming procedure.

Table 14.1: T score interpretation	
T score	*Interpretation*
0 to −1	Normal
1 to −2.5	Osteopenia
< −2.5	Osteoporosis
< −2.5 with fracture	Frank osteoporosis

(Source: World Health Organisation)

Management

Aims To prevent or reduce the level of osteoporosis.

General measures

Diet: High protein diet and adequate in calcium (milk and milk products)

Exercise: Regular exercise especially weight bearing

Stop smoking

Reduce alcohol intake

Calcium and vitamin D:

- Calcium (carbonate or lactate) 1–2 g o.d.
- Vitamin D: Alfacalcidol and calcitriol
- Alfacalcidol 0.25 μg–1.0 μg o.d.
- Calcitriol 0.25–0.5 μg o.d.

Analgesics

Specific measures:

I. Antiresorptives:

A. Hormone replacement therapy (HRT)

Indication: Postmenopausal osteoporosis

Drugs

1. Estrogens

Indication	Postmenopausal osteoporosis
	Intact uterus: Estrogen along with progesterone given to reduce chances of malignancy
	Hysterectomised: Estrogen given alone
Agents	• Natural estrogens: Estradiol, estrone, conjugated estrogens
	• Synthetic estrogens: Ethinyl estradiol, mestranol, stilbestrol
Dose	Ethinyl estradiol 0.05 mg t.d.s. Maint. 0.025 mg/day
	Conjugated estrogen 0.625 mg/day
	Estriol 4 mg/day for 2/52. Maint. 1–2 mg/day

2. Combined Estrogen + testosterone:

Indication	Postmenopausal osteoporosis
Agents	Mixogen (ethinylestradiol + methyltestosterone)
Dose	1–2 mg/day PO or 1 mL IM every 3–4 wks.
C/I	Breast cancer, vaginal bleeding, pregnancy, liver disease

3. Progestogens

Indication	Adjunct to estrogen replacement therapy (HRT) in menopausal women with an intact uterus
Agents	Norethindrone acetate
Dose	5–10 mg/day from 14th to 28th days of each cycle

4. Androgens

Indication	Hypogonadic androgen deficiency osteoporosis
Agents	Testosterone 25–50 mg IM twice weekly for 4–6 wks.
C/I	Suspected cases of breast or prostate carcinoma

B. Bisphosphonates

Indication	Postmenopausal, steroid induced and senile osteoporosis
Agents	• Alendronate 10 mg/day or 70 mg/wk.
	• Etidronate 400 mg/day for 2/52 followed by 11/52. Rept. 4 cycles/yr.
	• Other newer drugs: Ibandronate, risodronate and tiludronate

S/E: Esophagitis, gastritis and disturbance of bone mineralization

C. Calcitonin

Indication	Postmenopausal osteoporosis and osteogenesis imperfecta
Dose	100 units/day IM or s.c.

S/E: Flushing, local irritation, diarrhea

D. Thiazides

Indication	Hypercalciuria
Dose	Hydrochlorothiazide 25–50 mg/day 5.

II. Mineral supplements

Calcium supplementation

Indication	Postmenopausal and senile osteoporosis
Dose	Calcium (carbonate or lactate) 1000–2000 mg/day

Fluoride supplementation

Indication	Enhances bone formation
Dose	20–50 mg o.d.

Anabolic steroids

Indication	As an adjunctive therapy in the treatment of osteoporosis
Agents	Nandrolone decanoate (metadec) 25–100 mg every 3rd week IM
	Nandrolone phenylpropionate (durabolin, metabol) 25–50 mg/wk.IM
D/d	Osteomalacia and rickets
	In osteoporosis, there is a reduction in the bone mass and the mineral – matrix ratio is maintained, in contrast to osteomalacia and rickets – in which mineral – matrix ratio is disturbed due to reduced mineralization.

Frozen Shoulder (Periarthritis of Shoulder)

Definition	It is an inflammatory disorder of the soft tissues affecting the middle and the old aged.
Etiology	Traumatic: Fracture, dislocation, subluxation, rotator cuff tears
	Inflammatory: Rotator cuff tendinitis, supraspinatus calcification, bicipital tendonitis, glenohumeral arthritis, tuberculous
	Cardiovascular: Postmyocardial infarction
	Neoplastic: Lung tumors.
Diagnosis	Pain in the shoulder, which becomes worse at night
	Stiffness of the shoulder – increases with the passage of time
	Movements – painful and restricted.
Investigation	X-ray shoulder: Shows no abnormality
	In late stages: Calcified area may be seen in the region of supraspinatus tendon above head of humerus.

Management

Conservative treatment

Physiotherapy: Heat, e.g. infrared, short-wave diathermy, exercise, manipulation under anesthesia – in advanced cases

Analgesics

Intra-articular corticoids – for relief of shoulder pain and stiffness.

Surgical treatment: May be undertaken to remove the calcified deposit.

Refer: The patient to the orthopedic team.

Osteoarthritis (Degenerative Joint Disease)

Definition	It is defined as a chronic, progressive, arthropathy, characterized by degeneration of articular cartilage (architectural deterioration) and by formation (hypertrophy) of bone at the articular margins, and without systemic manifestations. It is the commonest type of arthritis the world over.
Etiology	Primary or idiopathic – commonly affecting the DIP joints
	Secondary – affecting any joint due to pre-existing joint disorders:

- Traumatic: Injury to articular cartilage due to:
  - Intra-articular causes, e.g. intra-articular fracture or dislocation
  - Extra-articular causes, e.g. bony block, torn muscle/tendon

  MOI: RSA, sports injury, fall from a height
- Inflammatory: Rheumatoid arthritis
- Infective: Septic arthritis, tuberculosis
- Endocrinal: Diabetes mellitus
- Metabolic: Hyperparathyroidism
- Neuropathic: Tabes dorsalis

Risk factors
- Advancing age: > 60 yrs.
- Overweight

- Wrong posture and misuse of the joint
- Strenuous exercises include regular use of stairs

Pathogenesis (Table 14.2)
- Synovitis: Hypersecretion of synovial fluid (SF), synovial membrane inflamed, e.g. thickened, hypertrophied
- Articular cartilage: Softened, roughened, wormed
- Synovial membrane: Inflamed, e.g. thickened, hypertrophied
- Subchondral bone: Sclerosis, ebunation, cysts formation
- Articular surfaces: Osteophytes
- Ankylosis: Bony.

Table 14.2: Pathogenesis of osteoarthritis			
Stage	Pathogenesis	Effects	Clinical (S/s)
I A	Synovitis	Hypersecretion – SF, Joint distension	Joint swelling, pain
		Synovium – thickened, hypertrophied	Disability
I B	Joint capsule, bursae ligaments	Capsulitis, bursitis, tendinitis, muscle spasm tendinitis	Movements painful, local tenderness
II	Cartilage	Roughened, worming	Movements painful and restricted
III	Bone (subchondral)	Sclerosis, eburnation, cysts and osteophytes	Pain, disability,
IV	Joint	Ankylosis (bony)	Movements restricted or absent

Diagnosis
- Age > 60 yrs.
- Onset – insidious
- Morning stiffness of joints
- Pain – presenting symptom: Dull aching, aggravated by joint use, weight bearing, relieved by rest
- Systemic manifestations – absent
- Swelling, or deformity
- Muscular wasting
- Crepitus
- Movements – painful and restricted.

Investigation X-ray shows: Asymmetric narrowing of the joint space
Osteophytes at joint margins
MRI studies – may reveal early changes, missed in X-rays
CT scan – indicated in cervical or lumbar spondylosis associated with neurologic manifestation.

Management

Aims
- To relieve pain

- To improve joint function
- To prevent deformities

Preventive treatment

Occupational therapy: Joint protection and conservation by:

- Avoiding joint stress, e.g. squatting, ascending/descending stairs, prolonged standing, long walks.

Conservative treatment

Physiotherapy Exercises – muscle strengthening exercises

- Active
- Passive
- Traction
- Heat, e.g. infrared, short wave diathermy
- Massage, e.g. stroking, compression
- Aid devices for ambulation, e.g. a walking stick or a walker, crutches, braces/belts, cervical collars
- Acupuncture and acupressure
- Yoga therapy

Medical treatment:

Drugs	Analgesics and non-steroidal anti-inflammatory drugs (NSAIDs)
Caution	Elderly patients are especially vulnerable to NSAID toxicity
I/A injection	Intra-articular steroids – for relief of pain:

- Hydrocortisone acetate 25 mg/mL + Lignocaine plain 1% 1 mL, Alt:
- Triamcinolone acetonide 40 mg/mL + Lignocain plain 1% 1 mL

Sodium hyaluronate 20 mg (2 mL) I/A Rpt b.i.w.

Caution	Not to be used frequently.

Surgical treatment

Indication	Persistent pain
	Reduction of activity
	Deformities
Surgery	Arthroscopic debridement: Excision of osteophytes, loose bodies, Synovectomy
	Reconstruction – debridement of the joint
	Arthroplasty – joint replacement
	Arthrodesis

Refer: The patient to the orthopedic team.

Ischemic Heart Disease (Arteriosclerotic Heart Disease)

Definition	It is the commonest cause of cardiovascular morbidity and mortality.
Etiology	Coronary artery disease (CAD).

Risk factors	Hyperlipidemia
	Diabetes mellitus
	Hypertension
	Past IHD
	Family history
	Smoking: Cigarette
	Obesity and overweight
	Physical inactivity, alcohol abuse.
Diagnosis	Age: > 60
	Sex: Men more affected than women
	Chest pain
	Breathlessness
	Headache
	Giddiness
	Difficulty in hearing, tingling sensations in ears
	Nausea, vomiting, sweating.
Investigation	Complete blood count
	Serum cholesterol
	Serum creatinine
	Serum glucose
	Serum calcium, potassium, magnesium
	Transaminases
	Uric acid
	ECG
	X-ray chest
	Treadmill test (TMT)
	Coronary angiography: To find the site and extent of narrowing.

Management

Preventive treatment

Avoid fried, fatty, fast food, and added salt
Avoid smoking of cigarettes
Avoid alcohol
Avoid/control obesity and over weight

General measures

Diet: Heart healthy diet, e.g. fruits and vegetables, salad
Lifestyle changes
Regular physical activity
Smoking cessation
Alcohol cessation

Medical treatment

Adequate treatment of hypertension and diabetes
Treatment of hyperlipidemias

Treatment of pathophysiology underlying the clinical manifestations of ischemic heart disease, e.g.

- Angina pectoris
- Acute myocardial infarction
- Coronary artery syndrome
- Heart failure
- Arrhythmias.

Surgical treatment: Coronary artery bypass grafting (CABG).

Refer: The patient to the cardiac team.

Hypertension in Elderly

Definition	Hypertension is a very common medical problem in the elderly. Number of elderly people is increasing due to improving health awareness. It is a major treatable cardiovascular risk factor. Hypertension increases with ageing. It occurs in more than two-thirds of individuals after the age of 65. Importance should be given to evaluate the comorbid conditions. It carries a very high risk for stroke and myocardial infarction.

Hypertension in elderly – defined as: BP > 160/100 mm Hg

Etiology	Primary and secondary
Primary or idiopathic	Cause unknown
Secondary	Atherosclerosis of renal arteries
	Acute and chronic glomerulonephritis
	Acute pyelonephritis
	Acute hydronephritis
	Cerebrovascular accident.
Risk factors	Age – a predictor of risk of subsequent CV mortality and morbidity
	Smoking
	Diabetes mellitus
	Dyslipidemia
	Family history of CVD, CVA, peripheral vascular disease
	Stress, anxiety.
Diagnosis	Age: > 65 years
	BP: > 160/100 mm Hg
	Headache
	Visual symptoms
	Palpitations
	Chest pain
	Difficulty in breathing
	Dyspnea on exertion
	Orthopnea
	Jugular venous distention
	Peripheral edema.

Investigation	Complete hemogram
	Lipid profile – HDL cholesterol, LDL cholesterol, triglycerides
	Serum creatinine and electrolytes – calcium, potassium
	Blood glucose
	Uric acid
	Urine examination
	ECG: Evidence of left ventricular hypertrophy increases risk of mortality in elderly
	CXR (X-ray chest)
Management	Treatment of hypertension, can significantly decrease the incidence of CV morbidity and improve quality of life in elderly patients.
Aim	To achieve BP of 140/90 mm Hg
Caution	Avoid volume depletion
General measures	
	Weight reduction
	Moderate physical exercise
	Avoid fried, fatty, fast food
	Take plenty of fruits, vegetables, salad
	Salt restriction
	Avoid smoking and alcohol
	Regular check-ups for BP, blood sugar and lipid profile
	Take regular prescribed medicines
Medical treatment	
	Antihypertensive therapy reduces the incidence of cardiovascular complications. Choice of antihypertensive medications should be based on patient's comorbidities and cost factor.
Drugs	Elderly patients who typically have low renin level, respond better to diuretics and CCB, while younger patients, who have high renin level, respond better to beta-blockers and angiotensin receptor inhibitors.
	Diuretics and CCB have been shown to reduce mortality and morbidity in elderly hypertensives.
Advantages	• Both groups of drugs are cheap and safe, and can be given o.d.
	• Medication with these, is the initial step of treatment.
Dose	Diuretics: Low dose of thiazide, e.g. hydrochlorthiazide 12.5 mg o.d.
	CCB: Nifedipine 30 mg o.d. or verapamil 90 mg o.d.
	Further medication of choice should be according to existing comorbid conditions.

Refer: The patient to the orthopedic team.

Chronic Pulmonary Disease

Described in appropriate section of Respiratory System Disorders.

References

1. David SG, Peter JW: Evaluation of dmentia. N Engl J Med 335:330–4;1996.
2. Evans DA, Funkenstein HH, Albert MS, Scherr PA, Cook NR, Chown MJ, et al. Prevalence of Alzheimer's disease in a community population of older persons: higher than previously reported. JAMA 262:2551–6;1989.
3. Bartus RT, Dean RL, Beer B, Lippa AS: The cholinergic hypothesis of geriatric memory dysfunction. Science. 217:408–414;1982.
4. Farlow MR: Alzheimer's Disease: Treatment update. CNS News. 5–12;2005.
5. Roy T, Dutt A, Chakraborty D, Biswas A: Dementia in India – A Critical Appraisal. JIMA Kolkata 103:154–160;2005.
6. Goldman SM, Tanner C: Etiology of Parkinson's disease. In: Jankovic J, (Ed). Parkinson's Disease and Movement Disorders. 3rd ed. Baltimore MD: Lippincott-Williams and Wilkins. 133–58;1998.
7. Tsui JK, Caine DB, Wang Y: Occupational risk factors in Parkinson's disease. Can J Public Health 90:334–7;1999.
8. Sengupta P, Mishra A, Ghosh B: Is Parkinson's Disease a Homogeneous Disorder. JIMA Kolkata 103:146–161;2005.
9. Campbell AJ, Reinken J, Allan Bc, Martinez GS: Falls in old age: a study of frequency and related clinical factors. Age Ageing 1981;10:264–70.
10. Guidelines' development group – Guidelines for the prevention of falls in people over 65. BMJ 49:664–72;2000.
11. Lach HW, Reed AT, Arfken CL, Miller JP, Paige GD, Birge SJ, et al: Falls in the elderly : reliability of a classification system. J Am Geriatr Soc 39:197–202;1991.
12. Dass CP, Joseph S: Falls in Elderly: JIMA Kolkata 103:136–144;2005.
13. Consensus development conference. Diagnosis, prophylaxis and treatment of Osteoporosis. Am J Med 90:107–10;1991.
14. Kapoor PS: Diagnosis, investigation and management of osteoporosis. The Indian Express 2002; 4 September.
15. Riggs BL, Hodgson SF, O'Fallon W.M. et al. Effect of fluoride treatment on Fracture rate in postmenopausal women with osteoporosis. N Engl J Med 327:802–9;1990.
16. Bhambhani M: Metabolic Bone Diseases. 14:29–34;2002.
17. Thornil TS: Shoulder pain-Manual of Rheumatology and Outpatient Orthopaedic Disorders. 3rd ed. Little, Brown and Company; 99–104.
18. Kapoor PS: Frozen shoulder. The Indian Express 2002; 6 November.
19. Joshi VR, Patel ND: Shoulder pain. J Gen Med 14: 35–37;2002.
20. Manek NJ, Lane NE: Osteoarthritis: current concepts in diagnosis and management. Am Fam Physician 61:1795–804;2000.
21. Hamerman D: Clinical implications of osteoarthritis and ageing. Ann Rheum Dis. 54:82–5;1995.
22. Kapoor PS: Osteoarthritis. The Indian Express 2002; 20 November.
23. Selwyn AP, Braunwald E: Ischemic heart disease. In: Wilson JD, Braunwald E. Isselbacher KJ, Petersdorf RG, Martin JB, Fauci AS, et al, editors. Harrison's Principles of Internal Medicine Vol 1. 12th ed. New York : McGraw-Hill. 964–71;1991.
24. Koppes G, McKiernan T, Bassan M, Froelicher VF: Treadmill exercise testing Part I and II. Curr Probi Cardiol 7:1–45;1977.
25. Resnick N: Geriatric Medicine. Harrison's Principles of Internal Medicine. New York: McGraw-Hill. 36–46;2001.
26. Sahoo R: Hypertension in the Elderly. CMJ 11:49–54;2005.
27. Sawhney JPS: Management of Hypertension. Family Medicine India 5:1–6;2001.

Skin Emergencies and Common Disorders

Common dermatoses
- Pruritus (itching)
- Pruritus ani and vulvae
- Acute urticaria and angioneurotic edema
- Atopic dermatitis (eczema)
- Psoriasis
- Seborrheic dermatitis
- Acne vulgaris
- Callosity
- Corn

Bacterial infections
- Boil
- Carbuncle
- Condyloma
- Erysipelas
- Cellulitis
- Decubitus ulcers (bedsores)

Fungal infections of skin
- Tinea capitis
- Tinea corporis
- Tinea cruris
- Tinea magnum and pedum

Viral infections
- Herpes simplex
- Herpes zoster
- Warts

Parasitic infections
- Scabies

Miscellaneous disorders
- Alopecia
- Keloids
- Hypertrichosis

Tumors of skin
- Benign – seborrheic warts
- Malignant – squamous cell carcinoma (epithelioma)
- Basal cell carcinoma (rodent ulcer)
- Malignant melanoma
- Paget's disease

Pruritus (syn. itching)

Definition	It is a sensation that initiates the urge to scratch. It is a modified type of pain, and is the commonest complaint of patients visiting dermatology department.
Etiology	Primary – idiopathic
	Secondary – hepatic or biliary disease, diabetes mellitus, nephritis, food and drug reaction, chemical irritants, stress, allergy, Hodgkin's disease.
Diagnosis	Itching
	Features of secondary disease.
Management	Removal of the cause
	Diet – avoid oily, hot, spicy foods

Proper hygiene

Daily baths, followed by dryness and use of talcum powder

Calamine lotion

Antihistaminic drugs

Corticosteroids.

Pruritus Ani and Vulvae

Etiology	Unknown.
Precipitating factors	Soaps, oils, colognes, douches, contraceptives, P/V exam, leucorrhea, diarrhea, worms, fungal infections, diabetes mellitus, psoriasis, seborrhea, hemorrhoids, unhygiene.
Diagnosis	Itching – mainly nocturnal
	Erythema.
Investigation	Hemogram, blood sugar, urinalysis.
Management	Diet – avoid hot, spicy junk foods
	Constipation – prevent/treat
	Proper hygiene
	Avoid irritant drugs
	Toilet of anus and vulva with savlon/dettol sol.
	Apply cream -- corticosteroid cream, calamine cream
	Antihistaminics.

Acute Urticaria and Angioneurotic Edema

Definition	A common inflammatory (allergic origin) condition of skin.
Etiology	Unknown – in majority of cases
	Allergy to foods or drugs:
	Foods: Fish, pork, egg, milk and milk products, fried and spicy foods, chocolate
	Drugs: Antibiotics (penicillin, sulphas), salicylates, opioids, NSAIDs, iodine, bromides, sera, vaccines, phenol, opium
	Infective: Bacterial, viral, parasitic
	Hepatitis – B.
Diagnosis	Itching, malaise, fever, nausea, vomiting, diarrhea
	Wheals – variable in size and shape, resolve within 24 hrs, may recur.
Investigations	CBC
	TLC and DLC – eosinophilia
	ESR
	C-reactive protein
	Skin prick test
	Complement fixation test
	LFT
	Stools examination – for worms.

Management
Emergency measures

> Airways maintenance – Endotrachial intubation, ventilator with oxygen
> Tracheostomy – may be required sometimes
> Drugs:
> Antihistaminics : Inj. epinephrine 0.3–1.0 ml of 1:1000 sol s.c. especially for laryngeal edema
> Corticosteroids
> IV fluids
> Local – antipruritic ointment

General measures

> Identify and avoid triggers
> Avoid spicy, hot, oily foods
> Avoid/less use of fish, pork, eggs, milk or milk products, chocolate
> Abstinence from use of unnecessary drugs/cosmetics.

Refer: The severe patient to the dermatology team.

Atopic Dermatitis (Eczema)

Definition — It is an inflammatory condition of the skin.

Etiology — Allergic – history (personal/family) of hay fever, asthma, eczema.

Diagnosis — Itching – mild to severe

Lesions – dry, leathery, lichenified, over face, neck, trunk, hands, feet.

Investigation — CBC

TLC and DLC – eosinophilia.

Management
General measures

> Avoid stress
> Diet – nutritious. Avoid spicy, oily, junk foods
> Avoid: Local irritants, e.g. exposure to irritating drugs, chemicals, soaps, fumes, leather shoes.

Specific measures

> Corticosteroids – triamcinolone 20 mg IM
> Local: Creames, ointments, lotions – containing antipruritic, lubricating, keratolytic agents.

Psoriasis

Definition — It is an acute or chronic inflammatory condition of the skin, characterized by silvery scales

Etiology — Unknown

May be a genetic disorder.

Precipitating factors — Trauma, irritation, stress.

Diagnosis	Itching
	Lesions – silvery scales on the scalp, knees, legs, elbows, forearm, chest, abdomen and back.
	Arthritis
	Stippled nails.
Management	Avoid irritating drugs/chemicals
	Warm baths, ultraviolet irradiation
	Corticosteroids:

- Triamicinolone 2.5 mg IM

  Local: Triamicinolone acetonide oint. or cream, b.i.d., Alt :
  Betamethasone valerate oint. or cream b.i.d., Alt :
  Calcipotriol ointment (Vitamin-D) – apply b.i.d.

- Ammoidine 0.7 mg/kg body wt. E.O.D. PO

  Local: Ammoidine cream or lotion – apply o.d.

Seborrheic Dermatitis

Definition	It is an acute or chronic dermatitis due to increased production of sebum
Etiology	Unknown
	May be a genetic disorder (hereditary)
Predisposing factors	Infective, nutritional, hormonal, and emotional – stress.
Diagnosis	Itching
	Lesions – dry scales or yellowish dandruff, on scalp, face, back, body folds.
Management	• Diet – avoid hot, spicy foods, sweets, alcohol
	• Proper rest, exercise, sleep, hygiene
	• Shampooing of hair with Selsun (selenium sulfide) lotion or shampoo, Dandruff plus, or Candid-TV,
	• Corticosteroid creams, lotions or solution.

Acne Vulgaris

Definition	It is a common inflammatory disorder of the sebaceous hair follicle, characterized by increased sebum excretion.
Etiology	Unknown
	May be a genetic disorder (hereditary).
Predisposing factors	• Infective – propionibacterium acnes
	• Cushing's syndrome
	• Sebaceous overactivity.
Diagnosis	Itching
	Lesions:
	• Blackheads (open comedons)
	• Whiteheads (closed comedones)

- Papules, pustules, nodules, or cysts, and scarring on the face, neck, chest, back, shoulders

Common in younger age

Commonest of all skin conditions.

Management	Aim is to prevent permanent scarring
	Diet: Avoid hot, spicy, fried foods, chocolate, nuts, alcohol, sweets
	Avoid unnecessary drugs especially iodides/bromides, oils, greases, cosmetics, irritable chemicals.
	Drugs: Antibiotics orally – tetracycline, trimethoprim, clindamycin
	Contraceptives orally – cyproterone with ethinylestradiol
	Corticosteroids – as anti-inflammatory
	Local: Tetmosol (sulfur) soap use
	Acne lotion – Retino-A lotion or cream or Benzoyl peroxide cream or lotion
	Extraction of blackheads with a comedo extractor.

Refer: The patient to a dermatologist.

Callosity
It is a localized hyperkeratosis.

Etiology	Chronic (prolonged) pressure or friction
	Occupational lesion – common in carpenters, Gardner's, violinist.
Diagnosis	Swelling over hand, finger, toes.
Management	Surgical – Excision with a sharp knife blade
	Apply betadine cream.

Corn
It is a callosity in which a cone-shaped horn projects into the corium.

Diagnosis	Pain – due to pressure of horn over the nerve endings
	Site – hard corns over bony prominences, precipitated by hard fitting shoes
	Soft corns – due to maceration by sweat, and are present in the interdigital clefts.
Management	Conservative treatment: Lysol application
	Surgical treatment: Excision (chiropod therapy).

Bacterial Infections of Skin
Boil (syn. Furuncle):   It is an infection of a hair follicle or a sebaceous gland.

Etiology	Bacterial infection – *Staphylococcus aureus*.
Diagnosis	Swelling, redness, tenderness, edema, pustule formation over top of swelling, which on bursting results in slough (infective gangrene).
Management	Analgesics, antibiotics, local antibiotic cream.

Carbuncle
It is an infective gangrene.

Etiology	Bacterial infection – *Staphylococcus aureus*.

Precipitating cause–diabetes mellitus.

Diagnosis	Swelling – hard, tender, red, vesicles, pustules, slough
	Fever, pain, malaise.
Management	Analgesics, antibiotics.

Condyloma

	Hypertrophy of epidermis.
Etiology	Syphilis.
Diagnosis	Swelling – fungating, sessile, raised, moist and sodden surface
	Site – angles of mouth, anus, vulva.
Management	Analgesics, antibiotics, surgical excision.

Erysipelas

It is a spreading acute inflammation of the skin and subcutaneous tissue, often following a scratch. It is extremely contagious, easily caught by contact with affected person.

Etiology	Bacterial infection – streptococci beta hemolytic.
Diagnosis	Rash: Rosy – red rash disappearing on pressure
	Pain, swelling, fever, chills, malaise.
Investigation	TLC and DLC – leukocytosis, ESR – raised.
Complications	May be fatal in very young and aged due to systemic toxemia.
Management	Rest, aspirin, antibiotics – penicillin.

Cellulitis

It is a spreading inflammation of skin and subcutaneous tissue, ending in suppuration, sloughing or gangrene. It affects deeper tissues comparative to erysipelas.

Etiology	Bacterial infection – streptococci, staphylococci, pneumococci.
Diagnosis	Fever – due to toxemia
	Swelling – hot, tender, brawny, edematous,
	Lymphadenitis.
Investigation	TLC and DLC – leukocytosis.
Management	Bed-rest, analgesics, antibiotics – penicillin.

Fungal Infections of Skin

Types	Tinea capitis, corporis, cruris, dermatophytosis, candidiasis.

Tinea Capitis (syn. Ringworm of Scalp)

Definition	An infection of scalp hair , occurring commonly in children.
Etiology	*Microsporum canis* and *Trichophyton*.
Transmission	Person to person contact, or by shared combs/hair brushes.
Diagnosis	Itching
	Lesions – round, grey, scaly patches on the scalp, present in solitary or multiple form
	Hair – brittle, discolored, hair loss.

Investigation   Microscopic examination of hairs – for organisms
                Cultural examination of hairs – for organisms.
Management   Self-limiting – may be
                Griseofulvin 0.25–0.5 g PO for 2/52.

Tinea Corporis (syn. Ringworm of body)

Definition   Lesions on exposed portions of the body, i.e. face, neck, arms.
Etiology   Dermatophyte fungi.
Diagnosis   Itching
                Lesions – clusters of rings of vesicles, asymmetrically distributed,
                      over exposed portions of the body.
Investigation   Microscopic examination – hyphae present
                Culture examination – confirms the diagnosis.
Management   Self-limiting
                Griseofulvin 0.5 g PO – for children
                          1.0 g PO o.d. – for adults
                Local – Oxiconazole cream or lotion
                      Povidone iodine cream or ointment.

Tinea Cruris (Jock itch)

Definition   Lesions on the groin and gluteal cleft.
Etiology   Dermatophyte fungi.
Diagnosis   Itching
                Lesions – erythematous macules with sharp margins, clear centres, in the
                intertriginus areas.
Investigation   Microscopic examination – hyphae present
                Culture examination – confirms the diagnosis.
Management   Griseofulvin 1 g PO o.d. for 1–2/52
                Local: Dusting powder
                      Oxiconazole cream or lotion.

Tinea Manum and Pedis (syn. Dermatophytosis)

Definition   Lesions on the palms and feet.
Etiology   Dermatophyte fungi.
Diagnosis   Itching
                Lesions.
Management   Griseofulvin 1 g PO o.d. for 1–2/52
                Local: Oxiconazole cream or lotion – apply b.i.d. or
                      Povidone-iodine cream or ointment – apply b.i.d.

Viral Infections of Skin
Herpes Simplex: It is an acute viral infection.

Etiology	Herpes virus.
Diagnosis	Neuralgia – burning and stinging
	Lesions – small, grouped vesicles over mouth, lips, genitals
	Lymph nodes (regional) – enlarged and tendered.
Investigation	CBC
	Tzanck test.
Management	
General	Remove the precipitating cause
	Local: Apply dusting powder, lotions
	Acyclovir cream – apply 4–5 times o.d. for 5–10 days.

Herpes Zoster (Shingles): It is an acute viral infection

Etiology	Virus identical with varicella virus.
Risk factors	Patients of Hodgkin's disease, lymphomas.
Diagnosis	Pain
	Lesions – grouped, tense, over face and trunk
	Lymph nodes (regional) – enlarged and tendered.
Investigation	CBC
	Varicella-zoster antibody test.
Management	
General	Analgesics – aspirin, paracetamol
	Hypnotics – barbiturates
	Corticosteroids – prednisone, triamcinolone.
Local	Povidone iodine oint. or crème

Wart

	It is a localized overgrowth of the epidermis.
Etiology	Viral infection.
Incubation	2–18/12
Diagnosis	Common in children
	Mostly present on the hands and are multiple.
Management	Curettage and cauterization of the crater.

Parasitic Infestations of Skin

Scabies

	It is a common skin disorder, affecting an entire family.
Etiology	Mite – *Sarcoptes scabby*.
Diagnosis	Itching – intense nocturnal.
	Lesions – vesicles and pustules in runs or galleries over sides of fingers and heels of palm, nipples, scrotum, buttocks.
Investigations	Microscopic study of mites, ova, black dots of feces.
Management	Scabicides: Kill the mites
	Agents: Lotions of benzyl benzoate, malathion, monosulfiram, lindane, crotamitons

Cream of permethrin

Advice: All members of affected family to be treated at same time

Method: To be applied to the whole body, below neck, at bedtime. Rept. for three consecutive nights

Oral ivermectin

C/I: Elderly and children.

Pediculosis	It is a common problem mostly found in children, more in girls.
Etiology	Parasite – *Pediculus humanus* (head lice).
Types	Pediculosis – capitis, corporis, pubis.
Transmission	By contact or shared – combs, towels, clothes.
Diagnosis	Itching
	Head lice – on skin or clothes
	Pyoderma.
Management	Advice: All members of affected family to be treated at same time
	Shampooning – with parasiticidal shampoos, on alternate days
	Wet combing of hair
	Pediculocides: Kill the lice
	Agents: Permethrin, phenothrin, lindane.

Miscellaneous Disorders of Skin
Hypertrichosis

Definition	It is defined as excessive hair growth on abnormal sites, and is a common disorder in females.
Etiology	Hereditary
	Nutritional
	Endocrinal
	Corticosteroids
	Metabolic
Diagnosis	Generalised hair growth (hirsutism)
	Localised hair growth – on ears, back.
Management	Shaving and applying of hair removal creme
	Drugs: Antiandrogens
	Electrolysis and diathermy – may destroy hair follicles permanently.

Keloids

Definition	It is defined as an overgrowth of fibrous tissue, occurring in the scars of burns, ulcers, vaccination, ear/nose piercing. It is not a tumor.
Etiology	Unknown – may be inheretid.
Diagnosis	Claw-like/finger-like processes – irregular, firm elevation of skin

Sites – face, neck, upper part of chest and abdomen

Itching.

Management | Excision
| Radiotherapy – pre- and postoperative.

Tumors of Skin

Benign

Seborrheic warts (syn. senile)

Originates from the skin as a pedunculated outgrowth.

Pathogenesis | It is a benign tumor – never undergoes malignant changes. Appears as a pedunculated outgrowth – like a finger or a cauliflower.
Etiology | Viral infection.
Diagnosis | Sites – trunk, neck, axilla
| Color – variable (pink, brown or black)
| Consistency – variable (soft or hard)
| Mobility – moves with the skin
| Painless.
Management | Not too unsightly or troublefree – no treatment required
| Too unsightly or troublesome – treated by:

- Cauterization: Chemical or electrical burning
- Cryosurgery: Freezing with CO_2
- Surgical removal – shaving with a scalpel.

Malignant

Squamous Cell Carcinoma (Epithelioma)

Originates from the prickle cell layer of the skin.

Pathogenesis | Appears as a small, hard, nodule, that ulcerates, forms a mass (cauliflower shape). It grows very rapidly.
Diagnosis | Sites: Exposed parts, e.g. lip, tongue, genitals (penis), anus
| Pain
| Lymphadenitis.
Complications | Metastasis – to regional lymph nodes, vital organs.
Investigation | CBC
| CXR
| Biopsy.
Management | Chemotherapy
| Radiotherapy
| Surgery.

Basal Cell Carcinoma (Rodent Ulcer)

Originates from the basal layer of the rete malpighii.

Pathogenesis	Appears as a small, red, hard, nodule, with shiny surface, that ulcerates. It grows slowly.
Diagnosis	Sites: Exposed parts, e.g. upper part of face
	Pain
	Lymphadenitis – not common.
Complications	Metastasis – rare to regional lymph nodes, vital organs.
Investigation	CBC
	CXR
	Biopsy.
Management	Chemotherapy
	Radiotherapy
	Surgery.

Malignant Melanoma

It is a highly malignant tumor of skin involving melanin producing cells.

Pathogenesis	Appears as a small, hard, black or brown nodule, that ulcerates.
Diagnosis	Sites: Exposed parts, e.g. hand, foot, anus, choroid of eye, mole
	Pain
	Lymphadenitis.
Complications	Metastasis – to regional lymph nodes, vital organs – liver, lungs.
Investigation	CBC
	CXR
	Biopsy.
Management	Chemotherapy
	Radiotherapy
	Surgery.

Paget's Disease

It is a malignant tumor of the apocrine sweat gland. It is an uncommon breast cancer.

Pathogenesis	The nipple and areola become red (rash), covered with scales. Later on the scales get detached and the nipple gets destroyed, disappears.
Diagnosis	Sites: Nipple, genitalia
	Itching
	Rash – resembling eczema
	Lymphadenitis.
Complications	Metastasis – to regional lymph nodes, vital organs – liver, lungs.
Investigation	CBC
	CXR
	Biopsy
Management	Chemotherapy
	Radiotherapy
	Surgery.

Practical procedures

Patch testing
Indications: Contact dermatitis
Skin biopsy
Indications: Inflammatory disorders
Tumors.

References

1. Domonkos A: Andrews' Diseases of the Skin. Saunders, 1971.
2. Rees B. Rees, Jr. Skin and Appendages. Current Medical Diagnosis and Treatment. Maruzen Asian Ed. 1975.
3. Gulhati CM: MIMS, Vol 28 No. 9, New Delhi, 2008.
4. Arora V: Drug Update, Vol 7 Issue-II, Sri Ganganagar, 2010.

Arthritis and Allied Rheumatic Emergencies

- Rheumatoid arthritis
- Ankylosing spondylitis
- Acute septic arthritis
- Acute gout
- Acute carpal tunnel syndrome
- Acute suppurative tendosynovitis

- Acute stenosing tenosynovitis (de Quervain's disease)
- Trigger finger and thumb
- Acute low backache
- Acute sciatica
- Prolapse intervertebral disc (PIVD)

Rheumatoid Arthritis

Definition   It is a chronic systemic inflammatory disorder of unknown etiology, characterized by symmetrical polyarthritis, joint destruction, deformity, disability, often leading to serious morbidity.

Epidemiology   Sex: Female: Male 3:1
               Age: 20–40 yrs, however, it may commence at any age.

Etiology   Unknown. May be due to autoimmunity, or infection.

Pathogenesis   (Table 16.1)

Acute phase   • Synovitis: Hypersecretion of synovial fluid (SF), synovial membrane inflamed, e.g. thickened, hypertrophied
               • Synovial membrane, capsule, ligaments, tendons – inflamed
               • Pannus formation
               • Articular cartilage – roughened, eroded, worn out

Chronic phase • Subchondral bone – eroded, sclerosis, ebunation, cysts formation
               • Articular surfaces: Osteophytes
               • Ankylosis: Fibrous

Diagnosis   Diagnostic criteria of rheumatoid arthritis (Table 16.2)
               • Onset of inflammatory signs: Usually insidious with prodromal symptoms of malaise, loss of weight, pain, fever, sweating or paresthesias (vasomotor disturbances) of hands or feet
               • Morning stiffness: Prolonged and aggravates post-strenuous activities
               • Pain: Mostly the main complaint, characteristic of periodical attacks
               • Polyarthritis: Usually of 3 or > joints (swollen/deformed)
               • Arthritis of small joints of hand and feet (wrist, MTP, PIP, ankle, MTP)

Table 16.1: Pathogenesis of rheumatoid arthritis

Phase	Pathogenesis	Effects	Clinical (S/s)
Acute A	Synovitis	Hypersecretion – SF, Joint distension,	Joint swelling, pain, disability
	Joint capsule, bursae, ligaments	Capsulitis, bursitis, tendinitis, muscle spasm tendinitis	Movements painful, local tenderness
	Pannus formation	Cartilage eroded, roughened, Bone erosion, ligaments and tendons erosion	Movements painful and restricted
Chronic	Organization	Ankylosis (fibrous)	Movements restricted or absent

- Subcutaneous nodules: Over bony prominences (points), in tendon sheaths or bursae
- Progression: It is centripetal and symmetrical

Investigation — CBC, ESR, TLC and DLC

Serological tests:

- Rheumatoid factor (latex particle agglutination): Usually positive
- Synovial fluid analysis: Immunoglobulin (quantitative) IgA, IgM, IgG

X-ray wrists and hands: Early changes seen are osteoporosis around the affected joint and erosion of cartilage at the periphery of the joint surface.

Management — The treatment is unsatisfactory. Till date any specific treatment of RA not available. The patient should be explained fully about RA being an incurable disease and that he/she better learn to live with it.

Conservative measures

Rest — Complete bed-rest indicated in patients with profound systemic and articular involvement

In mild cases – few hours rest may suffice, allowing patient to continue his/her routine work, while avoiding strenuous activities.

Table 16.2: Criteria for classification of rheumatoid arthritis

Criteria	Comment
1. Onset of S/S – insidious	Insidious with prodromal symptoms: fever, malaise, weight loss, sweating/paresthesia
2. Morning stiffness	Prolonged: For > 1 hr/day and for > 6/52
3. Polyarthritis of 3 or > joints	Joints swollen/deformed for > 6/52
4. Arthritis of small joints (hand/feet)	Wrists, MCP or PIP joints > 6/52, ankles, MTP or PIP joints > 6/52
5. Progression	Centripetal and symmetrical
6. Rheumatoid nodule	Subcutaneous nodule over bony points, in bursae and tendon sheaths
7. Radiographic changes	Osteoporosis, joint erosions
8. Serum rheumatoid factor	Usually positive

Heat and cold	Used for their muscle relaxant and analgesic effect

- Infra-red and short-wave therapy – very effective
- Even cold application helps in relief of pain.

Exercise	Active and passive.
Drugs	Analgesics:

Action : Analgesia

Agents : Paracetamol or dextropropoxyphene

S/E   : GI tract disturbances

Non-steroidal anti-inflammatory drugs (NSAIDs) with or without analgesics

Action : Analgesic and anti-inflammatory

Agents : Almost equally effective and it is advisable not to change the NSAIDs frequently, as response may take sometime to be seen

Caution : NSAIDs – may better be avoided

S/E   : GI tract disturbances

Corticosteroids:

Action : Anti-inflammatory

Agents : Cortisone, hydrocortisone, prednisone, prednisolone, triamcinolone, dexamethasone, betamethasone

Intra-articular steroids – helpful particularly in inflammation of selective joints

Intra-articular steroids – for relief of pain:

- Hydrocortisone acetate 25 mg/mL + Lignocaine plain 1% 1 mL , Alt :
- Triamcinolone acetonide 40 mg/mL + Lignocain plain 1% 1 mL

Sodium hyaluronate 20 mg (2 mL) I/A Rpt b.i.w.

Caution: Not to be used frequently.

Disease modifying therapy (DMARDs):

Action: Potential to modify the disease process favourably and thereby reduce the chances of joint destruction. These agents should start at earliest

Agents:

- Sulphasalazine 1–2 g t.d.s. PO Maint 0.5 g t.d.s.
- Methotrexate 7.5 mg weekly
- Cyclosporin
- Antimalarial agents – chloroquin, hydroxychloroquine
- Gold – lysosomal stabilizer, although exact mode of action unknown
  S/E: Monitor carefully for side effects of these DMARDs

Newer therapy:

- Anti-TNF alpha (tumor necrosis factor alpha) therapy
- Infliximab 5 mg/kg at weeks 0, 2, and 6.

Disadvantages: Very expensive, and under study

Physiotherapy and occupational therapy (rehabilitation):

Aims
- To control pain
- To prevent and correct deformity
- To improve joint function
- To maintain muscle strength.

Refer: The patient to medical outpatients or the GP.

Surgery   More effective in early disease when significant synovitis is present in single or few joints and in an advanced (late) disease. Though surgery cannot cure arthritis, it plays an important role especially in correcting the deformities and rehabilitating the patient.

Surgical procedures (options)

In early stages: Arthroscopy and arthroscopic debridement
                Synovectomy
                Tendon reconstruction

In later stages: Excision arthroplasty
                Arthrodesis
                Osteotomy
                Joint replacement:
- Unicompartmental joint replacement
- Hemiarthroplasty
- Total joint replacement, e.g. Total hip replacement
                                    Total knee replacement.

Refer: The patient to orthopedic team for surgical treatment.

Ankylosing Spondylitis (AS)

Definition   It is a crippling disease that affects mostly young men (20–40 yrs). It is a chronic inflammatory disease that affects mainly the axial skeleton (spine and sacroiliac joints) peripheral joints and extra-articular structures.

Etiology   Unknown.

Diagnosis   Low backache – pain may radiate down the thighs and legs
                Morning stiffness
                Difficulty in breathing
                Chest pain – due to restricted chest movements (expansion)
                Spine movements – painful and restricted
                Extra-articular s/s: uveitis, aortitis, pulmonary fibrosis, colitis, nephropathy

Investigation   CBC, ESR, TLC and DLC
                Rheumatoid factor
                Antinuclear antibodies
                C-reactive protein
                Uric acid
                Bone densitometry

X-ray SI joints and spine: Shows fuzziness or erosion of sacroiliac joints, narrowing of intervertebral spaces, ossification of ligaments, oseophytes formation, deformed joints in advanced cases.

MRI – confirms diagnosis

Management	No specific treatments known for this distressing condition.
Aims	To control pain
	To maintain joints mobility
	To prevent deformity formation

General measures

Rest	Bedrest
	Warm fomentation
	Deep breath exercises
Drugs	Analgesics
	NSAIDs: Indomethacin is drug of choice 25 mg t.d.s PO
	DMARDs – Sulphasalazine 1–2 g t.d.s. PO. Maint 0.5 g t.d.s. Alt:
	– Methotrexate 7.5 mg weekly
	Corticosteroids – to be used with caution of S/E
	Biophosphonates – helpful in managing osteoporosis
	Calcium – as dietry supplement
	Newer drugs: Very effective in severe AS
	Disadvantages: Very expensive, and under study

• Anti-TNF alpha (tumor necrosis factor alpha) therapy
• Infliximab 5 mg/kg at weeks 0, 2 and 6.

Physiotherapy	Exercises: Active – patient puts joints through range of motion
	Passive – someone puts joints through range of motion
	Isometric – muscle is contracted, but not shortened
	Isotonic – muscle is contracted and shortened
	Heat therapy: Infrared, shortwave diathermy
	Radiotherapy: Symptomatic relief
	S/E: High incidence of leukemia.

Surgical treatment: Indicated in severe flexion deformity of the spine.

Surgery	Osteotomy (wedge) of the spine
	Total hip arthroplasty.

Refer: The patient to the orthopedic team for surgical treatment.

Acute Gout

Definition	It is a metabolic disease resulting from the deposition of monosodium urate crystals in the synovial fluid and other tissues, due to disturbed purine metabolism or abnormal excretion of uric acid. Any abrupt change in the serum uric acid concentration may provoke an acute attack of gout.
Epidemiology	Male: Female ratio 9:1. Rare in premenopausal women
	Monoarthritis – 80%

Risk factors	Alcohol consumption
	Fasting
	Diet – purine rich foods, e.g. bacon, salmon, sweet breads
	Obesity
	Hypertension
	Lead exposure – occupational and environmental
	Trauma and surgery
	Drugs – thiazide diuretics.
Diagnosis	Pain:

- Site – MTP joint of great toe podagra) is the most susceptible joint. Other sites – feet, ankle, knees and fingers
- Onset – attack usually starts during night, and is moderate initially.
- Pain becomes persistently worse, continuous gnawing type.
- Intensity – agonizing pain accompanied by signs of inflammation, e.g. swelling, redness, warmth and tenderness
- Maximum inflammation develops within 1 day
  Fever – low grade
  Tophi – nodular masses of urate crystals deposited in soft tissues.

Investigation	CBC, ESR
	Serum uric acid – elevated
	Serum creatinine – elevated
	BUN
	Synovial fluid examination – urate crystals and leukocytes
	Aspiration of tophus – for study of urate crystals
	X-ray shows: Asymmetrical swelling (soft tissue) around a joint
	Subcortical cysts without erosions
	MRI.

Management

General measures

- Bed-rest
- Control of body weight
- Control over alcohol intake
- Diet – purine restricted diet, e.g. red meat, pulses, cheese
- Plenty of fluids orally
- Control of hypertension and hyperlipidemia

Specific measures

Drugs	NSAIDs: Fast acting drugs – currently the most favored treatment

- Indomethacin may be preferred 25–50 mg t.d.s.
- Naproxen 250–500 mg b.d.
- Diclofenac 50 mg b.d. or t.d.s.

Colchicine: PO 1.0 mg (0.5 mg tablets). Rept. 0.5 mg hourly till pain relief or toxicity (nausea/vomiting/diarrhea)

IV colchicine 2 mg in 10–20 ml saline

S/E: Nausea, vomiting, diarrhea

Uricosuric agents:

Action: Reduces serum uric acid by increasing renal excretion

- Allopurinol: 100–200 mg o.d. Maint 200–600 mg o.d. PO

  Indication: Recurrent attacks of gout

  S/E: Nausea, vomiting, diarrhea, skin rash

- Probenecid: 0.5 g b.d. PO

  Indication: Gout.

  C/I: Urine output < 1 ml/mt, renal calculi

- Corticosteroid agents:

  Action: Anti-inflammatory

  Indication: Used only when NSAIDs and colchicine non-effective

- Prednisone: 20–30 mg/day. I/A inj. – indicated in monarthric gout.

Refer: The patient to the orthopedic team.

Acute Carpal Tunnel Syndrome (syn. Tardy Median Nerve Palsy)

Definition	It is a space occupying lesion due to median nerve compression in the wrist at the level of carpal tunnel. It is a space occupying disorder, e.g. any condition that reduces the space of the carpal canal may initiate the symptoms.
Etiology	Traumatic: RSA, sports injury, falls, lifting heavy weight
	Inflammatory: Tenosynovitis
	Degenerative: Osteoarthritis.
Diagnosis	Usually a middle aged female
	Pain – severe, burning or severe pins and needles in the hand and fingers
	Paresthesiae in the median nerve distribution – may be chief symptom
	Morning stiffness of fingers
	Tinel's sign +ve.
Investigation	X-ray of hand – AP and LAT views.
Management	

Conservative treatment

Indication: Mild S/S present for < 2/12

Treatment: Inj. hydrocortisone 25–50 mg weekly into the carpal tunnel

Surgical treatment

Indication: Severe and progressive S/S

Procedure: Decompression of the tunnel by a longitudinal ventral incision (division of the deep transverse carpal ligament).

Refer: The patient to the orthopedic team for surgery.

Acute Suppurative Tendosynovitis

Definition	It is an acute inflammation of a tendon sheath.
Etiology	Traumatic: RSA, sports injury, falls
	Inflammatory: Wounds, bursitis, tuberculosis.
Diagnosis	Pain – severe
	Swelling
	Local tenderness
	Movements – painfull
	Sloughing of tendons.
Investigation	X-ray of hand – AP and LAT views
	CBC
	TLC and DLC.
Management	
Conservative	
	Antibiotics
	Analgesics
	Splintage of the affected part.
Surgery	Incision drainage of the affected tendon sheath.

Refer: The patient to the orthopedic team for surgery.

Acute Stenosing Tenosynovitis (de Quervain's disease)

Definition	It is a fibrous thickening of a tendon sheath, mostly the tendon sheaths of abductor pollicis longus and extensor pollicis brevis, at level of outer aspect of the radial styloid.
Etiology	Traumatic: RSA, sports injury, falls, lifting heavy weight
	Inflammatory: Bursitis
	Degenerative: Osteoarthritis.
Investigation	X-ray of hand – AP and LAT views.
Management	
Surgery	Incision of the thickened tendon sheath

Refer: The patient to the orthopedic team for surgery.

Trigger Finger and Thumb

Definition	It is a condition involving the flexor tendons of the finger or thumb.
Etiology	Thickening of flexor tendon or a constriction in the tendon sheath.
Diagnosis	Difficulty in flexing/extending the affected finger
	Snapping/triggering of distal joint (little force – suddenly releases the finger with a click)
	A nodule – palpated opposite the MP joint of the affected finger.
Investigation	X-ray hand – AP and LAT views.
Management	
Surgery	Slitting the fibro-osseous tunnel at the level of the constriction.
Post-care	Active exercises.

Acute Low Backache

Definition	It may be a symptom of various disorders. Low backache with or without referred pain along the distribution of the sciatic nerves, is often difficult to treat satisfactorily.
Etiology	Traumatic: RSA, sports injury, falls, lifting heavy weight
	Inflammatory: Osteomyelitis (bacterial, tubercular) discitis, sacrolitis
	Ankylosing spondylitis, spondyloarthropathies, prostatitis, endometritis, appendicitis, cholecystitis
	Endocrinal and metabolic: Diabetes, thyroid disorders, osteoporosis
	Degenerative: Spondylosis, spondylolisthesis, prolapsed disc
	Postural: Habitual, spinal deformity, e.g. kyphosis, scoliosis
	Neoplastic: Carcinoma colon
	Miscellaneous: Paget's disease, fluorosis.
Diagnosis	Pain: Lumbar or dorsal pain during the night
	Buttock pain if affecting right or left
	Heel pain
	Pain – may worsen on rest (inflammation)
	may worsen on activity (mechanical)
	may aggravates on coughing, sneezing
	may or may not radiate to the thigh, legs depending on whether there is compression of nerve roots
	Muscle spasm
	Deformity – kyphosis or scoliosis may be present
	Local tenderness
	Movements painful and restricted
	Neurological deficit – may or may not be present depending on whether there is compression of nerve roots
	Straight leg raising (SLR) test, and forward bending test.
Investigation	Hemogram, ESR, TLC and DLC, RA factor
	X-ray lumbosacral spine – AP and LAT views
	MRI
	Myelogram,
	CT scan.

Management

General measures

Bed-rest

Heat therapy – Infrared, shortwave diathermy

Traction, lumbar belt, braces

Analgesics, NSAIDs

Antibiotic – to control infection, if present.

Specific treatment

      Epidural block

      Treatment of the underlying cause.

Refer: The patients (with leg/legs weakness, altered perineal/perianal sensations, disturbed sphincter, fever, weight loss) to the orthopedic team.

Acute Sciatica

Definition	Few diseases cause more suffering and economic loss than sciatica. It is most resistant to treatment and is often difficult to treat satisfactorily, because its etiology may remain obscure even after careful physical and radiological examinations.
Etiology	Traumatic: RSA, sports injury, lifting heavy weight
	Inflammatory: Tuberculosis, spondylitis
	Infection of genitourinary, gastrointestinal, nervous system
	Endocrinal: Diabetes
	Neoplastic: Vertebral or pelvic tumors
	Degenerative: PIVD, spondylosis, spondylolisthesis.
Diagnosis	Pain down thigh and leg
	SLR test
	Forward bending test.
Investigation	Hemogram, TLC and DLC, ESR
	X-ray lumbosacral spine – AP and lateral views
	Myelography
	CT scan.

Management

General measures

      Bed-rest

      Heat therapy – infrared, shortwave diathermy

      Traction

      Lumbar belt

      Analgesics

      NSAIDs.

Specific treatment

      Treatment of underlying cause

      Surgery indicated only in limited cases: PIVD, spinal tumors.

Refer: The patient to the orthopedic team.

Prolapse Intervertebral Disc (PIVD)

Definition	It is the main cause of low backache and pain down thigh, legs. It commonly affects adults from 30 to 50, most often males. It results from compression upon nerve root or cord, by the backward protrusion of nucleus pulposus, due to weakning of posterior longitudinal ligament and the annulus fibrosus

as a result of trauma. The vast majority affect the disc between the L5 and S1 vertebrae. Disc between L4 and L5 is the next most vulnerable. The root of L5 or S1 is commonly affected.

Etiology	Traumatic – RSA, sports injury, fall from height, lifting heavy weight, injury by a lumbar puncture needle, degenerative.
Risk factors	Postural

Deformity, e.g. kyphosis, scoliosis

Spondylitis

Vertebral osteophytes

Violent actions – sneezing, coughing, lurching

Diagnosis   Symptoms are those of sciatica in most cases, depending on type of lesion (nerve root compression), e.g.

L5 lesions (L5 ruptured disc between L4 and L5):

- Pain: In the back, sacroiliac joint and hip, groin, thigh (posterolateral), outer calf, lateral malleolus, foot (dorsum), toes (1, 2, 3rd)
- Numbness: In the area of affected nerve, e.g. more medial over tibial region – extending over big toe, medial malleolus, and part of sole
- Local tenderness: Outer gluteal region and near fibular's head
- Weakness: Extensor of greater toe and foot
- Ankle jerk: Depressed
- SLR +ve

S1 lesions (S1 ruptured disc between L5 and S1):

- Pain in the sacroiliac joint, thigh (back), calf (back) to heel, sole (plantar surface) and toes (4th & 5th)
- Numbness: In the area of affected nerve, e.g. outer side of leg, foot, outer two toes and sole
- Local tenderness: Over sacroiliac joint, back of thigh and leg
- Weakness: Hamstrings, flexor of foot, flexor and abductors of toes
- Ankle jerk: Diminished or absent
- SLR +ve
- Lumbar curve: May be diminished or lost
- Prominent spinous processes (L3, 4, 5).

Investigation   Hemogram

ESR

Serum proteins

CSF examination

X-ray lumbar spine – AP and LAT views

Bone scans

MRI

CT scan.

Management

Conservative treatment

Bed-rest, heat therapy, massage, traction, lumbar belt, analgesics.

Surgical treatment: May be indicated in 10% of cases, when compression of nerve roots or spinal cord causes neurologic deficit.

Procedures
- Lumbar microdiscectomy – gold standard for treating disc prolapse, as it can be performed as an day care procedure, and has proven to be a safe and least traumatic procedure

Alternative surgical procedures:
- Laminectomy with or without arthrodesis spine
- Percutaneous lumbar discectomy – automated
- Percutaneous lumbar discectomy – endoscopic
- Percutaneous laser discectomy
- Microdiscectomy – transforaminal endoscopic
- Microdiscectomy – stereotactic lumbar

Future holds (procedures) in store:
- Artificial disc replacement or intervertebral disc transfer.

Refer: The patient to the orthopedic team.

Practical procedures/Investigations:
- Blood analysis:
  - ESR: SLE, tuberculosis
  - Blood uric acid: Gout
  - C-reactive protein: Inflammatory disorders
  - Complement fixation test
  - Immunological tests: Rheumatoid factor
  - Antinuclear antibody tests: SLE
- Synovial fluid analysis: Inflammatory, infective synovitis
- Biopsy:
  - Synovial: Rheumatoid arthritis
  - Renal: SLE, vasculitis
  - Lip: Sjögren's syndrome
- X-ray – AP and lateral views: Preferably of both sides for comparison, e.g. both hips, knees, ankles, feet, wrists, hands
- Ultrasound: Inflammatory – defining soft tissue structures
- MRI, CT scan: Inflammatory – defining soft tissue structures
- Arthroscopy: Inflammatory disorders

References

1. Bunch TW, et al: Synovial fluid complement: Usefulness in diagnosis and classification of rheumatoid arthritis. Ann Int Med 81:32;1974.
2. Johnson JS, et al: Rheumatoid arthritis, 1970–72. Ann Int Med 78:937;1773.

3. Nanavati N: Current Concepts in the management of rheumatoid arthritis. Journal of General Medicine 19–20;2002.

4. Sledge CB: Surgery for rheumatoid arthritis. Current Orthopaedics, 3,1;1989.

5. Agarwala S, Parasnis RN: Orthopaedicians and rheumatic diseases. Journal of General Medicine 14:55–60;2002.

6. Gokhale T, Hedge U, Jyotish CJ: Classification and diagnostic criteria for rheumatic diseases. Journal of General Medicine 14:7–14;2002.

7. Kapoor PS: Rheumatoid arthritis. The Indian Express 18 September, 2003.

8. Chaturvedi V: Ankylosing Spondylitis: A radical shift in management. Orthopaedics Today VI:42-48;2004.

9. Calabro JJ, Maltz BA: Ankylosing spondylitis. New England J Med 282:606;1970.

10. Kapoor PS: Ankylosing spondylitis. The Indian Express 4 June, 2003.

11. Engleman EP, Chatton MJ: Arthritis and allied rheumatic disorders. Current Medical Diagnosis and Treatment, 474–498;1975.

12. Russel ASA, Ansel BM: Septic arthritis. Ann Rheumat Dis 31:40;1972.

13. Pispati PK: Acute gout. Journal of General Medicine 14:27–28;2002.

14. Charnley J: Injuries of muscles and tendons. Bailey and Love's Short Practice of Surgery, 320-326;1965.

15. Frymoyer JW: Back pain and sciatica. N Engl J Med 318:291;1998.

16. Kapoor PS: Backache. The Indian Express 11 September, 2002.

17. Bell GR, Parkman RH: The conservative treatment of sciatica. Spine 9:54;1984.

18. Kapoor PS: The truth about sciatica. The Indian Express 30 October, 2002.

19. Rothman RC, Simeone F: Lumbar Disc Disease.Philadelphia. Saunders, 1975. 443–458.

20. Wilson DH, Harbaugh R: Microsurgical and standard removal of the protruded lumbar disc: A comparative study. Neurosurgery 8:422–427;1981.

21. Apostolides PJ, Jackobowitz R, Sonntag VK. Lumbar discectomy microdiscectomy: "the gold standard". Clin Neurosurg 43: 228-238;1996.

22. Silvers HR: Microsurgical versus standard lumbar discectomy. Neurosurgery 22(5): 837–841, May 1988.

23. Gulati Y: Lumbar microdiscectomy. Apollo Medicine 1;34–37, Sept 2004.

24. Mathews HH: Transforaminal endoscopic microdiscectomy. Neurosurg Clin N Am 7(1): 59–63, Jan 1996.

25. Kapoor PS: The role of immunological tests in routine synovial fluid analysis. Post Graduate Institute of Medical Education and Research, Chandigarh, 1973.

26. Regan JJ, Guyer RD: Endoscopic techniques in spinal surgery. Clinical Orthopaedics, 335:122;1997.

Oncological Emergencies

- Oncology emergency
  - Definition
  - Diagnosis
  - Management
- Classification of oncology emergencies and complications:
- Space occupying lesions:
  - Superior vena cava syndrome (SVCS)
  - Spinal cord compression (SCC)
  - Raised intracranial pressure (ICP)
- Metabolic disorders:
  - Tumor lysis syndrome
  - Hypercalcemia,

- Hyponatremia,
- Hyperuricemia
- GI tract disorders:
  - Acute intestinal obstruction
  - Acute bowel perforation
  - Acute enterocolitis
- UTI:
  - Acute hemorrhagic cystitis (acute abacterial cystitis)
- Bone disorders:
  - Bone marrow suppression

Oncology Emergency

Definition	Oncology emergency is defined as an acute, potentially life-threatening disorder, related directly/indirectly to malignancy or its management. It should be diagnosed and treated prompty.
Diagnosis	
General	Anorexia, loss of weight, thirst, constipation, fatigue, bodyaches, headache, drowsiness, confusion.
Local	
Breast	Swelling (mass), pain, nipple discharge, skin retraction, ulceration, lymphadenopathy
Lung	Pain, cough, dyspnea, hemoptysis, cyanosis, clubbing
GI tract	Nausea, vomiting, indigestion, dysphagia, constipation, diarrhea, pain abdomen, hematemesis, melena, jaundice
Gynecological	Pain, pelvic mass, P/V bleeding, P/V discharge, cervical erosion
Urological	Dysuria, hematuria, enlarged prostate
Head and neck	Pain, headache, hoarseness, deafness, cough, sinusitis, dysphagia
CNS	Headache, nausea, vomiting, convulsions

Musculoskeletal	Pain, swelling, deformity, restricted movement
Endocrinal	Headache, visual disturbance, hearing loss, hoarseness, nausea, vomiting, palpitations, hypertension, fatigue, polydipsia, polyuria, Mass – thyroid/pancreatic/adrenal
Risk factors	Smoking tobacco – cancer lung
	Alcohol abuse – cancer GI tract
	Diet – oral cancer due to chewing of betel nuts
	Ultraviolet light exposure – cancer skin
	Occupational – cancer skin due to lead poisoning
	– cancer lung due to radiation exposure
	X-rays exposure – cancer lung
Investigations	CXR: Cancer lung
	MRI: Cancer breast, gynecological, urological, CNS, head and neck
	CT scan: Cancer breast, lung, gynecological, urological, endocrinal, head and neck, bone, thyroid
	Ultrasonography: Cancer breast, GI tract, gynecological, urological
	Bronchoscopy: Cancer lung
	Endoscopy: Cancer GI tract
	Barium meal: Cancer GI tract
	Barium enema: Cancer colon, rectum
	Mammography: Cancer breast
	Tumor markers: CA15.3 for breast cancer, PSA for prostate cancer, CEA for GI tract cancers, CA119.9 for pancreatic cancer
Management	Chemotherapy
	Radiotherapy
	Surgery
	Steroid therapy – to reduce edema
	• Dexamethasone 2 mg/kg body weight
	• Betamethasone 10 mg IV. Rept. 4 mg IM every 6 hrly
	Hormonal therapy

Chemotherapy

Chemotherapy when used single or in combination with other therapies can eradicate the tumor (cure) in certain cases, or at least may reduce the tumor, thereby relieve the tumor produced symptoms and prolonging life.

Classification of Carcino-chemotherapeutic Drugs

1. Alkylating agents:

Cyclophosphamide (endoxan, cycloxan): Tab 50 mg, Inj. 200 mg/500 mg/1 g

Indications: Hodgkin's disease, leukemias, multiple myeloma, lymphosarcoma, breast cancer, lung cancer

Dose	Adult: 10–15 mg/kg IV every 7–10 days
	Children: 2–3 mg/kg/day PO or IV for 2/12
Use	In combination with surgery, radiotherapy
C/I	Hemorrhage – bladder
S/E	Pulmonary fibrosis, cystitis, cardiotoxicity

Chlorambucil (leukeran) Tab 2 mg, 5 mg
Indications: Lymphocytic leukemia, Hodgkin's disease, breast cancer

Dose	Adult: 0.1–0.2 mg/kg/day PO for 3–6/52
	Children: 0.1–0.2 mg/kg/day PO
C/I	Pregnancy, lactation
S/E	Pulmonary fibrosis, hepatotoxicity

Busulphan (myleran): Tab 0.5 mg, 2 mg
Indications: Leukemia

Dose	Adult: 2–8 mg/day (0.8 mg/kg) PO
	Children: 60 µg/kg/day PO
C/I	Pregnancy, lactation
S/E	Bone marrow depression

Melphalan (alkeran): Tab 2 mg, 5 mg, Inj. 50 mg

Indications	Multiple myeloma, malignant melanoma, breast cancer
Dose	6 mg o.d. for 2–3/52 or 10 mg o.d. for 1/52
C/I	Pregnancy, lactation
S/E	Allergic dermatitis, bone marrow depression, anemia

Mustine HCl (mustine HCl): Inj. 10 mg

Indications	Leukemia, Hodgkin's disease, bronchogenic carcinoma
Dose	0.1 mg/kg o.d. for 3–4 days. Infusion with 500 ml normal saline
C/I	Pregnancy, lactation
S/E	Nausea, vomiting, fever, bone marrow depression

Thiotepa   Inj. 15 mg vial

Indications	Breast cancer, urinary bladder cancer
Dose	0.3–0.4 mg/kg BSA IV weekly
C/I	Pregnancy, lactation
S/E	Fever, headache, rash, abdominal pain

2. Antimetabolites
   Folic acid analogs:
   Methotrexate (neotrexate, biotrexate) Inj. 50 mg/2 ml

Indications	Lymphocytic leukemia
Dose	20–40 mg/sq.m. twice weekly IV or IM Maint 15–30 mg/sq m/wk.
C/I	Pregnancy, lactation
S/E	Renal/hepatic impairment, bone marrow depression

Pyrimidine analogs

5-fluorouracil (fluracil): Inj. 250 mg/5 ml, Caps. 250 mg

Indications	Breast cancer, GI tract cancer
Dose	10–15 mg/kg IV o.d. for a week followed by 1 g weekly
C/I	Pregnancy, lactation
S/E	Dermatitis, chest pain, MI

6-mercaptopurine

Purine analogs

6-mercaptopurine (Puri-Nethol): Tab 50 mg

Indications:	Acute leukemia
Dose	Adult: 2.5 mg/kg o.d. PO
C/II	Pregnancy, lactation
S/E	Hepatotoxicity, bone marrow depression, skin rash, fever

3. Natural agents

 Vinca alkaloids:

Vincristine sulph (vincristine neocristin): Inj. 1 mg

Indications	Leukemia, lymphomas
Dose	Adult: 1.45 mg/sq.m. body surface area (BSA) IV weekly
	Children: 1.5 mg/sq m IV weekly
C/I	Charcot-Marie syndrome
S/E	Nausea, vomiting, dyspnea, hypotension/hypertension

Vinblastine sulph (cytoblastin): Inj. 10 mg

Indications	Hodgkin's disease
Dose	Adult: 5.5 mg/sq.m. BSA IV weekly
	Children: 5.0 mg/kg IV weekly
C/I	Leukopenia, infection
S/E	Dyspnea, bodyaches, leukopenia

Antibiotics

Actinomycin D

	Adult: 0.01 mg/kg/day IV for 5 days
	Children: 15 mcg/kg/day IV for 5 days

Bleomycin (bleocin): Inj. 15 mg

Indications	Malignant lymphoma, lung cancer, cervix cancer
Dose	15–30 mg IV or IV infusion twice weekly
C/I	Pregnancy, lactation
S/E	Pulmonary fibrosis, rash, renal/hepatic toxicity

4. Hormonal agents: Sex hormones and antagonists – especially for breast and prostate cancer

Aims	To control hormonal dependent neoplasms by depriving hormone stimulation

Agents

Androgens	Antiandrogens: Cyproterone acetate
Indication	Prostate cancer
Estrogens	Antiestrogens: Tamoxifen
Indication	Breast cancer
Progestins	Progestogens
Indication	Breast cancer

5. Adrenocorticosteroids:

Indication   Breast cancer
- Dexamethasone 2 mg/kg body weight
- Betamethasone 10 mg IV Rpt. 4 mg IM every 6 hrly
- Prednisone 60 mg o.d. PO for

Radiotherapy

Radiotherapy is an essential component of cancer therapy, along with surgery and chemotherapy. Together with surgery, radiotherapy currently remains the most cost-effective cancer treatment.

Purpose of radiotherapy: Curative or palliative

Aims
- To destroy cancer cells, with limited damage to surrounding normal cells
- Relief of pain and bleeding

Superior Vena Cava Syndrome (SVCS)

Etiology	Compression by enlargement/dilatation of trachea, lymph nodes, due to bronchogenic carcinoma, lymphoma, leukemia, Hodgkin's disease.
Diagnosis	Onset of symptoms – acute/subacute

- Dyspnea
- Flushing of face and neck
- Engorged veins – neck and arm veins
- Brawny edema
- Lymph nodes – enlarged
- Chest pain
- Sudden death – due to cardiovascular collapse

Investigation	CXR
	CT scan
	FNAC – CT guided
	Biopsy – lymph node
Management	Radiotherapy plus steroid coverage, Alt:
	Cyclophosphamide 10–15 mg/kg IV weekly plus steroid coverage
	Diuretic IV
	Chemotherapy – selective, i.e. as per type of tumor

Spinal Cord Compression (SCC)

Etiology Compression by a tumor – Carcinomas lung, breast, prostate, GI tract
– Multiple myeloma, lymphoma

Diagnosis Backache, weakness, numbness limb/limbs

Investigations CT scan
MRI

Management Steroid therapy – to reduce cord edema
- Dexamethasone 10 mg IV. Rept. 4 mg IM every 6 hrly for a week
- Betamethasone 10 mg IV. Rept. 4 mg IM every 6 hrly
- Prednisone 60 mg o.d. PO for a week
Surgery – decompression (laminectomy)
Radiotherapy
Chemotherapy

Raised Intracranial Pressure (RIP)

Etiology Primary – brain tumors (malignant)
Secondaries – carcinomas breast, lungs, thyroid, prostate

Diagnosis Headache, nausea, vomiting, visual disturbances, unconsciousness

Investigations CT scan, MRI

Management Steroid therapy – to reduce brain edema
- Dexamethasone 10 mg IV. Rept. 4 mg IM every 6 hrly
- Betamethasone 10 mg IV. Rept. 4 mg IM every 6 hrly
Mannitol IV
Anticonvulsant therapy
Surgery
Radiotherapy
Chemotherapy

Tumor Lysis Syndrome

Etiology Aggressive chemo-or radiosensitive tumors – causing renal failure, resulting in metabolic disturbances, e.g. hyperkalemia, hyponatremia, hypercalcemia and hyperuricemia (Table 17.1).

Hypercalcemia

Hypercalcemia is a common medical emergency, encountered in advanced cases of malignancy.

Etiology
- Carcinoma breast, lungs, thyroid, kidney
- Multiple myeloma

Diagnosis Nausea, vomiting, thirst, dehydration, polyuria, constipation, anorexia, muscular weakness, hangover, convulsions, coma

Table 17.1: Metabolic emegencies

Tumors	Metabolic disturbance	Emergencies
Leukemia, lymphoma, Multiple myeloma	Hyperkalemia	Impairs neuromuscular conduction, causing VF and cardiac arrest
Carcinoma lung, prostate, pancreas	Hyponatremia	Impairs plasma volume, circulatory failure, decrease in cardiac output
Carcinoma breast, lung, adrenal, renal, Multiple myeloma	Hypercalcemia	Impairs neuromuscular conduction, causing muscular weakness, stupor, coma
Leukemia, lymphoma, Multiple myeloma	Hyperuricemia	Impairs renal function, causing nephropathy, acute renal failure

Management

Emergency treatment due to malignancy:

1. IV fluids – Sodium chloride/sodium sulfate 3 L/msq/day
2. Cation exchange resins (Aluminum hydroxide) that bind potassium
3. Diuretics: Furosemide may/may not be given along sodium chloride
4. Corticoids – used in case of carcinoma.
   - Dexamethasone 2 mg/kg body weight, or
   - Prednisone 60 mg o.d. PO for a week
5. Mithramycin 25 μg/kg IV on alternate days for 2–4 doses
   Indication – severe hypercalcemia
6. Treatment of the cause

Refer: The severe patient to the medical team.

Hyponatremia

It is defined as decreased concentration of sodium (< 130 mEq/L in ECF)

Etiology	• Trauma incld. surgical trauma
	• Nausea, vomiting, diarrhea, excessive sweating in hot climate, intestinal obstruction, gastric aspiration, Addison's disease, nephritis
	• GI tract cancer
Diagnosis	Face drawn, sunken eyes, dry skin, tongue dry and coated, hypotension, dark colored urine of high specific gravity
Infants	Depressed anterior fontanelle
Investigation	Serum electrolytes
Management	Severe cases: Plasma or plasma expander
	Isotonic saline solution (0.9%) IV
	Less severe cases: Isotonic saline solution (0.9%) IV or Ringer's solution IV
	Treatment of the cause

Refer: The severe patient to the medical team.

Hyperuricemia

It is often observed in neoplastic patients receiving chemotherapy for cancer. As such hyperuricemia may be considered as a preventable complication rather than an acute medical emergency.

Etiology	Acute leukemia, lymphoma, multiple myeloma
Gout	
Diagnosis	Acute attack of monoarthritis – mainly the Ist MTP joint
S/S	Pain – agonizing, swelling, local tenderness, fever, hypertension
Investigation	Complete hemogram, serum creatinine, BUN, serum uric acid
	X-ray of affected joint: May show tophi
	MRI

Management

Emergency treatment

1. Aggressive hydration with IV fluids 3–4 L/day
2. Management of electrolyte imbalance – Sodium bicarbonate 6–8 g/day
3. Allopurinol 200 mg q.d.s. PO
4. Rasburicase 0.15–0.20 mg/kg body weight – for very severe cases
5. Emergency hemodialysis/or peritoneal dialysis

Acute Intestinal Obstruction

It is a common, serious, surgical emergency, that demands early diagnosis and treatment.

Etiology	Cancer – GI tract (gastric, pancreatic or large intestine)
Diagnosis	Pain abdomen – colicky in character
	Vomiting – frequency and type of vomitus, depending upon site of obstruction, i.e. to start with gastric contents, next small intestine (biliary) and lastly large intestine (fecal)
	Distension of abdomen – visible peristalsis may be present
	Tenderness – positive
	Rigidity – absent
Investigation	TLC and DLC: Leukocytosis – mild/absent
	Blood urea and electrolytes
	Serum amylase
	Plane X-ray abdomen: Shows gas shadows, fluid levels without any gas movement
	Ultrasound
	CT scan

Management

Conservative treatment

Ryle's tube aspiration – to relieve vomiting and distension
Maintenance of fluid and electrolytes balance
Antibiotics – Broad spectrum antibiotics
Flatus tube passage

Anticancer   Chemotherapy, surgery, and radiotherapy

Surgical treatment:

Indications   Failure of conservative measures

Fever – continuation

Leukocytosis

Bleeding per rectum

Mesenteric – secondaries

Parietal adhesions

Intussusception/volvulus

Refer: The patient to the surgical team.

Surgery   Relieving the obstruction and excision of gangrenous bowl and re-anastomosis.

Prognosis   Depends upon the causative factor and presence of strangulation.

Acute Bowel Perforation

Etiology   Perforation of tumor: Many tumors perforate during CT or RT, e.g.
- Carcinoma GI tract – stomach, colon, Hodgkin's disease, lymphoma Perforation of peptic ulcer

Acute Enterocolitis (Typhlitis)

It is an acute life-threatening inflammation of small and large intestines. Many patients with disseminated tumors have increased susceptibility to infection.

Etiology   Tumors: Acute leukemia, Hodgkin's disease, multiple myeloma

Infection – bacterial: *Esch. coli, Staphylococcus aureus/albus, Proteus, Pseudomonas,* typhoid

Amebic: *E. histolytica*

Diagnosis   Pain abdomen, distension, vomiting, diarrhea – profuse and watery

Fever

Local tenderness

Tachycardia, hypotension, shock

Investigations   TLC and DLC – leukocytosis

Stool examination – for membrane, leukocytes, gram – positive cocci

CT scan

Management   IV fluids and electrolytes

Blood/plasma transfusion

Corticosteroids – to combat shock

Antibiotics – BSA

Anticancer   Chemotherapy

Acute Hemorrhagic Cystitis (Acute Abacterial Cystitis)

Etiology   Tumors: Acute leukemia, lymphoma, multiple myeloma

Infection – due to *Esch. coli, Staphylococcus aureus/albus, Proteus, Pseudomons*

Predisposing factors	• Enlarged prostate, stricture urethra, stenosis extra urinary meatus
	• Pregnancy
	• Neoplasm – bladder tumor
	• UTI
	• Drugs: Cyclophosphamide, ifosfamide, sufosfamide
Diagnosis	Suprapubic discomfort, frequency, dysuria and urgency
	Severe cases – incontinence and hematuria
Investigations	Urine analysis – include culture and sensitivity test
	Cystoscopy
	CT scan of pelvis
Management	Hydration – plenty of fluids orally or IV infusion
	Blood transfusion/platelet transfusion
	Analgesics – pyridium orally
Anticancer	Chemotherapy

Bone Marrow Suppression

Etiology	Lymphoma, leukemia, Hodgkin's disease
	Chemotherapy
Diagnosis	Headache, nausea, vomiting, bleeding
Investigation	CBC, hemogram, BT and CT, ESR, platelet count
	CXR, X-ray of affected bone/bones, MRI, CT scan
Management	Hydration – plenty of fluids orally or IV infusion
	Blood transfusion/platelet transfusion
	Analgesics – pyridium orally
Anticancer	Chemotherapy

References

1. Keele CA, Neil E (editors): The Blood. Samson Wright's Applied Physiology, 10th ed., London, 1961.
2. Wintrobe MM, et al: Clinical Hematology, 7th ed. Lea and Febiger, 1974.
3. Perez CA, Brady LW, Helperin C, Schmidi-ulli-rich RK, (editors): Principles and Practice of Radiation Oncology, 4th ed. Philadelphia: Lippincott Williams and Wilkins 01–95, 2004.
4. Biswas LN, Deb AR, Pal S: Radiation Therapy: Experience in Indian Patients. JIMA Vol 103:09, 2005.
5. Yahalom J: Superior vena cava syndrome. In: DeVita VT Jr, Hellman S, Rosenberg SA (eds). Cancer, Principles and Practice of Oncology. 7th ed. Philadelphia: Lippincott Williams and Wilkins, 2273-80, 2005.
6. Bhuyan C, Saikia BJ, Choudhury N: Oncological emergencies – management guidelines for clinicians. JIMA Vol 103 No. 09, 474–78, 2005.
7. Sydney ES: Diagnosis and treatment of emergencies and complications of malignant disease. Current Medical Diagnosis and Treatment, 1975.
8. Gallagher C: Oncology. Hutchison's Clinical Methods. 21st ed. Saunders, London, 2003.

Emerging and Re-emerging Acute Infections

Emerging infections:
- HIV
- Hepatitis C
- Hepatitis E
- SARS
- Bird flu
- Chickungunia
- Swine flu
- Ebola virus
- Marburg virus
- Cholera
- Typhoid/paratyphoid fever

Re-emerging infections:
- Dengue
- Malaria
- Plague – bubonic (black death)
- Japanese B encephalitis

Contributing factors to Emerging/Re-emerging Infections

Sanitaion – poor

Envioronmental changes

Autoimmune – suppression

Antibiotics – resistance

Diagnostic modalities - advanced

HIV (Human Immunodeficiency Virus)

Definition   It is called 20th century plague, with fatal outcome – emerged as 2nd largest killer disease affecting human beings all over the world.

Etiology   Human immunodeficiency virus (HIV 1) of RNS-retrovirus group.

Transmission   Through sexual contact or by sharing articles with infected person.

Risk factors   Sex workers – especially childbearing mothers indulging in prostitution

Hetrosexual mothers with bisexual husbands, addicted mothers

Homosexuals with infected partners

Blood transfusion without testing for HIV

Drug abusers – sharing infected needles and by contacts with, e.g. saliva, tears, breast milk, blood, semen and vaginal secretions

Obesity and its accompaniment

Smokers

Nonalcoholic fatty liver disease

Hepatitis B and C.

Incubation	3 months to 5 yrs.
Diagnosis	Fever, headache, myalgia, arthralgia, fatigue, loss of weight, diarrhea, gastrointestinal bleeding, rashes, pneumonia.
Complications	Pneumonia, confusion, impaired mental status, encephalopathy, meningitis, stroke, retinitis, retinal necrosis, diarrhea.
Investigation	TLC and DLC – lymphopenia (< 2000/cmm)
	Platelet count – thrombocytopenia
	Raised levels of immunoglobulins – IgA, IgG, IgM
	ELISA test
	Culture of virus
	T cell growth factors.

Management

Prevention   Counseling of mothers (with AIDS) to change the lifestyle.
Screening of blood donors.

Specific
- No specific treatment either for HIV infection or the resulting immunodeficiency.
- At present, available therapy can neither eradicates the virus nor provides any definitive cure.
- Early diagnosis and control of infections by aggressive use of antibiotics may prolong the life of suffering child.
- Antiretroviral therapy (ART): Although ART does not cure HIV/AODS, but effective ART regimes inhibit the replication of HIV virus and reduces viremia to undetectable levels.

Many combinations of drugs are in use for therapy:
- Drugs: Peginterferon/interferon, zidovudin, ribavirin, ritonavir
- Chose the simplest regimen possible, reducing the dose frequency and no. of pills
- Chose the drugs with less no. of side effects

Monitor response by HIV copy no. and CD4 lymphocyte count

Drugs   Peginterferon alfa-2a 180 μg/wk., s.c. for 48/52
Interferon alfa-2a 3–4.5 mU t.i w., s.c. for 48/52
Zidovudine Adults: 500–600 mg o.d. PO in divided doses
                   Children >3 months old 180 mg/sq m q.d.s.
Ribavirin   Adults: 600 mg b.i.d. PO
Ritonavir   Adults: 600 mg b.i.d. PO
                   Children >2 yrs. 300 mg/sq m

Complications Treatment of the cause.

Refer: The patient/child to the medical/pediatric team.

Hepatitis C

Definition   Acute hepatitis C virus (HCV) is a major public health problem and a leading cause of death from liver disease

Etiology	HCV is an RNA virus of flavivirus group
Transmission	Blood transfusion – HCV infected blood or blood products
	Drug abuse – use of infected needles
	Sexual contact – with infected partner/partners
	Exposure – to infected blood/blood products and perinatal exposure
	Acupuncture, ritual scarification and tattooing
Incubation	6/52 to 6/12
Diagnosis	Fever, malaise, nausea, vomiting, pain abdomen, jaundice
	Liver – enlarged and tendered
	Splenomegaly – 20%
Investigation	Serological tests for anti-HCV:
	• HCV RNA – qualitative assay (amplification techniques–PCR and TNA)
	• HCV RNA – quantitative assay (PCR and DNA)
	HCV genotype determination (grades 6) – in all HCV infected patients, for purpose of duration of therapy and response
	Liver biopsy
Management	
Aim	To prevent complications of HCV infection
Treatment	
General	To reduce weight
	Avoid alcohol
Specific	Peginterferon/interferon alfa-2a with ribavirin yield better results
Genotype 1	Peginterferon alfa-2a 180 μg/wk. s.c. + ribavirin 1-1.2 g/o.d. PO × 48/52
	Interferon alfa-2a 3-6 mU s.c. t.i.w. + ribavirin 1-1.2 g/b.d. PO × 48/52
Genotype 2/3	Peginterferon/interferon alfa + ribavirin 0.8 g × 24/52
	Interferon alfa-2a 3 mU s.c. t.i.w. + ribavirin PO × 1 yr.
C/I	Not recommended for children < 3 yrs.

Hepatitis E

Etiology	RNA virus (single-stranded).
Transmission	Direct contact: Fecal-oral route
	Contaminated food and water.
Diagnosis	Incubation period: 15–60 days
	Fever, malaise
	Nausea, vomiting, anorexia, pain abdomen
	Urine – dark colored
	Jaundice – may appear
	Liver – enlarged and tendered
	Spleen – palpable.
Investigation	IgM antibodies to HEV.
Management	Disease is self-limiting and carrier state is unknown
	Vaccine – not available
	Passive immunization – not effective.

Rabies (Hydrophobia)

Etiology	Rabies virus of rhabdovirus group.
Pathology	Contamination of a wound with saliva of a rabid animal (usually a stray dog) results in multiplication of virus in the muscle, gets attached to it then ascends along axon to the spinal cord, further to neurons of brain, forming Negri body in the neurons, and destruction of neurons.
Diagnosis	Incubation period: 3–12 weeks
	Fever, malaise, headache
	Nausea, vomiting, anorexia
	Hydrophobia, dysphasia, anxiety
	Pain or paresthesia at site of wound
	Convulsions, paralysis
	Death.
Management	Rabies proves invariable fatal
	Inspite of intensive care, chances of survival are remote.
Prevention	Immunization of domestic dogs, cats and of veterinarians
	Human rabies immunoglobulin 20 i.u./kg body wt. IM. Max 1500 units

Treatment of complications

Secondary infections, pneumonia – treated by antibiotics

Encephalitis – treated symptomatically.

Prophylaxis	Toilet of wound with antiseptic fluids
	Debridement of wound
	Antibiotics
	Analgesics.
Emergency	Skillful ICU care, with special attention to the airway, oxygen therapy, control of seizures.

Severe Acute Respiratory Syndrome (SARS)

It is a newly recognized viral disease, originating in China.

Etiology	Coronavirus – RNA virus.
Transmission	By animals.

Mode of infection

By droplet infection

By direct contact

By fomites.

Diagnosis	Fever, cough, difficulty in breathing.
Investigation	CXR (X-ray chest) – shows bronchopneumonia.
Management	Antibiotic
	Antipyretic
	Antiviral – ribavirin 1–1.2 g in divided doses PO.

Refer: The patient to the medical team.

Bird Flu (Avian Influenza)

It is a contagious disease

Etiology	Virus H5N1
Transmission	Direct contact – with infected poultry or surfaces and objects contaminated by their feces and secretions
Pathogenesis	H5N1 is highly pathogenic viral strain, capable of jumping the species barrier and cause severe disease in humans with high mortality. Worse is that the avian virus is capable of cross-reacting with human influenza virus, leading to genesis of a new virus which may cause severe influenza epidemics in humans.
Incubation period	2–5 days. May be as high as 9 days
Diagnosis	Flu-like symptoms, e.g. fever, cough, sore throat, muscle aches, eye infections, pneumonia
Investigation	Throat and nasal swabs – for testing of H5N1 virus
	Blood for testing of H5N1 virus

Management

General measures

Isolation of the patient

Antipyretics and analgesics

IV fluids

Antiviral drugs   Effective against human infection are:

M2 inhibitors: Amantadine 100–200 mg o.d. PO for 5 days

Rimantadine 100–200 mg o.d. PO for 5 days

Neuraminidase inhibitors:

- Oseltamivir 75 mg b.i.d. PO for 5 days
  Children (1-12 yrs) 30–75 mg PO for 5 days
  Prophylaxis: 75 mg o.d. for 10 days within 2 days of exposure
- Zanimivir 10 mg (2 inhalations) b.i.d. for 5 days
  Prophylaxis: 10 mg o.d. for 10 days after exposure.

S/E	Drug resistant
	Psychiatric and neurologic disorders
	Nausea, vomiting, pain abdomen
	Allergic reactions
	Liver disorders.
Prophylaxis	Destruction of infected birds, full cooking of chicken, eggs.

Refer: The patient to the medical team.

Swine Flu (Pandemic Influenza)

It is very contagious viral disease

Etiology	Influenza A H1N1 virus
	Can cause severe worldwide epidemics or pandemics

Transmission	Human to human
	It is a respiratory infection that is spread through:
	Direct contact – with infected persons, e.g. cough, sneeze – infected droplets dispersed into the air or by touching surfaces/hands, being contaminated by infected droplets.
	Transmission between pigs and humans – currently no confirmation.
Incubation period	1–7 days
Diagnosis	Flu-like symptoms, e.g. fever with chills, cough, sore throat, running nose, difficulty in breathing, headache, nausea, vomiting, diarrhea, eye infections, rashes, night sweats, myalgia, arthralgia.
Categories	A. Mild fever, cough, sore throat with or without bodyache, headache, diarrhea and vomiting.
	B. High grade fever, severe sore throat, bodyache, diarrhea and vomiting
	C. In addition to symptoms of categories A & B, breathlessness, chest pain, drowsiness, hypotension, hemoptysis, bluish discoloration of nails, irritability and refusal to accept feed especially in younger children.
Complications	Pneumonia, ARDS, sinusitis, otitis media, croup, bronchitis, myositis, myocarditis, encephalitis, seizures, multiorgan failure, shock.
Risk factors	Extreme of age with pre-medical disorders are at higher risk of complications, e.g. CV, pulmonary, renal disorders, blood disorders, diabetes, neurological disorders, cancer, HIV/AIDS and pregnancy.
D/d	Common cold:
	Fever – is mostly high in influenza, as compared to common cold
	Constitutional symptoms – more severe in influenza
	Complications – may occur in influenza, while absent in common cold.
Investigation	
Aims	To establish geographic spread to new areas (with large scale community spread, it may not be possible/need to test all cases)
	To detect change in the character of the virus.
Tests	Only C category patients require testing:
	Viral culture – to detect live virus
	Viral antigen detection test
	Viral nucleic acid detection test.
Samples	Throat and nasal swabs – for detection of H1N1 virus
	Specimens to be collected (within 1–2 days of disease's onset) by hospital/clinic staff and transported in viral transport medium, on ice or in liquid nitrogen.
Methods	Antigen detection (rapid) tests:
	• Hemagglutination (HA) test,
	• Hemagglutination inhibition (HI) test
	Molecular detection tests: RT-PCR – most reliable test for influenza

Management

Non-pharmaceutical interventions

Aims	To contain a pandemic/to mitigate its impact
Preventive measures	• Cover your nose with disposable tissues/mask (N 95 triple layered), or with a hankie, while coughing or sneezing, or while attending to an infected/ill person
	• Avoid handshakes
	• Maintain personal hygiene, scrub hands clean with soap
	• Avoid close contact with people having cough and fever
	• Contact immediately GP in case of illness, fatigue or weakness
	• Avoid unnecessary air travels to places/countries, with widespread influenza infections
Triage during pandemic	Triage is used to identify salvageable individuals and provide them the critical/medical care (priortisation based on available resources) to ensure saving of as many lives as possible. Triage can be done at community level as well as hospital settings. GPs, health workers and trained health volunteers may screen patients and refer only the serious cases to AE units of hospitals.
Screening tool for triage	Developed by British Thoracic Society is CURB-65, e.g.
	C – consciousness
	U – blood urea
	R – respiratory rate
	B – blood pressure
	65 – aged > 65
Scoring	For every sign in CURB-65, a score of 1 given. Then add all scores.
	Score 2: Needs treatment in a hospital – as an OPD or indoor patient.
	Score 3–5: Needs hospital admission and may also need ICU treatment.
Emergency Care	Isolation of the patient – separation and movement restriction of an ill person. Isolation is voluntary, but can be enforced, if required.
	Place: In a hospital, or at home
	Quarantine of a person – who is not ill, but has been exposed to the infection. It may be done for an individual or community.
	Place: It can be done at home, or at a quarantine center
Measures	Airway maintenance
	• Ventilation (invasive mechanical) – for acute respiratory failure
	Breathing maintenance
	• Oxygen therapy – for respiratory distress, dyspnea
	Circulation maintenance
	Hydration – IV fluids
	Electrolyte balance
	Antipyretics and analgesics – paracetamol or ibuprofen
	Antibiotics – to control/prevent infections

Antiviral drugs	Help in reducing morbidity and mortality
Drugs	Antiviral drugs: Effective against human infection are:

M2 inhibitors: Amantadine 100–200 mg o.d. PO for 5 days

Rimantadine 100–200 mg o.d. PO for 5 days

Neuraminidase inhibitors:

- Oseltamivir 75 mg b.i.d. PO for 5 days
  Children (1–12 yrs) 30–75 mg b.i.d. PO for 5 days
  Prophylaxis: 75 mg o.d. for 10 days within 2 days of exposure
- Zanimivir 10 mg (2 inhalations) b.i.d. for 5 days
  Prophylaxis: 10 mg o.d. for 10 days after exposure.

S/E	Unnecessary use – especially in common cold, is a hazard and may develop resistance to the drug
	Psychiatric and neurologic disorders
	Nausea, vomiting, abdominal pain
	Allergic reactions
	Liver disorders.
Vaccines	Influenza virus vaccine 1 mg of 0.5 mL IM. Rept after 4/52
	Children (6 months–3 yrs) 1 mg of 0.25 mL IM.

Ebola Virus

Etiology	Is an acute febrile hemorrhagic disease caused by Ebola virus, morphologically similar to but antigenically distinct from the Marburg agent. Is a severe, often fatal illness, with a death of up to 90%. The illness affects humans and non-human primates (monkeys, gorillas and chimpanzees).
Virology	Ebola virus is one of three members of Filoviridee family (Filovirus), along with genus Marburg virus and genus Cuevavirus.

Genus Ebola virus comprises five distinct species:

- Bundibugyo ebolavirus (BDBV)
- Zaire ebolavirus (EBOV)
- Reston ebolavirus (RESTV)
- Sudan ebolavirus (SUDV)
- Taï Forest ebolavirus (TAFV).

Epidemiology	Discovered in 1976, during simultaneous outbreaks in southern Sudan and northern Zaire. The virus has resurfaced recently and has been spreading alarmingly to other western African countries and outside Africa to some European countries like Spain, France, Denmark, and Dallas in the USA (a Liberian Patient died from Ebola viral infection). There were 4,447 deaths out of 8914 of primary infections and a few secondary cases (doctors and paramedics). WHO warns of 10,000 new cases of Ebola every week, (with > 70% fatality rate) unless World steps up its response to avoid serious consequences. Many countries started arrival screenings.

Endemic	Prevalent mainly in southern Sudan, northern Zaire (Ebola named after the river in Zaire). Guinea, Liberia and Sierra Leone. Sporadic cases of disease also reported in some other countries like Spain in Europe, Dallas in the USA. Spread: That one ebola patient infects two people on average. Grim future: WHO warns of 10K new cases of Ebola every week in two months time, unless World steps up its response: Many countries have started arrival screenings.

Table 18.1: Ebola: A race against death

Infection rate (%)	Death rate (%)	No. of deaths (till date)
Sex M: 48.4 F: 51.6	> 50	4447 (70%) of 8914 infected
Age > 45: 25.4	< 15: 73.4	people
< 15: 13.8		

(*Source:* AFP, WHO/The New England Journal of Medicine)

Transmission	• Animals to humans: Close contact with blood, secretions, organs, or other body fluids of infected animals. • Humans to humans: Close and prolonged contact (nosocomial and community-acquired), through broken skin or mucous membranes with blood, secretions, organs or other body fluids of infected people or indirect contact with contaminated environments (health workers). • Semen of affected person up to 7/52 of recovery. • Health workers, laboratory technicians, doctors and paramedics (prone to infection) by ignoring to take precautionary measures • Exposure to the virus through disinfected rather than sterililized needles, played a role in transmission.
Pathogenesis	Maculo-papular rash leading to desquamation
Incubation period	2–21 days. The disease becomes contagious once the first symptoms appears
Diagnosis	Fever – abrupt onset of high fever, malaise, headache, fatigue, diarrhea, abdominal pain, vomiting, dehydration, loss of appetite, myalgias, lethargy. URC: Cough – dry hacking, pharyngitis Chest pain – pleuritic Skin rash – maculo-papular Hemorrhages – hematemesis, melena, nasal bleeding, bleeding gums, vaginal bleeding, metrorrhagia and abortion Thrombocytopenia, hypofibrinoginemia, hemolytic anemia Shock – due to massive blood loss Death – mostly occurs in 2nd week.
Investigation	TLC and DLC – neutrophil leukocytosis Elisa Antigen detection tests

	Serum neutralization test
	Reverse transcriptase polymerase chain reaction (RT-PCR) assay
	Electrone microscopy
	Virus isolation by cell culture and urine, semen, throat and rectal swabs (all samples to be handled and transported as per WHO guidelines)
D/d	Viral: Dengue fever, Marburg viral disease
	Bacterial: Shigellae, Salmonellae (typhoid fever), Meningeal, Plague
	Parasitic: Malaria
	Richettsial
Management	Preventive measures:
	Sunlight exposure – kills virus
	Hygiene – wash hands with soap
	Clothes – detergents in washing machines kill the virus
	Food – avoid raw meats, eat cooked foods
	Dead patients – handle with care while cremating/burying by using all bio-medicare
	Specific measures:
	Symptomatic as no effective treatment till date.
	Isolation of patient until virologically free of virus (approx. 3/52 post onset)
	Specific plasma antibodies
	IV fluids
	Blood transfusion
	Drugs (experimental): ZMapp, Avigan, TKM-Abola

Refer: The patient to the medical team

Marburg Virus

Etiology	Is an acute febrile systemic disease caused by Marburg virus, morphologically similar to but antigenically distinct from the Ebola agent. Is a severe, often fatal illness, with high mortality rate. The illness affects humans and non-human primates (monkeys, gorillas and chimpanzees).
Virology	Marburg virus is one of three members of Filoviridee family (Filovirus), along with genus Ebolavirus and genus Cuevavirus. The virus appears as an elongated filamentous particle (blister-like appearance). The virus is biosafety level 4 pathogen, and needs maximum biological containment facilities.
Epidemiology	Discovered in 1967, during simultaneous outbreaks in Marburg and Frankfurt, Germany, Belgrade and Yugoslavic, wherein laboratory technicians exposed to imported African green monkeys, got infected.
	Outbreaks also reported from Kenya. There were seven deaths out of 25 primary infections and six secondary cases (doctors and paramedics).
	Sporadic cases of disease also reported in some other African countries.
	A secondary case demonstrated Marburg virus (acquired by sexual

intercourse) in semen of a patient. The Marburg's natural reservoir is unknown.

Transmission	Animals to humans: Close contact with blood, secretions, organs, or other body fluids of infected animals.

- Humans to humans: Close and prolonged contact (nosocomial and community-acquired), through broken skin or mucous membranes with blood, secretions, organs or other body fluids of infected people or indirect contact with contaminated environments (health workers).
- Semen of affected person up to 7/52 of recovery.
- Health workers, Laboratory technicians, doctors and paramedics (prone to infection) by ignoring to take precautionary measures
- Exposure to the virus through disinfected rather than sterililized needles, played a role in transmission.

Pathogenesis	Lesions: In all organs, i.e. skin, lymphoid tissue, liver, lungs, brain, etc.

Skin: Maculo-papular rash leading to desquamation

Lymphoid tissue: Focal necrosis with degeneration

Liver: Eosinophilic cytoplasmic bodies

Lungs: Vascular lesions in arterioles – endarteritis

Brain: Multiple hemorrhagic infarcts with glial proliferation.

Incubation period	3–9 days. The disease becomes contagious once the first symptoms appear.
Diagnosis	Fever – abrupt onset of high fever, malaise, fatigue

Headache – abrupt onset, frontal and temporal regions

Diarrhea – watery, often severe, lethargy

Abdominal pain, vomiting, dehydration, loss of appetite

URC : Cough – dry hacking, pharyngitis, tonsillitis

Chest pain – pleuritic

Skin rash – maculo-papular, appears (5–7th day) on face, neck, arms

Hemorrhages – hematemesis, melena, nasal bleeding, bleeding gums, vaginal bleeding, metrorrhagia and abortion

Thrombocytopenia, hypofibrinoginemia, hemolytic anemia

Hepatomegaly, splenomegaly, lymphadenopathy

Psychological – dementation

Shock – due to massive blood loss

Death – mostly occurs in 2nd week.

Investigation	TLC and DLC – neutrophil leukopenia, atypical lymphocytes and neutrophils (Pelger-Huet), thrombocytopenia, hypoproteinemia

ESR - low

SGOT and SGPT – elevated

Antigen detection tests

Serum neutralization test

Reverse transcriptase polymerase chain reaction (RT-PCR) assay

Electrone microscopy

Lumbar puncture – normal or may be minimal pleocytosis

Virus isolation by cell culture and urine, semen, throat and rectal swabs (all samples to be handled and transported as per WHO guidelines)

D/d   Viral: Ebola viral disease, dengue fever

Bacterial: Shigellae, Salmonellae (typhoid fever), Meningeal, Plague

Parasitic: Malaria

Richettsial infection.

Management   Preventive measures:

Sunlight exposure – kills virus

Hygiene – wash hands with soap

Clothes – detergents in washing machines kill the virus

Food – avoid raw meats, eat cooked foods

Dead patients – handle with care while cremating/burying by using all bio-medicare

Specific measures:

Symptomatic as no effective treatment till date.

Isolation of patient until virologically free of virus (approx. 3/52 post onset)

Specific plasma antibodies

IV fluids

Blood transfusion

Drugs (experimental) : ZMapp, Avigan, TKM-Abola

Refer: The patient to the medical team.

Cholera

Definition	It is an acute epidemic disease.
Etiology	*Vibrio cholerae* or El Tor vibrios.
Transmission	By ingestion of contaminated food or drinking polluted water.
Endemic	Prevalent mainly in countries lacking modern sanitary techniques, e.g. regular testing and purification of water supplies and proper sewage disposal.
Incubation	1–5 days.
Diagnosis	Sudden onset of vomiting and severe diarrhea (rice water stools), dehydration, acidosis, hypokalemia, hypotension, subnormal temperature, rapid and shallow breathing, muscle cramps, sunken eyes, oliguria, shock, coma.
Investigations	CBC
	Hemogram – hemoconcentration
	Serum electrolytes, BUN
	Stool microscopy, stool culture.

Management

Preventive	Isolation of the patient
	Use only boiled water
	Avoid uncovered and uncooked fruits and vegetables.

Specific

Moderately ill   Monitor fluids input/output charts

Oral Rehydration Therapy (ORT):

- Oral rehydration salt solution (90 mEq/L of sodium) to be given in same volume as that lost.

Severely ill   IV fluids – Ringer's lactate sol. Or normal saline sol. (0.9% NaCl) @

         Adult: 50–100 mL/mt

         Children: <12 months @ 30 mL/kg/hr.

                 >12 months @ 70 mL/kg/6 hrs.

Start ORS sol. – when the patient can drink comfortably.

Drugs   Antibiotics:

- Tetracycline Adult: 0.5 g q.d.s. orally for 3–5 days

               Children: 12.5 mg/kg/dose q.d.s for 3 days

- Cotrimoxazole (Trimethoprim (TMP) + sulphamethoxazole (SMX)

               Adult: TMP 160 mg + SMX 800 mg b.d.orally

               Children: TMP 5 mg/kg/dose + SMX 25 mg/kg

               b.d. for 3 days

- Furazolidone Adult: 100 mg t.d.s./q.d.s. PO for 3–5 days

               Children: 5 mg/kg body wt. q.d.s. for 3 days

- Metronidazole Adult: 400–800 mg t.d.s. PO for 5–7 days

               Children : 35-50 mg/kg/day in 3 divide.

Prophylaxis   Cholera vaccine 0.5 mL IM or s.c. Rpt. 1 mL IM or s.c. after 1–4 wks.

Booster dose 0.5 mL during cholera's hazard.

Typhoid/Paratyphoid Fever

Serious infectious disease.

Etiology	Bacterial infection, e.g.
	Salmonella typhoid – typhoid fever
	Salmonella paratyphoid – paratyphoid fever.
Transmission	Source: Unhygienically prepared/undercooked food, contaminated milk, water, foods, and over-ripened fruits, vegetables
	Route: Fecal-oral – by ingestion of food contaminated by urine and feces of patients suffering from typhoid and of carriers (harbouring germs in their GI tract, gallbladder, or bone marrow.
Epidemiology	Endemic in tropical countries – due to poor hygiene/sanitation.
Incubation	14 days.
Diagnosis	Fever – temperature continues to rise – often to 41°C (105°F)
	Chills and sweating

Headache, vomiting

Constipation or diarrhea

Skin rash (red spots) – appears on 6th day of fever

Splenomegaly.

Complications Intestinal hemorrhage – due to perforation of the ulcerated intestine

Peritonitis

Shock

Death.

Investigations CBC

Hb and ESR

Blood culture – isolation and identification

Widal test.

Management

Prevention Do's:

- Maintain a high standard of personal hygiene – wash hands before and after meals
- Drink only bottled or boiled water
- Eat only thoroughly cooked food that is served hot

Don't:

- Avoid raw/undercooked seafood
- Avoid uncovered food served by street hawkers/unhygienic food joints
- Avoid tap water, ice-cubes, ice-creams, cut fruits.

Specific Antibiotics:

- Chloramphenicol 1 g PO q.d.s. – until fever disappears, or
- Ampicillin 100 mg/kg/day PO

Antipyretics

IV dextrose sol.

Treatment of complications.

Prophylaxis Typhoid vaccination:

Oral vaccine: 3 capsules taken over 5 days (days 1, 3, 5)

Injectable vaccine: 0.5 mL s.c. or IM. Rept after 4/52.

Dengue Fever (syn. Dengue Hemorrhagic Fever and Breakbone Fever)

It is an acute viral infection characterized by high fever and bodyaches (breakbone).

Etiology Arthropod-borne group of viruses.

Transmission Bite of Aedes aegypti mosquito.

Incubation 2–7 days.

Diagnosis Fever – high grade fever, chills, sore throat, headache, malaise

Severe bodyaches (deep muscle and joint pains)

Hemorrhagic phenomenon (crippled blood cells – bleeding gums, skin, intestine)

Rash (maculopapular, scarlatiniform, or petechial) starts on trunk, spreading out to face, arms and legs.

Acute abdominal pain, hepatomegaly

Shock.

Investigation	TLC and DLC: Leukopenia
	Platelet count – < 50000/cmm
	SGPT – levels elevated
	Blood culture
	Serological tests
	CXR (X-ray chest) – shows pleural effusion.
Management	No specific antiviral treatment. Treatment is supportive and symptomatic
	Hydrotherapy – to manage hyperpyrexia
	Drugs: Antipyretics and analgesics, e.g. paracetamol
	Maintenance of fluid intake. Promote oral fluid intake, preferably ORS or fruit juice
	IV fluids – to combat circulatory disturbance
	Blood transfusion or platelets suspended in plasma – for severe haemorrhage.
Shock	Monitor patient for dengue shock syndrome (DSS):

- IV fluids: Ringer's lactate, normal saline, or
5% dextrose @ 15 ml/kg over ½ hr.
- Oxygen therapy
- Check hematocrit – if rising, give plasma or 5% albumin @ 15 mL/kg
  – if hematocrit declining give blood transfusion
- Platelet transfusion – if coagulopathy results in severe bleeding.

Prevention	Keep a watch over water storage containers such as, overhead tanks, desert coolers, free of mosquitoes.

Acute (Severe) Malaria

Malaria continues to be a major killer of mankind – appx. 1 million die each year of malaria around the globe.

Etiology	*Plasmodium falciparum, P. vivax, P. ovale, P. malariae.*
Transmission	Bite of an infected female anopheline mosquito.

Manifestations of Severe Malaria (Pernicious Malaria)

- Cerebral malaria: This is the most dreaded complication of *P. falciparum* infection, caused by *Plasmodium falciparum, Plasmodium vivax* – very rare
- Severe anemia
- Acute renal failure
- Pulmonary edema or ARDS
- Hypoglycemia
- Hypotension

- Shock
- DIC
- Convulsions
- Acidemia
- Hemoglobinuria

Diagnosis   Onset – sudden
Fever – high fever for few days
Pallor, jaundice, anemia
Splenomegaly
Encephalopathy, neurological signs – variable, seizures
Intracranial pressure – elevated
Retinal hemorrhages
Hypoglycemia
Coma, death

Investigation   CBC, ESR
Hematocrit (PCV) 30%
Blood urea > 50 mg
Blood smear – thick blood film for diagnosis
              – thin blood film for identification of species
Immunological tests: Antigen detection by chromatography
                              by dipstick test
          Antibody detection by fluorescent microscopy

Management
Specific treatment (chemotherapy)
Aim   To save the patient's life
Drugs   Oral drugs: For uncomplicated malaria

- Chloroquine Adult: 1 g stat PO followed by 0.5 g at 6, 24 and 48 hrs.
                Children: 5 mg/kg infused over 4 hrs.
                      Rept three 8 hr infusions of 5 mg/kg each
- Pyrimethamine 1.25 mg/kg + sulfadoxine 25 mg/kg (single dose)
- Quinine   Adult: 300–600 mg t.d.s. PO for 7 days

Parentral drugs for complicated malaria:

- Quinine 20 mg salt/kg (loading dose) diluted in 10 ml/kg, 5–10% dextrose IV over 4 hrs. Rept after 8 hrs 10 mg salt/kg over 4 hrs.

Continue IV until patient can swallow oral:

- Artesunate 2.4 mg/kg IV bolus or IM (loading dose)
  Rept 1.2 mg/kg IV or IM after 12 hrs and then o.d. for 6 days
- Artemether 3.2 mg/kg IM (loading dose)
  Rept 1.6 mg/kg IM o.d. for 6 days

Supportive treatment
         Admit the patient

Nursing care

Sponging and fanning

NSAID drugs – indicated only in uncomplicated cases

Correction of fluid, acid, base and electrolyte disturbances

Treatment of complications

Refer: The patient to the medical team

Bubonic Plague (Black Death)

An acute disease transmitted to human beings by fleas from infected rats/wild rodents. Severe epidemics/pandemics raged through world (Europe and Asia) in 1340 and 1660 (In 14th century Europe about 25 million people, e.g. ¼th population died). Even now cases turn up in many countries.

Etiology	Pasteurella – *Yersinia pestis*, a gram–negative bacteria
Transmission	From rodent to rodant, and from rodent to human by the bites of fleas
Diagnosis	Fever/chills, headache, vomiting, thirst, malaise, bodyaches, delirium,
	Lymphadenitis (buboes) – cervical, axillary, or inguinal
	Septicemia, pneumonia (pneumonic plague – fatal)
	Purpuric spot (black plague) – appear over the skin
	Coma, death
Investigation	CBC
	Leukocytosis
	Smears – from bubo aspirates
	Cultures – from bubo aspirates, blood, or pus
	Agglutination tests
	CXR – pulmonary infiltration
Management	
Preventive	Rodent and flea control measures – total eradication not possible
Emergency	Airway maintenance

• Ventilation (invasive mechanical) – for acute respiratory failure

Breathing maintenance

• Oxygen therapy – for respiratory distress, dyspnea

Circulation maintenance

Hydration – IV fluids

Electrolyte balance

Antipyretics and analgesics – paracetamol or ibuprofen

Antibiotics – to control/prevent infections

Vaccine – partial immunization can be provided

Japanese Encephalitis (Japanese B Encephalitis)

It is an acute viral infection of the brain.

Etiology   Japanese encephalitis (JE) virus – of Flaviviridae family

Epidemiology   JE – leading cause of viral encephalitis in Asia and Far East

Transmission   Reservoirs – infected domestic swines and birds

                 Vectors – mosquito – Culex tritaeniorhynchus

                 Spread to humans – by the bite of mosquito

Incubation   5–15 days

Diagnosis   Fever, headache, nausea, vomiting, diarrhea, myalgia, followed by change in mental status, e.g. irritability, abnormal behavior, neurological deficit, e.g. hemiplegia, ocular palsy, convulsions, coma.

Investigations   IgM capture ELISA – to detect antibodies in serum/CSF

                 Immunofluorescence – to detect antigen

                 PCR – to detect nucleic acid

Management

Preventive   Early diagnosis and prompt treatment, e.g.

                 Availability of infrastructure of clinical management with standard operating procedure/guidelines

                 • Epidemic preparedness

                 • Integrated vector control method

                 • Vaccination – wherever feasible

Specific   No specific antiviral drug for JE

                 Symptomatic treatment

Prophylaxis   Active immunisation – live attenuated Sa-14-14-2 vaccine

                 Not recommended as a pandemic control.

References

1. Strader DB, et al: Diagnosis, management and treatment of Hepatitis C. HEPATOLOGY, Vol. 39, No. 4;2004.

2. Alter MJ. Prevention of spread of Hepatitis C. HEPATOLOGY, Vol. 36(suppl 1): 593–598;2002.

3. Pawlotsky JM. Use and interpretation of virological tests for hepatitis C. Hepatology 36 (suppl 1): S65-S73;2002.

4. Thomas DL. Hepatitis C and human immunodeficiency virus infection. Hepatology 36 (suppl 1): S201-S209;2002.

5. Rewari BB, Sukarma T: Emergencies in HIV medicine. JIMA, Vol. 107: 317–322;2009.

6. Wiwanitkit V: Leucocyte and Lymphocyte count in cases of bird flu infection in Thailand. JIMA, Vol. 106, 168–168;2008.

7. Special Articles: Sponsered by Deptt. of Health and Family Welfare, Govt. of India.

   • Epidemiology of seasonal, avian and pandemic influenza, 506–507

   • Case definitions for avian and pandemic influenza, 520–522

   • Clinical features of influenza, 524–526

- Laboratory diagnosis of influenza
- Case management for influenza

JIMA, Vol. 107;2009.

8. GrossmanM, Jawetz E: Infectious diseases: Bacterial: Cholera, plague and typhoid fever. Current Medical Diagnosis and Treatment, 811–823, Maruzen;1975.

9. Dhillon GPS, Raina VK: Epidemiology of Japanese encephalitis in context with Indian scenario. JIMA Vol. 106, 660–663.

10. Petersdorf R. Fever of unknown origion. An old friend revisited. Arch Intern Med 152:21;1992.

11. Rigau Perez JG, Clark GG, Gubler DJ, et al. Dengue and Dengue hemorrhagic fever. The Lancet 352:971–7;1998.

12. Mandell GL, Bennett JE, Dolin R. Principles and Practice of Infectious Diseases New York: Churchill Livingstone; 1995.

13. Tuberculosis in Children. Guidelines for diagnosis, prevention and treatment (A statement of the Scientific Committees of the IUATLD. Edited by Hershifield E.) Bulletin of International Union against Tuberculosis and Lung diseases. 66:61–7, 1991. WHO. Stop TB at source. WHO report on TB epidemic. Geneva 1995.

14. Looareesuwan S, Wilairatana P: Guideline in management of severe malaria. JIMA 10:628–31; 2000.

15. Warrel DA: Cerebral malaria: clinical features, pathophysiology and treatment. Ann Trop Med Parasitol 91:875–84;1997.

16. Dengue hemorrhagic fever. Diagnosis, treatment, prevention and control. 2nd ed. World Health Organization. Geneva 1997.

17. Rigau Perez JG, Clark GG, Gubler DJ, et al. Dengue and dengue hemorrhagic fever. The Lancet 352:971–7;1998.

Part III
Accident Emergencies

Section 19   MANAGEMENT OF MULTIPLE INJURIES

Management of Multiple Injuries

- Spinal contusion
- Management of spinal cord injuries
- Management of complications

Peripheral nerve injuries
- Neurapraxia
- Axonotmesis
- Neurotmesis

- Brachial plexus injuries
- Complete brachial plexus injuries
- Incomplete brachial plexus injuries
- Upper lesion (Erb Duchen)
- Lower lesion (Klumpke)

Limbs injuries:
- Management of fractures of the limbs

Management of Multiple Injuries

The survival of a patient with multiple injuries depends upon the judgement and planning of dealing surgeon, and readiness of hospital with adequate resuscitation facilities. Many improvements have been made in recent years, and subsequent development of accident and emergency (A&E) department, for the management of accident (multiple injuries) and emergency (medical/surgical).

Early Trauma Care
Ambulance Service

The management of patients with multiple injuries starts right from the site of accident. The ambulance attendants (professional staff members) are trained enough to bear the responsibility, until the patient reaches the hospital. The attendants record the site, date, and time of accident; position in which the patient was found, whether conscious or unconscious, drunk or sober, apprehensive, hostile, or cooperative, and the amount of bleeding observed/assessed (at the site and from soaked clothes). Management of the injured (resuscitation measures) should start immediately in an orderly manner (ABC of trauma management), i.e. airway and cervical spine control, breathing care, control circulation, combat shock, splint fractured limbs. The attendant is responsible for the comfortable transportation of patient to the hospital, is trained enough and well versed with resuscitation measures, that are continued uninterrupted until the patient reaches the A&E department, being informed in advance of the arrival of the injured patient.

Accident and Emergency Department
Trauma Team

The accident and emergency (A&E) team should consist of dedicated medical and nursing staff trained enough in accident and emergency care and well versed with resuscitation. Care of the patient in A&E requires regular assessment and monitoring especially the trends. This based on physical examination and use of various monitoring equipments. However, the equipments are not a substitute for good clinical skills. In fact accident and emergency care is labor intensive. Record all the monitoring on a pre-designed chart. The decision making in the A&E should proceed in the continuous manner of evaluation, intervention, and re-evaluation. A&E should have access to well-equipped laboratory facilities. Quick diagnostic tests especially for estimation of glucose. Electrolytes, proteins, blood counts, blood grouping, blood gas and cholesterol, etc. should be available. Portable X-ray unit and ultrasonography are desirable round the clock. Besides caring for clinical disorder, attention should also be paid towards diet, sedation, and control of infection. Also mandatory to communicate regularly with the relatives/attendants and apprise them of patient's condition.

Assessment of Injured Patient (Primary Survey) (Table 19.1)
Advanced Trauma Life Support (ATLS)

Triage (priority of treatment) In the management of multiple injuries (as per guidelines of ATLS course) priority of treatment is directed to life-threatening conditions such as airway obstruction, shock, or external hemorrhage, even before a detailed examination begins.

Aims of ATLS
- To provide an immediate treatment of patients with multiple injuries
- To standardize trauma resuscitation.

Table 19.1: Proforma for assessment of injured patients

Surname .... First name .... A&E no ....

Age/DOB .... Sex ....

Date ....

Son/daughter/wife of .... Time ....

Occupation .... Tel ....

Address ....

DOA .... DOD ....

Diagnosis ....

A&E consultant/dr.i/c ....

Complaints (symptoms) and their duration:

....

....

Preliminary (brief) History:

....

....

....

Preliminary (brief) examination:
Airway obstruction and cervical spine injury:

Breathless .... Gasping .... Cyanosis ....

Foreign bodies .... Blood .... Saliva .... Vomitus ....

Neck rigidity .... Tenderness ....

Deformity ....

Paresis of arm/and leg .... Movements ....

Breathing (respiration) disturbance:

Respiration .... Slow and shallow .... Slow and deep .... Noisy ....

Pulse .... BP .... SBP .... DBP ....

Temperature .... Subnormal .... High (> 40°C) ....

Circulation disturbance (hemorrhage and Shock)

Respirations .... Restlessness .... Thirst ....

Skin .... Cold clammy .... Pale ....

Disability syn. dysfunction of the CNS (assessment of conscious level):

Conscious level made by AVPU system:

Response .... Verbal stimulus .... Pain ....

Unresponsive .... Pupil .... Size ....

Reaction ....

Exposure: (Expose the patient completely)

X-ray cervical spine .... CXR .... X-ray pelvis ....

Detailed history (secondary survey):

....

....

....

....

....

Detailed examination:

Head injuries:

General physical examination:

Position .... Lying flaccid .... Curled up ....

Alert .... Unconscious .... Depth of unconsciousness........................

Eyes: .... Black eye .... Subconjunctival hemorrhage ....

Pupil: .... Dilated .... Pinpoint .... Equal ....

Vision .... Movements ....

Reacting to light .... Not-reacting to light ....

Eyes: .... Black eye ....

Subconjunctival hemorrhage ....

Bleeding/CSF: Nose .... Ear .... Mouth ....

Cranial nerves: Squint .... Facial palsy ....

Neck rigidity .... Movements ....

Limbs: Muscle power: RUL .... LUL .... RLL .... LLL................

      Sensations: RUL .... LUL .... RLL .... LLL ....

      Reflexes: RUL .... LUL .... RLL .... LLL ....

Local examination: (shave and clean the head)

Bruise .... Swelling .... Laceration ....

Fracture .... Simple .... Compound ....

Chest injuries:

General physical examination:

Position: Lying quite .... Retless ....

Dyspnea .... Cyanosis ....

Respiration: Abdominal .... Thoracic .... Movements ....

Local examination:

Wound: Penetrating .... Swelling .... Tenderness ....

Percussion: Resonant .... Cardiac dullness ....

Abdominal injuries: ....

General physical examination:

Position: Lying quite .... Restless ....

Respiration: Air hunger .... Movements ....

Local examination:

Distension .... Shifting dullness ....

Tenderness .... Rigidity ....

Liver: Tenderness .... Shifting dullness ....

Spleen: Tenderness .... Shifting dullness ....

Kidney: Tenderness .... Shifting ullness ....

Urinary bladder: Tenderness .... Shifting dullness ....

Stomach: Distension .... Shifting dullness ....

Large intestine: Peritonitis .... Surgical emphysema..

Spinal injuries:

Spinal column injuries: Fractures .... Fracture dislocation ....

Spinal cord injury: Paralysis ....

Limbs injuries:

Deformity .... Swelling .... Shortening ....

Wounds .... Tenderness .... Crepitus ....

Movements .... Shortning .... Abnormal mobility ....

Limbs: Muscle power: RUL .... LUL .... RLL .... LLL................

      Sensations: RUL .... LUL .... RLL .... LLL................

      Reflexes: RUL .... LUL .... RLL .... LLL................

Investigations

Features of ATLS
- Frequent re-evaluation of patient's condition
- Response to treatment
- A deteriorating condition necessitates a re-evaluation and treatment of 'ABC'.

Phases of ATLS
- Initial care
- Definitive care

Initial care (Diagnosis and Management of Life-threatening Entities)
Preliminary (Brief) History

Identification of a seriously injured patient relies on observation, history and physical examination (preliminary and detailed examination). At first contact (primary survey), the life-threatening entities, e.g. the ABCs (Airway's patency and cervical spine control, adequacy of breathing and circulation) are quickly assessed. If there is an abnormality in anyone of these, life support/resuscitation must be initiated immediately, followed by a quick assessment of the other two parameters, e.g. the D&E (dysfunction of the CNS, i.e. conscious level and exposure and environment). The finer points of history taking (secondary survey) including detailed examination may have to wait until later. Always suspect major injury in RSA and fall from a height.

History of accident

Inquire   From witnesses, ambulance crew, relatives or persons accompanying the patient:
- MOI: Was it vehicle accident or fall from a height?
- When, where and how did it happen? What happened next?
- Was it under influence of alcohol or drugs?
- Any seizure attack: Pre-/post-accident?

Preliminary (Brief) Examination

A. Airway obstruction

Etiology   Foreign bodies, blood, saliva, or vomitus.
             Cervical spine injury with or without paralysis

Diagnosis   Breathless or gasping, cyanosis
             Deformity
             Neck rigidity
             Local tenderness
             Paresis of arm and leg
             Movements – painful and restricted.

B. Breathing (respiration) disturbance

Etiology   Head injury
             Chest injuries
             Fracture ribs

Open chest wounds

Hemothorax

Tension pneumothorax

Flail chest

Cardiac tamponade.

Diagnosis   Breathless or gasping

Chest pain

Cyanotic or pale

Tachycardia, hypotension

X-ray chest, head, cervical spine – confirms clinical diagnosis.

C. Circulation disturbance (hemorrhage and shock)

Etiology   External or internal hemorrhage due to:

Fracture pelvis, chest, and abdominal injuries

Diagnosis   External hemorrhage is revealed type, while

Internal hemorrhage is concealed type.

Signs   Deep sighing respirations (air hunger)

Restlessness, thirst, pallor

Cold clammy skin – pallor or cyanotic

Tachycardia, hypotension

Unconsciousness – in case of shock.

D. Disability syn. dysfunction of the CNS (assessment of conscious level)

Etiology   Trauma – head injury

Infection

Diabetes

Psychiatric – epilepsy

Alcohol abuse, drug abuse – opiates, poisons

Shock

Diagnosis   Assessment of conscious level made by AVPU system, i.e.

Alert

Response to verbal stimulus

Response pain

Unresponsive to any stimulus

Pupil – size and reaction.

E. Exposure and environment

With the consent and co-operation of patient/attendant, clothing be removed as per requirements for examination, in a warm and well lit examination room, but subsequently cover the patient as much as possible, in order to decrease the anxiety and to prevent excessive heat loss.

F. Monitor vital signs

Pulse, BP, respiratory rate, temperature, ECG

Catheterization

IV lines,
Monitor input/output.

Management of Life-threatening Entities
A. Airway maintenance with cervical spine control

Maintenance of free airway is strongly stressed upon and should take the top priority treatment, as a life-saving measure. The treatment includes:

Basic management:

Airway (with cervical spine control):
Position of patient – supine, with tilting of head, and support of the jaw.
Immobilization of cervical spine – manually, sand bag, cervical collar.
Caution: Avoid tilting the head or moving the neck – in case of any suspicion of neck injury

- Removal of foreign bodies, blood clots, saliva, and vomitus from the mouth and nose by suction or manually.

Advanced management:

- Oxygen therapy – supply high flow oxygen by facemask. An apneic or hypoventilated patient requires bag and mask ventilation prior to the endotracheal intubation and IPPV
- Endotracheal intubation

Surgical management:

- Cricothyroidotomy
- Tracheostomy – indicated in head, chest, or upper abdomen injuries

B. Breathing (respiration) and ventilation control

Head injury: May lead to cessation of central control of breathing.
Management: Described in appropriate section of Head Injury.

Chest injuries

a. Open chest wounds – may be simple or complicated, due to direct violence, e.g. stab, bullet, or bomb shell fragments. Contusion and laceration of lung - common in chest wounds.
   Management:
   - To be covered with dressing pads and stitched later on, in order to prevent serious lesions like tension pneumothorax, an urgent surgical treatment is required after resuscitation.
   - Thoracotomy is indicated for uncontrollable bleeding.
b. Flail chest – due to severe violence, resulting in a flaccid unstable chest wall showing paradoxical movement, which produces faulty ventilation with anoxia, whereas impaired coughing causes collection of bronchopulmonary secretions.
   Management:
   - Oxygen, endotracheal intubation with positive pressure ventilation, deep breathing exercises, analgesics, antibiotics to prevent and control infection.
   - Urgent tracheostomy required – produces remarkable results.

c. Traumatic pneumothorax – penetrating chest wounds/blunt injury may produce pneumothorax (air in pleural cavity)

Management: Seal the wounds with dressing pad

d. Tension pneumothorax – is a life-threatening emergency

Management:

- To be treated on priority basis by immediate decompression, i.e. plunging an aspirating needle into the pleural cavity (needle thoracocentesis) through 2nd intercostals space, at the mid-clavicular level, to relieve air under tension. It is followed by introducing a catheter (chest drain) through the 4th intercostal space, at the mid-axillary line and connected to the suction apparatus.

e. Traumatic hemothorax – blood collects in the pleural cavity due to penetrating chest wounds, or from torn – heart, lungs, or blood vessels.

Management:

- Seal the wounds with dressing pads
- Repeated aspirations, and if fails then, intercostals tube with water seal drainage is indicated. If the bleeding persists, then:
- Thoracotomy is indicated.

f. Fractured ribs – due to direct violence, resulting in isolated fracture of ribs, with/without any associated complication.

Management: Treated by: Analgesics, intercostal blocks, strapping.

g. Stove in chest – roomy due to severe violence, resulting in multiple rib fractures and indentation of the chest wall and distressing paradoxical chest movement.

Management:

- Elevation of depressed chest wall by towel clips/clamps round the ribs.
- Endotracheal intubation and positive pressure ventilation
- Tracheostomy – if required.

h. Lung injuries: Contusion injuries resolve spontaneously, whilst lacerated injuries may require repeated aspirations/thoracotomy.

Antibiotics to prevent and control infection.

Deep breathing exercises.

Thoraco-abdominal wounds: Common in bomb blast injuries.

Management: Exploration to control bleeding.

Refer: The patient to the surgical team.

C. Circulation disturbance (hemorrhage and shock) control

External hemorrhage – controlled by direct pressure, e.g. sterile dressings, covered with a compression bandage. Failure of this, may require a tourniquet (preferably a pneumatic).

Internal hemorrhage – occurs in fracture pelvis, chest, abdominal injuries.

Hemothorax: Treated by repeated aspiration, catheterization, and if required thoracotomy.

Abdominal hemorrhage: Laparotomy is to be performed as an emergency.

General measures:

Monitor pulse, BP, respiration, temperature, ECG

Assess change in skin color, clamminess, conscious level

IV fluids – adult 1 L of 0.9% saline; children 20 mL/kg
Plasma expanders
Blood grouping and crossmatching
Blood transfusion
Catheterization
Monitor input/output.

Shock   **Described in Section 2 of General Symptoms.**

Detailed History (Secondary Survey)

History
* Of circumstantial events/environment related to injury
* Of allergies
* Of drugs/alcohol abuse
* Of seizure
* Of previous illness
* Of last meal

Detailed Examination

Includes a head to toe examination to identify other (specific) injuries. The patient is monitored throughout, and any deterioration necessitates a re-evaluation of 'ABC'.

Head injuries

General physical examination:

Position – lying flaccid/curled up

Level of consciousness – depth of unconsciousness

Respiration:
* Slow and shallow (concussion)
* Slow and deep, irregular, noisy (compression)

Eyes – black eye (local injury) or subconjunctival hemorrhage

Pupil response:
* Dilated, equal, reacting to light (concussion)
* Dilated, fixed, not-reacting to light (compression)
* Pinpoint, fixed, paralytic (hemorrhage)

Bleeding – nose/ear/mouth (# base of skull)

Hemoptysis

Temperature – subnormal (concussion) – rises > 40°C (hemorrhage)

Rigidity of neck – due to meningeal irritation (hemorrhage)

Cranial nerves – squint (injury 3rd/4th or 6th); facial palsy (7th nerve)

Muscle power of limbs – may be paralyzed

Reflexes

Local examination:

(Shave and clean the head)

Wound – scalp/head

Fracture – depressed

Swelling – hematoma

Rigidity of neck – due to meningeal irritation (hemorrhage)

Cranial nerves – squint (injury 3rd/4th or 6th); facial palsy (7th nerve)

Muscle power of limbs – may be paralyzed

Reflexes.

Chest injuries:

General physical examination:

Position – lying quite/restless and gasping

Dyspnea/cyanosis

Respiration – abdominal/thoracic

Chest movements – any restriction

Wound – penetrating (pneumothorax, surgical emphysema)

Swelling – surgical emphysema

Local examination:

Local tenderness

Percussion – resonant (surgical emphysema, pneumothorax)

Cardiac dullness – obliterated (pneumothorax)
      – increased (hemothorax)

Crepitus audible.

Abdomen and perineum injuries:

General physical examination:

Lying quite (peritonitis)

Restless (hemorrhage)

Respiration – air hunger (hemorrhage)

Movements of abdominal wall – abnormal

Local examination:

Distension

Local tenderness, rigidity, shifting dullness (as per seat of lesion)

Liver	Local tenderness, dullness – increased, shifting dullness
Spleen	Local ternderness, dullness – persistent over left side of abdomen, shifting dullness – over right side
Kidney	Swelling (fullness), local tenderness, dullness – lateral to erector spinae
Urinary bladder	Swelling (fullness), local tenderness, shifting dullness
Stomach	Rigidity – board-like, distension, shifting dullness
Large intestine	Peritonitis, surgical emphysema.
Spinal injuries	Spinal column injuries – fractures, fracture-dislocation
	Spinal cord injury – paralysis (meningeal hemorrhage).
Limbs injuries	Any deformity, swelling, wounds
	Local tenderness
	Pitting edema

	Muscle power, tone, reflexes, and sensations
	Pulses – peripheral
	Joints – movements
	Shortening.
Investigations	Specific investigations – as per presentation of each patient
	Complete blood count
	Serum proteins
	Serum electrolytes
	Serum alkaline phosphatase
	Blood cholesterol
	Blood sugar
	Blood grouping and crossmatching
	Blood urea
	Urine analysis
	ECG
	X-ray of affected region (chest, skull, abdomen, pelvis, and limb)
	Ultrasound – especially for abdominal injuries
	CT scan and MRI
	Angiography – indicated in pelvic injury, aortic injury
	Echocardiography

II. Definitive Care (Management of Specific Injuries)

The doctor incharge should plan the line of treatment in consultation with other specialists involved in the management of various lesions. It may be possible to manage all the injuries simultaneously but at times, these lesions to be dealt with, on priority basis, e.g. in a definite sequence. Compound fractures should preferably be treated along with head, neck, or chest injuries. Operative treatment for simple fractures may better be postponed to a later stage. But it is better not to postpone the corrective orthopedic measures for more than a day or so, in the patients who appeared unlikely to recover from their associated injuries.

Head Injuries Include scalp wounds and head injuries:

Scalp Wounds   Scalp wounds bleed profusely, as the blood vessels of scalp prevented from contraction due to firm adherence of vessel walls to the fibrous tissue of the scalp.

MOI	Direct violence – being hit by an object
	RSA.
Diagnosis	Bleeding scalp wound.
Management	Shaving of scalp and toilet of wound with antiseptic solutions
	Local anesthesia: Inj. xylocain 2%, local infiltration into the edges of the wound
	Debridement of the wound
	Apply artery forceps to the galea aponeurotica
	Stitching (interrupted stitches with black silk) of galea to galea and skin to skin

Apply firm bandage

Removal of stitches – after 7 days.

Head Injuries include injury to skull, brain, intracerebral vessels, separately or collectively.

MOI   Direct violence

RSA

Fall from a height.

Fractures of Skull

Types   Fractures of the vault and base of skull.

Fractures of Vault of Skull

MOI   Compression force – causes simple linear fissures.

Indentation force – causes simple or compound depressed fractures

Tangential force – causes compound fractures.

Mechanism of injury

Compression force – results in distortion of skull, while coming in contact with a hard flat surface, thereby causing displacement of brain, leading to severe cerebral injury.

Indentation force

Blows from large objects cause closed pond depressed fracture, dura remains intact, while blows from small objects cause compound depressed fractures, tearing both dura and brain tissue.

Tangential force

May tear apart a large segment of the bone, leaving dura mater intact. These are compound injuries, and injury to brain tissue is rare.

Diagnosis   Simple depressed fractures are rare

Swelling (hematoma) over the fracture site.

Compound fractures of the vault are common, variable in severity and mostly fatal injuries.

Hemiplegia may occur.

Lacerated scalp wound sometimes conceal the extent of fracture.

Investigation   X-ray skull – AP and lateral views to confirm the clinical diagnosis

CT scanning – to rule out any brain injury.

Management   It is a serious emergency and requires urgent surgical treatment, until and unless the patients condition warrants postponement.

First-aid treatment

Airway maintenance – by right posture

Endotracheal intubation, suction, and if required – tracheostomy.

Surgical treatment

Methods   Debridement of scalp wound, and if required, extend the wound to expose fully the fracture.

Burr-hole surgery – to remove loose bone fragments, wound stitched in layers

Reconstruction of skull defects – performed after an interval of 3–6 months period, by the use of plates, rib grafts, or acrylic inlay resin.

Refer: The patient to the surgical and neurosurgical team for surgery.

Fractures of Base of Skull

MOI	Compression force
	Indentation force
	Tangential force

Mechanism of injury

Fractures of base of skull are mostly produced by compression force and extension of fissures, extending from the vault fractures. The violent force extends into the weaker parts, e.g. middle ear fossae, air sinuses and finally into the foramina, exiting cranial nerves. Ring fracture occurs at the foramen magnum, by the indentation force of spinal column in Headon collisions – car accidents. Mastoid process is fractured by a tangential force.

Diagnosis   Discharge of blood, cerebrospinal fluid, or brain tissue.

Anterior fossa   Epistaxis – profuse and watery due to dilution with CSF or mixed with brain tissue.

Subconjunctival hemorrhage

Cranial nerves injury – 3rd, 4th or 6th nerve injury causing squint.

Middle fossa   Epistaxis – discharge blood mixed with CSF from the ear/mouth

Cranial nerves injury – facial (7th) nerve injury causing facial paralysis, while injury to auditory (8th) nerve causes deafness.

Posterior fossa Swelling at the nape of neck due to collection of blood.

Cranial nerve injury – injury to 9th, 10th, and 11th cranial nerves, injured at the jugular foramen.

Investigation   X-ray skull – to rule out an intracranial aerocele.

Management   Patient to be propped up in the bed, to combat the escape of CSF from the nose/ear

Antibiotics

Surgery   An early repair, to prevent occurrence of meningitis.

Refer: The patient to the surgical and neurosurgical team.

Brain Injuries

Mechanism of injury:

In any brain injury, the mechanism of injury is the same, e.g. displacement and distortion of the brain tissues, occurring at the time of injury. Brain is suspended inside the skull by slings formed by the cerebral vessels, and floats in the CSF anteroposteriorly. Lateral displacement of the brain is restricted by the falx cerebri (septum). Hence any direct blow on the front or backside of the head causes displacement of brain, resulting in the brain damage especially brainstem. Lateral blow may fracture the skull, but not enough displacement to cause severe brain damage.

Types of brain injury:

Cerebral concussion:

> Displacement of brain tissues is slight. There is a transient loss of consciousness or amnesia, without any brain tissue damage. In majority of patients, the recovery is complete.

Cerebral contusion

> Displacement of brain tissues is severe, resulting in tearing of brain tissue, especially brainstem. Loss of consciousness is prolonged and the recovery may be incomplete.

Cerebral laceration

> Displacement of brain tissues is more severe, resulting in more tearing of brain tissues.

Diagnosis
- Posture: Lying flaccid – a serious entity
  > Lying curled up – a non-serious entity
- Depth of consciousness: Conscious or unconscious
  - Conscious: History of prior unconsciousness – ICH
    Progressive deterioration of conscious level – brain compression
  - Unconscious: History of prior consciousness – extradural hemorrhage
  - Assessment of conscious level by:
    ◊ Using Glasgow Coma Scale (GCS), i.e. by observing three types of responses – eye opening, verbal and motor responses to the commands of speech and pain. Maximum score is 15. Any reduction in the score is an indication of a loss in the unconscious level. Alt:
    ◊ Using AVPU system, i.e. alert, responds or unresponsive to the commands of vocal and painful stimuli.
- Bleeding from nose/ears/mouth: In basal fracture of skull
- Vomiting
- Respiration: Rate: Slowed down
  > Rhythm: Irregular
- Pulse: Rate: Tachycardia
  > Rhythm: Thready
- BP: Hypotension followed by hypertension due to raised ICP.
- Pupil: Size and reactions
- Eye movements
- Neck rigidity: May be due to cervical spine injury, or cerebral irritation
- Muscle power: Loss of muscle power (paresis)
- Reflexes: Absent
- Sensations: Loss of sensations.

Investigations

> X-ray skull: AP and lateral views taken, to rule out any fracture, hemorrhage.

CT scanning: To identify and define the brain injury, and intracranial hematoma.

Lumbar puncture: Raised pressure in cerebral concussion.

Blood-stained cerebrospinal fluid – in cerebral laceration (subarachnoid hemorrhage).

Management

First aid treatment

Airway maintenance: Endotracheal intubation, or tracheostomy

Oxygen supply

Protection of the cervical spine

Bleeding control

Correction of hypovolemia, and resuscitation

Correction of hypovolemia, and resuscitation

Drugs – analgesics, antipyretics.

Refer: To neurosurgeon for persisting confusion, loss of consciousness, persisting coma, compound fractures, bleeding from nose/ears/mouth.

Definitive Treatment

Continuous observation of the patient to detect onset of complications, e.g. edema or hemorrhage, and to treat accordingly.

Monitor the pulse, BP, respiration, level of consciousness.

Nursing care to combat the neural lesion, by:

- Posture: Conscious patient – to be propped up, to relieve headache, while the unconscious patient – to be nursed on his/her side, to combat drowning of patient in his/her own secretions, e.g. saliva, blood, or vomitus.
- Repeated suctions to clear any secretions from throat or nose.

Catheterization – to relieve a distended bladder

Drugs: The fewer the better.

- In a conscious patient, aspirin to relieve any headache.
- In a serious patient, IV aminophylline 250 mg for its vasodilatation action, i.e. enhances blood supply to the ischemic brainstem and improvement of respiration by dilatation of bronchi.

Hypothermia – use of ice bags/cold sponging in brainstem lesions

Dehydration therapy – to relieve the high intracranial pressure, by use of 50 mL of 50% sucrose IV slowly Q.D.S.

Lumbar puncture – as a therapeutic measure to relieve high pressure.

A clear fluid with high pressure is indication of extradural hemorrhage, while a blood-stained fluid with high pressure, indicates cerebral lacerations.

Surgical treatment: A deteriorating level of consciousness, with development of paralysis, is indication of burr-hole exploration.

Refer: The patient to the surgical and neurosurgical team.

Intracranial Hemorrhage

Types	Extradural hemorrhage
	Subdural hemorrhage

Extradural Hemorrhage (Middle Meningeal)

MOI	Direct violence – blow from a stick, golf or cricket ball.
Mechanism of injury	Fracture of thin temporal bone, causing injury to the middle meningeal artery by the driven in dura. A short primary concussion occurs, followed by a lucid interval, e.g. intracranial hemorrhage collection and formation of a swelling underneath the temporal muscle.
	Finally there occurs cerebral compression especially of brainstem.
Diagnosis	Swelling – temporal region
	Confused, irritable
	Drowsiness
	Facial paralysis followed by paralysis of opposite arm and leg
	Pupils – dilated.
Management	It is an emergency and needs urgent operation – burr-hole exploration to relieve pressure.

Refer: The patient to the surgical and neurosurgical team for surgery.

Method	A burr-hole or trephine opening is made, to open the skull.
	The bleeder point is usually seen over the dura, which is secured by ligature or coagulated with diathermy
After care	Patient lying flat and carefully observed for improvement.
	If improvement is delayed or condition deteriorating then:
	Lumbar puncture is indicated.
	• Low pressure – inj. saline intrathecally, raises the pressure, and prevents coning formation of brainstem.

Subdural Hemorrhage

It is more common than extradural type of hemorrhage.

MOI	Direct violence
	RSA
	Fall from a height.
Mechanism of injury	Hemorrhage occurs due to rupture of connecting veins from cerebral hemispheres to the venous sinuses, due to displacement of brain especially brainstem inside the skull. Usually the superior cerebral veins are injured, causing hemorrhage, resulting in pressure over the cerebral hemispheres, with fatal results.
Diagnosis	Headache
	Confusion
	Hemiplegia
	Coma
	Pupils – dilated.

Investigation   X-ray skull
CT scan.

Management   Surgical treatment:

Method   Burr-holes made – to expose the dura
Opening of the subdural space, by incising the dura
Drainage of blood and clots from subdural space

After care   Patient lying flat with raised footend of bed to help in expansion of the brain.

Prognosis   The results are remarkable, if the surgery is performed before the formation of midbrain cone.

Refer: The patient to the surgical and neurosurgical team for surgery.

Chest injuries: Described in ATLS management

Abdominal Injuries

Types   Blunt injuries
Perforated (rupture) injuries.

MOI   Direct violence – hitting with a stick/rod/stone, stabbing, gunshot
RSA
Fall from a height.

Diagnosis   Signs of abdominal injuries are usually concealed and may require repeated examinations.

General S/S   Pain, local tenderness, abdominal rigidity, shifting dullness
Liver dullness – abstinence
Bruise over the abdominal wall or wound – may/may not
Internal hemorrhage – increasing pallor, restlessness, air-hunger, rising pulse, hypothermia, hypotension

Local S/S   Liver – local tenderness, shifting dullness and increased area of liver dullness
Spleen – local tenderness, muscle guard, shifting dullness, pain radiating to left shoulder
Kidney – fullness, shifting dullness, tenderness, hematuria
UB – local tenderness, shifting dullness, peritonitis
Stomach and small intestine – pain over epigastrium, vomiting, hemoptysis, local tenderness, muscle guard, shifting dullness
Large intestine – peritonitis, surgical emphysema.

Investigation   Ryle's tube aspiration
Hemogram
Blood grouping and crossmatching,
Blood urea
Serum electrolytes
Serum proteins

Urinalysis – catheterization to measure urine output

P/R – may show bleeding or a hematoma (boggy swelling)

P/V (if required as necessary) – may show bleeding

X-ray pelvis – to rule out pelvic fractures

CXR (sitting) – may show gas under the diaphragm

Plain X-ray abdomen – may show loss of psoas shadow and gas in the peritoneum

KUB

IVU – in suspected renal injury

Ultrasound – confirms diagnosis

CT scan – confirms diagnosis but time consuming

Diagnostic laparotomy

Diagnostic laparoscopy.

Management	
Emergency	Oxygen
	IV fluids – normal saline
	Blood transfusion
	Nasogastric (Ryle's) tube – for gastric aspiration
	Catheterization of bladder
Surgery	Laparotomy as an emergency procedure
Aim	To control the hemorrhage
Method	Repair:
Stomach	Repair of the perforation

Small intestine rupture: Simple closure of the perforation

Large intestine rupture: Exteriorisation is procedure of choice or closure of perforation followed by colostomy

Mesentery laceration: Resection of lacerated portion

Liver	Repair of the liver tear by mattress sutures parallel to tear
Kidney	Repair of the perforation
	Nephrectomy – indicated in severely damaged kidney, provided the contralateral kidney is healthy
Ureter	Uretero-ureteric anastomosis – for injury of one ureter
	Nephrostomy (bilateral) – for bilateral injury
Spleen	Splenectomy
Buttock	Debridement – to be undertaken first, in order to avoid hypotension
Ureter	Uretero-ureteric anastomosis – for injury of one ureter
	Nephrostomy (bilateral) – for bilateral injury
Spleen	Splenectomy
Buttock	Debridement – to be undertaken first, in order to avoid hypotension
	That may occur due to turning of the seriously injured patient.

Refer: The patient to the surgical team.

Shock: **Described in Section 2 of General Symptoms**

Spinal Injuries Always consider the possibility of spinal injury while managing patients with:

Major trauma – due to RSA/fall from height

Semi/unconsciousness

Neurological deficit.

Sites   Commonest sites: Cervical spine and dorsolumbar region.

Types   Stable and unstable injuries

A. Stable injuries   Posterior ligament complex and neural arch intact

Wedge (<20) fractures – commonest thoracolumbar injuries

B. Unstable injuries   Posterior ligament complex torn with/without fracture of neural arch or facet joints

Wedge (>20° or collapse of anterior margin – less than half of the posterior margin) fractures.

MOI   Fall from a height

Diving in shallow water

Fall of heavy weight on the back

RSA.

Mechanism of injury

Forces   Flexion, flexion rotation, hyperextension forces result in – sprains, fractures, dislocations, fracture dislocations, and paraplegia, depending upon the violence.

Management
Stable Fractures

Admit the patient – bed rest for 1/52

Analgesics

Physiotherapy – extension exercises for 4–6/52

Allowed up and home at 4–6/52.

Unstable Fractures with/without Neurological Deficit
First-aid treatment

Airway maintenance: Endotracheal intubation, or tracheostomy

Bleeding control

Drugs – analgesics, antipyretics

Spinal immobilization:

• Apply skull traction, maintaining traction, neck is slowly extended.

• Support neck with sand bags/apply a hard collar.

• Continue with traction.

Definitive Treatment

• Continuous observation – to detect onset of complications, e.g. cord damage, and to treat accordingly

- Monitor the pulse, BP, respiration
- Nursing care – to combat any neural lesion
- Catheterization – to relieve a distended bladder
- Dislocations/subluxation to be reduced by closed reduction (manipulation or traction) or by open reduction and internal fixation.

Surgical Treatment: Refer the patient to the orthopedic and surgical team for surgery:

Surgery	Arthrodesis: If no neurological deficit.
	If paraplegia – then arthrodesis is not required.
After care	Apply a cervical collar after 4 wks.

Sprains of Spine (Whiplash): These are common injuries of spine.

MOI	RSA.
Mechanism of injury	Sudden jerk leads to ligaments injury or muscles injury.
Diagnosis	Pain, swelling, local tenderness, movements – painful and restricted.
Investigation	X-ray spine – AP and lateral views.
Management	Rest
	Cold applications
	Massage
	Local infiltration of inj. xylocain 2%.

Dislocations   Dislocation alone can occur only in the cervical region, whereas in the dorsal and lumbar regions, always fracture-dislocations occur due to vertical or oblique directions of articular processes.

Dislocation between Atlas (C1) and Axis (C2)

MOI	Hanging by neck.
Mechanism of injury	Forward displacement of atlas following rupture of transverse ligament or fracture of odontoid process, death usually occurs due to injury to the brainstem and respiratory failure.
Management	If the patient survives, then under general anesthesia:
	Closed reduction: Flexion towards opposite side
After care	Skull traction, for one week, followed by plaster cast.

Refer: The patient to the orthopedic and surgical team for surgery.

Surgical treatment	
	ORIF (open reduction and internal fixation with plate and screws), if the conservative treatment fails
Aftercare	Head and neck in plaster cast (Minerva jacket).

Fractures of Spine

Types	Complete, incomplete, and compression fractures

Complete Fractures: Fracture-dislocations of the spine

MOI	Direct violence – at any level
	Indirect violence – flexion and rotation forces – commonly at C5 to C7, and L3 to L5 levels
Mechanism of injury	Dislocation occurs at disc level, along with fracture of vertebral body
Prognosis	Depends upon presence or absence of injury to the spinal cord and nerve root.

Incomplete Fractures

Fractures of the spinous and transverse processes
Fractures of the laminae
Fractures of the vertebral bodies (compression fractures)

MOI	Direct violence
	Stress fractures of the spinous processes
	Fall from a height
Diagnosis	Pain, local tenderness, movements – painful and restricted
	Fractures of spinous process: Common in dorsal region, due to greater length nad exposure to injury
	Fractures of transverse process: Occur commonly in lumbar region due to relatively greater length
	Fracture of lamina: May lead to compression of cord
	Compression fractures of vertebral bodies: May cause injury to the cord
Investigation	X-ray spine – AP and LAT views – collapse of the body and rarefaction.

Management

Conservative treatment – heat, massage, analgesics

Specific treatment

Incomplete fractures Traction for incomplete fractures

Closed reduction followed by traction

Complete fractures   Surgical treatment: ORIF, for complete fractures

Compression fractures plus/minus spinal cord or neural root injury: Arthrodesis.

Refer: The patient to the orthopedic and surgical team for treatment of complete and compression fractures.

Regional Spine Injuries
Cervical Spine Injuries

Types	Stable and unstable injuries
Stable injuries	Anterior wedge fractures of vertebral bodies, due to flexion injuries
Unstable injuries	Dislocation and fracture dislocations.

Classification of Cervical Spine Injuries

Flexion injuries

Flexion and rotation injuries

Extension injuries
Compression injuries.

Flexion and Flexion Rotation Injuries

MOI	RSA
	Sports injury – rugby, football, pole vaulting, and horse riding
	Fall from a height
	Diving head on into shallow water
	Fall of heavy weight on the back of head
Mechanism	Violence force acting on the back of head, leading to flexion of neck – causing stable anterolor wedge fracture of vertebral body, while posterior ligament complex and neural arch remain intact. Usually no neurological deficit occurs. In case of flexion/rotation injuries, the rotational force may cause unilateral dislocation of one facet joint – unstable injury.

Diagnosis

Stable wedge fracture: Pain, stiffness, movements – painfull and restricted

Unstable unilateral dislocation: Pain – radiating type, head slightly rotated and tilted away from locked facet.

Investigation	X-ray cervical spine – AP, LAT, and oblique views
	CT scan of cervical spine.

Management

Stable wedge fractures

Cervical collar for 6–8/52, followed by physiotherapy.

Unstable unilateral dislocation

Conservative treatment

Closed reduction: By manipulation, i.e. apply traction, maintaining traction, correct the rotation and then flexion, and finally bring the head into midline position followed by cervical collar or by skull traction followed by continuation of traction for 6–8/52.

Surgical treatment: **Refer:** The patient to the orthopedic and surgical team for surgery.

Indication	Failure of closed reduction and fixation
Method	ORIF (spinal plates and screws)
	Arthrodesis – if no neurological deficit
	Paraplegia – arthrodesis not required, if paraplegia is present
	Posterior ligament complex rupture – posterior arthrodesis is the treatment of choice.

Method of posterior arthrodesis:

Patient under general anesthesia – intubation

Patient turned to prone position

Midline incision – to expose the cervical spines

Torn posterior ligament is exposed

Adjacent spinous processes, laminae, and facet joints rawed

Spines wired together

Bone grafts placed on either side of spines.

After care   Continue with skull traction for 6 weeks, followed by a cervical collar.

Extension Injuries

MOI   RSA – in car accidents, e.g. forehead striking against the frontglass screen, dashboard.

Sports injury – boxing

Fall downstairs – forehead striking against ground.

Mechanism of injury   Hyperextension of neck leads to tearing of anterior longitudinal ligament, the cord may be stretched or kinked, causing neurological deficit

Diagnosis   History of injury, pain in the neck, weakness.

Investigation   X-ray cervical spine – AP and LAT views, show wedging of vertebra without narrowing of space.

Management   Extension injuries are stable.

Conservative   Treatment: Heat, analgesics, cervical collar.

Fractures of Atlas (C1)

MOI   RSA

Fall of a weight on the head

Fall from a height.

Diagnosis   Patient conscious or unconscious

Supports the head with hands

Pain – occipital region.

Investigation   X-ray cervical spine – AP view through the mouth and LAT view

CT scanning.

Management

Conservative treatment

Skull traction for 6/52

Analgesics

Surgical treatment   Arthrodesis

Indications   Failure of conservative treatment

After care   Cervical traction for 6 weeks, followed by collar for 2–3 months.

Refer: The patient to the orthopedic and surgical team for surgical treatment of patients, where conservative treatment fails.

Fractures of Axis (C2)

MOI   RSA

Flexion/extension injuries.

Diagnosis   An elderly patient, complaining of pain in neck, local tenderness, movements – painful and restricted

Investigation   X-ray cervical spine – AP and LAT views
                 CT scanning
Management
Conservative treatment
                 Skull traction for 4–6/52
                 Analgesics
                 Cervical collar
                 Minerva plaster jacket
Surgical treatment: Arthrodesis of spine.
Refer: The patient to the orthopedic and surgical team for surgical treatment of patients, where conservative treatment fails.

Compression injuries of cervical spine:
MOI   Fall of heavy weight on the head
                 Diving into shallow water
                 RSA.
Mechanism of neurological involvement
                 First of all the motor supply of upper limbs is affected, followed by that of lower limbs, next pain and temperature, and lastly touch sensation
Diagnosis   History of injury
                 Complaining of pain in neck
                 Local tenderness
Neurological assessment
                 A complete neurological examination, e.g.
                 Muscle power – testing of muscle power of upper and lower limbs
                 Sensations – testing of pin prick, touch, and temperature sensations
                 Reflexes – usually return within 4/52.
Investigation   X-ray cervical spine – AP and LAT views.
Management
Conservative treatment: Cervical traction for 6–8 weeks
Surgical treatment: Laminectomy – for removal of backward projecting bone fragments compressing cord.
Refer: The patient to the orthopedic and surgical team for surgical treatment of patients, where conservative treatment fails.

Fractures of Thoracic and Lumbar Spine
MOI   Fall from a height on to the toes
                 Fall of heavy weight over back of a stooping worker (mines)
                 Heavy weight lifting
                 RSA.
Mechanism of injury: Flexion and rotational forces.
Diagnosis   History of injury
                 Backache

Local tenderness

Movements – painful and restricted.

Investigation   X-ray – AP and LAT views.

Management

Conservative treatment

Bed-rest, analgesics

Plaster jacket with spine in extension

Physiotherapy.

Surgical treatment

Indication   Failure of conservative treatment

Methods   ORIF (Spinal plates and screws)

Arthrodesis.

Refer: The patient to the orthopedic and surgical team for surgical treatment of patients, where conservative treatment fails.

Spinal Cord Injury

Anatomy   The spinal cord ends at the level of lower border of 1st lumbar vertebra fracture-dislocations below this level are associated with injury to the cauda equina. Anatomical factors govern the extent of the cord and nerve lesion at different levels:

Cervical spine Horizontal articular processes and the large discs, yield high mobility with little resistance to even trivial forces, resulting in dislocation or fracture-dislocation.

Dorsal spine   Vertical articular processes, yield low mobility with great resistance to major forces resulting in fractures and cord injury as the spinal canal is narrow.

Lumbar spine Verticular, articular processes with great mobility, resulting in fracture-dislocations, due to flexion and rotation forces. Nerve lesions are rare, as the spinal canal is spacious.

MOI   RSA

Fall from a height

Mechanism of Injury

Acute flexion of spine causing long axis stretching of cord – resulting in concussion injury of cord.

Nipping of the cord by fractured fragment – resulting in crush injury of cord. Compression of cord by the protruded disc, due to acute flexion pathogenesis – resulting in paresis.

Lesions   Partial cord lesions: Show spastic paralysis in extension with exaggerated reflexes and extensor, plantar responses, and return of sensation. Urinary retention may persist for a longer period.

Complete cord lesions: Show spastic paralysis in flexion with flexor spasms, due to absence of inhibition of spinal flexor reflex arcs. The cord is irreparably damaged in.

Levels

Cervical:

Above C5 level	Paralysis of respiratory muscles, including diaphragm being supplied by the phrenic nerve (C4). There occurs sudden death.
At C5 level	Paralysis of arms, trunk, and legs. Patient breathes only with the aid of diaphragm, arms lie immobile against the trunk.
At C6 level	Arms abducted and externally rotated with forearm flexed and supinated, due to irritation of C5 segment.
At C7 level	Arms abducted and internally rotated with forearm flexed and pronated, due to irritation of C6 segment.
At C8 and T1 level	Paralysis of intrinsic muscles of the hand.
Below T1 level	Movements of arm – free down to finger tips

Dorsal:

At D2 level	Contraction of pupils, hyperaesthesia along the inner side of arms
Above D6 level	Paralysis of abdominal muscles

Lumbar

Above D12– L1 level :	Lumbar enlargement at this level contains center for nervous control of urinary bladder. Injury above this level prevents inhibitory impulses from cortex reaching the center, and thereby retention due to spinal shock, reflex micturition starts. Injury to this center or to nerves from it supplying the bladder (S2–3) leads to persistent retention due to paralysis of detrusor muscle.
Cauda equina	Just below level of cauda equina formation: Paralysis of legs and perineal muscles Anesthesia of perineum (saddle-shaped area) and legs Incontinence of urine and faeces.

Diagnosis

Neurological assessment

Complete neurological examination is conducted to find out any deficit, e.g.

Muscle power – testing of muscles below level of injury
Sensations – testing of pin prick and touch sensations
Reflexes

Lesions	Neuraprexia (syn. concussion): A temporary lesion, fully recoverable Axonotmesis: Rupture of axons within an intact sheath Neurotmesis: Partial or complete division of nerve

Spinal concussion (spinal shock)

Loss of all functions below the level of lesion, e.g.
Loss of voluntary movement
Loss of muscle tone
Loss of pain and temperature sensations
Loss of reflexes

Spinal Contusion

Stage of spinal shock: Complete flaccid paralysis below the level of lesion with urinary retention. Return of reflex activity.

Stage of septic complications.

Cord Injury

Complete transection of cord: Irrecoverable. Recovery of reflexes without muscle power, and sensations.

Incomplete transection of cord: Recovery possible – if there is any muscle power and sensations below level of lesion.

Injury to nerve roots/cauda equina: Potential recovery is there. Absence of reflexes.

Investigation X-ray spine – AP and LAT views show – wedging of vertebral body, no narrowing of disc space.

MRI/CT scanning

Management:

First aid treatment:

Position/posture: Cervical injuries: Head supported by sand bags

Dorsal and lumbar injuries: Patient in prone position

Analgesics: Inj. morphine – for relief of pain and anxiety

Prognosis Grave, if no recovery from spinal shock occurs within 48 hrs

Local treatment

Cervical injuries

Conservative treatment

Reduction by traction and manipulations, followed by skull traction for 1 wk

Minerva jacket: Plaster cast covering head, neck, and upper chest for four months.

Surgical treatmernt:

Laminectomy: Removal of protruding traumatic disc, pressing upon cord without a fracture

Indications Relief of pain due to nerve roots compression

Dorsal and lumbar injuries

Conservative treatment

Reduction by hyperextension in prone position.

Apply plaster from pelvis to axillae for 4–6/12.

Return of reflex activity

The period of spinal shock and flaccid paralysis persists for many days, following which lower motor neuron (LMN) lesion persists, due to injury of anterior horn cells, at level of lesion.

After care Partial or recoverable cord lesion: Adequate immobilization period, e.g. 2–4/12.

Complete cord lesion: Removal of plaster cast to avoid formation of bed-sores.

Management of complications: Death may occur due to following complications:

- Spinal shock: If present, then to be treated on priority basis
- Respiratory failure: Due to ascending edema
- Hypostatic pneumonia: Due to paralysis of abdominal and intercostal muscles.
- Urinary infection: Pyelonephritis.
- Bedsores: High protein diet – to combat protein loss from discharging sores. Good nursing care, e.g. regular change of bed sheets, turning to relieve pressure and toilet of skin with spirit and powder. Plenty of fluids.

Excision of sloughs, removal of sequestra.

- Urinary bladder: Lesions of bladder center cause permanent retention with overflow (incontinence)

Patient taught to evacuate the bladder by straining and by pressing the hand above the pelvis (over the bladder)

Indwelling catheterization – for 3–4/52, followed by automatic evacuation

Suprapubic cystostomy – carries the risk of infection and the method is demanding on staff

Physiotherapy:

- Chest: Deep breathing exercises and postural drainage
- Joints: Passive exercises with care to avoid risks of myositis ossificance

Assistance in sitting, standing, walking, use of wheelchair.

Rehabilitation – helping in return to work at earliest possible.

Peripheral Nerve Injuries

Types   Three types of injuries:
- Neurapraxia (concussion)
- Axonotmesis

Neurotmesis.

Neurapraxia	It is defined as a concussion injury.
MOI	Direct violence – stretch injuries
Mechanism of injury	There is a momentary loss of conduction. The nerve fibers and nerve sheath remain intact, and the recovery is almost complete.
Diagnosis	Loss of motor and sensory functions.
Investigation	Blood sugar – for diabetes mellitus
	Electrical reactions – no reaction of degeneration (RD).

Management

Conservative treatment

Immobilizing the limb in the position of relaxation of the affected muscle, by the use of splints, braces, etc.

Analgesics.

After care	Physiotherapy, e.g.

- Active and passive exercises
- Muscle stimulators.

Axonotmesis It is defined as rupture of axons within an intact nerve sheath.

MOI	Direct violence.
Mechanism of injury	Rupture of axons occurs within an intact neural sheath.
	Degeneration of ruptured axons occurs in distal segments, leading further to intraneural fibrosis, thereby affecting the conduction functions, followed by incomplete recovery.
Diagnosis	Loss of motor and sensory functions, e.g.
	Loss of muscle power, tone
	Loss of sensations – numbness
	Absent reflexes.
Investigation	Electrical reactions: Reaction of degeneration appears in the denervated muscles within two weeks.
Management	

Conservative treatment

Splints support to the paralyzed muscles of the affected limb

Passive exercises – to built up tone and muscle power

Massage

Analgesics.

Neurotmesis It is defined as partial or complete division of the neural sheath and fibres.

MOI	Direct violence – gunshot wounds; cut wounds; stab wounds
	RSA
	Fall from a height.
Mechanism of injury	In partial division, a lateral neuroma is formed at site of injury, whereas in complete division, a terminal neuroma is formed at the proximal segments end.
Diagnosis	Loss of motor and sensory functions.
Investigation	Electrical reactions: Reaction of degeneration appears in the denervated muscles within a short time.
Management	

Conservative treatment

Use of splints

Analgesics

Antibiotics.

Surgical treatment: Repair of injured nerve – nerve suturing.

After care	Physiotherapy.

Brachial Plexus Injuries

Types   Complete and incomplete injuries.

Complete Brachial Plexus Injury: Is a rare injury.

MOI   Direct violence.

Mechanism   Tearing of all the nerve roots, associated with fatal injuries of adjoining
of injury   vital structures.

Diagnosis   Complete paralysis of arm.

Investigation   X-ray – to rule out any fracture-dislocation.

Management

Conservative treatment: Use of splints and physiotherapy.

Incomplete Branchial Plexus Injury

MOI   Direct violence – cuts; stabs; and by blows with sticks, etc.

                  Fall from a height

                  Fall of heavy weight over shoulder

                  Obstructed labor – traction injury.

Mechanism   Usually the injury leads to traction or pressure lesions of
of injury   upper or lower parts of the plexus, e.g.

                  Upper lesion (Erb-Duchen)

                  Lower lesion (Klumpke**).**

Upper Lesion (Erb–Duchen)

Definition   It is defined as the upper lesion of brachial plexus, due to involvement of
                  C5 and C6 nerve roots.

MOI   Obstructed labor – traction force.

Mechanism   The injury is due to increased angle between the neck and shoulder, as
of injury   may occur during forced delivery of fetus, in obstructed labor, and also
                  by fall of a heavy weight over the shoulder.

Diagnosis   Arm – hanging by side of body and internally rotated

                  Elbow – fully extended

                  Forearm – fully pronated

                  Muscular wasting in lesions of long duration

                  Loss of muscle power

                  Loss of sensations and reflexes

Management

Conservative treatment

                  Immobilization of arm in relaxation position, by use of splints

                  Physiotherapy

Surgical treatment: Indicated in neurotmesis lesions.

Procedure: Exploration of brachial plexus. Suturing – difficult.

Lower Lesion (Klumpke)

Definition	It is the lower lesion of brachial plexus due to involvement of C8 and T1 nerve roots.
MOI	Fall from a height.
Mechanism of injury	The injury occurs due to forced hyperabduction of arm, when a falling person tries to hold an object, avulsing the nerve roots from the spinal cord.
Diagnosis	Deformity: Clawhand, e.g. extended first phalanx with flexed 2nd and 3rd phalanges Muscular wastings (late cases) of hand muscles Loss of sensations along inner side of forearm and hand (inner three and a half fingers).

Management:

Conservative treatment: Immobilization of arm in relaxation position, by the use of
Splints
Physiotherapy.

Surgical treatment

Indications	Neurotmesis lesions
Procedure	Exploration of brachial plexus.
Prognosis	Results of surgical treatment – not satisfactory.

Refer: The patient to the orthopedic and surgical team for surgery.

Management of Fractures of Limbs

In multiple injuries, it may be difficult to select particular methods of treatment, especially in cases where multiple fractures occur in the same limb. It may be difficult to follow the principles of reduction and fixation.

First-aid Treatment

Immobilization – by use of splints, or traction, to reduce pain and hemorrhage.
Compound fractures – covered with sterile dressing pads, to prevent/control infection.
Assessment – clinically and radiologically of fracture, e.g. site, pattern, displacement, angulation, rotation, and shortning to be noted.
Recording of involvement of skin, nerves, and blood vessels.

Local (Definitive) Treatment of Fractures

Principles	Reduction of fracture Immobilization (fixation) Rehablitation.

Reduction of Fractures

Anesthesia	Under general or local anesthesia reduction of displacement, angulation, or rotation of fragments is achieved.

Types   Closed or open reduction.

Methods   By traction force (manual)

                  By manipulation with hands

                  By continuous traction – skin or skeletal traction.

Immobilization (Fixation)

A. External fixation: By:

                  Splints – Thomas or Brawn splints

                  Plaster of Paris

                  Traction – fixed traction in a Thomas splint

                  External fixators.

B. Internal fixation: By:

                  Screws – cortical and cancellous : Self-tapping – Sherman and Lane

                                          : Require pretapping – AO series

                  Plate and screws

                  Intramedullary nailing

                  Interlocking nailing

                  Rush nails

                  Tension wires, percutaneous wires

                  Prosthesis, replacement arthroplasty.

Rehabilitation To send back the patient to his/her work, at the earliest possible.

Measures   Physiotherapy.

Resuscitation in Trauma

MOI   RSA

                  Fall from height

Management   Airway and cervical spine control:

                  • Immobilize the cervical spine with a collar

                  • Head – to be kept in neutral position

                  • Endotracheal intubation

                  • Cricothyroidotomy

                  Breathing assessment/control

                  Circulation control:

                  • IV fluids

                  • Blood transfusion

                  Drugs – described in appropriate section.

Shock   **Described in appropriate section III of General Symptoms.**

References

1. British Orthopaedic Association. Memorandum on Accident Services, 1959.
2. Clark R. 'Resuscitation and transfusion in severe injuries'. In: Modern Trends in Accident Surgery and Medicine. Ed. by Clarke R., Badger FG Sevitt S. London; Butterworths; 1959.
3. Robertson MA, Molyneux EM: Triage in the developing world – can it be done? Arch Dis Child 85:208–13;2001.
4. Hill G. A&E risk management. Medical Defence Union, London, 1991.
5. American College of Surgeons Advanced Trauma Life Support Course. American College of Surgeons, Chicago, Illinois, USA, 1989.
6. Murat JE, Huten, N, and Mesny, J: The use of Standardised assessment. Procedures in the evaluation of patients with Multiple Injuries. Archives of Emergency Medicine, 2, 11–15;1986.
7. United Kingdom Central Council (UKCC) Standards for Records and Records Keeping. 15–16 April, 1993.
8. Miller A. Closed injuries of the kidney, bladder, and posterior urethra. Proc R Soc Med 54, 563;1961.
9. Stevenson HM, and Richards, D: Discussion on non-penetrating injuries of the chest and abdomen. Proc. R Soc Med 54, 565–66;1961.
10. Walder DN: 'The Shocked Patient' Practitioner 187, 34;1961.
11. Radushkevich VP: 'Experience in the Combating of Shock and Terminal States' Sborn. Rab. Voronezhsk. Med. Inst. 30,15;1958.
12. Gentleman D, Dearden M, Midgley S, Maclean D: Guidelines for resuscitation and transfer of patients with serious head injury. BMJ 307:547–52;1993.
13. Isacsson G, Rich CL: Management of patients who deliberately harm themselves. BJ. 322: 213–15;2001.
14. Bailey and Love's Short Practice of Surgery: Cranio-Cerebral Injuries. 369–91.
15. Barnes R: Paraplegia in Cervical spine injuries. J Bone Jt Surg. 30B,234;1948.
16. Crooks F and Birkett, AN: Fractures and fracture-dislocations of the cervical spine. Brit. J Surg. 31,252;1944.
17. Cullen CH: Paraplegia in extension injuries of the spine. J Bone Jt Surg. 43B:600;1961.
18. Evans DK: Reduction of cervical dislocations. J Bone Jt Surg. 43B:552;1961.
19. Roaf R: A Study of the mechanics of spinal injuries. J Bone Jt Surg. 42B:810;1960.
20. Bohler L. The treatment of Fractures. 4th ed. Bristol; Wright, 1935.
21. Watson-Jones, R. Fractures and other bone and joint injuries. Edinburgh; Livingstone, 1952.
22. Wyatt JP, Illingworth RN, Robertson CE, Clancy MJ, Munro PT: Oxford Handbook of Accident and Emergency Medicine. 2nd ed. Oxford University Press, Oxford 2005.
23. Edhouse J, Wardrope J: Assessment of injured patients. Surgery International. 13,121–26;1997.

Part IV Surgical Emergencies

Orthopedic Emergencies

Traumatic:
- Fractures and dislocations:
  - Section A: General principles
  - Section B: Regional injuries
  - Section C: Practical procedures
- Fractures in children
- Traumatic disorders of joints:
  - Acute traumatic synovitis
  - Coccygodynea
  - Baseball pitcher's shoulder
  - Baseball pitcher's elbow
- Injuries of muscles and tendons:
  - Contusion
  - Rupture of muscles
  - Rupture of tendons:
  - Tendo-Achilles
  - Long head of biceps
  - Extensor pollicis longus
  - Supraspinatus
  - Avulsion of tendon – mallet finger
  - Sprains – tennis elbow, pulled elbow
  - Cut tendons – flexor and extensor

- Injuries of bursae:
  - Acute traumatic bursitis – tendo-Achilles bursitis
  - Chronic bursitis:
    - ◊ Housemaid's knee
    - ◊ Student's elbow
    - ◊ Baker's cyst
- Inflammatory:
  - Acute osteomyelitis
  - Acute suppurative arthritis
  - Wounds of joints
  - Ganglion
  - Traumatic myositis ossificans
  - Acute suppurative bursitis
  - Supraspinatus tendinitis
- Endocrinal and metabolic:
  - Osteoporosis
- Neoplastic:
  - Osteogenic sarcoma
  - Ewing's sarcoma
  - Multiple myeloma (plasma cell myeloma)
  - Secondary carcinoma of bone

Fractures and Dislocations

Section A   General principles
Section B   Regional injuries
Section C   Practical procedures

SECTION A: GENERAL PRINCIPLES

- Definition of fracture
- Cause/mode of injury (MOI)
- Types of fracture
- Pattern of fracture
- Diagnosis of fracture

- Investigations
- Treatment of fracture
- Treatment of life threatening situations
- First aid treatment
- Local treatment
- Reduction of fracture
- Fixation (immobilization) of fracture
- External fixation
- Internal fixation
- Implants
- Factors affecting healing of fracture
- Complications of fracture
- Fractures in Children
- References

FRACTURE

Definition   Is defined as break in the continuity of alignment of a bone.

Cause/mode of injury (MOI)

1. *Direct violence:* Fracture occurs at the site of impact, i.e. being hit by a falling or moving object.

   Example: Fracture skull vault due to fall of heavy weight

   Fracture of hand – being struck by a stick, etc.

2. *Indirect violence:* Fracture occurs away from the site of impact, i.e. twisting or bending force.

   Example: Fall on outstretched hand, causing fracture of clavicle.

3. *Muscular violence:* Fracture occurs due to sudden, violent muscular contraction.

   Example: Fracture patella due to violent contraction of quadriceps.

4. Stress (fatigue) fracture: Also known as march fracture.

   Common in army and police personnel, participating in long marches and prolonged standings.

   Example: Fracture of 2nd or 3rd metatarsals.

5. Pathological fracture: Fracture occurs in an abnormal or diseased bone. A little force may be sufficient to break the affected brittle, eroded, cystic bone.

   Example: Subtrochanteric fracture of femur due to secondary deposits.

Types of Fracture

1. *Simple fracture:* Also known as closed fracture. Skin is intact. The wound, if present, does not communicate with the fracture. Hence, chances of infection are rare.

2. *Compound fracture:* Also known as open fracture. Skin is broken. The wound communicates with the fracture. Hence chances of infection are common.

Types:

i. From without in – due to direct violence, contaminating wound, thereby entry of micro-organisms from outside.

ii. From within out – fractured bone pierces the skin. Chances of infection are comparatively less in this type.

Pattern of Fracture

1. *Transverse fracture:* Fracture at right angle to long axis of a bone. It is a stable fracture, no shortening, union favourable, and chances of early mobilization. Firm support required due to smaller area of bony contact.

   MOI: Mostly direct violence.

2. *Oblique fracture:* Fracture at an angle, less than right angle to long axis of a bone. Usually an unstable fracture, chances of displacement and shortening are common. Union may be earlier, due to larger area of bony contact. Proper reduction and firm support required.

   MOI: Mostly indirect violence.

3. *Spiral fracture:* Fracture occurs in a spiral form, across the bone. Usually an unstable fracture, chances of displacement and shortening are common. Union may be earlier, due to larger area of bony contact. Proper reduction and firm support required.

   MOI: Mostly indirect violence.

4. *Greenstick fracture:* Occurs in children. The bone bends, one cortex (convex side) breaks, while the other cortex (concave side) remains intact. No displacement. Healing is rapid, early mobilization.

   MOI: Direct or indirect violence.

5. *Hairline fracture:* Fracture may be complete or incomplete, no displacement, difficult to detect radiologically, repeated weekly X-rays and oblique view may reveal the fracture clearly. Healing is rapid, requiring mostly conservative treatment except fracture of scaphoid and fracture neck of femur.

   MOI: Mostly minimal violence.

6. *Single fracture:* The bone is fractured at one level.

   MOI: Mostly direct violence.

7. *Double fracture:* The bone is fractured at two different levels.

   MOI: Direct violence and fall from height.

8. *Comminuted fracture:* The bone is broken into more than two fragments. Greater comminution indicates severe violence, marked damage to adjoining muscles, tendons, nerves, vessels and skin.

   Comminuted fractures are mostly unstable and usually complicated ones.

9. *Butterfly fracture:* Is a comminuted fracture with a large butterfly type fragment.

10. *Impacted fracture:* In this type of fracture, one fragment is driven into the other fagment. Usually seen at junction of cortical and cancellous bones, i.e. end of the shaft or impaction of one cancellous fragment, i.e. fractures of vertebrae.

11. *Complicated fracture:* Also known as complex fracture. Fracture is associated with neurovascular, visceral injuries.
   Example: Fracture shaft of humerus with radial nerve injury.

12. *Pathological fracture:* Fracture occurs in an abnormal or diseased bone. A little force may be sufficient to break the affected brittle, eroded, osteoporotic, and cystic bone.

13. *Avulsion fracture:* Fracture occurs due to sudden, violent muscular contraction.
   Example:
   - Fracture patella, due to violent contraction of quadriceps.
   - Fracture tibial tuberosity, due to contraction of patellar tendon.
   - Fracture base of fifth metatarsal, due to contraction of peroneus bravis.
   - Fracture lesser trochanter, due to contraction of ilio-psoas.

14. *Intra-articular fracture:* Fracture involving a joint, causing irregularity of joint surface, leading to complication of stiffness of joint and finally to development of secondary osteoarthritis.

15. *Fracture-dislocation:* Joint dislocation, alongwith fracture of a bone of the joint.
   Example: Fracture dislocation of shoulder joint.
   Monteggia fracture-dislocation

Diagnosis of Fracture

Symptoms
1. Pain
2. Swelling
3. Difficulty/inability to move part

Signs
1. Deformity
2. Shortening
3. Local tenderness
4. Bone surface irregularity
5. Crepitus
6. Unnatural mobility
7. Loss of function
8. Wound
9. Shock

I. *Deformity:* Types: Displacement, angulation, and axial rotation
   Displacement: Is defined as shifting of distal fragment relative to proximal fragment. Displacement may be anterior/posterior/medial/or lateral. It may be partial or complete (no bony contact of fragments) and may lead to shortening, malunion, or nonunion due to interposition of soft tissues between fractured fragments.
   Angulation: It may be anterior/posterior/medial/or lateral, depending upon point of angle or position (tilt) of distal fragment. Angulation should never be neglected, as

deformity is regarded as sign of poor treatment. It may also interfere with normal functioning especially in upper limb, affecting pronation/supination.

Axial rotation: In this deformity, one fragment rotates on its long axis, relative to other fragment. It may or may not be associated with displacement or angulation. It may be detected radiologically, from the position of interlocking fragments, and from the differences in the relative diameters of the fragments.

II. *Shortening:* If present, is an important sign of fracture. Occurs due to overriding of fragments.

III. Local tenderness: In impacted fractures, local bony tenderness is the most important clinical sign while loss of function is the most important symptom.

IV. Bone surface irregularity: In the form of a gap, elevation, or a bend, if present, is a definite sign of a fracture.

V. Crepitus: While palpating or testing unnatural mobility, a crepitus or grating sensation may be felt or heard. Is also a definite sign of a fracture. It may also be positive in a haematoma, gas gangrene, surgical emphysema, and osteoarthritis.

VI. Unnatural mobility: Is elicited by moving one fragment against the other. If present, is a definite sign of a fracture, but to be elicited with great care to avoid occurrence of complications. It is absent in impacted fracture and greenstick fracture.

VII. Loss of function: There may be complete loss of function in a fracture case. Impacted fracture may present great difficulty in clinical diagnosis. X-ray is of great helpful in such cases.

VIII. Wound: If present may contain broken fragments, foreign body, blood clots, etc. There may be oozing of blood from the wound.

IX. Shock: If present, is a life threatening emergency, and to be managed on priority basis. It is oligaemic due to hemorrhage and vasoconstriction (to maintain peripheral vascular resistance).

Signs of shock: Unconscious

Air gasping or breathless

Pale, cyanotic

Hypotension.

Investigations   1. X-ray examination: Is the main investigation for confirming the clinical diagnosis of a fracture. X-ray of the affected bone taken, mostly in two planes (views), i.e. antero-posterior (AP) and lateral.

AP view: Reveals lateral or medial displacement, whereas lateral view reveals anterior or posterior displacement of distal fragment. Both views reveal upward or downward displacement.

Axial view: Required especially in fracture of calcaneum.

Oblique view : Required especially in fracture of scaphoid.

X-ray findings in a fracture, reveal :

i. Site and type of fracture.

ii. Displacement, angulation, rotation of fragments.

iii. Callus formation–sign of union.

iv. Sclerosis, rounding of fractured ends – sign of nonunion.

v. Avascular necrosis (AVN) of bone – decalcification of adjoining bones, while avascular necrotic bone preserves its density due to nonvascularization.

Examples:
- AVN of femoral head following fracture neck of femur.
- AVN of proximal fragment following fracture of scaphoid.

vi. Myositis ossificans is subperiosteal ossification, following fracture.

Example: Elbow fractures.

vii. Pathological fractures: X-ray may reveal the underlying pathological condition, responsible for erosion of bone, lowering the strength of bone – vulnerable to fracture even from trivial trauma.
- MRI of affected bone and joint
- CT scan of affected bone and joint

Management of Fracture

Principles of management of fracture:

I. Management of Life Threatening Situations

A. Airway obstruction

B. Breathing distress–tension pneumothorax, hemothorax, cardiac tamponade.

C. Bleeding (hemorrhage)

D. Chest injuries – flail chest

E. Head injuries and neurological disorders

F. Shock

G. Spine injuries

H. Abdominal injuries

I. Pelvis injuries

II. Management of Fracture

Principles:

1. Reduction of fracture
2. Fixation (immobilization) of fracture: External fixation and internal fixation
3. Rehabilitation

Management of Life Threatening Situations

Management of multiple injuries: Advanced trauma life support (ATLS)

1. Priority of treatment: In the management of multiple injuries, priority of treatment is directed to life threatening conditions such as airway obstruction, shock, or external hemorrhage, even before a detailed examination begins. The doctor incharge should plan the line of

treatment in consultation with other specialists involved in the management of various lesions. It may be possible to manage all the injuries simultaneously but at times, these lesions to be dealt with, on priority basis, e.g. in a definite sequence. Compound fractures should preferably be treated alongwith head, neck, or chest injuries. Operative treatment for simple fractures may better be postponed to a later stage. But it is better not to postpone the corrective orthopaedic measures for more than a day or so, in the patients who appeared unlikely to recover from their associated injuries.

Management: Described in the section – Management of Multiple Injuries: Advanced Trauma Life Support (ATLS)

Management of Fracture

I. First Aid Treatment

A. Relief from pain by:
1. Use of splints, slings, collars, braces, adhesive plaster strapping, traction
2. Analgesics: Inj. Morphine 10 mg IV. Repeat 8–12 hrly.
   Side effects: Nausea, vomiting, constipation, sedation, respiratory depression.
   Antidote: Inj. Nalorphine 5 mg IV + Inj. Stemetil or Inj. Perinorm
   Inj. Pethidine 50 mg IV. Repeat 8–12 hrly.
   Side effects: Addiction (dependence)
   Inj. Pentazocine 30–60 mg IM or IV. Repeat 3–4 hrly
   Side effects: Nausea, vomiting, dependence
B. Bleeding control – by bandaging of wound.
C. Infection control – by dressing of wound.

II. Local Treatment

A. Reduction of fracture: Closed and open reduction.
Indication: Correction of displacement, angulation, and rotation deformities.
Anesthesia : Local or general

Types of reduction: Closed or open

Closed reduction: Majority of fractures are reduced by this method.

Advantages
1. Relatively safe method. Chances of infection are less.
2. Relatively much cheaper.

Disadvantages
1. Failure of reduction sometimes due to interposition of soft tissues between fragments.
2. Failure to maintain reduction.
3. Prolonged immobilization.

Technique

1. By traction and manipulation by hands or
2. By traction

Open reduction: Should always be undertaken by a surgeon highly skilled in fracture management. Better to be avoided in children.

Indications

1. Failure of closed reduction.
2. Particular fractures – in need of perfect reduction and fixation, e.g. fracture neck of femur.
3. Compound fractures, complicated fractures.
4. Early mobilization required – especially in elderly patients.

Disadvantages

1. Relatively unsafe method. Chances of infection are more.
   Sometimes disastrous one, e.g. leading to gangrene, requiring amputation, or even death may occur.
2. Relatively much costlier method.

B. Fixation (immobilization) of fracture: External and internal fixation: Attention must be given not only to the broken bone, but also to the soft parts, while considering the correct method of fixation of each type of fracture.

External fixation:

i. Plaster of Paris: Is the most widely used form of fixation. Care should be taken of swelling, change in skin color, numbness, etc. following application of plaster – if present, then immidiately loosen the plaster by splitting, or remove/change the plaster.

ii. Traction: A. fixed traction – in a thomas splint or by continuous traction.

iii. Braces

iv. External fixator and ring fixator

Internal fixation:

By use of: Plates and screws, screws, intramedullary nailing and interlocking nailing, tension wires, percutaneous wires, etc.

Principles of Internal fixation of fractures:

1. Freedom from foreign body reaction: Implant should be biological inert, free from toxic reactions, inflammatory response, fibrous and giant cell reactions. These usually cause pain, swelling, and loss of function.
2. Freedom from rust: Implant should be made of high quality stainless steel etc., to avoid rusting of implant especially in compound fractures.
3. Freedom from mechanical failure: Implant should be lighter in weight, of great strength and of suitable design to match the shape and size of donor bone.

Materials commonly used are:

i. Stainless steel

  ii. Vitallium – alloys of chromium, cobalt, and molybdenum

  iii. Titanium

Advantages of Internal Fixation

  i. Firm fixation

  ii. Early weight bearing

  iii. Early return to work

Disadvantages of Internal Fixation

  i. Infection

  ii. Failure – due to faulty technique or faulty (wrong) selection of implant.

  iii. Failure – due to faulty selection of treatment (closed or internal fixation) for needs of each and every particular case.

Implants

1. Screws: Cortical and cancellous screws. Available in large range of lengths but restricted in range of diameters.

Types of screws:

A. Self-tapping screws: The screw cuts its own thread in the bone.

  Example: Sherman and Lanes screws.

  The screw has an OD (outside diameter) and a slot single, combination, or cruciate.

  Insertion: A hole is drilled through the bone, followed by driving in the screw, cutting its thread into the bone by its flutted end.

B. Screws which require bone to be tapped prior to insertion.

  Example: AO series screws.

  AO cortical screw has:

    i. An OD

    ii. A hexagonal socket

    iii. A buttress thread with pitch

  Insertion: A hole is drilled through the bone, followed by tapping with a corresponding tap and finally the screw is driven through.

C. Single cortical screw: Is a week internal support and requires external support, e.g. plaster of Paris or splint.

D. Cancellous screws: Indicated in cancellous bone. It does not require prior to tapping.

E. Locking screws: Cannulated, self-drilling, self-tapping screws

F. Dynamic hip screw (DHS)

2. Plates and screws

  i. Sherman plate: It is a light weight, comparatively of weaker strength plate, and requires external support.

  ii. Eggar plate: It is slotted, so that the screws are not fully tightened, allowing the bone ends to remain in contact. Requires external support.

  iii. Dynamic compression plate (DCP): It is slotted and tightening of plate is achieved by pinching of plate by the heads of screws.

iv. Nail/blade plate: It is being used in a fracture closer to a long bone's end.

Insertion: Nail or blade part is driven through the cancellous part, while the plate part is fixed with the cortical screws, to the shaft of the long bone.

v. Buttress plates, Y plates, Fracture plates, LC plates, cervical spine locking plates.

3. Intra-medullary nailing: For fractures of shafts of long bones, e.g. Kuntscher nail for fracture shaft femur.

4. Interlocking nails:
   Antegrade femoral nail (AFN)
   Proximal femoral nail (PFN)
   Distal femoral nail (DFN)
   Universal femoral nail (UFN) – Titanium solid nail
   Cannulated femoral nail (CFN)

5. Rush pins (nails) for fracture humerus, ulna, etc.

6. Spine system (Schanz screws) – for cervical spine surgery

7. Pedicle screw system – for low back surgery

Factors affecting Healing of Fracture

1. *Age:* Younger the patient, better are chances of early union of fracture. In children, union of fracture is faster, which slows down as the age advances. Also power of remodelling of fracture is stronger in children, while it decreases, as the child attains adolescence.

2. *Type of bone:* Healing in fracture of cancellous bone is comparatively earlier, than in fracture of cortical bone.
   Example: Fractures of os calcaneum and os vertebral bodies heal relatively earlier due to cancellous bone.

3. Distraction of bone ends due to:
   i. Interposition of soft tissues between bone ends.
   ii. Excessive traction force applied during immobilization period following reduction of fracture
   iii. Faulty internal fixation of fractures.

4. Movements at the fracture site: Faulty immobilization (fixation) of a fracture, resulting in movements at the fracture site, which in turn interrupts the vascularization of hematoma, leading to poor callus formation, and finally into delayed union, non-union.

5. Infection: May result in delayed or non-union, due to resorption of callus. Usually common in compound fractures and fractures treated by internal fixation. Rare in fractures treated by conservative measures.

6. Avascular necrosis of bone: Interruption of blood supply to the bone following fracture, may lead to avascular necrosis of the bone, due to rupture of vessels, supplying bone.

Example:

    i. Avascular necrosis of femoral head, following fracture neck femur.

    ii. Avascular necrosis of proximal segment of scaphoid following fracture scaphoid.

7. Quality of bone: Certain bones heal earlier than others following fracture, due to unknown factors.

    Example: Fracture clavicle – heals earlier in spite of uncontrolled movements at the fracture site.

    Fracture tibia–heals slowly in spite of firm fixation.

8. *Pathological fractures:* May heal slowly especially in case of primary and secondary malignant bone tumors, due to marked erosion of bone. On the other hand, union occurs without any delay, e.g. simple bone cyst.

9. *Intra-articular fractures:* Union is delayed due to dilution of hematoma by the sunovial fluid.

Complications of Fracture

General

1. *Shock*

Etiology	Oligaemic shock due to: Hemorrhage – external or internal
Diagnosis	Unconscious, breathless, pale, cyanotic, pupils – dilated, hypotension, pulse rapid
Management	On top priority basis. Measures:

    i. Airway maintenance: Position of head, removal of any foreign body, endotracheal intubation, ventilator – oxygen therapy

    ii. Breathing monitoring: Treatment of the cause, i.e. any chest injury, tension pneumothorax, hemothorax

    iii. Control of bleeding:

        By bandage, tourniquet, etc. for external hemorrhage

        By ligating torn vessel or soft tissue for internal hemorrhage

    iv. IV fluids – normal saline, dextrose

    v. Blood transfusion – if loss more than 1–2 liters

    vi. Plasma or plasma expanders – if loss less than 1 liter or if whole blood not available.

    vii. Drugs:

        Inj. Morphine 10 mg IV for relief from pain. Repeat after 8–12 hrly if required

        Inj. Hydrocortisone 100 mg IV to combat hypotension. Repeat 4 hrly.

        Inj. Ephedrine IV

    viii. Splintage of fractured bone, by use of splints, braces, arm slings, traction

2. *Hemorrhage*

Etiology	External or internal – due to rupture of vessels, soft tissues, bone fragments, etc. Bleeding may be extensive.

Management	External hemorrhage – control of bleeding by applying firm bandage, tourniquet
	Internal hemorrhage – control of bleeding by ligating the torn vessel, soft tissue repair.
	Blood transfusion, and if not available, then give plasma or plasma expander and IV saline.

3. Fat embolism

Etiology	Due to entry of fat particles from broken bone marrow, into the circulation. Is a serious, life threatening emergency. Commonly seen in fracture of femoral shaft, fracture pelvis, and fracture tibia.
Diagnosis	Confusion, irritation, or comatose, fever, Patechial hemorrhages in the skin, palate, conjunctiva, renal failure, death.
Management	Heparin IV, oxygen, IV fluids, monitoring vital signs

4. Hypostatic pneumonia

Etiology	May occur in an elderly patient, confined to bed, as commonly seen in fracture neck femur.
Diagnosis	Fever, chest pain, cough with expectoration, dyspnea, orthopnea, pulse rapid.
Investigations	Blood culture and X-ray chest – helpful in diagnosis.
Management	Make patient comfortable in the bed with support of back rest
	Oxygen therapy
	IV fluids
	Antibiotics
	Analgesics
	Expectorants
	Steam inhalation
	Monitoring – nursing care.

6. Acute renal failure

Etiology	Following fracture, due to shock, excessive bleeding, fat embolism
Diagnosis	Confusion, irritation, coma, fever, edema face and legs, oliguria
Investigations	Serum electrolytes, creatinine, ECG – to monitor potassium level
Management	Indwelling catheterization
	IV dextrose 20% slowly
	Antibiotics, heparinization.

Local Complications of Fracture

I. Early Complications

1. Arterial injury

Etiology	Blood vessels may be torn, or occluded by pressure of bone fragments, or spasm of vessels.
	Pathogenesis: Spasm of vessels leading to ischemia of muscles, necrosis, fibrosis, and contractures, e.g. Volkmann's ischemic contracture.

Examples: Brachial artery injury in a supracondylar fracture of humerus and popliteal artery injury in a fracture of lower end of femoral shaft.

Management   Post-reduction observation of fracture:

A. If pulse is doubtful, then: Check the reduction, loosen/remove the external fixation, e.g. POP/splint

B. Still no pulse, then: Inj. Papaverine.

C. Still no pulse, then: Exploration of artery

2. Nerve injury

Types of injuries

A. Neurapraxia (concussion): It is the commonest nerve injury and recovery occurs within a month or so.

B. Axonotmesis (lesion in continuity): It is rupture of axons within an intact neural sheath and recovery occurs within a few months.

C. Neurotmesis: It is complete division of nerve.

Examples: Radial nerve injury in fracture shaft humerus

Median and ulnar nerve injuries in supracondylar fracture of humerus

Management   Majority of nerve injuries are in continuity. After reduction of fracture or dislocation, recovery in nerve injuries, ususally starts after about 6–8 weeks, progressing satisfactorily thereafter.

During recovery period, the skin should be protected against trauma, burns, etc.

Joints to be mobilized by passive exercises. Prevent deformities, by use of splints, etc. e.g. cock up splint in wrist drop.

Surgical treatment:

Exploration – indicated in cases, where recovery is delayed or absent.

Primary suturing of nerves, if no infection.

Reconstructive surgery – where nerve repair not feasible.

3. Infection

Etiology   Infection in a compound fracture, or following ORIF of a fracture, may cause:

Osteomylitis – with discharging pus for a long period, in spite of use of antibiotics and surgical measures.

Gas gangrene – a highly serious life threatening emergency.

Management   Compound fracture:

Toilet of the wound with hydrogen peroxide and sterile fluids.

Debridement of wound and immobilization.

Antibiotics

Osteomyelitis:

Acute: Incision drainage of pus

Chronic: Saucerization, sequesterectomy, amputation

Gas gangrene: Oxygen, antibiotics, gas gangrene antitoxin, amputation

4. *Avascular necrosis of bone (AVN)*

Etiology   Is defined as death of bone due to interruption of blood supply (torn vessels) following a fracture or dislocation.

Example:
- Avascular necrosis of femoral head following fracture neck femur.
- Avascular necrosis of proximal segment of scaphoid following fracture waist of scaphoid.

Management   Firm fixation (ORIF) may help in recovery, but not always successful. In an established case – treatment of choice is THR, in case of AVN following fracture neck femur.

5. *Volkmann ischemic contracture (VIC)*

Etiology   Exact cause unknown. May be due to arterial spasm, following reduction of fractures.

Pathogenesis   Arterial spasm causes interruption of blood supply to muscles, resulting in necrosis, fibrosis, and finally to contractures

Examples: VIC of flexor group of muscles of forearm, following reduction of supracondylar fracture of humerus and fractures of forearm. Also seen in leg and calf

Diagnosis   Hand becomes white and numb

Radial pulse – absent

Failure to extend wrist and straighten fingers passively

Management
- Relax flexion at elbow and extend it beyond 90
- Exploration of artery
- Inj. Papaverine 2.5% sol. – to wash segment of artery in spasm
- Physiotherapy

6. *Tight plasters*

Diagnosis   Severe pain or numbness

Swelling of fingers/toes.

Skin of fingers/toes – Pale, white, or cyanotic

Management   *Preventive treatment:*

Elevate the limb

Watch circulation

Active exercises of fingers/toes

Specific treatment:

Split the plaster

Check circulation

Check reduction – clinically and radiologically.

7. *Slow: union*

Fracture takes comparatively longer time to unite wthout any change clinically or radiologically.

Management   Wait and watch for normal union, clinically and radiologically, periodically. No interference with reduction and fixation.

8. *Delayed: union* Fracture fails to unite within the specific time.

Radiologically, no callus visible, ends of bone fragments well defined, no sclerosis.

Management Continue the fixation.

Active exercises.

9. *Non-union:* Fracture fails to unite, and usually the end result of delayed union.

Etiology General: Old age, poor health, diseases like syphilis and tuberculosis.

Local: Delayed union, inadequate fixation, distraction, interposition of soft tissues between fragments, infection.

Diagnosis: Unnatural mobility at fracture site, after expiry of normal union period.

Radiologically: Sclerosis, rounding off bony ends, fracture line clearly visible, bony ends may be flared out

Management Internal fixation and bone grafting

10. *Malunion:* Fracture united in an abnormal anatomical position

Etiology Defective reduction and fixation

Diagnosis Deformity: Angulation or rotational deformity resulting in cosmetic effect and impaired functioning of the limb.

Shortening

Management If detected earlier, e.g. before union, the angulation may be corrected by wedging of plaster cast, and manipulation under anesthesia in late cases, e.g. after union of fracture – correction by osteotomy.

11. *Shortening*

Etiology Malunited fracture due to angular and rotational deformities

Oblique and spiral fractures and epiphyseal injuries

Diagnosis: Impaired functioning of the limb

Management Up to 2.5 cm – compensated by pelvis tilt

More than 2.5 cm – corrected by alteration of the footwear, e.g. raising by a wedge incorporated within the shoe

Corrective osteotomy for shortning due to marked angulation

12. *Joint stiffness*

Etiology Intra-articular, e.g.

A. Fibrous adhesions

B. Injury to articular cartilage

C. Prolonged immobilization

Extra-articular, e.g.

A. Injury to joint capsule, ligaments, tendons, muscles, etc.

B. Fibrosis

Mechanical obstruction, e.g.

A. Intra-articular fractures

B. Myositis ossificans.

Management   *Preventive treatment:*
First aid splintage, before reduction
Perfect reduction
Adequate fixation
Elevation of limb
Active exercises.
Specific treatment :
- Physiotherapy
- Surgical treatment, i.e. correction of the cause.

13. *Myositis ossificans*

A bony mass appears in the tissues near a joint, resulting in restricted movements due to mechanical obstruction

Etiology   Repeated manipulations for reduction of fracture

Pathogenesis   Hematoma formation in the muscle, leading to bone formation as a result of calcification and ossification of this hematoma

Example: Myositis ossificans of brachialis muscle at the front of elbow joint, following reduction of supracondylar fracture

Investigation   X-ray confirms diagnosis

Management   Early excision: Yields poor results, with recurrence
Late excision: Yields good results, with less chances of recurrence

14. *Osteoarthritis*

Degeneration of joint, following fracture

Etiology   Intra-articular fractures
Injury to articular cartilage, capsule, ligament
Avascular necrosis
Infection
Malunion

Management   Treatment of the cause
Physiotherapy: Shortwave therapy, infra red therapy, exercises
Intra-articular injections of hydrocortisone with xylocain (Lidocaine) 2% –once or twice a week
Surgical measures:
- Synovectomy
- Excision osteophytes
- Arthroscopy
- Reconstruction
- Total joint replacement
- Arthrodesis.

15. *Sudeck's dystrophy*

Etiology   Unknown
May be due to sympathetic response to fracture.

Diagnosis:
- Painful, restricted movements.
- Swelling of hand and fingers
- Skin – warm and shining
- Tenderness present over wrist and metacarpals.

Investigation   X-ray: Shows fracture united, osteoporosis, mottling of carpus

Management
- Anti-inflammatory analgesics
- Physiotherapy

16. Bed sores

Etiology   Due to local pressure by ridges, produced by uneven application of a bandage, loose plaster, infection, and malnutrition.

Diagnosis   Pain, discomfort, edema, gangrene

Management   Cut a window in the plaster cast AS dressings.

17. Visceral complications

  i. Rupture of urethra or bladder in fracture pelvis
  ii. Rupture of kidney, spleen, liver, intestine, etc. due to local trauma, e.g. compression of abdomen in RSA.
  iii. Paralytic ileus:

Etiology   Frequently seen following fracture pelvis or lumbar spine.

Diagnosis   Distension abdomen, absent bowel sounds, vomiting, constipation

Investigation   Serum electrolytes

Plain X-ray abdomen

Abdominal paracentesis

Laparotomy

Laparoscopy

Management   Nasogastric suction

IV fluids

18. Cast syndrome

Etiology   Plaster jackets, hip spicas, or plaster beds

Diagnosis   Vomiting

Constipation

Abdominal distension

Management   Removal of plaster

Nasogastric suction

IV fluids.

Fractures in Children

Principles of Fracture Treatment in Children

Childhood fractures are different from adult fractures, and also the principles of treatment are quite different. The treatment of fractures in children is simple as compared to complex one in adults.

Principles

1. Delayed union: Absent in children, due to remarkable osteogenic activity.

2. Deformity: It is rare in children, due to great power of remodeling.

3. Shortning of limb: Self-correctable, due to stimulation of growth.

4. Joint stiffness: It is rare.

5. Manipulation of greenstick fracture: It is easier, due to strong periosteum.

6. Immunity of certain bones: Fracture spine rare, paraplegia unknown, fracture pelvis rare.

7. Problematically childhood fractures:

   i. Supracondylar fracture of humerus – associated with vascular injuries.

   ii. Fracture of capitellum – associated with late cubitus valgus and ulnar nerve palsy.

   iii. Separation of lower femoral epiphysis – causing gangrene of foot, due to pressing of popliteal vessels.

References

1. Bohler, L (1935) The treatment of Fractures. 4th ed. Bristol, Wright.

2. Watson-Jones, R (1952) Fractures and other Bone and Joint Injuries. Edinburgh, Livinstone.

3. Advanced Life Support Working Group. European Resuscitation Council Guidelines 2000 for Adult Advanced Life Support. Resuscitation 2001:48:211–21.

4. Campbell, WC (1956) Operative Orthopaedics, Kimpton.

5. Clarke, R (1959) Resuscitation & Transfusion in Severe Injuries. In Modern Trends In Accident Surgery and Medicine. Ed. By R Clarke, FG Badger & S Sevitt, London Butterworths.

6. Nicholas, TH & Rumer, GF (1960) Emergency Airway – A Plan of Action. J Amer Med Ass 174, 1930.

7. McRae R, (1984) Practical Fracture Treatmant. Edinburgh, Churchill Livingstone.

8. Pediatric Life Support Working Group. European Resuscitation Council Guidelines 2000 for advanced pediatric life support. Resuscitation 48:231-4:2001.

9. Principles and Practice of Pediatric Surgery. Vol I: Trauma:357–509. Keith T Oldham, Paul M Colomham, Robert P Folgia, Michel A Skinner.

Section B: Regional Injuries

Upper Limb Injuries
Injuries about the Shoulder Girdle

1. Fractures of clavicle

2. Dislocation of acromioclavicular joint

3. Dislocation of sternoclavicular joint

4. Fracture of scapula

5. Dislocation of shoulder joint

6. Fracture-dislocation of shoulder joint

7. Old un-reduced dislocation of shoulder joint

8. Recurrent dislocation of shoulder joint

9. Shoulder cuff injuries

10. Fractures of greater tuberosity

11. Fracture neck of humerus

12. Fracture shaft of humerus

Fractures of Clavicle

Sites	Fracture occurs commonly at the junction of middle and outer thirds, and may also occur in the middle third.
MOI	Fall on the outstretched hand – commonest cause
	Direct violence
	RSA
	Sports injury.

Diagnosis

Patterns

In children	Greenstick fracture – no deformity,
	Local tenderness present,
	Reluctance to move the arm.
In adults	Separation of bony ends
	Elevation of proximal end by the pull of sternomastoid,
	Displacement of outer end – downwards, forwards, and inwards by the pull of pectoralis,
S/S	Pain, local tenderness, bony irregularity, crepitus, unnatural mobility at fracture site.
Investigation	X-ray clavicle – AP view.

Management

Greenstick fracture in children

Cuff and collar sling

Analgesics

Refer: To the next fracture clinic.

Fractures in Adults

Conservative treatment

Apply figure of 8 bandage or a clavicle brace

Cuff and collar sling or arm pouch

Analgesics

Refer: To the next fracture clinic.

Surgical treatment: **Refer** the patient to the orthopedic team for surgery.

Surgery	ORIF – Medullary fixation with 2 medullary pins, Alt:
	– Plate and screws
Indications	• Failure of conservative treatment, e.g. persistent separation of fragments
	• Neurological due to pressure exerted by displaced fragment upon the brachial plexus
	• Ligament injury (coracoclavicular) by distal fragment
After care	Arm supported in an arm pouch for 1–2/52.
	Removal of pins after 8–12/52

Dislocation of Acromioclavicular Joint

MOI   Fall on the outstretched hand.

Pathogenesis   Dislocation occurs due to tearing of acromioclavicular ligament, coronoid and trapezoid ligaments, while subluxation occurs due to tearing of acromioclavicular ligament only.

Diagnosis   Prominence of acromial end of clavicle

                     Local tenderness

                     Movements of the joint – painful and restricted.

Investigation   X-ray clavicle (focusing acromioclavicular joint) – AP view.

Management

Subluxation   Arm supported in an armpouch for 4/52

                     Active exercises of fingers, and elbow.

Dislocation   Surgical treatment

Refer: The patient to the orthopedic team for surgery.

Surgery   ORIF, e.g. coracoclavicular screwing and repair of coronoid and trapezoid ligaments or

                     Acromionectomy.

After care   Arm supported in an arm pouch for 6/52

                     Active exercises of fingers, wrist, and elbow.

Dislocation of Sternoclavicular Joint

MOI   Fall on the outstretched hand

                     Direct violence.

Diagnosis   Sternal end of clavicle – prominent,

                     Local tenderness,

                     Movements of shoulder – painful and restricted.

Investigation   X-ray clavicle (focusing sternoclavicular joint) – AP view.

Management

Subluxation   Arm pouch for 2–3/52

                     Active exercises of fingers, wrist, and elbow.

Dislocation

Conservative treatment

                     Closed reduction and applying a figure of 8 bandage.

Surgical treatment; **Refer** the patient to the orthopedic team for surgery.

Surgery   ORIF:

                     • Open reduction and fixation with fascia lata, Alt:

                     • Plating (Hook plate)

After care   Arm pouch or a sling for 2/52

                     Active exercises of fingers and elbow

Fractures of Scapula

Sites	Common sites are neck and body of scapula.
MOI	Direct violence.
Diagnosis	Flattening and drooping of shoulder
	Lengthening of arm
	Local tenderness
	Movements of shoulder painful and restricted.
Investigation	X-ray scapula – PA view.
Management	

Conservative treatment

> Warm fomentation
> Massage – with warm oil or an anti-inflammatory creme
> Strapping – adhesive
> Analgesics
> Arm pouch for 2–3/52
> Active exercises of fingers, wrist, elbow

Surgical treatment: **Refer** patient to orthopedic team for surgery.

Surgery	Open reduction
Indication	• Dislocation of shoulder plus fracture neck of humerus.
	• Drooping of shoulder.
After care	Physiotherapy

Dislocation of Shoulder Joint

Types	Anterior and posterior dislocations
	Anterior dislocation: Common type – head lies in front of glenoid.
MOI	Fall on the outstretched hand.
Diagnosis	Flattening of the shoulder
	Prominent acromion, fullness in the deltopectoral groove
	Loss of resistance beneath the acromion.
Investigation	X-ray shoulder joint – AP and LAT views.
Management	Closed reduction under anesthesia.
Methods	Kocher's and Hippocratic methods.
Kocher's	Apply traction, continuing traction gradually rotate the arm externally once the dislocation is reduced, then bring the arm across the chest, and finally rotate the arm internally. The dislocation is reduced now.
After care	Strapping arm the front of chest.
	Arm sling for 4/52 and active exercises of fingers, wrist, and elbow.
Hippocratic	Surgeon places his heel of foot into the axilla of patient, keeping full care not to injure the side of chest wall, the head of humerus is levered back into its position.
After care	Same as for Kocher's method.

Fracture-dislocation of Shoulder

Types	Dislocation of shoulder plus fracture neck of humerus
	Dislocation of shoulder plus fracture greater tuberosity.

Dislocation of Shoulder Plus Fracture Neck of Humerus

MOI	Fall on the outstretched hand
	Direct violence.
Diagnosis	Swelling, local tenderness, crepitus
	Passive movement of arm minus that of head of humerus.
Investigation	X-ray shoulder – AP and LAT views.
Management	

In elderly patient: Only arm sling and active exercises advisable.

In younger patient: Open reduction is usually indicated, as closed reduction fails due to difficulty in controlling small sized upper fragment.

After care	Arm sling and active exercises of fingers, wrist, and elbow.

Dislocation of Shoulder Plus Fracture Greater Tuberosity

MOI	Fall on the outstretched hand, or direct violence.
Diagnosis	Swelling, local tenderness, crepitus
	Movements (esp. abduction) – painful and restricted.
Investigation	X-ray shoulder – AP and LAT views.
Management	Same treatment as for dislocation of shoulder.
	Apposition occurs when dislocation is reduced.
Surgery	ORIF – of fracture greater tuberosity with a screw
Indication	Marked displacement of fracture

Refer: The patient to the orthopedic team for surgery.

Old Unreduced Dislocation of Shoulder

Management	< 6/52 – closed reduction and arm sling.
	> 6/52 – physiotherapy in elderly and open reduction in younger

Refer: The patient to the orthopedic team for surgery.

Recurrent Dislocation of Shoulder

MOI	Repeated dislocation of shoulder occurring, due to little trauma, and many a times, the patient may be able to reduce dislocation, himself or herself.
Pathology	There may be following pathological lesions:

- Bankart lesion
- Flattening of posterolateral aspect of head
- Rounding of glenoid margin
- Defective shoulder cuff includes capsule.

Investigation	X-ray shoulder – axial view.

Management

Surgical treatment: **Refer** the patient to the orthopedic team for surgery.

Surgery   Surgical repair: Types of repair:

Bankart' repair Anchoring the glenoid labrum and the anterior capsule to the glenoid cavity by mattress sutures passed through holes in the rim.

Putti-plat repair Restricting the external rotation by overlapping and shortning the subscapularis tendon and overlapping and tightening the capsule

Bone-block repair

                 Buttress the joint by fixing a bone graft to the glenoid

After care   Immobilization – arm kept in internal rotation for 4/52, followed by exercises.

Shoulder Cuff Injuries

Anatomy   Shoulder cuff comprises – tendons of supraspinatus, teres minor, and infraspinatus.

MOI   A little trauma may cause tears (lesions) in the degenerated shoulder cuff. These lesions are:
                 • Supraspinatus tendonitis,
                 • Rupture of supraspinatus tendon,
                 • Calcification of supraspinatus tendon,
                 • Subdeltoid bursitis.

Diagnosis

Supraspinatus tendonitis (painful arc syndrome):

                 Pain appears in the shoulder over an arc – 60 to 120° of abduction, with freedom from pain on movement outside limits of that range.
                 Tenderness over greater tuberosity, i.e. insertion of supraspinatus.

Rupture of supraspinatus tendon

                 Pain and tenderness over greater tuberosity
                 Abduction painful at 90°.

Calcification of supraspinatus tendon

                 Pain in the shoulder
                 Stiffness
                 X-ray shows calcified deposit above head.

Subdeltoid or subacromial bursitis

                 Pain in the shoulder
                 Tenderness over greater tuberosity
                 Painful restricted abduction.

Management

Conservative treatment

                 Short-wave diathermy or infrared fomentation plus analgesics
                 Intra-articular inj. hydrocortisone with lignocaine 2%, plus exercises.

Surgical treatment: **Refer** the patient to the orthopedic team for surgery.

Surgery   Repair of the lesion – especially in the young patient.

Fracture Neck of Humerus

Definition	Fracture line passes through the surgical neck, and rarely through the anatomical neck.
Patterns	Greenstick fracture – in children
	Impacted (abduction and adduction) fracture – in adults
	Unimpacted fracture.
MOI	Fall on the outstretched hand, or direct violence.
Diagnosis	Patient supports the arm with the other hand,
	Local tenderness,
	Deformity.
Investigation	X-ray shoulder – AP view.

Management

Conservative treatment

Impacted fracture: Arm sling or cuff and collar sling for 4/52

After care – physiotherapy

Unimpacted fracture: Closed reduction and arm sling

After care	Physiotherapy.

Surgical treatment: **Refer** the patient to the orthopedic team for surgery.

Surgery	Internal fixation with:

- Rush pinning/ender nailing, Alt:
- Plate and screws – locking compression plate (LCP)

After care	Physiotherapy.

Fracture Shaft of Humerus

MOI	Fall on the outstretched hand, or direct violence.

Pathogenesis

In fractures of proximal third: Proximal fragment adducted due to pull of pectoralis

In fractures of middle third: Proximal fragment abducted due to pull of deltoid.

Diagnosis	Patient supports the arm with the other hand
	Deformity – mostly angulation
	Local tenderness
	Unnatural mobility.
Complication	Radial nerve palsy (wrist drop) may accompany the fracture.
Investigation	X-ray humerus – AP and LAT views.

Management

Conservative treatment

U-plaster method

Apply a U-slapped plaster slab, starting from axilla, to under the elbow, to the top of shoulder, supported by elastic crepe bandage.

Hanging cast method

The weight of the limb plus that of plaster, reduce fracture and maintain reduction. It may lead to non-union due to distraction.

After care   Cuff and collar sling. Union normally occurs in about 6–8/52.

Surgical treatment: **Refer** the patient to the orthopedic team for surgery.

Surgery   Internal fixation

Indications   Patient–bedridden

Patient double/comminuted fracture

Radial nerve palsy

Compound fracture.

Methods   Rush pinning/Ender nailing – antegrade or retrograde

Intramedullary nailing – solid humeral nail (UHN), PHN

Interlocking nailing under C-arm supervision

Interlocking nailing (open) without C-arm supervision

Plate and screws.

Management of complications of internal fixation

Non-union   ORIF plus bone grafting.

Radial nerve   Usually the recovery begins 8/52 after the injury

palsy   Provide the patient with a wrist drop splint and regular physiotherapy

Wait for 8/52.

Exploration of radial nerve – if no evidence of recovery

References

1. Charnley J. The Closed Treatment of Common Fractures. Churchill Livingstone, Edinburgh (Recently reprinted by the John Charnley Trust), 1968

2. McRAE R, Esser M: Practical Fracture Treatment, 4th ed. Churchill Livingstone, Edinburgh, 2002.

3. Gille J, et al. Hook plate for medial clavicle fracture. Indian Journal of Orthopaedics, Vol 44-2, 221–223; 2010.

4. Throckmorton T, Kuhn JE. Fractures of the medial end of the clavicle. J Shoulder Elbow Surg, 16:49–54;2007.

5. Vander Griend R, Tomasin J, Ward Ef. Open reduction and internal fixation of humeral shaft fractures: results using AO plating techniques. J Bone Joint Surg (Am) 68A: 430–3;1986.

6. Stern PJ, Mattingly DA, Pomeroy DL, et al. Intramedullary fixation of humeral shaft fractures. J Bone Joint Surg (Am) 66A: 639–46;1984.

7. Rommens PM, Blum J, Runkel M. Retrograde Nailing of Humeral Shaft Fractures. Clin. Orthop. 350: 26–39;1998.

8. Robinson CM, Bell KM, Court Brown CM, et al. Locked nailing of humeral shaft fractures: experience in Edinburgh over a two year period. J Bone Joint Surg (Br) 74B: 558–62;1992.

Injuries about the Elbow

- Fractures in children:
  - Supracondylar fracture
  - Lateral condyle fracture
  - Medial epicondyle fracture
  - Lateral epicondyle fracture
  - Fracture neck of radius

- Fractures in adults:
  - Fracture of lower end of humerus (Y or T shaped)
  - Fracture of capitellum
  - Fracture of olecranon
  - Fracture head of radius
- Dislocations and fracture-dislocations: May occur in any age.
- Injuries of muscles and tendons: Tennis elbow (lateral epicondylitis)

Supracondylar Fracture of Humerus

Definition	It is one of the commonest fracture of childhood, involving distal end of humerus.
Pattern	Fracture line is proximal to trochlea and capitulum.
Types	Posterior – common type and Anterior – rare type.
MOI	Fall on the outstretched hand.
Diagnosis	Deformity – distal fragment is displaced backwards, upwards, and outwards Swelling Local tenderness Olecranon, medial and lateral epicondyles – preserve their relation Shortning of the arm Movements at the elbow painful and restricted.
Investigation	X-ray elbow – AP and LAT views.
Complications	• Injury to brachial vessels • Injury to ulnar, median, or radial nerves • Movements of elbow – painful and restricted • Malunion • Cubitus valgus or varus • Volkmann's ischemic contracture • Myositis ossificans.

Management

Conservative treatment: Closed reduction under C-arm supervision

Anesthesia	General
Method	Traction is applied to extended elbow – to disengage fragments Correction of lateral displacement Maintaining traction in the length of arm, flex the elbow. Forward drawing of posterior displaced lower fragment – into line with axis of humerus Finally flex the elbow to 60–70° – to lock reduced fragments by taught triceps Check the radial pulse before applying plaster slab for 6–8 weeks
Remanipulation	In case of previous poor reduction

After care   Admit the child for overnight stay in the hospital, for observation of circulation. Elevate the arm. Cuff and collar sling.

Surgical treatment: **Refer** the child to orthopedic team for surgery.

Indication   Failure of conservative treatment

                 Instability

Surgery   Internal fixation – Rush pin/Ender nails

                 Followed by plaster fixation.

Refer: The child to next fracture clinic.

Fracture of Lateral Condyle

Definition   It is the commonest epiphyseal injury around the elbow in children.

Pattern   The detached fragment (incld. Capitellum and half of trochlea) is displaced and rotated by forearm extensors and lateral ligament. It is an intra-articular fracture, therefore accurate reduction is essential.

MOI   Fall on the outstretched hand or fall on the point of olecranon.

Diagnosis   Swelling,

                 Deformity – cubitus valgus

                 Local tenderness,

                 Movements at elbow – painful and restricted.

Investigation   X-ray elbow – AP and LAT views.

Complications   Non-union, deformity – cubitus valgus, late ulnar nerve palsy

Management

Surgery   Internal fixation: Kirschner wires – is the treatment of choice.

                 Followed by plaster fixation.

Refer: The child to orthopedic team for surgical treatment.

Fracture of Medial Epicondyle

MOI   Fall on the outstretched hand or direct violence.

Diagnosis   Swelling

                 Deformity – cubitus valgus

                 Local tenderness

                 Movements at elbow – painful and restricted.

Investigation   X-ray elbow – AP and LAT views

                 Absence of medial epicondyle from its normal position

                 Inclusion of fragment inside the joint.

Management

Conservative treatment: Closed reduction under general anesthesia

Method   Forced valgus, supination, extension, dorsiflexion of wrist

                 Followed by plaster fixation.

Refer: The child to next fracture clinic.

Surgical treatment

Surgery   Internal fixation – Kirschner wire fixation
                 Followed by plaster fixation.
Indication   Failure of conservative treatment.
Refer: The child to orthopedic team for surgical treatment.

Fracture of Lateral Epicondyle
MOI   Fall on their outstretched hand or direct violence.
Diagnosis   Swelling
                 Local tenderness
                 Movements at elbow – painfull and restricted.
Investigation   X-ray elbow – AP and LAT views.
Management   Closed reduction and plaster cast for 3–4/52.
Refer: The child to next fracture clinic.

Fracture Neck of Radius
Pattern   Usually a greenstick fracture.
MOI   Fall on the outstretched hand – drives the capitellum against head of
                 radius.
Diagnosis   Swelling
                 Local tenderness
                 Movements at elbow – painful and restricted.
Investigation   X-ray elbow – AP and LAT views.
Management
Conservative treatment
                 For little/no tilt: Cuff and collar sling and analgesics
                 For marked tilt: Manipulation (traction, pronation, supination) under
                 anesthesia.
Surgical treatment: **Refer** the child to the orthopedic team for surgery.
Surgery   • Open reduction
                    Indication: Failure of conservative treatment
                             Marked displacement
                 • Excision of radial head
                    Indication: Danger of cubitus valgus development.

Fracture of Lower End of Humerus (Intercondylar)
Pattern   T or Y shaped fractures of lower end of humerus.
MOI   Fall on the point of elbow, the olecranon wedges into lower end of humerus,
                 causing separation and comminution.
Diagnosis   Swelling, deformity, local tenderness, crepitus, unnatural mobility,
                 movements at elbow – painful and restricted.
Investigation   X-ray elbow – AP and LAT views.

Management
Conservative treatment
Indication   Comminuted fracture
Method   Closed reduction and plaster (POP) cast
Refer: The patient to next fracture clinic
Surgical treatment: **Refer** patient to orthopedic team for surgery.
Indication   Non-comminuted fracture
Surgery   Internal fixation: Plate and screws (LCP), Rush pin/Ender nail, or screws.
                 POP cast – knuckles to above elbow.
After care   Physiotherapy.

Fracture of Capitellum
MOI   Fall on the outstretched hand, causing fracture of the capitellum by an upward thrust transmitted by the radial head.
Diagnosis   Swelling, local tenderness, movements at elbow painful and restricted.
Investigation   X-ray elbow – AP and LAT views.
Management
Conservative treatment
Method   Closed reduction and plaster applied to extended elbow.
Refer: The patient to next fracture clinic
Surgical treatment: **Refer** the patient to the orthopedic team for surgery.
Surgery   Internal fixation – Smile pins and plaster cast for 4–6/52
After care   Physiotherapy.

Fracture of Olecranon
MOI   Direct violence – fall on the point of elbow
                 Indirect violence – fall on the outstretched hand
                 Avulsion injury – caused by triceps contraction.
Diagnosis   Swelling, local tenderness, bone irregularity, movements at elbow – painful and restricted.
Investigation   X-ray elbow – AP and LAT views.
Management
Conservative treatment
Method   Plaster cast above elbow for 6–8/52
Indication   Hairline and undisplaced fracture.
Refer: The patient to next fracture clinic.
Surgical treatment: **Refer** the patient to the orthopedic team for surgery.
Surgery   ORIF
Indications   Displaced closed fractures (transverse, oblique, comminuted)
                 Open fractures
Methods   Displaced closed fractures:
                 • Zuelzer hooked plate and screws

- Croll olecranon screw
- Lag screw
- Tension band wiring (Kirschner wires, rush pin)

Open fractures:
- Clamp cum compressor device

After care   Physiotherapy.

Fracture Head of Radius

MOI   Fall on the outstretched hand.
Types   Chip fracture involving less than one-third of periphery
                    Comminuted fracture of whole head.
Diagnosis   Swelling
                    Local tenderness
                    Movements at elbow – painful and restricted.
Investigation   X-ray elbow – AP and LAT views.
Management
Conservative treatment
Indication   Chip fractures
Method   Plaster cast above elbow

Refer: The patient to next fracture clinic.

Surgical treatment: **Refer** the patient to the orthopedic team for surgery.

Indication   Comminuted fractures
Surgery   Excision of radial head.
After care   Physiotherapy.

Dislocation of Elbow

Age   May occur in any age.
Types   Posterolateral – commonest type
                    Anterior – rare type.

Posterior Dislocation

MOI   Fall on the outstretched hand.
Diagnosis   Deformity – Olecranon displaced up
                        – Relationship of olecranon, medial and lateral epicondyles
                            disturbed, i.e. almost at same level
                    Shortening of forearm
                    Movements at elbow – painful and restricted.
D/d   Supracondylar fracture of lower end of humerus.
Investigation   X-ray elbow – AP and LAT views.
Management
Conservative treatment

Method   Closed reduction under general anesthesia
After care   Cuff and collar sling for 3/52

Anterior Dislocation

Associated with olecranon fracture.
MOI   Fall on the elbow.
Management
Conservative treatment
Indication   Dislocation of elbow
Method   Closed reduction.
Surgical treatment: **Refer** the patient to the orthopedic team for surgery.
Surgery   ORIF
Indication   Fracture of olecranon
Method   Fixation with:
                • Screw, or
                • Tension wire, or
                • Croocked plate and screws.
Followed by   Plaster in extension of elbow for 4/52.
After care   Physiotherapy.

Tennis Elbow (Lateral Epicondylitis)

Definition   It is a very common disorder of unknown pathogenesis.
Etiology   Traumatic: RSA, sports injury, direct violence.
MOI   Abrupt pronation of the forearm, causing strain on the extensor aponeurotic
                fibres.
Diagnosis   Pain – over the outer aspect of the elbow
                Local tenderness – over lateral epicondyle
                Movements – passive pronation to the full extent exaggerate pain.
Investigation   X-ray elbow – AP and LAT views.
Management
Conservative   Heat – IR or SWD
                Elbow support
                Local – inj. hydrocortisone 25–50 mg + inj. lignocain 2%.
Surgery   Release of extensor aponeurosis.
Refer: The patient to the orthopedic team for surgery.

References

1. Attenborough CG. Remodelling of the humerus after supracondylar fractures in children. J Bone Jt Surg. 35B:3;1953.
2. Dunn N. Fractures of the olecranon. Brit Med J. 1:214;1939.
3. Eastwood WJ. T-shaped fracture of the humerus. J Bone Jt Surg. 19:364;1937.
4. Jackobsson A. Fracture of the capitellum of the humerus in adults. Acta Orthop. Scand. 3:184;1957.

5. Kundu ZS et al. Management of open olecranon fractures using clamp cum compressor device. Indian Orthopedics, Vol 43-1:50–54;2009.
6. Jeffory CC. Fractures of the head of the radius in children. J Bone Jt Surg. 32B:314;1950.
7. Seddon HJ. Volkmann's Contracture. J Bone Jt Surg. 38B:152;1956.
8. Boyd DW, Aronson DD. Supracondylar Fracture Humerus, Ulnar Nerve, Iatrogenic Injury. J Orthop Trauma. 19:158–163;2005.

Forearm Bones Injuries

- Monteggia fracture dislocation
- Galeazzi fracture dislocation
- Fracture both bones forearm
- Isolated fracture radius
- Isolated fracture ulna

Monteggia Fracture Dislocation

Pattern	Fracture of ulna with dislocation of radial head.
Types	Anterior – common type – Posterior – rare type
Anterior type	Dislocation of radial head forwards along with anterior angulation of fractured ulna
Posterior type	Dislocation of radial head backwards along with posterior angulation of fractured ulna.
MOI	Fall on the outstretched hand or direct violence.
Diagnosis	Deformity, local tenderness, movements – painful and restricted esp. pronation and supination.
Investigation	X-ray forearm includes elbow and wrist – AP and LAT. views.
Management	

Surgical treatment: **Refer** the patient to the orthopedic team for surgery.

Surgery	ORIF of fractured ulna (plating or rush pin).

Anterior Monteggia

	ORIF of fractured ulna (plating or rush pin)
	Reduction of radial head is achieved by pressing backwards over head of radius.
	For unstable radial head – fixation with percutaneous K-wire.
After care	Forearm and elbow immobilized in supination and flexion, by plaster for 6/52.

Posterior Monteggia

	ORIF of fractured ulna (plating or rush pin)
	Reduction of radial head is achieved by pressing forwards over head of radius, with elbow in extension position.
After care	Forearm and elbow immobilized in supination and extension, by plaster for 6/52, followed by physiotherapy.

Galeazzi Fracture Dislocation

Definition	Fracture of radius with dislocation of inferior radioulnar joint.
MOI	Fall on the outstretched hand or direct violence.
Diagnosis	Swelling, local tenderness, movements at wrist – painful and restricted.
Investigation	X-ray forearm include elbow and wrist – AP and LAT views.
Management	

Surgical treatment: **Refer** the patient to the orthopedic team for surgery.

Surgery	ORIF of fractured radius (plating of radius)
Method	Reduction of radius is followed by spontaneous reduction of ulna while inferior radioulnar joint does not require any opening.

Note: All fracture-dislocations of radial shaft, best treated by ORIF.

Postoperative	Plaster slab for 6–8/52.
After care	Physiotherapy.

Fracture both Bones Forearm in Children

Pattern	Mostly greenstick fractures.
MOI	Fall on the outstretched hand or direct violence.
Diagnosis	Swelling, local tenderness, resents moving arm.
Investigation	X-ray forearm includes elbow and wrist – AP and LAT views.
Management	

Undisplaced greenstick fracture: Closed reduction and POP cast

Anesthesia	General.
Method	Closed reduction of angulation deformity.
	Usually the deformity is overcorrected, to prevent recurrence of angulation, due to sagging.
After care	Plaster cast for 4–6/52, followed by physiotherapy.

Displaced fracture: Closed reduction of angulation and rotation, under the C-arm (traction and correction of displacement).

Surgery	**Refer** the patient to the orthopedic team for surgery.
Surgery	ORIF
Indication	Failure of closed reduction.
Postoperative	Plaster slab with flexed (90°) elbow, for 4–6/52.
After care	Physiotherapy.

Fracture Both Bones Forearm in Adults

MOI	Direct violence or fall on the outstretched hand
Diagnosis	Deformity – angulation, rotation
	Shortening
	Unnatural mobility
	Loss of function.
Investigation	X-ray of forearm includes elbow and wrist – AP and LAT views.

Management   ORIF is treatment of choice in adults.

Conservative treatment: Closed reduction under C-arm supervision.

Indications   Elderly patient

Undisplaced fractures

Multiple injuries.

D/Adv.   Difficulty in reduction

Failure to maintain reduction

Displacement – marked

Rotational deformities – common

Volkmann ischemic contracture – common.

Surgical treatment: **Refer** the patient to the orthopedic team for surgery.

Surgery   ORIF – Plating of both fractured bones or

– Plating of radius and nailing of ulna

Method   Apply a tourniquet

Exposure (Henry) Radius – anterior incision

Ulna – posterior incision

Postoperative   Plaster cast for 6–8/52.

After care   Physiotherapy.

Isolated Fracture of Radius

Pattern   Fracture of radius, without involvement of inferior radioulnar joint, is a rare entity.

MOI   Direct violence.

Diagnosis   Swelling, tenderness, movements at wrist – painful and restricted.

Investigation   X-ray forearm includes wrist and elbow – AP and LAT views.

Management

Surgical treatment: **Refer** the patient to the orthopedic team for surgery.

Surgery   ORIF of fractured radius (plating).

Indication   ORIF of fractured radius, as it is difficult to prevent angulation of distal fragment towards ulna by muscle pull, if treated by closed reduction and plaster.

Postoperative   POP for 6–8/52.

After care   Physiotherapy.

Isolated Fracture of Ulna

Pattern   Mostly greenstick fractures.

MOI   Fall on the outstretched hand or direct violence.

Diagnosis   Swelling, tenderness, bone irregularity, ulnar angulation.

Investigation   X-ray forearm includes elbow and wrist – AP and LAT views.

Management

Conservative   Displacement slight: Plater in mid-pronation for 8–10/52.

Surgical treatment: **Refer** the patient to the orthopedic team for surgery.

Surgery   ORIF

Indication   Displacement/angulation marked

Postoperative   POP for 6–8/52.

After care   Physiotherapy.

References

1. Holdsworth F. Fractures of the radius and ulna. Modern Trends in Orthopaedics, 3:84;1962.
2. Moore JR. The closed fractures of the long bones. J Bone Jt Surg. 42A:869;1960.
3. Evans EM. Fractures of the radius and ulna. J Bone Jt Surg. 33B:548;1951.
4. Knight RA , Purvis GD. Fractures of both bones of the forearm in adults. J Bone Jt Surg. 31A:755;1949.
5. Robertson RC. Intramedullary fixation of fractures of the forearm. Amer J Surg. 85:496;1953.
6. Smith H, Sage FP. Internal fixation of fractures of the radius and ulna. J Bone Jt Surg. 41B:172;1959.

Injuries about the Wrist and Hand

Closed Hand Injuries:

- Colles' fracture
- Smith's fracture (syn. reversed Colles' fracture)
- Barton's fracture
- Slipped radial epiphysis
- Fracture of the radial styloid
- Scaphoid fracture
- Lunate dislocation
- Bennett's fracture dislocation
- Metacarpal fractures
- Rupture of ulnar collateral ligament (Gamekeeper's thumb)
- Fractures of phalanges
- Mallet finger

Open hand injuries

Colles' Fracture

Definition   It is defined as a fracture of radius within 2.5 cm of the wrist and usually occurs in old ladies. Shortening of radius causes subluxation of the inferior radioulnar joint and a prominent ulnar styloid.

MOI   Fall on the outstretched hand.

Diagnosis   Deformity – dinner fork, i.e. lower end of radius is displaced backwards, radially and rotated. Radial and ulner stylosis processes are on same level.

Investigation   X-ray forearm includes wrist – AP and LAT views.

Management   Closed reduction under general anesthesia.

Method   The assistant holds the arm above the flexed elbow. The surgeon grips the patient's wrist with one hand above and the other below the level of fracture, changing hands accordingly to suit patient's left or right wrist. For patient's left wrist, surgeon places palm of his left hand on the palmar surface of patient's wrist above level of proximal fragment, the palm of his right hand is then applied to the dorsal surface of patient's wrist distal to level of fracture.

Steps	i. Disimpaction of distal fragment: Surgeon applies traction with the right hand, in line of forearm, and increases the deformity a little by extending the wrist.
	ii. Palmar flexion: Maintaining traction to disengage the fractured fragments, the distal fragment is flexed gently, followed by direct pressure exerted by right hand on the dorsal surface of distal fragment, while in the opposite direction, by left hand on the ventral surface of the proximal fragment.
	iii. Maintaining traction, the patient's wrist is promoted by surgeon by pronating his own right hand, while maintaining his left hand stationary, to prevent proximal fragment from following the distal fragment.
	iv. Ulnar deviation of patient's wrist is the final movement.

Postreduction position: Palmar flexion, ulnar deviation, and pronation.

Immobilization The reduction is maintained by applying plaster slab to the dorsal and radial surfaces cf the wrist, and the plaster extends from the level of metacarpal heads to the elbow – below its crease in front while up to olecranon level posteriorly

After care Elevate the hand in a cuff and collar sling,
Watch the circulation for any impairment, i.e. any swelling of fingers, numbness or severe pain in the fingers
Active exercises of fingers, thumb, elbow, and shoulder
Anti-inflammatory analgesics

Refer: The patient to next fracture clinic.

Removal of cast: After 6–8/52, followed by physiotherapy.

Complications:

i. Malunion
   Management: Physiotherapy. Surgery – rarely indicated
ii. Rupture of extensor pollicis longus
   Management: In elderly – physiotherapy
iii. Sudeck's atrophy:
   S/S: Swelling of fingers, skin of hands – warm and tendered, movements – painful and restricted.
   X-ray – shows osteoporosis.
   Management: Physiotherapy.

Smith's Fracture (syn. Reversed Colles' Fracture)

MOI	Fall on the back of hand.
Diagnosis	Deformity – in the opposite direction to that of Colles' fracture, i.e. lower end of radius is displaced forwards – in front of lower end of radius, and tilted anteriorly (posterior angulation)

Fracture – usually impacted

Investigation	X-ray forearm includes wrist – AP and LAT views
Management	Closed reduction under general anaesthesia
Method	Disimpaction of fragments: Apply traction to the supinated arm
	Dorsiflexion: Maintaining traction to disengage the fractured fragments, the distal fragment is extended gently, followed by direct pressure exerted by right hand on the ventral surface of distal fragment, while in the opposition direction, by left hand on the dorsal surface of the proximal fragment.
Immobilization	The reduction is maintained by applying plaster slab to the dorsal and radial surfaces of the wrist, and the plaster extends from the level of metacarpal heads to above elbow.
After care	Elevate the hand in a cuff and collar sling,
	Watch the circulation for any impairment, i.e. any swelling of fingers, numbness or severe pain in the fingers
	Active exercises of fingers, thumb, elbow, and shoulder
	Anti-inflammatory analgesics.

Refer: The patient to next fracture clinic.

Removal of cast: After 6–8/52, followed by physiotherapy.

Barton's Fracture

Definition	It is a type of Smith's fracture, involving only the anterior part of radius.
Diagnosis	Deformity, pain, swelling, local tenderness, movements of wrist – painful and restricted.
Investigation	X-ray forearm includes wrist – AP and LAT views.
Management	

Conservative treatment

Closed reduction as for Smith's fracture.

Immobilization: As for Smith's fracture.

Surgical treatment: **Refer** the patient to the orthopedic team for surgery.

Surgery	ORIF (screw – cancellous, or buttress plate).
Indication	Failure of closed reduction.

Slipped Radial Epiphysis

Definition	Common in adolescence and in childhood, is the counterpart of Colles' fracture.
MOI	Fall on the outstretched hand or direct violence.
Diagnosis	Deformity: Displacement of distal radial epiphysis along with a small piece of metaphysic (Salter-Harris injury).
Investigation	X-ray wrist – AP and LAT views.
Management	Closed reduction and plaster fixation (same as for Colles' fracture).

Refer: The child to the next fracture clinic.

Fracture of the Radial Styloid

MOI	Fall on the outstretched hand
	Engine (generator, pump, auto) starting handle– backfires.
Diagnosis	Deformity – slight displacement
	Engine (generator, pump, auto) starting handle– backfires.
Diagnosis	Deformity – slight displacement
	Local tenderness
	Movements at wrist – painful and restricted.
Investigation	X-ray wrist – AP and LAT views.

Management

Conservative treatment

Closed reduction and plaster fixation (same as for Colles' fracture).

Surgical treatment: **Refer** the patient to the Orthopedic team for surgery.

Surgery	ORIF (screw – cancellous, or buttress plate).
Indication	Failure of closed reduction.
After care	Physiotherapy.

Scaphoid Fracture

Definition	Commonest bone to be fractured in the wrist.
MOI	Fall on the outstretched hand in an elderly woman
	Engine (generator, pump, auto) starting handle – backfires.
Diagnosis	Pain – outer aspect of wrist
	Fullness of snuff-box
	Local tenderness
	Movements at wrist – painful and restricted.
Investigation	X-ray wrist – AP, LAT, and oblique views
	Certain cases – fractures become visible only after 2–3/52.

Management

Conservative treatment

Every case of sprained wrist – should be suspected as case of fracture scaphoid, even if the X-ray being negative, and should be treated with the wrist in plaster cast (scaphoid cast) and X-ray repeated after 3/52, to confirm diagnosis of scaphoid fracture.

Method	Cock-up plaster cast for 8–10/52:
	Position: Patient keeps the hand – as if holding a glass
	Cast:

- Plaster cast includes metacarpal bone of thumb
- Embraces sides of forearm and wrist – to prevent lateral displacement
- Not to interfere with free movements of fingers.

After care	Physiotherapy.

Surgical treatment: **Refer** the patient to the orthopedic team for surgery.

Surgery	ORIF (cancellous screw fixation).
Indication	Displaced unstable fracture of scaphoid
	Failure of conservative treatment
Complications	
Non-union	Symptomless or wrist pain, difficulty in performing work.
Management	Symptomless – active exercises
	Symptoms (marked):

- Early case: Screw fixation plus bone grafting
- Late case: Excision radial styloid

Sudeck's atrophy: Pain, swelling, local tenderness, painful and restricted movements of fingers and wrist

Management	Analgesics
	Immobilization of wrist – 2–3/52.
After care	Physiotherapy – active exercises.
Osteoarthritis	Pain, swelling, painful and restricted movements of fingers and wrist
Management	Analgesics and physiotherapy.

Dislocation of Lunate

MOI	Fall on the outstretched hand.
Diagnosis	Pain, swelling, local tenderness.
Investigation	X-ray hand includes wrist – AP and LAT views.
Management	Closed reduction under general anesthesia.
Method	Apply traction to the supinated wrist
	Extend the wrist, maintaining traction
	Apply pressure over the lunate – bone reduces (click sound)
	Flex the wrist
	Apply plaster cast with wrist in flexion for 2/52, followed by plaster cast with wrist in neutral position for another 2/52.
After care	Physiotherapy – active exercises.

Bennett's Fracture-dislocation

Definition	It is an intra-articular fracture through the base of first metacarpal. The shaft is dislocated laterally by the unopposed action of the abductor pollicis longus.
MOI	Fall on the outstretched hand or
	Direct violence or
	Forced abduction of thumb.
Diagnosis	Pain, swelling, local tenderness, painful and restricted movements of the thumb.
Investigation	X-ray thumb – AP, LAT, and oblique views.
Management	
Conservative treatment	
	Closed reduction under anesthesia. Reduction is easy but is difficult to maintain.

Method	Apply traction to the thumb, followed by abduction of thumb and then apply pressure over the outer aspect of base of thumb
	Plaster fixation – including MP joint of thumb, for 5–6/52.
After care	Physiotherapy.

Surgical treatment: **Refer** the patient to the orthopedic team for surgery.

Indication	Closed reduction is easy but is difficult to maintain.
Surgery	ORIF – intramedullary or percutaneous Kirschner wires
	Plaster cast (Colles type slab).
After care	Physiotherapy.

Fractures of Metacarpals

MOI	Sports injury, e.g. boxing – knuckles striking face.
	Direct violence.
Diagnosis	Pain, swelling, local tenderness, bone irregularity.
Investigation	X-ray hand – AP and LAT views.
Management	

Conservative treatment

Indication	Undisplaced fractures
Method	Plaster fixation (Colles type slab) for 3–4/52.
After care	Physiotherapy – active exercises.

Surgical treatment: **Refer** the patient to the orthopedic team for surgery.

Indication	Displaced fractures:
Surgery	ORIF – intramedullary (single/multiple) Kirschner wires, Alt:
	– percutaneous Kirschner wires
	Plaster cast (Colles type slab).
After care	Physiotherapy

Fracture Neck of Fifth Metacarpal

MOI	Sports injury – boxing
	Direct violence, e.g. fighting – clenched fist meeting resistance.
Diagnosis	Deformity – angulation
	Pain, local tenderness, movements painful.
Investigation	X-ray hand – AP and LAT views.
Management	

Conservative treatment

| Indication | Angulation – slight/moderate. |
| Method | Closed reduction and plaster slab for 4/52. |

Surgical treatment: **Refer** the patient to the orthopedic team for surgery.

| Indication | Angulation – marked |
| Surgery | ORIF (percutaneous/intramedullary Kirschner wiring). |

Rupture of Ulnar Collateral Ligament (Gamekeeper's Thumb)

| MOI | Forced abduction. |

Diagnosis	Deformity – persistent flexion of terminal phalanx
	Pain, local tenderness, movements of thumb painful and restricted especially grasping.
Investigation	X-ray of thumb – AP and LAT views.
Management	

Conservative treatment

Indication	Incomplete tear or undisplaced avulsion fracture
Method	Plaster fixation (scaphoid type cast) for 6/52.

Surgical treatment: **Refer** the patient to the orthopedic team for surgery.

Indication	Complete tear or rotated fracture
Surgery	Repair of torn ligament and open reduction of fracture
	Plaster fixation (scaphoid type cast) for 6/52.
After care	Physiotherapy – active exercises

Fracture of Phalanges

MOI	Direct violence, e.g. – by a hammer's blow or
	Crush injury – pressed by a door/window-sash.
Diagnosis	Deformity – angulation
	Pain, swelling of finger, local tenderness, bone irregularity, movements – painful and restricted.
Investigation	X-ray hand (focusing affected finger) – AP and LAT views.
Management	Fractures of phalanges are difficult to treat, due to involvement of flexor tendon sheath.

Conservative treatment

A. Fracture of proximal and middle phalanges

Methods	Closed reduction and fixation with:
	Splintage – aluminium splints covered with foam-plastic or rolled bandage held in the palm or
	Plaster slab (volar) for 3/52.

Surgical treatment: **Refer** the patient to the orthopedic team for surgery

Surgery	Intramedullary Kirschner wires.
After care	Physiotherapy – active exercises.

B. Fracture of terminal phalanx

Surgery	Toilet of wound, debridement and suturing, followed by:
	Strapping of finger to adjacent normal finger or
	Splintage – aluminium splints covered with foam-plastic.

Mallet Finger

MOI	Forced flexion of finger from extension position. The extensor tendon tears its attachment to the phalanx (avulsion injury).

Diagnosis   Deformity – persistent flexion of terminal phalanx
                   Loss of extension of terminal phalanx.
Investigation   X-ray hand – AP and LAT views.
Management
Conservative treatment
                   Apply splint in hyperextension (DIP joint) for 5/52.
Surgical treatment: **Refer** the patient to the orthopedic team for surgery.
Surgery   Arthrodesis in extreme cases of failure.

Trigger Finger

Definition   It is a condition affecting the flexor tendons of the finger or thumb.
Etiology   Thickening of flexor tendon/constriction in the tendon sheath
Diagnosis   Difficulty in flexing/extending the affected finger
                   Little force – suddenly releases the finger with a click
                   A nodule – palpated opposite the MP joint of the affected finger.
Investigation   X-ray hand – AP and LAT views.
Management
Surgical treatment: **Refer** the patient to the orthopedic team for surgery.
Surgery   Slitting the fibro-osseous tunnel at the level of the constriction.
Post-care   Active exercises.

Open Hand Injuries

Types   Cuts, lacerations, injection injuries
                   Crush injuries
                   Compound injuries
                   Burns injuries.
MOI   Direct violence, e.g. – by a hammer's blow or
                   Crush injury – pressed by a door/window-sash
                   RSA.
Diagnosis   History of injury
                   • Mode of injury
                   • Time of injury
                   • Any first-aid treatment received
                   • Any food taken and when it was taken
                   Examination.
Investigation   X-ray examination.
Management
Aims   To prevent infection
                   To promote primary healing
                   To salvage injured parts.
Treatment
Drugs   Antibiotics, inj. tetanus toxoid
                   Analgesics.
Surgical treatment: **Refer** the patient to the orthopedic team for surgery:

Anesthesia	General or regional block.
Tourniquet	Required during:

- Toilet of wound
- Examination of wound's depth
- Repair of deep structures

Caution	Tourniquet to be used as briefly, when the viability of skin is questionable.

Shave and prepare: Shave the surrounding uninvolved skin

Toilet of wound: With antiseptic (betadine) solution, followed by saline irrigation

Debridement	Excision of dead skin
Removal	Of foreign material
Bleeders	Clamped
Repair	Tendons: Flexor tendons – primary suturing
	Extensor tendons – primary suturing
	Nerves: Clean wounds – primary suturing
	Crush injury – secondary suturing
	Skin: Clean wounds – primary suturing
	Infected wounds – secondary suturing
	Fractures: Clean wounds – primary procedure
	Infected wounds – late reconstructive surgery
After care	Physiotherapy after 3/52.

Refer: The patient to the orthopedic team for surgery.

References

1. Holdsworth F. Fractures of the radius and ulna. Modern Trends in Orthopaedics. 3:84;1962
2. Furlong R. Injuries of the hand. Boston, Little, Brown, and Co, 1957
3. Riordan, Daniel C. Emergency treatment of compound injury of the hand. Orthopedics 1:30;1957
4. Milford L. Hand surgery. Cambell's Operative Orthopaedics. IGAKU Shoin LTD. Tokyo,1965

Lower Limb Injuries

Fractures of Pelvis and Hip
Fractures of Pelvis

Principles	• Pelvic ring: The pelvic ring is formed by union of two halves of pelvis to the sacrum by the sacroiliac ligaments posteriorly, and by the symphysis pubis anteriorly. This pelvic ring protects the pelvic organs.

- Fractures of pelvic ring at two different levels, lead to marked separation of the ring, while isolated fractures are mostly stable injuries.
- Internal hemorrhage: Blood vessels supplying pelvis (richly supplied), are prone to injury, by the fractures. Hemorrhage is mostly severe, leading to oligemic shock.
- Visceral injury: Fractures of pelvis often cause damage to the male urethra or urinary bladder and rarely to the rectum.

Types of pelvic fractures:
>   i. Fractures of iliac crest
>   ii. Fractures of true pelvis

Fractures of Iliac Crest

Pattern	These are stable fractures, due to support from muscles on the inner side (iliacus) and outer side (glutei).
MOI	Fall from height
	Direct violence.
Diagnosis	Pain, swelling, local tenderness.
Investigation	X-ray pelvis –AP view.
Management	Bed-rest
	Analgesics
	A wide cloth support to the pelvis is sufficient for 2–3/52.

Fractures of True Pelvis

Pattern	Fractures can occur at two levels on the same side or on the opposite side.
MOI	RSA
	Fall from height or fall downstairs.
Diagnosis	Local signs: Bruising over the ileum, groin, or perineum
	Local tenderness
	Bone irregularity.

Signs of visceral complications:
   i. Urethral injury: Blood per urethra, perineal hematoma, distended bladder
  ii. Bladder injury: Suprapubic tumor like mass, strangury, local tenderness
 iii. Rectal and vaginal examinations – helpful in diagnosis.

Investigation	X-ray pelvis – AP view.
	Hemogram, PCV, blood electrolytes,
	BUN, blood sugar, serum proteins,
	Blood grouping and crossmatching.

Management

General or first-aid treatment
>   Treatment of shock (if present):
>   Airways maintenance, oxygen therapy
>   IV fluids, blood transfusion, plasma or plasma expander
>   Inj hydrocortisone IV,
>   Inj ephedrine – if required urgently
>   Inj morphine or pethidine or pentazocine, or tramadol
>   Bed-rest
>   Traction.

Local treatment Closed reduction and traction or
>   Closed reduction and plaster hip spica.

Surgical treatment: **Refer** the patient to the orthopedic team for surgery.

Surgery	ORIF (plating and screws)
Indications	Associated bladder injury
	Early mobilization desirable.
After care	Walking prohibited for 2–3/12.

Fracture of Sacrum

MOI	Direct violence – fight, kicks
	Fall from height
	RSA.
Diagnosis	Swelling, local tenderness, bone irregularity.
Investigation	X-ray sacrum – AP and LAT views.
Management	Symptomatic:

- Bed-rest for 2–3/52
- Analgesics: Paracetamol, NSAIDs, PO or IM
- Local block – Inj. lignocaine 2% infiltration

Fracture of Coccyx

MOI	Direct violence – fight, kicks
	Fall from height
	RSA.
Diagnosis	Pain – while sitting, aggravates on coughing or defecation
	Swelling, local tenderness, bone irregularity.
Investigation	X-ray pelvis focusing coccyx – AP and LAT views.
Management	Symptomatic:

- Bed-rest for 2–3/52
- Analgesics: Paracetamol, NSAIDs, PO or IM
- Local block – inj. lignocaine 2% infiltration

Traumatic Coccydinea

History of direct violence or RSA

No fracture

Pain – usually severe

Local tenderness

Investigation	X-ray pelvis – AP view
Management	

Conservative treatment

Symptomatic treatment, e.g.

Bed-rest, heat, seitz baths, analgesics

Local block – inj. lignocaine 2% infiltration

To sit on an inflated tube.

Surgical treatment: Excision in extreme cases.

Fracture Neck of Femur

Types	Intracapsular and extracapsular.

Intracapsular Fractures of Femoral Neck

Types
: Subcapital and transcervical.
Femoral head ischemia – more common in the subcapital than in transcervical.

MOI
: Indirect violence – missing a step in an elderly patient.
Direct violence – RSA, fall from height in young adults

Pathogenesis
: In elderly, trivial trauma to the osteoporotic bone.
In young adults and children, high velocity trauma to the normal healthy bone.

Diagnosis
: Age: Common in elderly and uncommon in young adults
- An elderly lady (common) unable to bear weight after fall
- Lower limb lies externally rotated (as if paralyzed)
- Shortening of limb
- Elevation of greater trochanter – as confirmed by:

    A. Bryant's triangle: Patient lies supine. Three lines drawn on both sides: One from anterior superior iliac spine, vertically down to the bed, second horizontally from top of greater trochanter to join first line at right angle and third from anterior superior iliac spine to top of greater trochanter.

    Interpretation: Comparative decrease of second line indicates upward elevation of greater trochanter.

    B. Nelaton's line: Patient turned to healthy side. Measuring tape is placed from anterior superior iliac spine to the ischial tuberosity.

    Interpretation: Normally the tape (vide this line) touches the top of greater trochanter, and any upward displacement is demonstrated.
- Loss of function.

Grading
: Garden: Grade I and II – undisplaced fractures
  Grade III and IV – displaced fractures
Pauwels': Based on Pauwels' angle formed by the fracture line with the horizontal plane, e.g.
Type I ($< 30°$)
Type II ($30–50°$)
Type III ($> 50°$).

Complications
: Non-union and avascular necrosis (AVN).

Investigation
: Hemogram, serum electrolytes, serum proteins, BUN.
Blood grouping and crossmatching,
Urine analysis
ECG.

X-ray pelvis – AP view, to study type of fracture and distorted Shenton's line.

X-ray of affected hip – LAT view, to study angulation of head over neck, and fragmentation

CXR – PA view to rule out any pathology

Management   Has evolved significantly.

Conservative treatment

Closed reduction and

Immobilization in POP hip spica in abduction and internal rotation (Whitman abduction plaster)

Complications   Non-union, bedsores, respiratory and CV complications, disuse osteoporosis.

Surgical treatment: **Refer** the patient to the orthopedic team for surgery.

Surgery   Is treatment of choice.

Methods
• Open reduction and internal fixation (ORIF)
• Arthroplasty:
  – Hemiarthroplasty:
    ◊ Unipolar cementless (Austin Moore, Thompson)
    ◊ Bipolar cemented/cementless
  – Total hip replacement (THR):
    ◊ Cemented, hybrid, or cementless
  – Osteotomy and internal fixation (double angle barrel plate)

Open Reduction and Internal Fixation (ORIF)

Indication   Younger patient

Methods
• Cannulated hip screws/cancellous partially threaded screws
• Cannulated screws/cancellous partially threaded screws, with fibular strut graft
• Sliding hip screw (SHS)
• Moore/knowles pins: Choice for children.

Prosthesis Replacement (Medullary/Stem syn. Femoral Endoprosthesis)

Indication   Elderly patient

Method   Excision of the femoral head, and replacement with a Thompson or Austin Moore prosthesis:

After care   Breathing exercises, starting on the same day of operation
Quadriceps, toes, ankle exercises – first day onwards

Follow-up visit   2–3/12. If satisfactory, then next visit after one year and so on for 5 yrs, with periodical check X-rays.

Bipolar Cemented Hemiarthroplasty

Indications   Displaced femoral neck fracture in elderly.

Total Hip Replacement (THR)

Indications
- Inherent complications, e.g. fixation failure, non-union, and AVN
- Elderly: Especially subcapital fracture of femoral neck
- Middle age: ORIF failure, non-union, AVN

Advantages
- Mobilization – early weight bearing
- Postoperative complications – minimal
- Rehabilitation – early rehabilitation

Types   Cemented and uncemented.

Hybrid Total Hip Replacement

Indication   Younger patients
AVN

Osteotomy

Indications   Viable option to aid union in non-union or neglected cases of femoral neck fracture.

Aims   To change the line of weight bearing
To convert shearing force across fracture line into compression force.

Types
- Subtrochanteric displacement osteotomy (McMurray)
- Abduction osteotomy (Pauwel's) using DCP.

Subtrochanteric Displacement Osteotomy (McMurray)

Method
- Osteotomy made just proximal to the lesser trochanter
- Distal figment displaced – beneath the femoral head
- Fixation of osteotomy – with a plate and screws.

Abduction Osteotomy (Pauwel's)

Method
- Osteotomy made at the intertrochanteric level
- Lateral wedge – removed
- Fixation of osteotomy – with an angle blade plate (DCP).

Management of Complications
Non Union

Etiology
- Inadequate immobilization (failure of internal fixation)
- Ischemia of femoral head – due to disruption of blood supply

Management

Head viable   Treatment of choice is:
- Subtrochanteric displacement osteotomy:
  – McMurray – no longer in vogue or
  – Pauwel's valgization osteotomy
- Nailing and bone grafting (Peg graft) in younger patient

Head non-viable Either treatment is:
- Prosthesis or
- Total hip replacement (THR)

Surgical treatment: **Refer** the patient to the orthopedic team for surgery.

Avascular Necrosis (AVN)

Etiology
: In majority of patients, the cause is interruption of blood supply due to rupture of blood vessels by the fracture

Management
: In elderly: THR is the treatment of choice

In younger: – Preventive, e.g. prompt reduction, stable fixation
                  – Osteotomy

Extracapsular Fractures or Trochanteric Fractures

Definition
: Any fracture from the extracapsular part of the femoral neck to a point 5 cm (2 inches) distal to the lesser trochanter.

Types
:
- Intertrochanteric: Fracture line extending from greater trochanter to lesser trochanter, along the intertrochanteric line. Reduction – simple and easily maintained.
- Pertrochanteric (comminuted fractures): Main fracture along the intertrochanteric line along with multiple fractures in the cortex. Reduction is difficult to achieve.
- Subtrochanteric: Fracture of the trochanter extending from lesser trochanter to 5 cm distally, into the femoral shaft. Reduction is difficult to achieve and maintained.

Classification
: Stable: Undisplaced, non-comminuted, intertrochanteric fractures
Unstable:
- Displaced, comminuted, pertrochanteric fractures
- Subtrochanteric fracture extending into femoral shaft
- Reverse oblique fracture
- Trochanteric fracture (comminuted) extending into femoral neck
- Trochanteric wall (lateral) fracture.

Principles
:
- Problem is of survival – as these fractures occur in comparatively older age, and longer period of immobilization.
- Fractures occur in the cancellous bone, therefore chances of early union of fracture are comparatively better due to:
  - Safe blood vessels – hence no chances of avascular necrosis
  - Adequate size of neck and head fragments – good fixation
- Non-union – extremely rare
- Early weight-bearing possible – postinternal fixation
- Early mobilization – postinternal fixation.

MOI
: Indirect violence, i.e. missing a step by an elderly patient
Direct violence.

Diagnosis	An elderly lady
	Lower limb externally rotated
	Shortning of limb
	Local tenderness
	Loss of function.
Investigation	X-ray Hip – AP and lateral views to confirm type of fracture.
Management	

Conservative treatment: If patient is unfit (unwilling) for surgery

| Treatment | Bed-rest, fixed traction (in Thomas splint). |

Surgical treatment: Refer the patient to the orthopedic team for surgery.

Surgery	Internal fixation is treatment of choice.
Methods	• SP nail plate
	• McLaughlin nail plate
	• Sliding compression screws:
	– Dynamic hip screw (DHS)
	– Dynamic condylar screw (DCS) – blade plate (95°)
	• Intramedullary nailing (IMN) with sliding hip screws (SHS)
	– Proximal femoral nail (PFN)
	– Gamma nail
	– Ender nails
	• Arthroplasty (bipolar or total hip replacement)
	• External fixator.
Indications	Stable fracture: DHS – is the gold standard
	Unstable fracture: DHS with modification, or IMN with SHS
	IMN or arthroplasty
	DHS – yields poor results
	DCS – sparingly used in reverse oblique fracture.
	– used in subtrochanteric fracture

Dynamic Hip Screw (DHS)

Indication	Intertrochanteric fracture – stable and unstable (moderate)
Types of DHS	• Long barrel plate: For larger femoral head and neck length
	• Short barrel plate: For shorter femoral head and neck length

Intramedullary Nailing (IMN)

| Advantages | Reduction (closed) easy, short invasive surgery, less blood loss, early mobilization and reduced mechanical (fixation) failure. |
| Disadvantage | Mechanical (fixation) failure, pain in the thigh, stiffness, deformity, nail extrusion. |

Arthroplasty (Bipolar or Total Hip Replacement)

| Indication | Pathological fractures, neglected fractures, fixation failure |
| Advantages | Pain relief, early mobilization, lower revision rates |

Disadvantages Extensive surgery,
                Cemented implants.

External Fixation

Indication   Poor risk patients
Disadvantage   Infection
Alternative   Sliding hip screw (SHS).

Complications of fixation of trochanteric fractures:

Minimal as compared to intracapsular fractures.
- Nail breakage – due to faulty fixation
  Management: Replacement of broken nail
- DHS failure – due to faulty placement in neck and head
  Management: Revision surgery
- Shortening – due to medial shifting of shaft (comminuted fracture)
  Management: Fixation of trochanteric fragment with screw
- Non-union – due to faulty implant/bony failure
  Management:
  – Revision surgery, e.g. removal of implant and fixation in valgus plus bone grafting
  – THR – in elderly patients
- Malunion (varus and external rotation) – due to faulty fixation
  Management: Valgus osteotomy.

Slipped Upper Femoral Epiphysis

Occurs in adolescence

Etiology   Hormonal imbalance – Frohlich syndrome, gigantism
                History of trauma.
Diagnosis   Adolescent, fatty, sexually immature, pain in groin or knee, limp
                Leg – externally rotated
                Movement (internal rotation) – painful and restricted.
Investigation   X-ray hip – AP and LAT views, to confirm slip especially in LAT view
                X-ray normal Hip – AP view, for comparison purpose.
Management   Reduction and pinning
                Osteotomy – for deformed late cases.
Complications   Avascular necrosis:
Prevention   Avoid forced manipulation to correct deformity
Surgical treatment: Osteotomy – indicated in established cases.

Dislocation of Hip

Types

Posterior type Commonest type. The femoral head is displaced on to the dorsum ilii
Anterior type   Very rare type. The femoral head is displaced to the side of the symphysis pubis (pubic type) or under the adductor muscles (obturator type)

Central type	It is a rare type. The femoral head is pushed through the broken acetabulum.
MOI	• RSA (car accident, i.e. dashboard dislocation – force being transmitted up the femoral shaft). • Fall of heavy weight over the back of a stooping person, e.g. mines accidents. • Fall from a height.

Diagnosis

Posterior dislocation

- Attitude: Flexion, adduction and internal rotation
- Shortening of limb
- Loss of resistance in Scarpa's triangle
- Absence of femoral pulse
- Hip rigidity
- Movements of hip – painful and restricted
- X-ray hip – AP view confirms the diagnosis.

Anterior dislocation

- Attitude: Flexion, abduction and external rotation
- Lengthening of limb
- Loss of resistance in Scarpa's triangle
- Absence of femoral pulse
- Hip rigidity
- Movements of hip – painful and restricted
- X-ray hip – AP view confirms the diagnosis.

Central dislocation

- Greater trochanter – moves towards pelvis
- Hip rigidity
- Movements – painful and restricted
- Rectal examination – feel the head moving, on moving thigh
- X-ray pelvis – AP view confirms the diagnosis.

Investigation	X-ray pelvis focusing the dislocated hip – AP view confirms the clinical diagnosis and type of dislocation.

Management

Conservative treatment: Closed reduction is treatment of choice.

Method	Anesthesia: General • Place the patient flat on a mattress on the floor • An assistant steadies the iliac crest • The surgeon flexes the knee and hip at right angles, the femur is lifted vertically up with great force intaining the upward pull, the limb is rotated internally and externally, the femoral head snaps into its socket.
Check X-ray hip	AP view (if reduction achieved without C-arm' use).

| After care | • Fixed traction in a Thomas splint – for 4/52, followed by: Physiotherapy for 2/52 and that being followed by weight bearing. In case of fracture of acetabular rim, weight bearing allowed after 8/52 of injury. |
| | • Bigelow's method: Hip is flexed, abducted, externally rotated, extended and finally kept in neutral position. |

Surgical treatment: **Refer** the patient to the orthopedic team for surgery.

| Surgery | ORIF |
| Indication | For a large fragment of acetabulum |

Complications of Dislocation of Hip

Unreducible Dislocation: Due to interposition of soft tissue (labrum) or bony fragment into the acetabulum

| Management | Closed reduction under general anesthesia with full muscle relaxation. If closed reduction fails, then open reduction is indicated |

Fracture Acetabular Rim: Fracture of posterior lip of acetabulum

| Management | Closed reduction followed by fixed traction in a Thomas splint for 4/52, followed by physiotherapy for 2/52. |
| | Weight bearing after 8–10/52 of injury. |

Surgical treatment: **Refer** the patient to the orthopedic team for surgery.

| Surgery | ORIF |
| Indication | For a large fragment of acetabulum |

Fracture Neck Femur

Management	Surgery is treatment of choice:
	• In elderly patient: Prosthesis (Thompson or Austin Moore)
	• In middle aged: Total hip replacement (THR)
	• In younger patient: ORIF

Slipped Upper Femoral Epiphysis

| Management | **Refer** the patient to the orthopedic team for surgery (ORIF). |

Trochanteric Fracture Hip

| Management | **Refer** the patient to the orthopedic team for surgery (ORIF). |
| Methods | DHS or PFN |

Fracture of Femoral Shaft

| Management | **Refer** the patient to the orthopedic team for surgery (ORIF). |
| Method | Reduction of dislocation hip, followed by ORIF of fractured femoral shaft |

Fracture of Patella

| Management | **Refer** the patient to the orthopedic team for surgery. |
| Method | Reduction of dislocated hip, followed by surgical treatment of fractured patella, i.e. tension wiring or excision, depending upon type of fracture. |

Sciatic Nerve Palsy

Management

Conservative   Majority of patients with sciatic nerve palsy are best treated by conservative measures, i.e. use of foot drop splint, and physiotherapy

Surgical treatment: **Refer** the patient to the orthopedic team for surgery.

Method   Exploration of nerve, indicated rarely.

Avascular Necrosis of Femoral Head

Management   **Refer** the patient to the orthopedic team for surgery.

Method   Total hip replacement (THR)

Osteoarthritis Hip

Etiology   Avascular necrosis of femoral head

Intracapsular fracture neck of femur

Management   **Refer** the patient to the orthopedic team for surgery.

Method   Total hip replacement (THR)

Old Unreduced Dislocation of Hip

Management

Conservative   Closed reduction (manipulation) within a week or

Skeletal traction for 3–4/52.

Surgical treatment: **Refer** the patient to the orthopedic team for surgery.

Method   Open reduction – if conservative treatment fails

Osteotomy – after 1/12.

References

1. Addison J. Prosthetic replacement in the primary treatment of fracture of femoral neck. Proc R Soc. Med 52:908;1959.
2. Charnley J. The treatment of fractures of the neck of the femur by compression. Acta Orthop. Scand 30:29;1961. Blocky NJ and Purser DW. The treatment of Displaced fractures of the neck of the femur by compression. A Preliminary report. J Bone and Jt Surg 39B:45;1957.
3. Charnley J. Total hip replacement by low friction arthroplasty. Clin Orthop 72:7–21;1970.
4. Eftekhar NS. Principles of total hip replacement. St. Louis Mosby, 1978.
5. Oh I, Harris WH. A cement fixation system for total hip arthroplasty clin orthop 164:221–229;1982.
6. Claffey TJ. Avascular Necrosis of the Femoral Head. An Anatomical Study. J Bone Jt Surg 42B: 802;1960.
7. Coleman SS, Compere CL. Femoral neck fractures, pathogenesis of avascular necrosis, Non-union, and Late Degenerative Changes. J Bone Jt Surg 39A:1419;1957.
8. Crawford HB. Conservative treatment of impacted fracture of the femoral neck. A report of fifty cases. J Bone Jt Surg 42A:471;1960.
9. Garden RS. Low-angle fixation in fractures of the femoral neck. J Bone Jt Surg 43B:647;1961.
10. Phemister DB. The recognition of dead bone based on pathological and X-ray studies. Ann Surg 72, 466 (1949) Treatment of Necrotic Head of Femur in Adults. J Bone Jt Surg 31A:55;1920.
11. Trueta J. The normal vascular anatomy of the human femoral head during growth. J Bone Jt Surg 35B:442;1957.
12. Kulkarni GS, et al. Intertrochanteric fractures. Indian Journal of Orthopaedics Vol 40:1;2006.

13. Marya SKS, et al. Failed fixation; Trochanteric Fracture: Revision hip arthroplasty. Indian Journal of Orthopaedics Vol 8:3;2004.

14. McRae Ronald. Practical fracture treatment. Churchil Livingstone, 1984

15. Crenshaw AH. Campbell's Operative Orthopaedics Vol 1. CV Mosby Co. Tokyo, 1965.

16. Rains AJH, et al: Bailey and Love's short practice of surgery 13th ed. H.K. Lewis and Co. Ltd., London, 1965.

17. Babhulkar SS. Management of trochanteric fractures. Indian Journal of Orthopaedics Vol. 40 No. 4:210–17;2006.

18. Sandhu HS, et al: Femoral neck fractures. Indian Journal of orthopedics Vol. 42 No.1:1–2;2008.

19. Thuan V Ly, Swiontkowski MF. Management of femoral neck fractures in young adults. Indian Journal of Orthopaedics. Vol. 42 No. 1:3–12;2008.

20. Singh MP, et al. Femoral neck fractures in young adults: Osteosynthesis and primary valgus osteotomy using broad DCP. Indian Journal of Orthopaedics. Vol. 42 No. 1:43–48;2008.

21. Marya SKS, et al. Prosthetic replacement in femoral neck fracture in the elderly: Results and review of the literature. Indian Journal of Orthopaedics. Vol. 42 No. 1:61–67;2008.

22. Gupta DK, Agarwal P. Fibular osteosynthesis in neglected femoral neck fractures. Indian Journal of Orthopaedics. Vol.40 No. 2, 97–99;2006.

23. Kulkarni GS, et al. Intertrochanteric fractures. Indian Journal of Orthopaedics. Vol. 40 No.1, 16–23;2006.

24. Singh AK, et al. Management of trochanteric fractures. Indian Journal of Orthopaedics. Vol.40 No. 2, 100–102;2006.

25. Halder SC. The gamma nail for peritrochanteric fractures. J Bone Joint Surg Br, 74: 340–4;1992.

Fractures of Femur and Injuries about Knee

1. Fractures of femoral shaft
2. Fractures of upper 3rd of femur
3. Supracondylar fracture of femur
4. Femoral condylar fractures
5. Fractures of patella
6. Dislocation of knee
7. Internal derangements of knee (IDK)
   i. Injury to collateral ligaments – commonly medial
   ii. Injury to neniscus or cartilage – commonly medial
   iii. Injury to cruciate ligaments
   iv. Injury to infrapatellar pad of fat
   v. Fracture of tibial spine
   vi. Loose bodies.

Fractures of Femoral Shaft

Sites	Fractures of upper 3rd
	Fractures of middle 3rd
	Fractures of distal 3rd
MOI	Fall from height
	RSA
	Crush injuries.

Diagnosis   Deformity:

In fractures of proximal 3rd:

Proximal fragment – flexed by iliopsoas, abducted by glutei, everted by external rotators.

Distal fragment – adducted by adductors, upwards by hamstrings and quadriceps, everted by weight of limb

In fractures of middle and distal 3rd: Backward angulation, shortening by quadriceps and hamstrings

Local tenderness

Unnatural mobility

Loss of function.

Investigation   X-ray thigh including knee and hip – AP and LAT views

Hemogram, serum electrolytes, proteins, blood urea,

Blood grouping and crossmatching.

Management

Aims of treatment: Three main aims:

- Restoration of alignment – is essential as malalignment results in undue strain upon the knee joint, and later on development of osteoarthritis
- Restoration of length – by prevention and correction of shortening due to contraction of powerful muscles of thigh
- Prevention of knee stiffness – by prevention and correction of the adhesions of soft tissues especially the extensor mechanism.

Conservative treatment: Traction, and hip spica

Traction and countertraction: To prevent and correct shortening.

Traction   It is applied to the distal fragment and countertraction and is applied to the proximal fragment, to prevent the trunk and pelvis following the traction force and to prevent the recurrence of shortening.

Methods of applying traction and countertraction:

Fixed traction   Traction is applied by tying the cords to the foot end of the Thomas splint, which is passed over the limb, so that padded ring of splint rests against the ischial tuberosity, which provides countertraction.

Types of traction

Skin traction   Indicated in children and younger patients, using adhesive plaster (traction sets include adhesive tapes, traction cords, spreader bar).

Skeletal traction   Indicated in older patients and where heavy traction is required, using a Steinmann pin.

Gallows traction   Indicated in children below the age of 5 years, using strapping, and the legs are hung up by overhead pulley, so that buttocks are lifted up from the bed. The child's weight acts as countertraction.

Continuous traction (syn. balanced traction): More comfortable and precise method.

It is attached to the limb by skin or skeletal traction, which is applied to the pulleys of Bohler Brawn splint.

Hip spica	Indicated in a fretful child, and in a compound fracture.
Method	Hip spica to include – from nipple line to the injured leg – up to toes and normal leg – above knee.

Surgical treatment: **Refer** the patient to the orthopedic team for surgery.

Indications	• Failure of closed reduction
	• Multiple fractures
	• Early mobilization required.
Methods	• Intramedullary nailing
	• Intertlocking nailing under C-arm
	• Interlocking nailing (open) without C-arm
	• Plating and screws.

Intramedullary Nailing (IMN)

Advantages	Reduction (closed) easy, short invasive surgery, less blood loss, early mobilization and reduced mechanical (fixation) failure.
Disadvantage	Mechanical (fixation) failure, pain in the thigh, stiffness, deformity, nail extrusion.

Refer: The patient to the orthopedic team for surgery.

Management of Special Situations
Fractures of Femur and Tibia in the Same Leg

Management	Conservative treatment: Closed reduction of tibial fracture and below knee plaster cast, incorporating a Steinmann pin (skeletal traction) through tibial tubercle, using Thomas splint, for reduction and immobilization of femoral fracture.

Surgical treatment: Refer the patient to the orthopedic team for surgery.

Surgery	Intramedullary nailing of femur and plating of tibia.

Pathological Fracture

Management	Refer the patient to the orthopedic team for surgery.
Surgery	Intramedullary nailing and bone grafting.

Vascular Injury

Management	Refer the patient to the orthopedic team for surgery.
Surgery	Intramedullary nailing of femur followed by vessel repair.

Nerve Injury

Management	Majority of nerve lesions are in continuity and are recoverable. In case of compound fractures, where nerve division is suspected, treatment required is nerve exploration and internal fixation of femoral fracture.

Fractures of Femoral Neck and Shaft

Management　Refer the patient to the orthopedic team for surgery.

Surgery　Proximal femoral nailing (PFN) is the treatment of choice.

Fracture of Femoral Shaft and Dislocation of Hip

Management　Refer the patient to the orthopedic team for surgery

Surgery　Reduction of dislocated hip, followed by internal fixation of femur.

Fracture of Upper Third

Management　Refer the patient to the orthopedic team for surgery.

Surgery　Intramedullary nailing and traction in a Thomas splint.

Complications of Fractures of Femur

   i. Shock (oligemic) – described in General Section

  ii. Embolism (fat) – described in section

     Management: Heparin (IV), oxygen, IV fluids, monitoring vital signs

 iii. Delayed union:

     Management: Prolonged immobilization

 iv. Non-union:

     Management: Refer the patient to the orthopedic team for surgery.

     Surgery: Intramedullary nailing and bone grafting.

   v. Malunion

     Management: Refer the patient to the orthopedic team for surgery.

     Surgery: Corrective osteotomy/osteoclasis.

 vi. Knee stiffness

     Cause:

- Quadriceps tethering – leading to adherence to fracture site
- Intra-articular fractures – leading to adhesions formation or formation of a mechanical block
- Prolonged immobilization – especially in delayed union

     Management: Physiotherapy – active exercises, SWD/IR

 vii. Shortening:

     Management: Up to 2.5 cm (1") – corrected by shoe modification

                       > 2.5 cm (1") – corrected by surgery, i.e. osteotomy

Refer: The patient to the orthopedic team for surgery.

Supracondylar Fracture of Femur

MOI　　　　　RSA

　　　　　　　Direct violence.

Diagnosis　　Deformity – angulation

　　　　　　　Swelling

　　　　　　　Local tenderness

Movements – painful and restricted

Shortening.

Investigation   X-ray thigh including knee – AP and LAT views.

Management

In children   Minimal displacement in majority of cases.

Conservative treatment

Closed reduction and a cylinder plaster, walking with crutches, weight bearing after formation of callus.

In adults   Distal fragment is angulated posteriorly by pull of gastrocnemius.

Conservative treatment

Traction to the limb with knee in flexion by bending the Thomas splint at the fracture level.

After care   Active exercises of the knee.

Surgical treatment: **Refer** the patient to the orthopedic team for surgery.

Surgery   ORIF:

Implant: Distal femoral nail (DFN), blade plate, or nail plate.

DFN   It is available in diameters of 9 mm (solid) and 10, 11 mm (cannulated) and in long and short version, with distal locking options. DFN short has 2 ML holes for proximal locking while the DFN long has 2 AP and 1 ML proximal locking holes.

Femoral Condylar Fractures

Patterns of fracture:

    i. Unicondylar fracture without displacement

    ii. Unicondylar fracture with displacement

    iii. T or Y shaped intercondylar fracture

    iv. Comminuted fracture

    v. Intra-articular condylar fracture.

MOI   Direct violence.

Diagnosis   Swelling, deformity, local tenderness,

Movements of knee – painful and restricted.

Investigation   X-ray knee – AP and LAT views.

Management

Unicondylar Fracture without Displacement

Conservative treatment: Traction for 4–6/52, followed by physiotherapy.

Unicondylar Fracture with Displacement

Surgical treatment: **Refer** the patient to the orthopedic team for surgery.

Surgery   Dynamic compression plate (DCP/DCS).

T or Y Shaped Intercondylar Fracture
Conservative treatment: Traction and manipulation
Surgical treatment: **Refer** the patient to the orthopedic team for surgery.
Surgery: ORIF – DCP/DCS.

Comminuted Fracture
Conservative and surgical treatment – both have reservations.

Intra-articular Condylar Fracture
MOI	Compression forces, i.e. femoral condyle is sheared off by tibia.
Diagnosis	Swelling, local tenderness
	Movements of knee – painful and restricted.
Investigation	X-ray knee – AP and LAT views.
Management	Being an intra-articular fracture, the fracture sometimes fail to unite, due to dilution of fracture hematoma by the synovial fluid.

Surgical treatment: **Refer** the patient to the orthopedic team for surgery.
Surgery	ORIF – reduction and fixation with cancellous screws and a cylinder plaster.
After care	Weight bearing allowed after 6/52
	Till then non-weight bearing walking in crutches.

Fractures of Lateral Tibial Condyle (Bumper Fracture)
MOI	RSA – an abduction strain, forces the leg into valgus.
Pattern	

  i. Vertical splitting of lateral tibial condyle caused by lateral femoral condyle, driven down into the tibial head.
  ii. Depressed lateral tibial condyle along with fracture of neck of fibula. It is the commonest condylar fracture.
  iii. Comminuted fracture of lateral tibial plateau.

Diagnosis	Swelling, local tenderness, movements of knee – painful and restricted.
Investigation	X-ray knee – AP and LAT views.
Management	
Conservative treatment	Closed reduction and immobilization in a plaster cylinder for 4–6/52, followed by physiotherapy

Surgical treatment: **Refer** the patient to the orthopedic team for surgery.
Surgery	ORIF (screw/screws, horizontally placed studding with nut bolts)
Indication	Displaced fracture.

Fracture of Medial Tibial Condyle   It is a rare injury.
MOI	RSA – an adduction strain, forces the leg into varus.
Diagnosis	Swelling, local tenderness,
	Movements of knee – painful and restricted.
Investigation	X-ray knee – AP and LAT views.

Management

Conservative   Closed reduction and immobilization in a plaster cylinder for 4–6/52,
treatment   followed by physiotherapy.

Fractures of Patella

Fracture of the patella is the commonest fracture around the knee.

Pattern of fractures

- Vertical fracture
- Transverse fracture
- Comminuted (stellate) fracture
- Avulsion fracture of upper pole
- Avulsion fracture of lower pole.

MOI   Direct violence

               Indirect violence, i.e. by a violent contraction of the quadriceps.

Diagnosis

Vertical fracture: Swelling, local tenderness, movements painful and restricted.

Transverse fracture: Swelling, local tenderness, gaping between two fragments, movements
– painful and restricted.

Comminuted fracture

               Mostly a compound fracture, articular surface of patella is damaged beyond
               repair, patella appears broader, and fragmented with grating on movement,
               swelling, local tenderness, and the movements of knee – painful and restricted.

               Avulsion fracture of upper pole: A distinct gap between the tendon and
               the patella.

               Avulsion fracture of lower pole: A distinct gap between the ligament and
               its bony attachment.

Investigation X-ray knee – AP and LAT views.

Management   Conservative and surgical treatment.

Vertical Fracture

               Splintage of leg in full extension

               Internal fixation – if articular surface is irregular.

Transverse Fracture: ORIF of fracture patella and repair of torn quadriceps

Methods of repair

- Tension band wiring
- Figure of 8 wiring
- Vertical screw/screws

Comminuted Fracture: Partial patellectomy and repair of torn quadriceps

Avulsion fracture: Surgical repair.

Refer: The patient to the orthopedic team for surgery.

After care   Physiotherapy – active exercises, SWD, or IRD.

Dislocation of Knee

MOI	RSA
	Sports injury.
Diagnosis	Deformity
	Swelling, local tenderness
	Movements of knee – painful and restricted.
Investigation	X-ray knee – AP and LAT views.
Management	
Conservative treatment	Closed reduction under general anesthesia, followed by traction for 3/52, followed by 3/52 in a plaster cylinder.

Surgical treatment: **Refer** the patient to the orthopedic team for surgery.

Surgery: Open reduction – if closed reduction fails

After care: Physiotherapy – active exercises, SWD/IRD.

Internal Derangements of Knee (IDK)

Definition	IDK includes following:

- Injury to collateral ligaments – commonly medial
- Injury to meniscus or cartilage – commonly medial
- Injury to cruciate ligaments
- Injury to infrapatellar pad of fat
- Fracture of tibial spine
- Loose bodies.

Injury of Collateral Ligaments

MOI	Traumatic – forced abduction to the extended leg.
	RSA
	Sports injury – especially common in footballers.
Mechanism of Injury	Medial one – commonly injured: Usually associated with injury to the medial meniscus, due to attachment of its deeper fibers to meniscus. With further continued strain, the cruciate ligament especially the anterior one may rupture.
Diagnosis	Pain, tenderness over bony attachments of the ligament, movements of knee (esp. abduction) – painful and restricted.
Investigation	X-ray knee – AP and LAT views, to rule out any bony lesion
	MRI
	Arthroscopy (endoscopy) – diagnostic
Management	
Conservative	Analgesics,
	SWD/IRD, local massage
	Elastic crepe bandage/knee cap/brace
	Plaster cylinder with knee flexed at 20°
	Bed-rest for 2/52.

Surgical	**Refer** the patient to the orthopedic team for surgery.
Surgery	Repair of collateral ligament
	Meniscectomy
	Repair of anterior cruciate ligament (ACL).

Injury of Medial Meniscus

MOI	Traumatic – RSA
	Sports injury – especially common in footballers.
Mechanism of injury	The flexed knee is subjected to rotational and abduction strains. The knee momentarily opens upon the medial side, the meniscus is sucked inside and gets nipped between the condyles of femur and tibia, resulting in a tear. Repeated strains lead to a 'Bucket handle' tear.
Diagnosis	Common in footballers and mine workers
	Pain, tenderness over joint line – midway between patellar and medial collateral ligaments, history of locking of knee, followed by sudden unlocking and effusion
	Local tenderness
	McMurray's test – positive.
Investigation	X-ray knee – AP and LAT views, to rule out any bony lesion
	MRI
	Arthroscopy (endoscopy) – diagnostic
Management	
Conservative	Analgesics
	Elastic crepe bandage/knee cap/brace
	SWD/IRD, local massage
	Plaster cylinder with knee flexed at 20°
	Bed-rest for 2/52.
Surgical	**Refer** the patient to the orthopedic team for surgery.
Surgery	Meniscectomy – in confirmed cases
Method	Endoscopic or open surgery

Injury to Lateral Meniscus

It is a rare injury.

MOI	Sports injury.
Management	Analgesics,
	SWD/or IRD,
	Knee cap.

Cysts of Lateral Meniscus

Diagnosis	Pain on the lateral side of knee
	A round hard swelling over lateral side of knee.
Management	**Refer** the patient to the orthopedic team for surgery.
Surgical	Excision of cyst.

Injury to Cruciate Ligaments
Anterior Cruciate Ligament (ACL) Injury

MOI	Direct violence.
	Traumatic – RSA, sports injury, fall from height.
Pathogenesis	Isolated tears are uncommon, and usually associated with tears of medial collateral ligament and/medial meniscus.
Diagnosis	Anterior cruciate ligament (ACL) – commonly injured
	Pain, swelling, tenderness,
	Movements: Abnormal forward/backward movements of tibia over femur
	Knee can be hyperextended.
Investigation	X-ray knee – AP and LAT views, for any bony lesion
	MRI.
	Arthroscopy (endoscopy) – diagnostic
Management	
Conservative	Analgesics
	Elastic crepe bandage/knee cap
	Plaster cylinder with knee flexed at 20°, for 6/52 – if anterior tibial spine is intact.
	Bed-rest for 2/52.
After care	Physiotherapy.
Surgical	**Refer** the patient to the orthopedic team for surgery.
Surgery	• ORIF (screw fixation) – if anterior tibial spine is fractured.
	• Re-attach/ACL replacement (tendon of semitendinosus) is the treatment of choice – if ACL is avulsed.
	• Repair of associated tears of medial collateral ligament and media meniscus.

Posterior Cruciate Ligament (PCL) Injury

MOI	Direct violence.
Pathogenesis	Tibia is forced backwards.
Diagnosis	Abnormal backward movement of tibia over femur.
Investigation	X-ray knee – AP and LAT views, for any bony lesion
	MRI
	Arthroscopy (endoscopy) – diagnostic
Management	Same as for ACL injury.

Injury to Infrapatellar Pad of Fat

MOI	Traumatic – when hypertrophied, may be nipped in between the femur and tibia during extension of the knee.
Diagnosis	History of pain and locking of knee without being followed by sudden unlocking (cf. medial meniscus injury).
	Local tenderness over sides of ligamentum patellae.

Investigation   X-ray knee – AP and LAT views, for any bony lesion
                  Arthroscopy (endoscopy) – diagnostic
Management   **Refer** the patient to the orthopedic team for surgery
Surgery   Excision of hypertrophied fat – by endoscopic surgery

Fracture of Tibial Spine

It is a rare injury, mostly found in children.

MOI   Traumatic – RSA, sports injury.
Mechanism   Fall on the bent knee with a violent twist of tibia over the femur
Diagnosis   Pain, swelling, tenderness, restricted extension of knee.
Investigation   X-ray knee – AP and lateral views.
Management
Conservative
Indication   Undisplaced fracture
Treatment   Aspiration of knee
                 Elastic crepe bandage/knee cap/brace, or
                 Plaster cylinder
                 Bed-rest for 2/52

Surgical treatment: **Refer** the patient to the orthopedic team for surgery.

Indication   Displaced fracture
Surgery   ORIF of fragment with a screw, or
                 Excision of fragment.

Loose Bodies

MOI   Direct violence
Diagnosis   History of locking at different angles each time
Investigation   X-ray knee – AP and LAT views
                 Arthroscopy (endoscopy) – diagnostic
Management
Surgery   Sugical removal – by endoscopic or by open surgery.

Refer: The patient to the orthopedic team for surgery.

References

1. Attenberg AR, Shorkey RL. Blade-plate Fixation in Non-union and in Complicated Fractures of the Supracondylar Region of the Femur. J Bone Jt Surg 31A:312;1949.
2. Apley AG. Fracture of the Lateral Tibial Condyle Treated by Skeletal Traction and Early Mobilisation. J Bone Jt Surg 38B,699;1956.
3. Bradford CH, et al. Fracture of the Lateral Tibial Condyle. J Bone Jt Surg 32A,39;1950.
4. Campbell Operative Orthopaedics. 9th Ed. Vol I-IV. S. Terry Canale, Kay Daugherty, and Linda Jones. Mosby, 1998.
5. Charnley JC, Baker SL. Compression Arthrodesis of the Knee. A Clinical and Histological Study. J Bone Jt Surg 34B:187;1952.
6. Duthie HL, and Hutchinson JR. The Results of Partial and Total Excision of the Patella. J Bone Jt Surg 40B:75;1958.

7. Hohl M, and Luck JV. Fractures of the Tibial Condyle. J Bone Jt Surg 38A:1001;1956.
8. Jackson JP, and Waugh WL. Tibial Osteotomy for Osteoarthritis of the Knee. J Bone Jt Surg 43B: 114;1961.
9. Krettek C, Manss J, Konemann B, et al. Deformation of Femoral Nails with Intramedullary insertion. J Orthop. Res 16(5):572–5;1998.
10. Krettek C., Konemann B., Miclau T., et al. A New Technique for the Distal Locking of Solid AO Unreamed Tibial Nails. J Orthop Trauma 11 (16):446–51;1997.
11. Meyers MH., and McKeever FM. Fracture of the Intercondylar Eminence of the Tibia. J Bone Jt Surg 41A:209;1959.
12. O Donoghue DH. Surgical Treatment of Fresh Injuries to the Major Ligaments of the Knee. J Bone Jt Surg 32, 725 - (1955) An Analysis of End-results of Surgical Treatment of Major Injuries to Ligaments of the Knee. J Bone Jt Surg 37A:1;1950.
13. Palmar I. Fracture of the Upper end of the Tibia. J Bone Jt Surg 33B:160;1951.
14. Shorbe HB, Dobson CH. Patellectomy (Repair of Extensor Mechanism) J Bone Jt Surg 40A:1281;1958.
15. Smillie IS. Injuries of the Knee Joint. Edinburgh ; Livingstone, 1951.
16. Wilson EF. Repair of Cruciate Ligaments. J Bone Jt Surg 43B:342;1961.
17. Bohler L, Bohler J. Kuntscher's Medullary Nailing. J Bone Jt Surg 31A:295;1949.
18. Dehne E., Immermann EW Dislocation of Hip Combined with Fracture of Shaft of Femur on same side. J Bone Jt Surg 33A:731;1951.
19. Slee GC. Fractures of Tibial Condyles. J Bone Jt Surg 37B:427;1955.
20. Locking Compression Plate – LCP – A New AO Principle; Injury Volume 34, Supplement 2, November, 20–30;2003.
21. Shetty MS, Kumar A, Kanthi KG: Locking Compression Plate – LCP – A Boon in Traumatology.
22. Kulkarni GS, et al. Intertrochanteric fractures. Indian Journal of Orthopaedics. Vol. 40 No.1, 16–23;2006.
23. Singh R, et al. Titanium elastic nailing in pediatric femoral diaphyseal fractures. Indian Journal of Orthopaedics. Vol. 40 No.1:29–34;2006.
24. Shekhar L, Mayanger JC. A clinical study of Ender nails fixation in femoral shaft fractures in children. Indian Journal of Orthopaedics. Vol. 40 No.1:16–23;2006.
25. Kapoor SK, et al. Expandable self-locking nail in the management of closed diaphyseal fractures of femur and tibia. Indian Journal of Orthopaedics. Vol. 43 No.3:264–270;2009.
25. Kapoor SK, et al. Expandable self-locking nail in the management of closed diaphyseal fractures of femur and tibia. Indian Journal of Orthopaedics. Vol. 43 No.3:264–270;2009.

Fractures of Tibia and Fibula

1. Fractures in children
2. Fractures in adults
3. Compound fractures
4. Fracture both bones of leg

Principles

Mechanisms of tibial injury

- Prone to torsional forces, causing oblique and spiral fractures.
- Prone to infection, as one-third of tibia is subcutaneous.
- Prone to Volkmann ischemic contracture due to injury to the popliteal artery in fractures of upper one-third.

- Prone to develop osteoarthritis of ankle and knee, as a result of angulation deformity commonly seen in fractures of both bones.
- Prone to delayed/non-union, as a result of poor blood supply, especially of distal one-third.

Fractures in Children
Greenstick Fractures

MOI   RSA, falls from a height and direct violence.
Diagnosis   Swelling, local tenderness, resents moving leg
Investigation   X-ray leg including ankle and knee – AP and LAT views
Management
Conservative treatment
                   Plaster cast – from groin to toes, with knee slightly flexed, for 4/52
After care   Apply elastic crepe bandage for 1/52 after removal of plaster cast.

Displaced Fractures of Tibia

Management   Closed reduction
Method   Traction, manipulation, and plaster cast above knee for 6/52.
After care   Same as for greenstick fractures.

Fractures in Adults

MOI   RSA, sports injuries, direct violence.
Diagnosis   Swelling, local tenderness, bone irregularity.
Investigation   X-ray leg including ankle and knee – AP and LAT views.
Management
Conservative treatment: Closed reduction
Method   Traction, manipulation and plaster cast from groin to toes for 8–10/52
After care   Check X-ray, and if fracture united, then partial weight bearing with the help of crutches for 2/52, followed by full weight bearing.

Surgical treatment: **Refer** the patient to the orthopedic team for surgery.
Indications
- Displaced fractures
- Open tibial diaphyseal fractures
- Unstable closed fractures
- Comminuted fractures of tibia with small medullary canals.

Methods
- Intramedullary nailing:
  - Universal tibial nail (UTN) and TEN.
- Plating and screws – dynamic compression plate (DCP)

Universal Tibial Nail (UTN)

Indications
- Open tibial diaphyseal fractures
- Unstable closed fractures
- Comminuted fractures of tibia with small medullary canals.

Features
- 9° proximal bend for easy insertion
- Proximal locking holes (1 dynamic and 1 static ML holes)
- Distal locking holes (2 ML and 1 AP hole)

Titanium Elastic Nail (TEN)

Indications   Diaphyseal fractures of long bones with narrow medullary canal, i.e. lower limb in pediatric patients and in small-stature patients.

Features
- Available in 2 to 4 mm diameters (color-coded)
- Tip of nail is curved for easy insertion.

Compound Fractures

Management
- Debridement and toilet of wound
- Stable fracture: Apply a plaster cast above knee
- Unstable fracture and wound clean: ORIF
- Unstable fracture and infective wound: External fixator application (allows free dressings).

Fractures Both Bones of Leg

MOI   RSA
Fall from height
Direct violence

Diagnosis   Deformity – angulation and rotation, loss of function.

Investigation   X-ray leg includes ankle and knee – AP and LAT views.

Management

Conservative treatment: Closed reduction and plaster cast above knee.

Surgical treatment: **Refer** the patient to the orthopedic team for the surgical treatment of displaced fractures.

Surgery
- Intramedullary nailing
- Intramedullary interlocking nailing under C-arm, is treatment of choice
- If fracture can be reduced easily without exposing the fracture site
- Intramedullary interlocking (open) nailing without C-arm or X-ray
- Plating and screws – Dynamic compression plate (DCP)

After care   Weight bearing in plaster for 4–6/52.

Ununited Tibial Shaft Fracture

Etiology   An intact fibula associated with a tibial shaft fracture, increases the incidence of delayed union.

Diagnosis   Pain, swelling, local tenderness at the fracture site (>20/52 period)
X-rays: Showing delayed union/non-union

Management   Fibulectomy (partial).

References

1. Rahman MM, Taha WS, Shaheen MM. A simple technique for distal locking of tibial nails. Injury 29(10)789–90;1998

2. Krettek C, Konemann B, Miclau T, et al. A New Technique for Distal locking of Solid AO Unreamed Tibial Nails, 1997

3. Moore JR. The Closed Fracture of the Long Bones. J Bone Jt Surg 42A:869;1960

4. Nicoll EA. The Treatment of gaps in Long Bones by Cancellous Insert Grafts. J Bone Jt Surg 38B:70;1956. Personal communication (1960)

5. Butt MF, et al. Partial resection of fibula in treatment of ununited tibial shaft fractures. Indian Journal of Orthopaedics Vol 40 No.4 247–49;2006

Ankle

Anatomy	• Ankle joint resembles a mortise, e.g. tenon joint of a carpenter. The tenon is talus, whereas the mortise is formed by inferior articular surface of tibia and medial and lateral malleoli.
	• The lateral malleolus of fibula is firmly attached to the tibia by anterior and posterior tibiofibular ligaments.
	• The ankle is firmly supported by the deltoid ligament on medial side and lateral ligament on the lateral side.
	• Ankle joint transmits more weight than any other body joint. It is therefore a very stable joint, with limited mobility.
Movements	
At ankle	Flexion (plantar flexion)
	Extension (dorsiflexion)
At subtalar	Inversion
	Eversion
At mid-tarsal	Abduction
	Adduction of forefoot.

Injuries about the Ankle

1. Pott's fracture
2. Ankle dislocation
3. Ankle sprain

Pott's Fracture

Definition	It is a fracture-dislocation of the ankle joint and requires accurate reduction and fixation.
MOI	RSA
	Direct or indirect violence. Various patterns of Pott's fracture occur as a result of different types of violence.
Mechanisms	Various patterns of Pott's fracture occur as a result of different types of violence. As per classification of Lauge-Hansen:
	• Supination/external rotation
	• Supination/adduction
	• Pronation/external rotation
	• Pronation/abduction
	• Pronation/dorsiflexion.

Types	1st degree: Fracture of one malleolus
	2nd degree: Bimalleolar fracture
	3rd degree: Bimalleolar fracture + fracture of the 3rd malleolus, i.e. posterior part of the inferior articular surface of tibia.
Diagnosis	Pain, difficulty in walking, swelling, local tenderness
	Deformity,
	Movements of ankle – painful and restricted.
Investigation	X-ray ankle – AP and LAT views.
Management	
Aims	• To restore the normal ankle mortice
	• To restore the weight bearing alignment of the ankle, i.e. ankle should be at a right angle to the long axis of the leg
	• To restore the contours of the articular surfaces.

Conservative treatment

Type I (1st degree): Heat – SWD or IRD, ellastic crepe bandage, or adhesive plaster, analgesics, rest.

Type II (2nd degree): Below knee plaster cast for 4–6/52.

Type III (3rd degree): Manipulation of ankle, followed by plaster cast for 4–6/52.

Surgical treatment: **Refer** the patient to the orthopedic team for surgery.

Indications: Failure of conservative treatment, to achieve the above said aims especially in the following:

- Fracture medial malleolus – displaced
- Bimalleolar fractures
- Trimalleolar (Cotton) fractures

Surgery	ORIF
Methods	Screw – Long self-tapping (Sherman)
	– Cancellous screw
	– Lag screw with washer
	Plate (Zuelzer) and screws

Ankle Dislocation

Ankle dislocation without fracture is very rare.

MOI	RSA
	Sports injury
	Fall from height
Diagnosis	Pain, swelling, local tenderness, deformity, movements at the ankle – painful and restricted.
Investigation	X-ray ankle – AP and lateral views.
Management	Closed reduction under anesthesia, followed by POP cast.
After care	Check X-ray

Refer: The patient to the orthopedic team.

Foot Injuries

Include

1. Fractures of talus
2. Fractures of calcaneus
3. Rupture of Tendo-Achilles
4. Fracture of fifth metatarsal
5. Fractures of metatarsals
6. Dislocation of phalanges
7. Dislocation of toes
8. Crush injuries of the foot.

Fractures of Talus
Fracture of the Neck of Talus

Fracture neck of talus is the commonest amongst fractures of the talus.

MOI	RSA, sports injuries, fall from a height.
Mechanism	Fracture of neck of talus occurs as a result of dorsiflexion and upward force resulting in shearing of talar neck by the sharp anterior articular surface of the tibia. The continuing dorsiflexion force results in four types of injuries, e.g.
Type I	Undesplaced fracture of the talar neck.
Type II	Displaces fracture of the talar neck with subluxation or dislocation of the subtalar joint.
Type III	Fracture talar neck with subluxation or dislocation of subtalar and ankle joints.
Type IV	Fracture talar neck with subluxation or dislocation of subtalar, ankle and talonavicular joints.
Diagnosis	Pain, difficulty in walking, swelling, local tenderness. Movements of ankle – painful and restricted.
Investigation	X-ray foot includes ankle – AP, oblique and LAT views.

- AP and oblique views: To assess the congruity of the ankle mortise.
- Lateral view: To visualize the fracture line and to assess subtalar joint.

Management

Conservative treatment

Type I	Below knee plaster cast for 8–10/52. Non-weight bearing with crutches till the healing of fracture.
Type II and III	Closed reduction (foot is plantar flexed and everted) under anesthesia. Below knee plaster cast, 8–10/52, Non-weight bearing with crutches till the healing of fracture
After care	Physiotherapy

Surgical treatment

Refer: The patient to the orthopedic team for surgery.

Indication
- Type II and III: Failure of conservative treatment
- Type IV

Surgery	ORIF: Open reduction and pinning of the talonavicular joint.
	• Screws: (2 parallel screws) cortical or cancellous (cannulated)
	• K-wire + 1 screw
After care	Physiotherapy

Complications of Fracture Neck of Talus

Avascular necrosis	Leading to osteoarthritis of the ankle joint
	Management: Arthrodesis of ankle joint.
Malunion	Due to reduction failure
	Management: Arthrodesis – subtalar or tripple
Pott's fracture	Malleolar fractures may complicate fracture neck of talus.
	Management: ORIF – of malleolar fracture is treatment of choice.
Osteoarthritis	Due to avascular necrosis or malunion
	Management: Arthrodesis of ankle joint is treatment of choice
Osteomyelitis	Following compound fractures or surgery
	Management: Debridement, antibiotics, talectomy, arthrodesis or amputation.

Fracture of Body of Talus

MOI	RSA, fall from a height, sports injuries.
Pattern	Fracture of upper articular surface of the talus
	Vertical fracture – splitting, without disturbing the ankle or subtalar joints.
Management	Same as for type I – talar neck fracture,
	For displacement – reduction and cross-screwing,
	For comminuted fracture – reconstruction is indicated.

Fracture of Calcaneus

MOI	Fall from a height, mine explosions.
Mechanism	The degree of displacement depends upon the force of violence.
	Sometimes there is no displacement, i.e. if fallen height is comparatively small. With greater fallen height, there may occur flattening and widening of calcaneum, with involvement of subtalar joint.
Diagnosis	Swelling, broadening of heel, local tenderness,
	Movements: Inversion and eversion at the subtalar joint – painful and restricted.
Investigation	X-ray foot – AP and LAT views.
Management	If no displacement: Below knee plaster cast for 6/52.
	If marked displacement: Closed reduction and below knee plaster cast for 8/52, followed by physiotherapy.
Avulsion fracture	ORIF (screw fixation) and below knee plaster cast for 8–10/52, followed by weight bearing and physiotherapy.

Rupture of Tendo-Achilles

MOI	Sports injury, i.e. jumping or sprinting,
	Direct violence, i.e. cut/crush injuries.

Diagnosis	A gap in the tendon above its insertion,
	Weakness of plantar flexion.
Management	**Refer** the patient to the orthopedic team for surgical treatment.
Surgery	Repair of torn tendon, followed by a long leg plaster cast, with knee and ankle in flexion, for 3/52. After 3 weeks, apply a below knee plaster cast for another 3/52, with ankle at right angle.
After care	Physiotherapy.

Fracture of Fifth Metatarsal

MOI	It is an avulsion fracture of base of fifth metatarsal due to sudden contraction of peroneus brevis muscle, as a result of inversion strain.
Diagnosis	Pain, local tenderness
	Movements of adduction and abduction – painful and restricted.
Investigation	X-ray foot – AP and LAT views.
Management	

Conservative treatment:

> Heat – SWD/IRD
> Elastic crepe bandage
> Analgesics
> Plaster cast below knee for 3/52 – in severe cases.

Refer: The patient to the next fracture clinic.

Fracture of Metatarsals

MOI	Crush injury, i.e. – falling of heavy weight on the foot or – vehicle wheel running over the foot.
Diagnosis	Pain, swelling,
	Local tenderness
	Movements – painful and restricted.
Investigation	X-ray foot – AP and LAT views.
Management	

Conservative treatment

> Heat – SWD/IRD
> Elastic crepe bandage
> Analgesics
> Walking plaster shoe – in severe cases.

Refer: The patient to the next fracture clinic.

Surgical treatment: **Refer** the patient to the orthopedic team for surgery.

Surgery	ORIF (open reduction and K-wire fixation).

March Fracture (syn. Fatigue Fracture)

Usually fracture neck of second metatarsal.

MOI	Repeated stress, as seen commonly in army and police recruits.

Diagnosis	Pain
	Local tenderness.
Investigation	X-ray foot – AP and LAT views.
Management	Conservative treatment:
	Rest
	Elastic crepe bandage
	Analgesics
	Plaster shoe in severe cases

Refer: The patient to the next fracture clinic.

Dislocation of Toes

MOI	RSA, sports injuries.
Diagnosis	Pain, difficulty in walking, deformity, local tenderness.
Investigation	X-ray toe.
Management	Closed reduction (by traction) and
	Immobilization by strapping to the adjacent normal toe.

Phalangeal Fractures

MOI	RSA
	Sports injury
	Fall of heavy weight on the foot.
Diagnosis	Pain, difficulty in walking, swelling, wound.
Investigation	X-ray foot – AP and LAT views.
Management	Conservative treatment:
	Toilet of the wound
	Debridement of wound
	Immobilization of toe – by adhesive strapping to adjacent toe or a walking plaster with toe platform for 4/52.

Refer: The patient to the next fracture clinic.

Surgical treatment: **Refer** the patient to the orthopedic team for surgery.

Surgery	ORIF (open reduction and Kirschner wire fixation) of fracture.

Crush Injury of the Foot

MOI	RSA
	Fall of heavy weight on the foot.
Diagnosis	Pain
	Difficulty in walking
	Wound.
Management	Toilet of the wound
	Debridement of wound
	Dressing

Antibiotics

Analgesics.

Surgical treatment: ORIF (open reduction and K-wire fixation) of fractures.

Refer: The patient to the next fracture clinic.

References

1. Hawkins LG: Fractures of the neck of the talus. J Bone Joint Surg 52A:991–1002;1970.
2. Canale ST, Kelly FB Jr.: Fractures of the neck of the talus. J Bone Joint Surg 62A:97–102;1980.
3. Krishna EK, Malhotra R: Fractures of the neck of talus: Current concepts. Orthopaedics Today Vol. III No. 4: 236–241.
4. Blair HC: Comminuted fractures and fracture dislocations of the body of the astragalaux. Am J Surg 59:37–43;1943.
5. Rose GK: Ankle Injuries. Modern Trends in Orthopaedics 3:155–186;1962.
6. McRae R: Practical fracture Treatment. Churchill Livingstone, Edinburgh 1984.

Traumatic Disorders of Joints

Acute Traumatic synovitis of Knee

MOI	Direct trauma
	Aseptic penetrating wounds – include surgical interventions.
Diagnosis	Swelling, pain, tenderness, movements – painful and restricted.
Investigation	X-ray of the joint MRI/CT scan
	CBC.
Management	
Conservative	Bed-rest
	Immobilization of joint – by applying Buck's traction
	Ice/warm moist packs – for relief of pain
	Analgesics.
Surgical	Aspiration of knee
	Application of elastic crepe bandage.

Refer: The patient to orthopedic team – for treatment of any tear, e.g. IDK

Internal Derangements of Knee (IDK)
Described in Fractures of Femur and Injuries about Knee

Coccygodynea

Etiology	Traumatic – arthritis of sacrococcygeal joint
	Spasmodic
	Functional.
Diagnosis	Low backache, local tenderness.
Investigation	CBC
	X-ray pelvis – AP view.

Management
Conservative   Warm fomentation
                Analgesics – NSAID's
                Inj. hydrocortisone with 2% lignocain.
Surgery   Coccygectomy.
Refer: The patient to the orthopedic team for surgery.

Baseball Pitcher's Shoulder

Etiology   Occupational – repeated strains
                Sports injury.
Diagnosis   Pain – referred to deltoid region, tenderness, movements of shoulder
                painful and restricted.
Investigation   CBC
                X-ray shoulder – AP and lateral views.
Management
Conservative   Warm fomentation
                Analgesics – NSAIDs
                Inj. hydrocortisone with 2% lignocain.
Surgery   Exploration.
Refer: The patient to the orthopedic team for surgery.

Baseball Pitcher's Elbow

Etiology   Occupational – repeated strains
                Sports injury.
Diagnosis   Pain – over front of medial humeral condyle, tenderness, swelling,
                movements of elbow painful and restricted.
Investigation   CBC
                X-ray elbow – AP and lateral views.
Management
Conservative   Warm fomentation
                Analgesics – NSAIDs
                Inj. hydrocortisone with 2% lignocain.
Surgery   Excision of osteophytes – from origin of common flexor muscles, olecranon
                and olecranon fossa.
Refer: The patient to the orthopedic team for surgery.

Injuries of Muscles and Tendons

Contusion
MOI   Direct trauma.
Diagnosis   Pain, swelling (hematoma), tenderness.
Investigation   X-ray of the affected part.
Management   Rest, elastic crepe bandage, analgesics.

Rupture of Muscles

MOI	Direct trauma
	Indirect trauma – stumbling, sports injury.
Diagnosis	Quadriceps muscle – commonly injured
	Pain, visible gap, tenderness, movements painful and restricted.
Investigation	X-ray of the affected part.
Management	
Conservative	Warm fomentation
	Analgesics – NSAIDs
	Elastic crepe bandage.
Surgery	Repair with mattress stitches.

Rupture of Tendons

Rupture of Achilles tendon

MOI	Direct trauma
	Sports injury.
Diagnosis	Commonest tendon rupture
	Pain, visible/palpable gap, plantar flexion – painful and restricted.
Management	
Surgical	Early suture of the Achilles tendon.

Refer: The patient to the orthopedic team for surgery.

Rupture of Long Head of Biceps

MOI	Direct trauma
	Degenerative – osteoarthritis of shoulder.
Diagnosis	Swelling – prominent on flexing the elbow.
Investigation	X-ray shoulder.
Management	
Conservative	Warm fomentation
	Analgesics – NSAIDs
	Elastic crepe bandage.
Surgery	Repair – exploration of shoulder, excision of I/A part of tendon and fixation of proximal end of distal segment of tendon into bicipital groove.

Refer: The patient to the orthopedic team for surgery.

Rupture of Extensor Pollicis Longus

MOI	Direct trauma
	Degenerative – sequel of post Colles' fracture.
Diagnosis	Inability to extend the terminal joint of thumb.
Management	
Surgery	Tendon transferring (extensor indices proprius into it).

Refer: The patient to the orthopedic team for surgery.

Rupture of Supraspinatus

MOI	Direct trauma
	Degenerative – osteoarthritis of shoulder.
Diagnosis	Swelling – prominent on flexing the elbow
	Pain, disability.
Investigation	X-ray shoulder.

Management

Conservative	Warm fomentation
	Analgesics – NSAIDs
	Inj. hydrocortisone with 2% lignocain
	Aspiration and needling of calcified deposits.
Surgery	Excision of adhesions and manipulation of shoulder
	Excision of calcified deposits
	Repair of tears
	Acromionectomy.

Refer: The patient to the orthopedic team for surgery.

Avulsion of Tendon–Mallet Finger

MOI	Direct trauma.
Diagnosis	Deformity – persistent flexion of terminal phalanx, due to rupture of extensor tendon near its insertion
	Movement – active extension of terminal phalanx absent.

Management

Conservative	Splintage – in a position of right angled flexion at the PIP joint, with hyperextension at the TIP joint.
Surgery	Fowler operation – releasing central slip of extensor expansion from middle phalanx.

Refer: The patient to the orthopedic team for surgery.

Aftercare	Splintage for 3/52 – in a position of PIP joint in 30° flexion and TIP joint in hyperextension.
	Active exercise of finger.

Sprain of Ankle

MOI	RSA
	Sports injury
	Developmental – ladies wearing high heels.
Mechanism	Inversion injuries of the ankle – lead to tearing of tibiofibular ligament.
Diagnosis	Pain, swelling, tenderness, limp, movements – painful and restricted.
Investigation	X-ray ankle – AP and lateral views.

Management

Conservative	Heat – IR or SWD
	Elastic crepe bandage/ankle support
	Local – inj. hydrocortisone 25–50 mg + Inj. lignocain 2%.

Surgery   Fixation – cross-screwing.
Refer: The patient to the orthopedic team for surgery.

Cut Tendons – Flexor and Extensor

MOI   Direct trauma
                     Occupational – industrial hazards.
Mechanism   Flexor tendons – retract within tendon sheaths
                     Extensor tendons – retract little within paratenon (connective tissue)
Management
Conservative   Toilet of the wound
                     Debridement of the wound
                     Suturing the skin.
Surgery
Primary suturing
Indications   Clean wound and of < 6 hrs duration,
                     Uncomplicated – intact skin, no neurovascular deficit
                     Flexor tendons injury
Secondary suturing
Indications   Contaminated wound and of > 6 hrs duration
                     Extensor tendos injury
Techniques   • End-to-end suture (Bunnell crisscross stitch) – at the volar surface of
                       hand or wrist
                     • End to side anastomosis – for tendon transfers
                     • Double right angled suture – to suture severed ends without any
                       shortening
                     • Roll stitch – to suture extensor tendons near the MP joints
                     • Attachment of tendon.
Refer: The patient to the orthopedic team for surgery.

Injuries of Bursae
Acute traumatic Bursitis
Tendo-Achilles Bursitis

MOI   Direct trauma
                     Sports injury
                     Infection.
Diagnosis   Pain, swelling, tenderness, limp, movements of ankle painful.
Investigation   CBC
                     X-ray ankle – AP and lateral views.
Management
Conservative   Rest, warm fomentation, elevation, immobilization of the affected part,
                     analgesics, antibiotics
                     Aspiration and inj. hydrocortisone with lignocain 2%.
Surgery   Excision of entire bursa.
Refer: The patient to the orthopedic team for surgery.

Chronic Bursitis
Housemaid's Knee

MOI	Recurrent injuries
	Infection.
Mechanism	Repeated friction/pressure.
Diagnosis	Pain, swelling, tenderness, limp, movements of knee painful.
Investigation	CBC
	X-ray knee – AP and lateral views.
Management	
Conservative	Rest, warm fomentation, elevation, immobilization of the affected leg.
	Aspiration and inj. hydrocortisone with lignocain 2%.
Surgery	Excision of entire bursa.

Refer: The patient to the orthopedic team for surgery.

Student's Elbow (Olecranon Bursitis)

MOI	Recurrent injuries
	Infection.
Mechanism	Repeated friction/pressure.
Diagnosis	Pain, swelling, tenderness, limp, movements of elbow – painful.
Investigation	CBC
	X-ray elbow – AP and lateral views.
Management	
Conservative	Rest, warm fomentation, elevation, immobilization of the affected arm.
	Aspiration and inj. hydrocortisone with lignocain 2%.
Surgery	Excision of entire bursa.

Refer: The patient to the orthopedic team for surgery.

Inflammatory
Acute Osteomyelitis (Acute Pyogenic Infection of Bone/Acute Osteitis)

Etiology	Bacterial infection, e.g. *Staphylococcus, Streptococcus, Pneumococcus, Meningococcus, Gonococcus, Haemophilus influenzae*, gram-negative bacilli.
Transmission	Direct: Compound fractures
	Indirect: Hematogenous – through bloodstream.
Diagnosis	Age – common in children
	Bone – tibia, femur, humerus are commonly affected
	Site – bone ends (metaphysis)
	Onset – sudden
	Pain – severe
	Fever with chills
	Swelling
	Skin – hot, red

	Local tenderness – over the bone
	Swelling of joint – absent initially, may present later on
	Movements – free initially, and later on may be painful and restricted.
Investigation	Hemogram
	TLC and DLC – leukocytosis
	ESR – raised
	Blood culture
	X-ray: Normal in early cases. Later on there occurs rarefaction of the metaphysis, and subperiosteal bone formation.
Complications	• Septic arthritis
	• Deformity/shortening.
Management	
Conservative	Bed-rest
	Immobilization – by splint, traction
	Elevation of the part
	Warm fomentation
	Antibiotics
	Analgesics
	Fluids – orally or IV.
Surgery	Incision and drainage of abscess.
Indications	Swelling (overlying)
	Acute local tenderness – persisting for > than 24 hrs
	Fever – persisting for > than 24 hrs

Refer: The patient to the orthopedic team.

Acute Suppurative Arthritis

Etiology	Bacterial infection, e.g. Staphylococcus, Streptococcus, Pneumococcus, Meningococcus, Gonococcus, *Haemophilus influenzae*, gram-negative bacilli.
Diagnosis	Onset – sudden
	Pain – severe
	Fever with chills
	Swelling of joint
	Skin – hot, red
	Local tenderness
	Movements – painful and restricted.
Investigation	Hemogram
	TLC and DLC – leukocytosis
	ESR – raised
	Blood culture

Synovial fluid analysis: Leukocytosis

Smear and culture study of causative organism

X-ray: Normal in early cases, but later on shows demineralization, bony erosion, narrowing of joint space, osteomyelitis.

Management

General measures

Bed-rest

Immobilization of joint by splint, traction

Elevation of the part

Warm fomentation

Antibiotics

Analgesics

Fluids – orally or IV.

Surgical measures

Aspiration of joint.

Incision and drainage.

Refer: The patient to the Orthopedic team.

Acute Suppurative Tenosynovitis

Described in Section 16 of Arthritis and Allied Rheumatic Emergencies.

Acute Stenosing Tenosynovitis

Described in Section 16 of Arthritis and Allied Rheumatic Emergencies.

de Quervain's Disease

Described in Section 16 of Arthritis and Allied Rheumatic Emergencies.

Trigger Finger/Thumb

Described in Section 16 of Arthritis and Allied Rheumatic Emergencies.

Acute Carpal Tunnel Syndrome

Described in Section 16 of Arthritis and Allied Rheumatic Emergencies.

Ganglion

Etiology   Traumatic

Degenerative (collagen).

Diagnosis   Age – common in adults

Sex – common in females

Site – common on the dorsum of wrist and foot.

Management
Conservative   Aspiration and inj. of a sclerosing agent
                    Strapping.
Surgical   Excision.
Postoperative: Chances of recurrence.

Acute Rheumatic Myositis
Described in Section 16 of Arthritis and Allied Rheumatic Emergencies.

Traumatic Myositis Ossificans
Sites   Branchialis muscle – following fracture/dislocation of elbow
                    Quadriceps muscle – following direct contusion.
Etiology   Passive stretching exercises.
Diagnosis   Swelling of elbow/knee
                    Stiffness of the elbow/knee.
Investigation   X-ray of elbow/knee – AP and lateral views.
Management
Conservative   Cuff and collar sling/knee cap or brace
                    Avoid strenuous exercises/work – weight lifting or massage.
Surgical   Excision of matured myositis.
Refer: The patient to the orthopedic team.

Acute Suppurative Bursitis
Etiology   Traumatic – penetrating wounds
                    Infective.
Diagnosis   Site – prepatellar
                    Swelling of knee
                    Tenderness
                    Movements – painful and restricted.
Investigation   X-ray of knee – AP and lateral views.
Management
Conservative   Rest, warm fomentation, analgesics, antibiotics.
Surgical   Drainage.

Acute Rheumatoid Arthritis
Described in Section 16 of Arthritis and Allied Rheumatic Emergencies.

Acute Gout
Described in Section 16 of Arthritis and Allied Rheumatic Emergencies.

Ankylosing Spondylitis
Described in Section 16 of Arthritis and Allied Rheumatic Emergencies.

Acute Low Backache
Described in Section 16 of Arthritis and Allied Rheumatic Emergencies.

Acute Sciatica
Described in Section 16 of Arthritis and Allied Rheumatic Emergencies.

Periarthritis of Shoulder
Described in Section 14 of Geriatric Emergencies

Supraspinatus Tendinitis

Etiology	Traumatic
	Infective
	Degenerative
Diagnosis	Swelling of knee
	Tenderness
	Movements – painful and restricted (painful arc).
Investigation	X-ray of knee – AP and lateral views.
Management	
Conservative	Rest, warm fomentation, analgesics, antibiotics, inj. hydrocortisone
	Manipulation – after few days.

Prolapse Intervertebral Disc (PIVD)

It is the main cause of low backache and pain down thigh, legs. It commonly affects adults from 30 to 50, most often males. It results from compression upon nerve root or cord, by the backward protrusion of nucleus pulposus, due to weakening of posterior longitudinal ligament and the annulus fibrosus as a result of trauma. The vast majority affect the disc between the L5 and S1 vertebrae. Disc between L4 and L5 is the next most vulnerable. The root of 5th lumbar or 1st sacral is commonly affected.

Etiology	Traumatic – RSA, sports injury, fall from height, lifting heavy weight, injury by a lumbar puncture needle
	Degenerative.
Risk factors	Postural
	Deformity, e.g. kyphosis, scoliosis
	Spondylitis
	Vertebral osteophytes
	Violent actions – sneezing, coughing, lurching.
Diagnosis	Symptoms are those of sciatica in most cases, depending on type of lesion (nerve root compression), e.g.
L5 lesions	Pain: In the hip, groin, thigh (posterolateral) outer calf, lateral malleolus, foot (dorsum), toes (1, 2, 3 rd)
	Numbness: In the area of affected nerve, e.g. more medial over tibial region – extending over big toe, medial malleolus, and related part of sole.

Local tenderness: Outer gluteal region and near fibular's head.

Weakness: Extensor of greater toe and foot

Ankle jerk: Depressed

SLR: Positive

S1 lesions	Pain: In the sacroiliac joint, thigh (back), calf (back) to heel, sole (plantar surface) and toes (4th and 5th).

Numbness: In the area of affected nerve, e.g. outer side of leg, foot, outer two toes and sole.

Local tenderness: Over sacroiliac joint, back of thigh and leg.

Weakness: Hamstrings, flexor of foot, flexor and abductors of toes

Ankle jerk: Diminished or absent

SLR: Positive

Lumbar curve: May be diminished or lost

Prominent spinous processes (L3, 4, 5).

Investigation	Hemogram, ESR, serum proteins,

CSF examination,

X-ray lumbar spine – AP and LAT views

Bone scans

MRI

CT scan.

Management

Conservative treatment

Bed-rest

Heat therapy, massage

Traction

Lumbar belt

Analgesics.

Surgical treatment: May be indicated in 10% of cases, when compression of nerve roots or spinal cord causes neurologic deficit.

Procedures
- Microsurgical arthroscopic lateral-approach laser-assisted fluoroscopic discectomy – gold standard for treating disc prolapse, as it can be performed as an day care procedure, and has proven to be a safe and least traumatic procedure. Alt.:
- Laminectomy with or without arthrodesis spine
- Percutaneous lumbar discectomy – automated
- Percutaneous lumbar discectomy – endoscopic
- Percutaneous laser discectomy
- Microdiscectomy – transforaminal endoscopic
- Microdiscectomy – stereotactic lumbar
- Artificial disc replacement or intervertebral disc transfer – future holds (procedures) in store.

Refer: The patient to the orthopedic team

Osteoporosis

Described in Section 14 of Geriatric Emergencies

Osteogenic Sarcoma

Definition	It is a highly malignant tumor originating from osteoblastic cells of bone.
Incidence	Most frequent.
Age	2nd and 3rd decades.
Bones	Large tubular bones, e.g. distal femur, proximal tibia and humerus.
Site	Metaphysis of long bone, growth being checked by the epiphyseal plate from spreading to epiphysis. Post fusion, the growth spreads to the epiphysis and articular cartilage.
Spread	Tumor may be central or commonly eccentric, destroys the cortex and produces marked periosteal reaction. An early systemic spread to lungs – causes blood-stained pleural effusion.
Properties	Osteogenic or osteolytic.
Etiology	Unknown.
Possibility	May be related to the sites of growth.
Diagnosis	Pain – precedes swelling, visible distended skin veins, tenderness, palpable bony hard fusiform swelling – commonly seen in the region of knee or shoulder.
Investigation	CBC
	X-ray – diagnostic. The lesions variable from sclerotic to lytic, are fairly large, located in the metaphysis, abolishing bone architecture, and new bone formation (subperiosteally) – resulting in stripping of periosteum (Codman's triangle and Sun-rays appearance) PET-CT scan.
	CXR – pleural effusion
	Biopsy – to be performed with great care (risk of dissemination).
Management	
Surgical	Amputation (as high as possible) – is the treatment of choice.
	Femur/tibia – hind-quarter amputation or disarticulation through hip
	Humerus – fore-quarter amputation or disarticulation through shoulder joint
	Radiotherapy – controversial. Radiotherapy to both lungs along with amputation may affect survival rate.
	Chemotherapy – in combination with amputation may be beneficial
	Agents: – Methotrexate 12–15 g/m^2 PO or IM
	– Doxorubicin 60–75 mg/m^2 IV. Rept. every 3/52.
Prognosis	Poor.

Ewing's Sarcoma

Definition	A highly malignant tumor originating from reticuloendothelial system.
Incidence	Rare.

Age	2nd decade (5–20 yrs).
Bones	Large tubular bones of lower limb or pelvis, or any bone.
Site	Diaphysis of long bones.
Properties	Tumor may be osteolytic or osteoblastic.
Etiology	Unknown.
Diagnosis	Pain, fever, tenderness, palpable bony hard swelling.
Investigation	CBC
	X-ray – diagnostic. Marked diffuse rarefaction of the shaft, with subperiosteal deposition of bone in layers (onion effect)
	PET-CT scan
	CXR
	Biopsy.
D/d	Chronic osteomyelitis.
Management	Is highly unsatisfactory.
Radiotherapy	Highly sensitive to RT. Little effect on distant metastasis.
	RT in combination with CT yields better result.
Surgical	Amputation – rarely indicated in failure cases of RT and CT.
Prognosis	Poor.

Multiple Myeloma (Plasma Cell Myeloma)

Definition	A malignant tumor of hematopoietic origin (malignant proliferation of plasma cells) that involves > 10% of bone marrow.
Etiology	Unknown.
Diagnosis	Age – usually appears in 6th and 7th decades of life and is rare in < 40 yrs.
	Race – seen in all races.
	Sex – twice common in males
	Severe bone pain – aggravated by motion
	Bones are involved in 90% of patients – skull, pelvis, spine, ribs and femurs
	Pathological fractures
	Fever
	Fatigue, thirst, loss of weight, anemia.
Investigation	CBC
	Anemia – normocytic, normochromic type
	Rouleau formation – marked
	ESR – greatly elevated
	TLC and platelet count – normal
	Serum alkaline phosphatase – elevated
	Serum globulin – elevated
	Urine – appearance of Bence Jones proteose – precipitates on addition of nitric acid and disappears on warming
	X-ray – diagnostic, e.g. shows multiple punched out areas

MRI – highly accurate in detecting an early epidural involvement

Bone marrow (aspiration) biopsy – shows sheets of plasma cells with large nuclei and nucleoli.

D/d   Connective tissue disorders.

Chronic infections.

Skeletal metastasis.

Amyloidosis – always associated with plasma cell neoplasia.

Abnormal gamma globulin products, especially those of Bence Jones type, are directly involved in these tissue (amyloid) infiltrates.

Management   No effective treatment known and the disease is always fatal.

General measures

Aims   Relief from pain and reduction of tumor masses

Ambulation of patient to combat negative calcium balance

Prevention of exposure to trauma to avoid occurrence of the pathological fractures.

Treatment   Blood transfusion – to combat anemia

Analgesics – for control of pain

Chemotherapy (alkylating agents):

- Melphalan (alkeran) – most effective agent available.
  Dose: 6 mg o.d. PO, for 2–3 weeks
  Maintenance dose: 1–4 mg o.d. every 4 weeks along with
  Prednisone 2 mg/kg
- Cyclophosphamides 50–100 mg PO 1–3 times o.d. along with
  Vincristine 1.4 mg/sq.m weekly

Radiotherapy – for control of pain and for reducing tumor mass

Surgery   Decompression with radiotherapy – for cord compression

Stem cell transplantation (SCT) – for selective patients.

Refer: The patient to the oncology and medical team.

Prognosis   Average survival time after diagnosis is 2 years. Occasionally a patient may live for many years in apparent remission.

Secondary Carcinoma of Bone

Definition   It is the most frequent malignant bone tumor. It is commoner than primary bone tumor.

Incidence   Common.

Age   Above 40 yrs.

Bones   Vertebrae, pelvic bones, femurs, humerus.

Site   Spine, pelvis, thighs and arms.

Properties   Tumor may be osteolytic or osteoblastic.

Etiology   Metastasis from primary growth in breast, bronchus, thyroid, prostate, and kidney.

Diagnosis	Pain – very severe, swelling, pathological fracture – may be found.
Investigation	CBC
	Serum acid phosphatase estimation
	X-ray – diagnostic. Shows irregular destruction of bone without surrounding reaction, while sclerosis in case of metastasis from carcinoma prostate
	CXR
	Mammography CT scan
	US abdomen and pelvis
	Biopsy.
Management	Is highly unsatisfactory.
Radiotherapy	Sensitive to radiotherapy.
	RT in combination with CT yields better result
Surgical	• Orchidectomy combined with estrogen therapy – in case of secondary deposits from carcinoma prostate
	• Thyroidectomy combined with radioactive iodine – in case of secondary deposits from carcinoma thyroid
	• Mastoidectomy combined with testosterone – in case of secondary deposits from carcinoma breast.
Prognosis	Poor.

References

1. Bunch TW, et al: Synovial fluid complement: Usefulness in diagnosis and classification of rheumatoid arthritis. Ann Int Med 81:32;1974.
2. Johnson JS, et al: Rheumatoid arthritis, 1970-72. Ann Int Med 78:937;1773.
3. Gokhale T, Hedge U, Jyotish CJ: Classification and diagnostic Criteria for Rheumatic Diseases. Journal of General Medicine 14:7–14;2002.
4. Kapoor PS: Rheumatoid arthritis. The Indian Express 18 September, 2003.
5. Chaturvedi V: Ankylosing spondylitis: A radical shift. In: Management. Orthopaedics Today VI:42; 2004.
6. Calabro JJ, Maltz BA: Ankylosing spondylitis. New England J Med 282:606;1970.
7. Kapoor PS: Ankylosing Spondylitis. The Indian Express 4 June;2003.
8. Engleman EP, Chatton MJ: Arthritis and allied rheumatic disorders. Current Medical Diagnosis and Treatment, 474–498;1975.
9. Russel ASA, Ansel BM: Septic arthritis. Ann Rheumat Dis 31:40;1972.
10. Joshi VR: ACR criteria for classification of acute gouty arthritis. Journal of General Medicine 14;2002.
11. Pispati PK: Acute gout. Journal of General Medicine 14;2002.
12. Frymoyer JW: Back pain and sciatica. N Engl J Med 318:291;1998.
13. Kapoor PS: Backache. The Indian Express 11 September;2002.
14. Bell GR, Parkman RH: The conservative treatment of sciatica. Spine 9:54;1984.
15. Kapoor PS: The truth about sciatica. The Indian Express 30 October;2002.
16. Rothman RC, Simeone F: Lumbar Disc Disease. Philadelphia. Saunders, 443–458;1975.
17. Wilson DH, Harbaugh R: Microsurgical and standard removal of the protruded lumbar disc: A comparative study. Neurosurgery 8: 422-427;1981.

18. Apostolides PJ, Jackobowitz R, Sonntag VK. Lumbar discectomy microdiscectomy: "the gold stand microdiscectomy: "the gold standard". Clin Neurosurg 43: 228–238;1996.

19. Silvers HR: Microsurgical versus standard lumbar discectomy, Neurosurgery 22(5): 837-841, May 1988.

20. Gulati Y: Lumbar microdiscectomy. Apollo Medicine 1; 34–37, Sept 2004.

21. Mathews HH: Transforaminal endoscopic microdiscectomy. Neurosurg Clin N Am 7(1): 59–63, Jan 1996.

22. Sledge CB: Surgery for rheumatoid arthritis. Current Orthopaedics, 3,1. 1989.

23. Regan JJ, Guyer RD: Endoscopic techniques in spinal surgery. Clinical Orthopaedics, 335, 1.

Orthopedic Practical Procedures
Joint Puncture

Indications

Diagnostic   Aspiration of joint and physical, microscopical and bacteriological examinations of the aspirated fluid

Therapeutic: To administer intra-articular drugs

To relieve tension by withdrawing: Fluid (synovitis), blood (hemophilia, trauma) and pus (septic).

Joints

Shoulder joint
- Enter the needle just lateral to the tip of the coracoid process and push in a direction backwards, upwards, and outwards, or
- Enter the needle just lateral to the angle formed by the junction of the acromion with the spine of the scapula.

Elbow joint
- Flex the elbow to a right angle, with the forearm semi-pronated, enter the needle just proximal to the radial head, in a direction directly forwards, i.e. just below the ulnar (better) or radial styloid process and push in at right angle to the process.

Hip joint
- Enter the needle at a point 5 cm below the anterior inferior iliac spine and push in upwards, backwards and medially, or
- Enter the needle from the side just above the upper border of the greater trochanter and push in direction of inwards and upwards in a line parallel with femoral neck.

Knee joint
- Enter the needle through the vastus lateralis, and push in direction of inward and backward, or
- Enter the needle on either side of the ligamentum patellae below the patella, and push directly backwards in an upward direction.

Ankle joint
- Enter the needle just below the tip of either malleolus and push in an upward direction, so that it enters the joint between malleolus and articular surface of the talus.

Lumbar Puncture

Site   L4–L5 intervertebral space.

Indication	Diagnostic and therapeutic purposes
C/I	Papilledema – may cause herniation of medullary cone (fatal)
	Lumbar spine disorders
	Skin infections
Method	• Hold the child in sitting/lateral recumbent position, with neck flexed to the chest and knees flexed to abdomen
	• Sterile the area (3rd–4th intervertebral space)
	• Local anesthesia (1% lignocain) given
	• Introduce a lumbar puncture needle with stylet in position, through skin, between spines, through ligamentum flavum
	• Withdraw the stylet, collect the CSF, replace the stylet and then withdraw the needle
	• Seal the puncture site with Tinc. Benzoin co.

Arthroplasty

Definition	Arthroplasty is a reconstructive procedure to restore joint motion and function of the muscles, ligaments and other soft tissues controlling it or function of a joint. Over the years, many different types of hip arthroplasties have been described.
Joints	Most suitable for hip, knee, elbow and TM joints.
Indications	Traumatic – to relieve pain
	Infective – infective arthritis, tubercular arthritis
	Inflammatory – RA
C/I	Tuberculosis – causing ankylosis in a single joint
	Shortening – by growth impairment (due to injured epiphysis)
	Osteoporosis – severe
	Osteomyelitis – causing extensive sclerosis of bone
	Age – young children
	Occupation – workers doing strenuous work
Techniques	Variable as per anatomy and physiology of the joint.
Aims	• To relieve/reduce joint pain
	• To restore/improve joint function
	• To correct deformity
	• To construct a new joint in an ankylosed joint
	• To fashion new joint articular surfaces – post-ankylosis
	• To restore soft tissue structures (cosmetic adjustment).

Hip Arthroplasty

Types	• Resection (fashioning) arthroplasty
	• Interposition arthroplasty:
	– Soft tissues (muscle and fascia lata)

- Cups arthroplasties:
  - Unipolar (vitallium cup)
  - Bipolar (double cup/surface replacement)
- Total hip replacement (THR)
- Hybrid total hip replacement.

Resection (Fashioning) Arthroplasty

Example   Girdlestone pseudoarthrosis
Indication Degenerative disease of the hip, tuberculous arthritis, and septic arthritis.

Interposition Arthroplasty

- Interposition of soft tissues, e.g. muscle and fascia lata between articular surfaces
- Interposition of a cup between femoral head and acetabulum

Surface Replacement (Double Cup) Arthroplasties

Example   Vitallium cup arthroplasty. Two metallic cups fixed with acrylic cement, one on to the femoral head and other into the acetabulum.
Indication Painful hip, chronic arthritis, fracture neck femur: Rarely used currently, due to high rate of failures.
Hemiarthro- Using a metallic cup mounted on a short-curved intramedullary stem. The
plasty   femoral head not resected but reamed to fit within the thin-walled metal cup.
Indication Rarely used currently, due to high rate of failures.

Unipolar (Femoral) Prostheses

Example   Moore (long stem) and Thompson (short stem) metallic prostheses
Indication Fracture neck femur, degenerative arthritis.

Total Hip Replacement (THR)

Indications
- Inherent complications, e.g. fixation failure, non-union, and AVN
- Elderly: Especially subcapital fracture of femoral neck
- Middle age: ORIF failure, non-union, AVN

Advantages
- Mobilization – early weight bearing
- Postoperative complications – minimal
- Rehabilitation – early rehabilitation

Types   Cemented and uncemented.
Preoperative planning
Exposure   Lateral, anterolateral, or posterior approach
           Femoral neck resection
           Femoral preparation
           Acetabular preparation

Acetabular cementing and pressurization
Acetabular implantation
Trial reduction
Further femoral preparation
Femoral cementing
Stem implantation
Reduction – by gental delivery of head into the acetabulum
Check X-ray.

After care | Breathing exercises, starting on the same day of operation
Quadriceps, toes, ankle exercises – first day onwards.

Follow up visit 2–3/12. If satisfactory, then next visit after one year and so on for 5 yrs, with periodical check X-rays.

Dynamic Hip Screw (DHS)

Indication Intertrochanteric fracture – stable and unstable (moderate)

Advantages
- Simple, predictable, highly successful procedure
- Shearing force converted into compression force by the SHS screw
- Mobilization – early
- Mechanical failure – less

Disadvantage
- Fixation failure: Sliding of the screw
- Implant cutting of osteoporotic bone
- Danger of lateral wall fracture.

Types of DHS
- Long barrel plate: For larger femoral head and neck length
- Short barrel plate: For shorter femoral head and neck length

Technique

Anesthesia General

Position Patient is placed supine on the orthopedic table

Reduction Indication: Displaced fracture

Closed reduction: By traction in neutral position, and slight internal rotation

Open reduction: Indicated in failure of closed reduction

Exposure Lateral approach

Fixation With a long barrel standard plate and 32 mm thread length screw

Neck shaft angle (barrel and plate): 135°

After care Same as for intracapsular fractures.

Arthroscopy (Endoscopy) and Arthroscopic Surgery

It cannot be emphasised too strongly that arthroscopic surgery should only be attempted by surgeons who have total confidence in their arthroscopic technique.

Types Diagnostic and operative (surgical).

Indications Diagnostic:

Preoperative assessment of internal derangement of knee

Postoperative assessment of problems, e.g. persistent symptoms

	Operative:
	Synovial biopsy, synovectomy, adhesions and ankylosis – release, excision of fat-pad, removal of loose bodies, foreign bodies, trimming, shaving, drilling of articular cartilage of patella, femur, tibia, meniscectomy Prolapse intervertebral disc (PIVD).
Techniques	Single and double puncture techniques
Method	Preoperative:

General or local anesthesia

Examination under anesthesia

A tourniquet applied – for knee procedures

Skin preparation and draping of the part

Distension of the joint – with irrigation fluid

Approaches: Anterolateral, central, anteromedial, posteromedial, insertion of the arthroscope:

- Knee flexed to 90°
- A 5 mm incision made with blade at a point 2 mm above the anterior horn of lateral meniscus, close to patellar tendon.
- A sharp trocar, locked into the arthroscope sheath, pushed upwards, medially and backwards towards intercondylar notch.
- Patella lifted by the tip of the sheath, and the scope passed into the suprapatellar pouch, as the knee straightened.
- Assembly of the scope – by insertion of the telescope and attachment of the light cable and irrigation tube.

Examination	The examination made in chronological manner, e.g.

- Suprapatellar pouch
- Patellofemoral joint
- Medial compartment
- Intercondylar notch
- Lateral compartment
- Posteromedial compartment
- Posterolateral compartment
- Use of percutaneous needles and blunt hooks to manipulate structures.

Post-care	A single stitch of monofilament nylon through skin and subcutaneous tissues and a sterile gauze dressing applied.

Intramedullary Nailing (IMN)

Advantages	Reduction (closed) easy, short invasive surgery, less blood loss, early mobilization and reduced mechanical (fixation) failure.
Disadvantages	Mechanical (fixation) failure, pain in the thigh, stiffness, deformity, nail extrusion.
Technique	
Anesthesia	General

Position	Patient is placed supine on the orthopedic table.
Reduction	Under C-arm. Closed reduction: By traction in neutral position, and slight internal rotation
Exposure	Lateral approach
Incision	Just proximal to greater trochanter
Fixation	IMN with SHS and distal interlocking screws
After care	Same as for intracapsular fractures.

References

1. Charnley J: Total prosthetic replacement of the hip. Triangle 8:211;1968.
2. Oh I, Harris WH: A cement fixation system for total hip arthroplasty. Clin Orthop 164:221–229;1982.
3. McGinty JB, Matza RA: Arthroscopy of the knee. Evaluation of an out-patient procedure under local anaesthesia. Journal of Bone and Joint Surgery 60A:787–789;1978.
4. Zaman M, Leonard MA: Meniscectomy in children: A study of fifty-nine knees. Journal of Bone and Joint Surgery 60-B:436;1978.
5. Oretorp N, Gillquist J: Transcutaneous meniscectomy under arthroscopic control. International Orthopaedics Today 3:19–25;1979.
6. Dandy DJ, Jackson RW: Arthroscopic Surgery Knee. Churchill Livingstone, 1981.
7. Bhan S, Pankaj A: History and evolution of hip arthroplasty. Orthopaedics Today 1:24–30;2004.

Abdominal Emergencies

Symptoms and signs (non-specific manifestations)

Abdominal emergencies:

- Traumatic:
  - Abdominal injuries:
    - ◊ Blunt injuries
    - ◊ Perforated (rupture) injuries
- Inflammatory:
  - Acute abdomen (acute abdominal pain):
  - Intra-abdominal causes
  - Extra-abdominal causes
- Acute appendicitis:
  - Types: Non-obstructive and obstructive type
  - Perforated appendix
  - Appendicitis in children
  - Appendicitis in elderly
  - Differential diagnosis of acute appendicitis
  - Appendicectomy
  - Indications for emergency operation (stopping of delayed treatment)
  - Management of appendicular abscess
  - Interval appendicectomy
- Acute cholecystitis

- Acute pancreatitis
- Injury of intestine
- Acute intestinal obstruction
- Acute intussusception
- Ruptured ectopic gestation
- Acute ureteric colic
- Acute peritonitis
- Acute pyelonephritis
- Acute salpingitis

Liver disorders

- Injuries of liver
- Wounds of liver

Hernia

- **Strangulated inguinal hernia**
- **Strangulated femoral hernia**
- **Strangulated para-umbilical hernia**

Practical procedures:

- Plane X-ray abdomen
- Ultrasonography
- MRI
- CT scan
- Radionuclide scintigraphy (nuclear medicine)
- Laparotomy

Symptoms and Signs (Non-specific manifestations)

Symptoms   Pain abdomen

Distension abdomen

Nausea, vomiting, diarrhea, constipation

Dysphagia

Flatulence

Indigestion

Hiccups

Heart burn

	Hematemesis
	Bleeding per rectum
	Melena
Signs	Jaundice
	Skin rashes
	Clubbing of fingers
	Liver/spleen – normal or enlarged.

Signs
- Hematemesis
- Bleeding per rectum
- Melena
- Jaundice
- Skin rashes
- Clubbing of fingers
- Liver/spleen – normal or enlarged.

Investigations
- TLC and DLC: Leukocytosis
- Serum amylase – raised: Acute pancreatitis
- Urine analysis – albumin and casts: Acute intestinal obstruction
- Diastage index rise: Acute pancreatitis
- Stools: Color, odor, occult blood, fecal fat
- X-ray (plain) abdomen: Multiple levels of gas and fluid: Acute Intestinal obstruction
- Endoscopy: Eesophagus, stomach, duodenum
- Barium meal: Dysphagia, gastric and duodenal ulcers
- Barium enema: Intestinal obstruction
- Proctoscopy: Anal fissure, polyps, hemorrhoids
- Sigmoidoscopy: Polyps, proctitis, amebic dysentery, carcinomas
- Ultrasonography: Pyloric stenosis, intussusception, appendicitis, cholelithiasis, cirrhosis liver, liver abscess
- MRI: Tumors of liver, pelvis, imaging bile duct and pancreatic duct
- CT scan: Staging patients with cancer of esophagus, stomach, pancreas
- Needle biopsy: For histological study
- Cholecystography: Gallbladder disorders include stones
- Laparotomy: Confirms clinical diagnosis.

Abdominal Injuries

Types
- Blunt injuries
- Perforated (rupture) injuries.

MOI
- Direct violence – hitting with a stick/rod/stone, stabbing, gunshot RSA, sports injury, fight
- Fall from height.

Diagnosis
- Pain, local tenderness, abdominal rigidity, shifting dullness
- Liver dullness abstinence
- Bruise over the abdominal wall or wound – may/may not internal hemorrhage – increasing pallor, restlessness, air-hunger, rising pulse, hypothermia, hypotension.

Signs
- Liver: Local tenderness, shifting dullness and increased area of liver dullness
- Spleen: Local tenderness, muscle guard, shifting dullness, pain radiating to left shoulder
- Kidney: Fullness, shifting dullness, tenderness, hematuria
- UB: Local tenderness, shifting dullness, peritonitis

Stomach and small intestine: Pain over epigastrium, vomiting, hemoptysis, local tenderness, muscle guard, shifting dullness

Large intestine: Peritonitis, surgical emphysema.

Investigation	Blood for grouping and crossmatching
	CXR (sitting) – may show gas under the diaphragm
	Plain X-ray abdomen – may show loss of psoas shadow and gas in the peritoneum
	X-ray pelvis – may show a pelvic fracture
	Ultrasound – confirms diagnosis
	CT scan – confirms diagnosis but time consuming.
Management	
Emergency	Airway care, oxygen therapy
	IV fluids – normal saline
	Blood transfusion
	Nasogastric (Ryle's) tube – for gastric aspiration
	Catheterization of bladder
Surgical	**Refer** the patient to the surgical team.
Surgery	Laparotomy as an emergency procedure
Aim	To control the hemorrhage
Method	Repair:
Stomach	Repair of the perforation

Small intestine rupture: Simple closure of the perforation

Large intestine rupture: Exteriorisation is procedure of choice, Alt:

Closure of perforation followed by colostomy

Mesentery laceration: Resection of lacerated portion

Liver	Repair of the liver tear by mattress sutures parallel to tear
Kidney	Repair of the perforation
	Nephrectomy – indicated in severely damaged kidney, provided the contralateral kidney is healthy
Ureter	Uretero-ureteric anastomosis – for injury of one ureter
	Nephrostomy (bilateral) – for bilateral injury
Spleen	Splenectomy.

Acute Abdomen

Definition	It is defined as any condition resulting in severe abdominal pain.
Classification	
Visceral pain	Due to spasm or distension:
	• Intermittent and gripping (colicky) type due to spasm or
	• Continuous type due to distension, mostly referred to area of distribution of same somatic nerves
Examples	Acute appendicitis

	Acute renal colic
Parietal pain	Due to irritation of peritoneum by blood or exudates
	Pain is continuous, burning and localized type
Example	Pain at the site of inflamed area
Torsional pain	Due to pull or twisting of mesentery
Example	Torsion of ovary, spleen.

Etiology
Intra-abdominal Causes

Inflammatory	• Acute appendicitis
	• Acute pancreatitis
	• Acute cholecystitis
	• Acute salpingitis
	• Acute peritonitis
	• Acute diverticulitis
Perforation	• Peptic ulcer
	• Typhoid ulcer
Obstruction	• Acute intestinal obstruction: Due to obstruction:
	• In the lumen: Gallbladder stones, worms, fecolith
	• In the wall: Intussusception, growth, fibrous strictures
	• Outside wall: Hernias, adhesions, tumors, paralytic ileus, embolism, thrombosis of mesenteric vessels
Hemorrhage	• Rupture of ectopic pregnancy
	• Rupture of spleen
Torsion of pedicle	• Twisted ovarian cyst
Spasmodic (colics)	• Renal
	• Biliary
	• Appendicular
	• Intestinal

Extra-abdominal Causes

Respiratory	• Pneumonia, pleurisy, pneumothorax, Pott's disease
CVS	• Pericarditis, CAD, angina pectoris, aneurysm of aorta
Pediatrics	• Acute appendicitis
	• Acute intussusception
	• Acute intestinal obstruction
	• Acute peritonitis
Diagnosis	Pain:
	• Intermittent, gripping type of colics
	• Continuous, burning type of perforated peptic ulcer
	• Agonising type of acute pancreatitis and torsion, etc.

Pressure gives relief in colics, while aggravates in inflamed cases

Vomiting: Appears soon after pain: Acute appendicitis, pancreatitis, biliary and renal colics

Appears simultaneously with pain: Acute intestinal (small) obstruction

Absent/late appearance: Large intestinal obstruction

Frequency: Constant, frequent and perfuse: Acute intestinal obstruction and acute pancreatitis

Constipation: It is the usual feature in acute abdomen

Micturition: Anuria, dysuria (strangury): Acute renal colic, acute peritonitis, acute appendicitis

Swelling

Local tenderness

Rigidity

Shifting dullness

Hypotension: Intestinal hemorrhage, shock.

Investigation Special	CBC
	TLC and DLC: Leukocytosis
	Serum amylase–raised: Acute pancreatitis
	Urine analysis: Albumin and casts: Acute intestinal obstruction
	Diastage index rise: Acute pancreatitis
	Stools: Color. odor, occult blood, fecal fat
	X-ray (plain) abdomen: Multiple levels of gas and fluid: 　　　　　　　　　Acute intestinal obstruction
	Endoscopy: Esophagus, stomach,
	Ultrasonography: Pyloric stenosis, intussusception, appendicitis, cholelithiasis
	MRI: Tumors of liver, pelvis
	Laparotomy: Confirms clinical diagnosis.
Management	
Emergency	Airway care, oxygen therapy
	IV fluids – normal saline
	Blood transfusion
	Nasogastric (Ryle's) tube – for gastric aspiration
	Catheterization of bladder
Surgical	**Refer** the patient to the surgical team.

Acute Appendicitis

Definition	It is defined as inflammation of the vermiform appendix.
	It is one of the most frequent causes of acute abdomen.
	It is more common in young males, although sex is no bar.
Etiology	Exact cause unknown.
	Contributory etiological factors:
	Obstruction of appendicular lumen due to:
	• Fecoliths, foreign body, worms – ring/threadworms, stricture

- Abuse of purgatives
- Non-vegetarian diet – rich in meat
- Familial tendency.

Bacteriology	Mixed infection
	Mostly *E.coli*, streptococci, *Cl. welchii*.
Pathogenesis	Types: Non-obstructive and obstructive types.

- *Non-obstructive type:* Inflammation of mucous membrane and lymph follicles, is gradual in onset, and terminates in one of following, i.e. resolution, ulceration, suppuration, fibrosis, gangrene, and finally into localized peritonitis. It is less serious than obstructive type, due to release of inflammatory products into cecum.
- *Obstructive type:* Less common than non-obstructive type, and is more serious in nature. The appendix becomes highly inflamed, i.e. swollen, red, later on green, gangrenous, perforated, finally generalized peritonitis.

Diagnosis	Age – common in young children, although age is no bar
	Pain abdomen
	Nausea, vomiting, anorexia, constipation
	Fever – low grade.

Non-obstructive type

Pain abdomen – initially around umbilicus, or in the epigastrium (dull aching and constant visceral pain – due to distension of appendix)

Pain later on shifts to the right iliac fossa (localized, somatic pain – due to irritation of parietal peritoneum by inflamed appendix).

Nausea, vomiting, anorexia

Fever – low grade

Pulse – rise in pulse rate

Constipation/diarrhea and high fever in children

Local tenderness at McBurney point

Rigidity

Swelling – appear after 3–4 days.

Obstructive type

Pain abdomen – severe, colicky, abrupt onset

Vomiting – common

Tenderness – right iliac fossa.

Perforated appendix

Pain disappears temporarily but followed by features of spreading peritonitis:

- Pain and vomiting aggravate
- Pulse rate – rises
- Temperature – subnormal
- Abdominal movements – restricted
- Auscultation – silent abdomen.

Appendicitis in Children

Constitutional disturbances – more marked in children than in adults

Vomiting or diarrhea – may precede the pain

Pain abdomen – usually colic type

Temperature – high

Pulse rate – high

Appendicular mass – rare, due to short omentum and poor

Inflammatory response.

Incidence of perforation and peritonitis – more.

Appendicitis in Elderly

Incidences of gangrene, perforation, and peritonitis, are comparatively more due to arteriosclerosis of appendicular artery.

Clinical picture resembles subacute intestinal obstruction

Pulse and temperature – often normal

Abdominal signs – mild

Rigidity – absent or slight, due to lax abdominal wall.

Investigation

TLC: Leukocytosis

DLC: Neutrophils – increase

Plane X-ray abdomen: Insignificant in early cases

Ultrasonography

CT scan.

D/d

List of conditions causing abdominal pain is endless (vast) as appendicitis may simulate these disorders.

Acute Cholecystitis

Steady severe pain in the right hypochondrium

Murphy's sign positive: Examiner's fingers pressed over the right costal margin, at the outer border of rectus, and the patient is asked to take a deep breath, resulting in the gallbladder to descend and hit the examining fingers. The patient winces – confirming inflamed gallbladder.

Boas' sign positive: Pain radiating through to right scapula

Retching/noisy vomiting

Jaundice – may be positive

Ultrasound and IV cholecystography confirm diagnosis

Acute Intestinal Obstruction

Pain – continuous colicky type around umbilicus

Vomiting

Plane X-ray abdomen – shows fluid levels

Acute Salpingitis

Discharge – per vaginum

Dysmenorrhea

Burning micturition

Per vaginum (P/V) examination – confirmatory

Acute Pancreatitis

Pain in the epigastrium – with back radiation, and abrupt onset

Nausea, vomiting, cyanosis

Local tenderness positive

Distention, fever

Leukocytosis

Acute Intussusception

A healthy baby – suddenly screaming, followed by

Vomiting

Constipation, followed by passage of blood and mucous per rectum

Lump in the abdomen

Barium enema study: Shows a typical pincer-like ending of the barium enema

Ruptured Ectopic Gastation

Sudden colicky pain over the hypochondrium

Fainting, collapse

Vomiting

History of missed periods

Blood-stained discharge per vaginum

Twisted Right Ovarian Cyst

Severe pain abdomen, referred to loin

Rising pulse rate

Temperature – unchanged

Right Ureteric Colic

Pain in the loin, referred to groin

Urinary symptoms

Local tenderness positive in the right iliac fossa

Plane X-ray abdomen: Shows right ureteric stone

Urine – microscopic examination: Reveals RBC and a deposit

Acute Right Pyelonephritis

Pain abdomen

Polyuria

Local tenderness

High fever

Pyuria

Management: Treatment of choice is appendicectomy.

Refer: The patient to the surgical team for surgery.

Surgery	Appendicectomy
Techniques	Open surgery (Grid-Iron)
	Laparoscopic surgery (minimum invasive)

Appendicectomy

It should preferably be performed as an emergency operation, at an early stage, before formation of a localized mass

Anesthesia	General
Technique	Open surgery
Incision	Grid-Iron incision is made with its center over McBurney's point, right angles to a line joining anterior superior iliac supine to umbilicus
	External oblique muscle incised in length of incision
	Internal oblique and transversus abdominis muscles separated in layers
	Peritoneum is opened
	Appendix is delivered into the wound
	Mesoappendix is clamped and severed and separated from appendix
	Appendix is crushed near its junction with cecum
	A ligature is passed around crushed portion, close to cecum
	A purse-string suture inserted into caput caeci
	The stump is invaginated while purse-string suture is tied, burying the appendicular stump.

Management of Appendicular Mass

For an appendicular mass, treatment of choice is conservative, i.e. Ochsner–Sherren regimen. The fact is that nature has localized the lesion, it is dangerous to perform surgery at this stage – due to the difficulty in finding an intact appendix and possibility of fistula formation.

But to be operated at any time, in case of failure to control infection.

Actually the conservative treatment is simply postponement of the operation and not a substitute for operation.

Management of Cases by Delayed Treatment

History (noting of onset of attack in hours, e.g. 5, 10, 20 hrs and so on)

Recording of signs – in diagrammatic form

Rigidity is indicated by shading

Lump – drawn near to scale

Monitoring pulse every 2 hrly, and temperature every 4 hrly

Recording for any vomiting
Water 30–50 c.c. hrly PO
Monitoring IV fluids daily
Assessment of electrolytes daily
Warm fomentation
Fetus tube passage
Antibiotics.

Emergency Operation (Stopping of delayed treatment)

Indications	Rising pulse rate
	Pain abdomen
	Nausea, vomiting, diarrhea
Surgery	**Refer** the patient to the surgical team for surgery – appendicectomy as soon as possible after complete resolution of the mass.

Appendicular Abscess

Definition	Failure of resolution of an appendicular mass, indicates pus within the mass.
Management	**Refer** the patient to the surgical team for surgery.
Surgery	Incision drainage of appendicular abscess
Indications	Swelling – not reducing after 5th day of treatment or increasing
	Temperature – continuously > 38°C for days.
Anesthesia	General
Technique	Retrocecal and subcecal appendicular abscesses: To be drained extra-peritoneally
	Pre- or post-ileal abscesses: To be drained intraperitoneally
	Pelvic abscess: To be drained into rectum.

Interval Appendicectomy

Indication	A post-drained appendicular abscess
Interval	Usually 3/12 after drainage of an appendicular abscess.

Acute Cholecystitis

Definition	It is defined as inflammation of gallbladder, associated with gallstones
Etiology	Gallstones blocking cystic duct
	Vascular abnormalities of bile duct
	Pancreatitis.
Pathogenesis	Obstruction of cystic duct leads to inflammation, distention of gallbladder, ischemia, gangrene, and finally perforation and localized abscess
Diagnosis	Severe pain in the right hypochondrium, radiating to the top of right shoulder
	Nausea, vomiting, dyspepsia
	Jaundice – may be present

	Fever
	Respiratory rate – increased
	Local tenderness, rigidity.
Investigation	TLC – leukocytosis
	Serum bilirubin and lipase – increased
	Serum transaminase and alkaline phosphatase – increased
	Plane X-ray abdomen – show gallstones
	Ultrasound
	IV cholangiography.
D/d	Acute pancreatitis
	Acute appendicitis
	Peptic ulcer with perforation
	Acute hepatitis

Management

Conservative treatment

Rest: To inflamed gallbladder and biliary system by:

- Gastric aspiration for 3–5 days
- Nothing by mouth
- IV dextro-saline sol
- Daily assay of electrolytes

Sedatives: Atropine – most effective, Alt:

- Pethidine 100 mg IV or IM, no morphine

Anticholinergic: To reduce gastric and pancreatic secretions.

- Propantheline given

Diet: Depending upon improvement of overall clinical condition, the Ryle's tube is removed, fluids given orally followed by fat-free diet

Antibiotics:

- Benzathine penicillin 0.5 mU o.d. IM
- Ampicillin 250–500 mg t.d.s. Children 125–250 mg
- Cefazolin 25–100 mg/kg o.d. IM or IV children 25–50 mg/kg o.d.
- Cefotaxime 1–2 g b.i.d. IM or IV
- Kanamycin 0.5–1 g o.d.
- Broad spectrum antibiotics IV drip

Surgical treatment:	**Refer** the patient to the surgical team.
Indications	Pulse rate and temperature not falling, and persisting pain
	Uncertainty about the diagnosis
	Frequency of perforation of gallbladder
Surgery	Cholecystectomy to be performed as an emergency procedure.
Technique	Laparoscopic surgery.

Acute Pancreatitis

Definition	It is defined as inflammation of the pancreas. It is a serious disorder, with high mortality.

Etiology	Unknown
	Mainly associated with disease of biliary tract
	May occur in association with:

- Hyperparathyroidism
- Hyperlipidemias
- Alcoholism
- Vascular disease

Pathogenesis	The exact pathogenesis is unknown. There occurs acute edema and cellular infiltration, leading to necrosis of acinar cells, hemorrhage, fat necrosis.
Diagnosis	History of alcohol abuse
	Onset – abrupt following a heavy meal
	Pain (agonizing) over the epigastrium – with back radiation
	Nausea, vomiting, constipation, fever, sweating
	Local tenderness, abdominal rigidity
	Shock
Investigation	TLC and DLC: Leukocytosis
	Serum amylase estimation: Elevated
	Serum calcium level: Falls below 7 mg/100 ml, may cause death
	Plane X-ray abdomen: Shows gallstones
	Diagnostic laparotomy
D/d	Acute cholecystitis
	Acute intestinal obstruction
	Acute renal colic
	Acute peptic ulcer with perforation.

Management

Preventive treatment

Stop drinking alcohol

Stop taking large meals or foods containing high fat content

Correction of associated etiological factors.

Conservative treatment: It is treatment of choice.

Bed-rest

Withhold fluids and food orally

Nasogastric aspiration – continuously

Monitor vital signs ½ hrly during acute phase

Analgesics: Atropine sulfate 0.4–0.6 mg s.c. as antispasmodic

- Tramadol 100 mg IM/IV for relief of pain or pentazocine 40 mg IM
- Morphine should not be given as it increases spasm of sphincter of Oddi

IV plasma followed by dextrosaline

IV calcium gluconate 10 mL of 10% sol o.d.

Antibiotics:
- Benzathine penicillin 0.5 mU o.d. IM
- Ampicillin 250–500 mg t.d.s. children 125–250 mg
- Cefazolin 25–100 mg/kg o.d. IM or IV children 25–50 mg/kg o.d.
- Cefotaxime 1–2 g b.i.d. IM or IV
- Kanamycin 0.5–1 g o.d.
- Broad-spectrum antibiotics IV drip

Specific treatment	
Surgical	Surgery is contraindicated, except that when diagnosis in doubt, patient very ill despite conservative treatment, and an associated disorder present. Once diagnosis is confirmed, it is better to close the abdomen rather than manipulation of pancreas, that may increase the mortality. An associated cholecystitis is indication for immediate cholecystectomy.

Refer: The patient to the surgical team.

Prognosis	Recurrences are common
	Mortality rate in acute hemorrhagic pancreatitis is high, especially in presence of hepatic, cardiovascular, or renal involvement.
Convalescent care	
Diet	Bland diet. Avoid fried junk food and spices
	Plenty of fluids, between meals
Alcohol	Forbidden
Antispasmodic	Belladona extract 15 mg T.D.S. or
	Atropine sulphate 0.4–0.6 mg T.D.S.
Antacids	Given hrly until the attack subsides

Acute Intestinal Obstruction

	It is a common, serious, surgical emergency, that demands early diagnosis and priority treatment.
Types	Dynamic – increased peristalsis acting against an obstruction, i.e. in the lumen by a bolus of undigested food, feces, or a gallstone in the wall, i.e. by an inflammatory stricture outside the wall, i.e. by hernia or adhesions
	Adynamic – cessation of peristalsis, resulting in loss of propulsive force i.e. paralytic ileus.
Etiology	Obstruction of lumen by: A bolus of undigested food, hard feces, gallstones
	Inflammatory strictures of the wall
	Hernia or adhesions outside wall
	Peristalsis inhibition, i.e. paralytic ileus.
Diagnosis	Pain abdomen – colicky in character
	Vomiting – frequency and type of vomitus, depending upon site of obstruction, i.e. to start with gastric contents, next small intestine (biliary) and lastly large intestine (fecal).
	Distension of abdomen – visible peristalsis may be present
	Tenderness – positive
	Rigidity – absent.

Investigation	Plane X-ray abdomen: Shows gas shadows, fluid levels without any gas movement
	TLC and DLC: Leukocytosis – mild/absent.
D/d	Acute appendicitis
	Acute cholecystitis
	Acute renal colic
	Acute pancreatitis
	Acute salpingitis
Management	Conservative treatment:
	Ryle's tube aspiration – to relieve vomiting and distension
	Maintenance of fluid and electrolytes balance
	Antibiotics

- Benzathine penicillin 0.5 mU o.d. IM
- Ampicillin 250–500 mg t.d.s. Children 125–250 mg
- Cefazolin 25–100 mg/kg o.d. IM or IV. Children 25–50 mg/kg o.d.
- Cefotaxime 1–2 g b.i.d. IM or IV
- Kanamycin 0.5–1 g o.d.
- Broad-spectrum antibiotics IV drip

Flatus tube passage

Surgical treatment

Indications	Failure of conservative measures
	Fever – continuation
	Leukocytosis
	Bleeding per rectum

Refer: The patient to the surgical team.

Surgery	Relieving the obstruction and excision of gangrenous bowel and reanastomosis.
Prognosis	Depends upon the causative factor and presence of strangulation.

Acute Intussusception

Definition	A part of the gut gets invaginated into adjacent one – mostly the proximal into the distal.
Etiology	Idiopathic
Factors	Polyp, inverted Meckel's diverticulum, carcinoma.
Diagnosis	A healthy baby – suddenly screaming, followed by vomiting, constipation, followed by passage of blood and mucous per rectum.
	Lump in the abdomen.
Investigation	Plain X-ray abdomen – may show gas shadows in the small gut
	Barium enema study – shows a typical pincer like ending of the barium enema.
Management	Surgery is treatment of choice. **Refer** the patient to the surgical team

Surgery	Operative reduction
After care	Gastric aspiration – for 12–24 hrs.
	Dextrose saline IV or s.c. with hyaluronidase
	Orally fluids/mother's milk on the 2nd day

Acute Salpingitis
Described in Section of Gynecology and Obstetrics Emergencies.

Acute Ectopic Gestation
Described in Section of Gynecology and Obstetrics Emergencies.

Twisted Ovarian Cyst
Described in Section of Gynecology and Obstetrics Emergencies.

Acute Peritonitis

Definition	It is defined as inflammation of the peritoneum. It is a serious disorder, with high mortality.
Etiology	Bacterial infection, i.e. *E. coli*, *Cl. welchii*, Kleb., pneumococci.
	Source of infection, e.g. perforation of GI tract
	Penetrating wound of abdominal wall
	Inflamed appendix
	Intestinal obstruction
	Cholecystitis
	Salpingitis
	Twisted ovarian cyst
Diagnosis	Pain abdomen
	Vomiting
	Fever
	Rigidity of abdominal wall
	Local tenderness
Management	Fowler's position
	Rest to GI tract by:

- Nothing by mouth
- Water intake PO 1 Oz (30 cc)/hr (to be aspirated later on)
- Gastric aspiration via Ryle's tube
- IV fluids and electrolytes

Blood transfusion – if Hb < 70%, plasma transfusion

Antibiotics:

- Benzathine penicillin 0.5 mU o.d. IM
- Ampicillin 250–500 mg t.d.s. Children 125–250 mg
- Cefazolin 25–100 mg/kg o.d. IM or IV. Children 25–50 mg/kg o.d.
- Cefotaxime 1–2 g b.i.d. IM or IV
- Kanamycin 0.5–1 g o.d.
- Broad-spectrum antibiotics IV drip

Treatment of cause

Complications Acute intestinal obstruction

Paralytic ileus

Abscess

Refer: The complicated patient to the surgical team.

Acute Ureteric Colic

Etiology Renal calculus

Diagnosis Pain (agonizing) in the loin, referred to groin

Nausea, vomiting, sweating, hypothermia

Tachycardia

Urinary symptoms – stranguary, hematuria, pyuria, anuria

Local tenderness, abdominal rigidity

Investigation Urine – microscopic examination reveals RBC and a deposit

Plain X-ray abdomen – shows ureteric stone

Pyelography – to visualize the calculus not seen in plain X-ray

Cystoscopy – confirms the diagnosis

CT scan

Management

Conservative Plenty of fluids PO or IV fluids

Antispasmodic

Instrumentation Ureteric catheterization

Surgery Meatotomy

Ureteric lithotripsy – for ureteric stones

Laparoscopic – ureterolithotomy

Laser – for ureteric stones

Dialysis Anuria – persistent.

Refer: The patient to the surgical and dialysis teams.

Acute Pyelonephritis

More common in females, especially soon after marriage and during pregnancy

Diagnosis More common on the right side

Nausea, vomiting, headache

Pain (severe) abdomen

Fever – high

Polyuria with burning pain

Local tenderness, abdominal rigidity

High fever

Pyuria

Investigation   Urine analysis incld.C/S

Management	Alkalinization of the urine:
	IV 10 mL sodium bicarbonate + 10 mL sodium lactate
	Antispasmodic
	Plenty of fluids PO
	Antibiotics:

- Norfloxacin 400 mg b.i.d. PO for 7–10 days
- Nitrofurantoin 50–100 mg q.d.s. PO for 7–10 days.

INJURIES OF LIVER

Liver Rupture

Definition	Is an acute emergency that demands priority attention and treatment.
MOI	Direct – crush injury
	Fall from a height
	Violence – hit by a stick or an iron rod
Pathogenesis	Tears in the liver – found in autopsy report (death case). Mostly tears found on anterior or superior surface
	Rupture of right lobe – more common than left lobe
Diagnosis	Signs of hemoperitoneum with localizing signs of pain abdomen, tenderness, and rigidity in the RUQ, increased area of liver dullness and shifting dullness
Investigation	CBC– leukocytosis or leukopaenia, ESR – raised
	Serum electrolytes estimation
	X-ray abdomen
	CT scan
Management	
General treatment	
	Maintain fluid and electrolyte balance
	Nothing by mouth until acute symptoms have subsided
	IV dextrose infusion
	Blood transfusion – of cardinal importance
	IV potassium supplementation
Specific treatment	
	Surgery: Laparotomy

Refer: The patient to the medical and surgical team.

Wounds of Liver

Definition	Is an acute emergency that demands priority attention and treatment.
MOI	Direct – gunshot injuries and stab wounds
Diagnosis	Appearance:

- Quite – peritonitis
- Restless – hemorrhage

Pulse – rapid

Respiration – high

Rigidity – cogwheel rigidity of the limbs

Pain abdomen

Tenderness, and rigidity in the RUQ, increased area of liver dullness and shifting dullness

Convulsions

Coma, death may occur.

Investigation CBC – leukocytosis or leukopaenia, ESR – raised

Serum electrolytes estimation

CT scan: Diagnostic

Management

General treatment

Maintain fluid and electrolyte balance

Nothing by mouth until acute symptoms have subsided

IV Dextrose infusion

Blood transfusion

IV potassium supplementation

Specific treatment

Surgery: Laparotomy

Refer: The patient to the medical and surgical team.

Hernia

Definition Is defined as protusion of a viscus or portion of a viscus through an abnormal opening. Hernia constitutes a major health problem, irrespective of country, race, or socioeconomic status, and repair of inguinal hernia is one of the commonest surgical procedures worldwide.

Site May occur in any part of the body – external abdominal (commonest).

External abdominal hernia – protusion of a viscus, mostly within a peritoneal sac, through an abdominal wall's weak region.

- Inguinal hernia
- Umbilical hernia/paraumbilical hernia

Femoral hernia

Obturator hernia

Hiatus hernia

Diaphragmatic/epigastric hernia

Hernia in pregnancy

Types Reducible

Irreducible/unreducible (complicated reducible)

Obstructed (complicated irreducible)

Strangulated (complicated irreducible)

Incarcerated (obstructed or strangulated)

Inflammed.

Strangulated Inguinal Hernia

Definition	Is defined as a complicated irreducible inguinal hernia, whereby impaired blood supply to its contents result in imminent gangrene.
	Incidence: Femoral hernia more likely to strangulate, although inguinal hernia is four times more common. May occur at any time during life, and in both sexes. Indirect inguinal herniae strangulate more commonly than direct ones (wide neck of sac).
	Constricting agent: Neck of sac, external abdominal ring, adhesions within sac.
	Contents: Small intestine, omentum, or both, rarely large intestine.
Etiology	Unknown. Incidence: high during infancy, females to males 5:1.
Pathogenesis	(Intestinal obstruction + irreducibility + impaired circulation): Intestinal obstruction and impaired blood supply (initially impeded venous return), intestinal wall congested, serous fluid discharged into sac, intestine appears purpled in color, increased intestinal pressure causing strangulated loop distended, increased venous stasis causing impaired arterial blood supply, sub-serosal acchymoses, blood effusion into the loop, serosa covered by fibrinous exudates, intestinal walls become flabby and friable, due to loss of tone, intestinal vitality lowered, favoring bacterial migration through intestinal wall into fluid in the sac, gangrene of rings of constriction – become deeply furrowed and greyish/greenish, resulting in perforation of intestinal wall. The strangulated mesentery becomes congested and hemorrhagic, its vessels thrombosed, gangrenous, resulting in peritonitis.
Diagnosis	Pain abdomen: Abrupt, paroxysmal, localized over hernial site initially, generalized abdominal pain supervenes sooner, pain increasing in intensity, and with onset of gangrene ameliorates
	Vomiting: Forcible, often repeated
	Abdominal distension – pain ceases (grave significance).
	Hernia: Tense, extremely tender, cough impulse absent.
Varieties	• Strangulated partial enterocele (Richter's hernia): Portion of intestine's circumference involved, usually complicates femoral hernia, local signs of strangulation mostly not visible – vomiting once or twice, colic occurs, diarrhea, or delayed constipation
	• Strangulated omentocele: recurrent attacks of abdominal pain missing, vomiting and constipation mostly absent, delayed gangrene, abscess formed, general peritonitis.
Investigation	CBC, PT, MNPT, INR, Blood sugar
	LFT profile
	PAC serology panel
	RFT
	CK-MB
	CXR

Ultrasound abdomen

ECG

Echocardiography

TMT

PGT

Complications Intestinal perforation, sepsis, gangrene.

Management Emergency surgery.

Pre-operative measures:

Muscular relaxation: By nursing in a warmed bed.

Congestion reduction: By elevation of foot end of bed.

IV fluids

Gastric aspiration

Pre-medication

Surgery: Inguinal herniotomy and herniorrhaphy.

Methods: Open mesh repair v/s laparoscopic procedure

Strangulated Femoral Hernia

Definition Is defined as a complicated irreducible femoral hernia, whereby impaired blood supply to its contents result in imminent gangrene.

Incidence: Femoral hernia more likely to strangulate, although inguinal hernia is four times more common. Femoral hernia is 3rd most common type of hernia, incisional hernia being 2nd. Femoral hernia is very rare before 15th year, female to male ratio is 2:1, more prevalent in the multiparae.

Constricting agent: Neck of sac, external abdominal ring, adhesions within sac.

Contents: Small intestine, omentum, or both, rarely large intestine.

Etiology Unknown

Pathology That the hernia passes down the femoral canal to the saphenous opening, thereby directed forwards due to fascial attachment to the circumference of saphenous opening, pushing the cribriform fascia before it, then curves upwards towards inguinal ligament. The hernia is narrow while in the femoral canal (inelastic), while after passing through saphenous opening becomes enlarged due to laxity of groin tissues. Fully distended femoral hernia assumes shape of a retort, irreducible and apt to strangulate.

Pathogenesis Femoral hernia strangulates frequently and develops gangrene rapidly, due to narrow, unyielding femoral ring, in majority of cases obstructing agent is the narrow neck of femoral sac. Richter's hernia occurs frequently. Obstruction + irreducibility + impaired circulation: Obstruction and impaired blood supply (initially impeded venous return), the strangulated hernia becomes congested and hemorrhagic, vessels thrombosed, gangrenous, resulting in peritonitis.

Diagnosis	Incidence: very rare in younger age (<15 yrs).
	Site: Right side affected more than left side 2:1, and bilateral (20%)
	Symptoms: Less pronounced than of inguinal hernia
	Pain: Dragging type, pain increasing in intensity, ameliorates with onset of gangrene
	Swelling: Commonest complaint, below inguinal ligament
	Local tenderness
	Vomiting: Forcible, often repeated
	Abdominal distension: Pain ceases (grave significance).
	Hernia: expansile cough impulse.
Investigation	CBC, PT, MNPT, INR, blood sugar
	LFT profile
	PAC serology panel
	RFT
	CK-MB
	CXR
	Ultrasound abdomen
	ECG
	Echocardiography
	TMT
	PGT
Complications	Intestinal perforation, sepsis, gangrene.
D/d	Strangulated inguinal hernia (swelling above inguinal ligament).
	Psoas abscess: Fluctuating swelling
	Psoas bursitis: Less apparent with flexed thigh
	Obturator hernia
Management	Emergency surgery (herniorrhaphy).
	Pre-operative measures:
	Muscular relaxation: By nursing in a warmed bed.
	Congestion reduction: By elevation of foot end of bed.
	Femoral trus: highly unsatisfactory (encourages strangulation)
	IV fluids
	Gastric aspiration
	Pre-medication
	Surgery: Herniotomy and herniorrhaphy.
	Methods: Lockwood (low operation)
	McEvedy (high operation)
	Lotheissen (inguinal operation)
	Lotheissen (modified operation).

Strangulated Para-umbilical Hernia

Definition	Is defined as a complicated irreducible para-umbilical hernia, whereby impaired blood supply to its contents result in imminent gangrene, due to narrow neck and fibrous edge of linea alba.
	Incidence: Para-umbilical hernia occurs more commonly in adults, and female to male ratio is 5:1, more prevalent in the obese and flabby multiparae.
	Constricting agent: Narrow neck of sac and fibrous edge of linea alba.
	Contents: Greater omentum, small intestine, and/or portion of transverse colon.
Etiology	Unknown
Pathology	That the hernia enlarges, becomes rounded or oval, passes downwards, the sac becoming loculated due to adherence of its fundus to omentum.
	Fully distended para-umblical hernia become irreducible due to omental adhesions within the sac, apt to strangulate and gangrene.
Pathogenesis	Para-umbilical hernia strangulates frequently and develops gangrene rapidly, due to narrow, unyielding narrow neck of sac.
	Obstruction + irreducibility + impaired circulation: Obstruction and impaired blood supply (initially impeded venous return), the strangulated hernia becomes congested and hemorrhagic, vessels thrombosed, gangrenous, resulting in peritonitis.
Diagnosis	Incidence: Common in adults, women to men 5:1
	Site: Just above or below the umbilicus
	Symptoms: Less pronounced than of inguinal hernia
	Pain: Dragging type, pain increasing in intensity, ameliorates with onset of gangrene
	GI tract: Intestinal colic due to intestinal obstruction, NVD
	Swelling: Commonest complaint, below inguinal ligament
	Local tenderness
	Abdominal distension – Pain ceases (grave significance).
	Hernia: Expansile cough impulse.
Investigation	CBC, PT, MNPT, INR, Blood sugar
	LFT profile
	PAC serology panel
	RFT
	CK-MB
	CXR
	Ultrasound abdomen
	ECG
	Echocardiography
	TMT
	PGT

Complications Intestinal perforation, sepsis, gangrene.
D/d   Strangulated inguinal hernia (swelling above inguinal ligament)
               Psoas abscess: Fluctuating swelling
               Psoas bursitis: Less apparent with flexed thigh
               Obturator hernia
Management   Emergency surgery (herniorrhaphy).
               Pre-operative measures:
               Muscular relaxation: By nursing in a warmed bed.
               Congestion reduction: By elevation of foot end of bed.
               Femoral trus: Highly unsatisfactory (encourages strangulation)
               IV fluids
               Gastric aspiration
               Pre-medication
               Surgery: Herniotomy and herniorrhaphy.
               Methods: Mayo's operation (early cases).
                        Paul-Mikulicz (gangrenous cases).

Practical Procedures
Ultrasonography
Most frequently employed non-invasive imaging technique.

Technique   It consists in transducer translating reflection of sound waves from interfaces
               in tissues into cross-sectional images of normal and abnormal anatomy.
Indications   Pyloric stenosis, intussusception, appendicitis, cholelithiasis.

Magnetic Resonance Imaging (MRI)
Technique   MRI yields images reflecting magnetic differences in body tissue rather
               than difference in X-ray absorption or acoustic reflection. Images are
               obtained in the sagittal, coronal, and axial planes.
Indications   Detecting metastasis
               Assessment for intra-abdominal structures and great vessels.

Computer Tomography (CT) Scan
Technique   It consists in obtaining digitalized cross-sectional images by rapid bursts
               of X-rays during one revolution of both tube and detectors which are on
               opposite sides of patient to be scanned. It allows only limited assessment
               of cardiac structures.
Indications   Evaluation of trauma
               Detecting metastasis.

Nuclear Medicine (Radionuclide Scintigraphy)
Advantage   Nuclear medicine procedures are safe, reproducible and cost-effective.

| Technique | Special imaging devices like gamma cameras and computer system give static or dynamic images. Different compounds labeled with isotope technetium – 99m, utilized to evaluate various organ/ system |

GIT ^{99m} Tc-sulfur colloid orphytate (oral)

Musculoskeletal ^{99m} Tc-MDP

CVS ^{99m} Tc-RBC

GUS ^{99m} Tc-DTPA

Oncology ^{99m} Tc-MDP, 201 thalidium chloride.

Premedication Sedation and immobilization required.

Indication To obtain functional information about various organ systems.

Acute abdomen.

Laparotomy

It is an emergency (diagnostic and therapeutic) procedure

Indications Abdominal injuries

Acute abdomen

Tumors.

Laparoscopy

Technique Under anesthesia, the laparoscope is inserted through small key hole opening. The procedure allows visualization of the organs.

Indications Acute abdomen

Chronic cholecystitis

Removal of tumors.

Other Surgical Procedures

Described in appropriate surgical disorders.

References

1. De Dombal FT: Acute abdominal pain. Scand J Gastroenterol (Suppl) 14:29;1979.
2. Lee PWR: The plain X-ray in the acute abdomen: A surgeon's evaluation. Br J Surg. 63:763;1976.
3. Silen W: Cope's early diagnosis of the acute abdomen. 17th ed. London, Oxford Press, 1987.
4. Staniland JR et al: Clinical presentation of acute abdomen. Study of 600 patients. Br Med J. 2:393; 1972.
5. Valman HB: Acute abdominal pain. Br Med J. 282:1858;1981.
6. Butler C: Surgical pathology of acute appendicitis. Hum Patol 12:870;1981.
7. Schwartz SI et al: Principles of surgery, 5th ed. New York. McGraw-Hill, 1989.
8. Silen W: Cope's Early Diagnosis of the Acute Abdomen. 17th ed. London, Oxford, 1987.
9. Swash M: Hutchison's Clinical Methods 21st Ed. Saunders, London, 2002.

Gynecology and Obstetric Emergencies

Symptoms and signs (non-specific manifestations)
- Gynecology and obstetrics emergencies:
- Vaginal bleeding:
  - Abortion or miscarriage
  - Hydatidiform mole
  - Acute ectopic gestation
  - Antepartum hemorrhage (APH):
    ◊ Accidental hemorrhage (placental abruption)
    ◊ Inevitable hemorrhage (placenta previa)
  - Postpartum hemorrhage (PPH)
  - Abnormal premenopausal uterine bleeding
  - Postmenopausal bleeding
- Vaginal discharge:
  - Leukorrhea
- Vomiting in pregnancy:
  - Hyperemesis gravidarum (pernicious vomiting of poregnancy)
- Acute disorders of menstruation:
  - Premenstrual tension syndrome
  - Primary dysmenorrhea
  - Metrorrhagia
- Traumatic:
  - Injuries to the genital tract:
    ◊ Obstetric injuries
    ◊ Coitus injuries
    ◊ Direct trauma injuries
    ◊ Foreign bodies and instruments injuries
    ◊ Burns injuries
- Inflammatory:
  - Acute salpingitis
  - Acute endometritis
  - Acute cervicitis

- Acute infections:
  - Acute gonorrhea
  - Puerperal pyrexia
- Acute backache in pregnancy
- Toxemias of pregnancy:
  - Pre-eclampsia and eclampsia
  - Essential hypertension in pregnancy
  - Renal disease (nephritis) in pregnancy
- Prolapse uterus (procidentia)
- Endometriosis and adenomyosis
- Gynecologic oncology:
  - Uterine fibroids
  - Carcinoma uterine cervix
  - Twisted (torsion) ovarian cyst
  - Practical procedures:
    ◊ Forceps
    ◊ Cesarean section
    ◊ Episiotomy
    ◊ Induction of labor
    ◊ Induction of premature labor
    ◊ Induction of abortion
    ◊ Dilatation and evacuation (D&E)
    ◊ Dilatation and curettage (D&C)
    ◊ Dilatation of cervix
    ◊ Hysterotomy
    ◊ Cervical cauterization
    ◊ Cervical biopsy
    ◊ Endometrial biopsy
    ◊ Hysterectomy
    ◊ Hysteroscopy
    ◊ Laparoscopy
    ◊ Imaging modalities:
       Plain X-ray abdomen and pelvis

CXR	Transabdominal
Hysterosalpingography	Transvaginal
Hysterosonography/ultrasonography (US)	CT scan
	MRI

Symptoms and Signs (Non-specific manifestations)

Majority of gynecology and obstetric patients, visiting A&E department complain of:

Acute abdominal pain

Vaginal bleeding

Vaginal discharge

Vomiting – during pregnancy

Acute Abdominal Pain

Etiology

A. Gynecology and obstetric causes:

Acute ectopic pregnancy

Acute salpingitis

Torsion ovarian cyst, torsion uterus

Dysmenorrhea

Dysparunia

B. Surgical causes

Acute appendicitis

Acute intestinal obstruction

Acute pancreatitis

Acute cholecystitis

Acute peptic ulcer

Vaginal Bleeding

Etiology

Obstetrical causes

A. In early months of pregnancy (1st and 2nd trimester)

Abortion

Hydatidiform mole

Ectopic gestation

B. In later months of pregnancy (final – 3rd trimester):

Antepartum hemorrhage (APH):

- Accidental hemorrhage (placental abruption) due to premature separation of normally situated placenta
- Inevitable hemorrhage (placenta previa) due to separation of placenta situated in the lower uterine segment

C. During and post-labor

Postpartum hemorrhage (PPH)

Gynecological causes

> Uterine fibroids
> Endometriosis
> Hormonal imbalance
> Cervical erosion
> Cervical polyp
> Cancer cervix

Diagnosis   Past and family history of bleeding per vaginum

> Distension of abdomen
> Pain abdomen with/without vaginal bleeding
> Local tenderness
> Shifting dullness.

Investigation   Complete hemogram

> Blood grouping and crossmatching
> TLC and DLC, ESR, BT and CT
> Urine analysis:
> P/V examination: Avoid vaginal examination (only in theatre)
> Vaginal smears
> Plane X-ray abdomen
> US, CT scan and MRI – as per requirement.

Management

Conservative treatment

> Admit the patient
> Position – Trendelenburg
> IV fluids
> Blood transfusion
> Analgesics and antibiotics
> Hormonal therapy

Surgical treatment: **Refer** the patient to the gynecology and obstetric team for:

Surgery   Dilatation and currettage (D&C). If D&C fails, then Alt.:

> Hysterectomy – especially in postmenopausal cases.

Abortion or Miscarriage

Definition   Interruption of gestation, before the fetus becomes viable, i.e. before 28/52, and thereafter, until full time, being termed as premature labor.

Etiology   Ovular defects: Due to parental disorders

> Uterine defects
> Chromosomal defects
> Placenta and membranes defects
> Immunological factors

Direct trauma, i.e. – instrumentation, RSA and falls

Poor ill-health, malnourishment

Maternal infections – localized acute infections

Advancing age

Endocrinal disturbances, i.e. diabetes mellitus

Hypothyroidism

Poisoning – lead, quinine, ergot, phosphorus, mercury.

Types of Abortions

Threatened

Inevitable: Complete, incomplete and septic

Missed

Habitual or recurrent

Criminal (septic).

Diagnosis   History (incld. S/S) of pregnancy

S/S   Pain abdomen, vaginal bleeding, dilated os and protrusion of the ovum

D/d of different types of abortions

Threatened Abortion: Every abortion is to be considered as threatened, until and unless proved as inevitable.

S/S   Not severe, i.e.

Bleeding – slight and not severe

Pains – mild backache/dull pain.

Inevitable Abortion: It is defined as the clinical abortion, and being considered as inevitable (certain to happen) due to escape of liquor amni or protusion of ovum through the external os.

S/S   Bleeding – excessive

Pains – severe

Dilatation of os by two fingers or more.

Complete Abortion: All of conceptus (fetus, membranes, and decidua) is expelled during first 10/52.

S/S   Of pregnancy disappear

Bleeding per vaginum – occurs, followed by:

Pains (cramps).

Incomplete Abortion: It is defined as an abortion, where the entire products of conception are not expelled due to firm attachment of placenta. Fetus escapes due to rupture of membranes, while placenta remains with parts of membranes and decidua.

S/S   Commonest type during 0–20/52

Pains – subside after expulsion of fetus, while bleeding – continues

Os – remains patent.

Septic Abortion: It is defined as an abortion due to infection of remaining contents inside the uterus, as a result of failure in their expulsion/removal

S/S   Fowl smelling discharge per vaginum after few days

Fever – due to sepsis

         pain abdomen – mild to severe

P/V: Purulent vaginal discharge, tender uterus. Once the contents removed, the discharge ceases, os closes, and condition improves.

Missed Abortion: It is defined as an abortion, where the dead fetus is retained inside the uterus for a variable period.

S/S   Symptoms of abortion appear and disappear, without expulsion of concepts.

S/S of pregnancy disappear

Vaginal discharge

Bleeding and pain – absent

After few weeks, dry-shrivelled conceptus (caverneous mole) is expelled.

Habitual Abortion: It is defined as an abortion, where a woman aborts several times(three or more abortions) due to congenital abnormalities of uterus, retroverted uterus, cervical erosion, cervical polyp, thyrotoxicosis, etc. The woman does not like to have any treatment in her anxiety to have a child.

S/S   Anemia

Palpitation

Investigation   Hemogram – shows anemia

ESR – raised

TLC and DLC – leukocytosis

Cervical/vaginal swab – for culture sensitivity test

Urine analysis includes culture

Pregnancy tests – remain positive for couple of days after fetal death

Plane X-ray abdomen – in late abortion: Shows fetal skeleton and intra-uterine gas

USS – to exclude ectopic gestation and to indicate fetal viability.

D/d   Ectopic pregnancy

Hydatidiform mole.

Complications

Hemorrhage – major cause of maternal death

Infection – especially in criminally induced abortion

Salpingitis, peritonitis, septicemia – causes of death

Perforation of uterus.

Management

Emergency treatment: If abortion has occurred after Ist trimester:

Admit the patient

IV fluids

IV oxytocin in drip – to induce uterine contraction, in order to control blood loss and to help in expulsion of clots and tissues.

Prostaglandins – IM/IV/intra-amniotic, especially in 2nd trimester

- Misoprostol is of choice – cheap, easily available and easy to use.
  Dose: 400 μg sublingual/oral/vaginal. Rpt. 6 hrly up to 4 doses.
- Inj. ergometrine – 500 μg IM, given only in complete abortion

Blood transfusion – to combat shock due to blood loss.

General treatment

Bed-rest

Sedatives

Contraindications for coitus and douches

Antibiotics – especially in septic abortions.

Surgical treatment

Refer: The patient to the gynecology and obstetric team for:

Surgery   Dilatation and evacuation (D&E) to remove the retained concepts

Preoperatively   Start IV oxytocin drip, to avoid uterine penetration.

Management of Different Types of Abortion
Threatened Abortion

Conservative treatment

Bed-rest

Sedatives – diazepam 5–10 mg o.d. PO

- Pentazocine 30–60 mg IM/IV/s.c. 4 hrly.

Progesterone – role is controversial: To be reserved for confirmed cases of progesterone deficiency

Light diet

Liquid paraffin

Avoid sexual intercourse for 2–3/52

Avoid undue exertion

Avoid unnecessary P/V examination

Progress   Many patients – eventually abort.

Inevitable Abortion

Conservative treatment

Normally no treatment required. Nature does the work

Drug: Ergometrine 0.5 mg IM followed by 0.5 mg b.d. PO

Surgical treatment: **Refer** the patient to the gynaecology and obstetric team for surgery.

Indications	Hemorrhage – severe, continuing
	Ovum protruding through the Os
	Infection
Surgery	Dilatation and curettage (D&C)
	IV fluids, blood transfusion.

Septic Abortion Usually incomplete type
Conservative treatment

> Admit the patient
> IV fluids, blood transfusion
> Vaginal swab for culture sensitivity test
> Antibiotics
> Analgesics/hypnotics

For gas gangrene

> Oxygen therapy, antibiotics, blood transfusion, IV fluids

Medical methods

Drugs	Ethacridine – emcredil
	Prostaglandins – prostodine
Doses	Emcredil 0.1% sol. (extraocular instillation) transcervically + prostodin 0.25 mg IM every 3 hrs. Max 10 doses

Surgical methods: **Refer** the patient to the gynaecology and obstetric team for surgery.

| Surgery | Dilatation and curettage (D&C) |

Missed abortion
Conservative treatment

> IV fluids
> IV oxytocin drip
> Antibiotics
> Analgesics/hypnotics

Surgical treatment: **Refer** the patient to the gynaecology and obstetric team for surgery.

Surgery: Avoid surgical treatment. If at all required, then D&C is of choice.

Hydatidiform Mole: It is a degenerative disorder of chorion, characterized by the chorionic villi, forming clusters of varying sized cysts, distended with fluid.

Etiology	Exact cause is unknown.
Predisposing	Age > 30 yrs
	Malnourishment
	Maternal immune mechanism – disturbed
	Past history of hydatidiform moles.
Diagnosis	Amenorrhea – of a short period
	Uterus – comparatively larger for duration of pregnancy.
	Bleeding per vaginum at 6–8/52, irregular in character
	Nausea, vomiting – excessive

Investigations

FSH and LT estimation – titer elevated

Vaginal smear examination – shows cell groupings

X-rays abdomen and pelvis

Ultrasonography

CT scan after 3rd month – shows a honeycomb appearance of uterine contents.

D/d

Hyperemesis gravidarum

Hydramnios

Uterine tumors

Threatened/complete abortion.

Management

Conservative treatment

Admit the patient

IV fluids

Blood transfusion

Antibiotics.

Surgical treatment

Surgery

Dilatation and suction evacuation

D&C: Contraindicated, e.g. risk of perforation of uterus, Alt.:

Hysterotomy

Hysterectomy.

Refer: The patient to the gynaecology and obstetric team for surgery.

Acute Ectopic Gestation

Definition

Any pregnancy occurring from fertilization of the ovum outside uterine cavity (tubal, ovarion, abdominal) is defined as ectopic gestation.

Majority are tubal.

Etiology

Unknown.

Predisposing factors:

Traumatic: Abdominal surgical trauma (tubal surgery)

Inflammatory: Salpingitis, peritonitis

Neoplastic: Pelvic tumors.

Diagnosis

Acute abdominal pain

Bleeding per vaginum (irregular)

Swelling in the hypogastric region (adnexal mass palpable behind uterus)

Local tenderness

Investigation

Hemogram – shows anemia

TLC and DLC – Leukocytosis, serum amylase – elevated

Hormonal tests:

• Pregnancy test – positive/negative

• Serum beta-hCG level – slow rise

Plain X-ray abdomen – shows a pelvic mass

Ultrasonic scanning – diagnostic in early pregnancy

Laparoscopy (diagnostic) – to confirm suspected ectopic gestation.

Complications	Hemorrhage (excessive bleeding per vaginum)
	Shock.
D/d	Acute appendicitis
	Acute pancreatitis
	Acute intestinal obstruction
Management	
Emergency	Admit the patient
	Position – Trendelenburg
	Monitor vital signs
	IV fluids
	Blood transfusion
	Oxygen therapy
	Analgesics – Inj. tramadol HCl IM or IV
	Antibiotics
Surgical	**Refer** the patient to the gynaecology and obstetric team.
Aim	To stop bleeding by removal of products of conception
Procedures	Laparoscopic surgery – removal of products of conception
	– ligation of bleeders

Indication: Esp. indicated, when other tube is absent or diseased

Procedures: Salpingectomy – indicated, if tube is totally damaged

Salpingotomy

Hysterectomy – for interstitial and corneal gestation.

Laparoscopy (diagnostic).

Antepartum Hemorrhage (APH)

Definition	Hemorrhage in later months of pregnancy (final 3rd trimester).
Types	Accidental antepartum hemorrhage
	Inevitable antepartum hemorrhage (placenta previa).

Accidental Antepartum Hemorrhage

Definition	It is defined as bleeding after 28th week of pregnancy, or during 1st and 2nd stages of labor (prior to baby's birth) due to premature separation of normally placed placenta (situated within upper uterine segment).
Etiology	Unknown in majority of cases.
Precipitating	Multiparae
factors	Uterine fibroids
	Congestive heart failure
	Toxemia of pregnancy – essential hypertension
	Anemia

	Trauma: History of accidents – falls, etc.
	Smoking.
Diagnosis	Bleeding per vaginum
	Pain abdomen – severe
	Swelling
	Local tenderness
	Tachycardia
	Hypotension
	Shock.
P/V	Avoid vaginal (P/V) examination – until she is in operation theatre with readiness for cesarean section
Investigation	Hemogram
	Blood grouping and crossmatching
	Urine – albuminuria.

Management

Conservative treatment

Admit the patient

Treatment of shock

IV fluids, blood transfusion

Oxygen therapy

Morphine 10–40 mg IM or diamorhine 10–25 mg s.c., Alt.:

Tramadol HCl 100 mg IM or IV

Shift the patient to operation theatre – if bleeding continues.

Surgical treatment: **Refer** the patient to the gynaecology and obstetric team for immediate delivery in severe cases.

Surgery	Amniotomy (rupture of membranes) Alt.:
	Cesarean section – seldom carried out.
	Inj. ergometrine IM and oxytocin infusion for 2–3 hrs after delivery.

Inevitable Antepartum Hemorrhage (Placenta Previa)

Definition	Bleeding after 28th week of pregnancy, due to the separation of a placenta situated in the lower uterine segment. Uncommon type.
Etiology	Low implantation of ovum due to late growth of trophoblast.
Precipitating factors	Multiparae than primigravidae
	Elder women
	Previous cesarean section
	History of placenta previa.
Diagnosis	Bleeding – severe
	Abdominal examination: Presenting part high and not engaged
	Malpresentations
P/V	Avoid P/V examination – as may cause severe bleeding.

Investigation	Hemogram
	Blood grouping and crossmatching
	Ultrasound scanning
	MRI – helpful in posterior placenta previa.
Management	Admit the patient
	Morphine 10–40 mg IM or diamorphine 10–25 mg s.c., Alt:
	Tramadol HCl 100 mg IM or IV
	IV fluids, blood transfusion
	Monitor the patient
	Shift the patient to operation theatre – if bleeding continues.

Surgical treatment: **Refer** the patient to the gynecology and obstetric team for
Immediate delivery in severe cases.

Procedures	• Amniotomy (rupture of membranes), Alt:
	• Cesarean section – safest method of child's delivery
	IM ergometrine and oxytocin infusion for 2–3 hrs after delivery.

Postpartum Hemorrhage (PPH)

Definition	Excessive bleeding during 3rd stage, i.e. before expulsion of placenta and during first 6 hrs after delivery, while bleeding occurring later than 6 hrs after delivery is called puerperal hemorrhage.
Etiology	Traumatic – injuries during delivery
	Atonic uterus (inertia)
	Blood – coagulation disorders.
Predisposing factors	Multiparity – over distension of uterus
	Malnourishment
	APH
	Obstructed labor
	Mismanagement of 3rd stage
	Initiation/augmentation of fast delivery by oxytocin
	Uterine fibroids.
Diagnosis	Bleeding per vaginum
	Pallor, restlessness, fainting
	Pulse – fast, shock
	Hypotension.
Management	It is a serious emergency and to be treated on priority basis.
Aims	Stimulation of inert uterus to retract
	Removal of uterine contents
	Prevention of blood escape – mechanically.

Emergency treatment

Admit the patient

Oxygen – by facemask

IV lines set up

Blood – for grouping and crossmatching, hemogram, BT and CT

Maintain blood volume – give IV Hartmann's, dextrose saline, or normal saline, or Hemaccel – plasma expander

Blood transfusion

Oxytocin 0.5 ml (5 i.u.) IV infusion @ 1–3 mU/min, immediately post-delivery.

Ergometrine 0.2 mg IM at end of 3rd stage

Monitor BP, pulse, electrolytes, input/output.

Refer: The patient to the gynaecology and obstetric team for:

Control of bleeding promptly by

Manual removal of placenta

    Anesthesia – general

    Position – lithotomy

    Toilet of vulva with antiseptic solution

    Pass gloved right hand gently into uterus, edge of placenta sought for, the left hand on the abdomen – pressing fundus down

    Placenta separated and removed, followed by inj. ergometrine

    After bleeding is controlled, it is advisable to give oxytocin infusion to maintain uterine contraction.

Packing of uterus:

    Anaesthesia – general

    Position – lithotomy

    Toilet of vulva with antiseptic solution

    Catheterize the bladder

    Cervix pulled down by sponge holding forceps

    Packing of uterus and vagina, tightly with sterile gauze

    Antibiotics

    Removal of packs after 24 hrs.

Hysterectomy:

Indications   Bleeding persists

               Placenta accreta

Treatment of traumatic PPH

    Stitching of tears of vulva and vagina, ligation of bleeding arteries.

Abnormal Premenopausal Uterine Bleeding

Definition   Excessive or continuing uterine bleeding during or between periods.

Etiology

During periods

    Menorrhagia (hypermenorrhea) due to:

    Myoma, endometriosis, hypertrophic uterus, blood disorders

    Polymenorrhea – bleeding occurring > once every 24 days

Between periods

Metrorrhagia (irregular bleeding at times other than the normal menstrual period) due to:
- Ovulation bleeding
- Anovulatory bleeding
- Estrogen therapy
- Endometritis
- Tuberculosis
- Hypothyroidism
- Cervical polyps
- Uterine fibroids
- Carcinoma uterine cervix

Diagnosis
History of LMP and PMP

History of any medication received – especially estrogen

Abdomen distension, shifting dullness, edema legs

Local tenderness

Discharge per vaginum.

Investigation
Hemogram, BT and CT

ESR

TFT

Urine analysis

Vaginal smears – for cytological and bacteriological study

Plain X-ray abdomen – to study for any fluid, tumor

Ultrasonography

Hysterosalpingography

Cervical biopsy and curettage study.

Complications Anemia, infection, infertility.

Management

Emergency treatment

Admit the patient

Position – Trendelenburg position

Morphine 10–40 mg IM or diamorhine 10–25 mg s.c., Alt:

Tramadol HCl 100 mg IM or IV

NSAIDs – Mefanamic acid – to reduce blood loss

Danazol – to reduce blood loss. C/I: Pregnancy.

IV fluids, blood transfusion.

Surgical treatment: **Refer** the patient to the gynecology and obstetric team for:

Procedures
Dilatation and curettage (D&C): Is treatment of choice, Alt:

Hysterectomy: Indication: If D&C fails to stop bleeding, women > 40 yrs of age

Pos care
Hormonal therapy: Following D&C, for couple of months:
- Estrogens and progesterones – to control hypermenorrhea.

Post-menopausal Vaginal Bleeding

Definition   Vaginal bleeding that occurs > 6/12 post-menstrual cessation during or between periods.

Etiology   Traumatic

Hormonal imbalance – estrogens misuse

Blood disorders

Polyps, cervical erosions, uterine fibroids, prolapse uterus

Carcinoma – cervical, endometrium

Diagnosis   Bleeding per vaginum – spotting or profuse bleeding

Pain abdomen

Local tenderness.

Investigation   Vaginal fluid examination – for cytologic and bacteriologic study

Aspiration biopsy or suction curettage.

Management   Admit the patient

IV fluids

Antibiotics

Sedatives.

Surgical treatment: **Refer** the patient to the gynaecology and obstetric team for:

Procedures   • Dilatation and curettage, Alt:

           • Hysterectomy – if D&C fails to stop bleeding.

Vaginal Discharge
Leukorrhea (Leucorrhoea)

Definition   White or yellowish vaginal discharge. May occur at any age. It is not a disease, but manifestations of ovulation.

Etiology   Traumatic

Infective:

• *Trichomonas vaginalis*

• *Haemophilus vaginalis*

• *Candida albicans*

• *N. gonorrheae*

Inflammatory

Hormonal disturbance, stress

Neoplastic – benign or malignant.

Diagnosis   Vaginal discharge – with discomfort

Itching, irritation, burning sensation

Dysparunia.

Investigation   Hemogram, TLC and DLC

Vaginal smear – for cytologic and bacteriologic study

Examination of a hanging drop preparation.

Management

Preventive treatment

Use of condom during sexual intercourse. Better avoid coitus till full recovery.

Proper hygiene

Avoidance of extramarital sex

Antibiotics.

Specific treatment: Treatment of causative organism:

A. *Trichomonas vaginalis:*

Metronidazole (flagyl) 200 mg t.d.s. for 1/52 PO

Husband should also take the same course

Tinidazole tab 2 g as single dose or 150 mg b.i.d. PO

Topical providone-iodine (betadine) 200 mg vaginal pessaries

1–2 pessaries per vaginum at night for 2/52

B. *Candida albicans* (thrush) – whitish discharge:

Application of gention violet 1–2% sol, locally to vulva, vagina and cervix b.i.w. for 2–3/52

Condom protection

Mycostatin (nystatin) 0.1 mU vaginal pessaries (suppositories)

1–2 pessaries per vaginum at night for 2/52

Clotrimazole 100 mg vaginal pessaries at night for 1/52

C. *Haemophilus vaginalis:*

Co-trimoxazole (sulphamethoxazole 400 mg+trimethoprim 80 mg) 1 Tab b.i.d. for 1–2/52

Clotrimazole 100 mg vaginal pessaries at night for 1/52

Ampicillin 500 mg q.d.s. for a week PO.

Surgical treatment: **Refer** the patient to the gynecology and obstetric team for:

Procedures Cauterization

Cryosurgery

Bartholinectomy

Vomiting in Pregnancy
Hyperemesis Gravidarum (Pernicious Vomiting of Pregnancy)

Definition It is defined as persistent, severe vomiting and nausea during pregnancy. It may be fatal, if not treated adequately. It is an exaggeration of normal morning sickness.

Etiology Unknown.

Predisposing factors: Physiological and psychological factors.

Diagnosis Vomiting

Nausea – morning sickness

	Onset – commonly during 5–6/52 of pregnancy
	Dehydration, loss of weight
	Jaundice, hemorrhage
	Anuria
	Convulsions, blindness, coma.
Investigation	Hemogram – hemoconcentration, PCV
	Serum electrolytes – Na, K increased, serum proteins decreased
	BUN – increased
	Urine – Ketoneuria, proteinuria
	Fundus examination: Retinal hemorrhages and
	Retinal detachment
	Thyroid function tests (TFTs) – to rule out thyroid dysfunction
	Liver function tests (LFTs) – to rule out liver dysfunction
	Ultrasound – to confirm intrauterine pregnancy.
D/d	Gastric disorders, cholecystitis, hyperthyroidism, diabetes
	Intestinal obstruction, poisoning, infection.
Management	
Conservative	Admit the patient, complete bed-rest
	Nothing by mouth for 48 hrs.
	IV fluids – 5% dextrose saline or normal saline
	Maintenance of electrolyte balance
	Ryle's tube feeding – liquid diet followed by dry diet
Drugs	• Metoclopramide HCl. (perinorm) 10 mg o.d./or t.d.s. IV or IM
	• Prochloperazine (stemetil) 5 mg b.d./or t.d.s. IM.

Obstetric treatment: **Refer** the patient to the gynecology and obstetric team.

Indications	Convulsions, blindness, jaundice, hemorrhage, anuria
Procedure	Termination of pregnancy, i.e. therapeutic abortion
Prognosis	Intractable hyperemesis gravidarum is fatal both to mother and fetus.

Acute Disorders of Menstruation
Premenstrual Tension Syndrome

Definition	It is a monthly abnormality, characterized by retention of fluid and overactivity. It occurs in about 80% of women, mainly during middle age.
Etiology	Exact cause unknown.
Precipitating factors	
	Over-reaction to onset of menstruation
	Hormonal imbalance – hypersecretion of estrogen, progesterone, adrenal corticosteroids
Diagnosis	Young (30–40 yrs) unmarried are more prone
	Psychological – anxiety, stress, agitation, depression, feeling of insecurity
	Nausea, vomiting, diarrhea, constipation

	Headache, backache
	Breast tenderness, weight gain.
Investigation	Hemogram
	Blood sugar – hypoglycemia may be present
	Urine analysis.
D/d	Hyperthyroidism, hyperinsulism, hyperaldosteronism.
Management	
Conservative	Support and reassurance, positive thinking, stress management
	Diet – salt restricted, high protein diet, vitamin B$_6$
	Diuretics along with sedatives for agitated patients, and diuretics along with stimulants for depressed patients
	Hormone therapy: Progesterone supplements
	Estradiol – implants or patch therapy
	Gonadotrophin releasing hormone (GnRH).
Surgery	Ovariectomy and hysterectomy – indicated only in severe cases.

Refer: The patient to the gynecology and obstetric team for surgery.

Primary Dysmenorrhea

Definition	Painful menstruation.
Etiology	Cause unknown.
Predisposing factors	Psychological – usually associated with emotional stress
	Hormonal imbalance – progesterone withdrawal
Diagnosis	Pain abdomen (cramps) – lower abdominal pain
	Nausea, vomiting, headache
	Local tenderness
	Breast engorgement
	Pelvic heaviness
	Irritation
P/R	To rule out any malposition of the genital tract.
P/V	To be avoided in young unmarried patients
Investigation	Hemogram, ESR, C-reactive protein
	Ultrasound, laparoscopy, hysteroscopy.
D/d	Acute pain abdomen.
Management	
Conservative treatment	
	Bed-rest, warm bottle fomentation
	Analgesics:
	• Aspirin, NSAIDs PO
	• Atropine 0.3–0.6 mg IM, Alt:
	• Tramadol HCl 50–100 mg b.i.d. PO or 100 mg IM/IV

Oral contraceptives – to suppress ovulation
- Diethylstilbestrol 0.5 mg orally OD for 14 days beginning Ist day of period or methyltestosterone 5 mg t.d.s, 5th to 10th day for 2–3 months.

Surgical treatment: **Refer** the patient to the gynecology and obstetric team.

Surgery   Dilatation of cervix – indicated in married older women
Pre-sacral sympathectomy – indicated if repeated dilatations fail
Hysterectomy – as a last alternative/choice.

Metrorrhagia

Definition   It is defined as an acyclic bleeding from the uterus. It may be intermittent or continuous, and is superimposed on a normal menstrual cycle (during intervals between menstrual periods).

Etiology   Hormonal changes – triggering ovulation
Neoplastic – carcinoma cervix, endometrium, cervical polyps, cervical erosion, tumors of vagina and vulva.

Diagnosis   Bleeding per vaginum – mid-menstrual
Pain abdomen – cramps
Anxiety, stress.

Investigations   CBC
BBT charting
PAP smear examination
D&C – endometrial curettage
Ultrasonography
Hysteroscopy.

Management

General   Assurance to patient – to alleviate her anxiety
Drugs – combined oral contraceptives.

Emergency   IV fluids, blood transfusion

Refer: The patient to the gynecology and obstetric team for surgery.

Surgery   D&C – treatment of choice
Hysterectomy – indicated in intractable bleeding in women >age 50.

Injuries to the Genital Tract

Types   Obstetric injuries – common during childbirth
Gynecological injuries – rare
Traumatic injuries – rare.

MOI   Obstructed labour – causing tears of perineum, vagina, cervix, uterus
Coitus (esp. forced one, e.g. rape case) – causing tears of hymen, vagina, perineum
Antenatal – tear of uterus due to rupture of a previous cesarean section scar
Direct – falls astride gates, stairs, chairs, automobiles
Foreign bodies/instrumentation – vaginal tears by use of pencil, knitting needle, sound, bougies, for attempted criminal abortion

Burn injuries – by use of chemicals (e.g. lysol), douching at high temperature, or by cautery/diathermy during cervical cauterization

Induction of labor by oxytocin drip.

P/V	Under anesthesia and with great care – to feel the rent.
Management	
Preventive	Good obstetric practice: Most of the obstetrical injuries are preventable, e.g. by recognising the probable causes of obstructed labor during pregnancy and timely treated by cesarean section.
Specific	Hemorrhage – control by packing
	IV fluids, blood transfusion
	Analgesics.
Surgery	**Refer** the patient to the gynecology and obstetric team for surgery.
	Tears/lacerations – suturing under anesthesia
	Foreign bodies – removal under anesthesia
	Burns – extensive scarring requires cosmetic surgery
	Perforation of uterus – small perforation requires repair
	– large perforation requires hysterectomy (laparoscopic surgery).

Acute Salpingitis   It is a common gynecologic problem and may be unilateral or bilateral.

Etiology	Bacterial infection: Gonococci, streptococci, tubercular
	Forceps delivery
Diagnosis	Severe abdominal pain in the hypogastrium, non-radiating
	Fever – high with chills
	Leukorrhea
	History of abortion
Investigation	TLC and DLC – leukocytosis
	ESR – raised
	Culture of vaginal discharge
D/d	Acute appendicitis
	Acute ectopic gestation
	Acute intestinal obstruction

Management

Conservative treatment

Antibiotics
- Ampicillin 250–500 mg t.d.s.
- Cefazolin 25–100 mg/kg o.d. IM or IV
- Cefotaxime 1–2 g b.i.d. IM or IV
- Kanamycin 0.5–1 g o.d.
- Broad spectrum antibiotics IV drip
- Metronidazole (flagyl) 400 mg b.i.d. PO for 1/52
- Antitubercular drugs for tubercular salpingitis:
  - Streptomycin 1 g o.d. IM for 3/12

– Isoniazid 150–300 mg o.d. PO for 3/12
– PAS 10–20 g o.d. PO for 3/12 ·

Analgesics   Analgesics/hypnotics

Surgical treatment: **Refer** the patient to the surgical team for surgery.

Indications   For failure of conservative treatment

Surgery
- Incision drainage – of pelvic abscess
- Dilatation and curettage – of excessive bleeding per vaginum
- Excision – of tumor

Acute Endometritis

Definition   Inflammation of the endometrium of the uterus.

Etiology   Infective – due to septic abortion, gonorrhea, puerperal sepsis, instrumentation, IUC devices.

Diagnosis   Fever – high
Vaginal discharge – purulent
Menstruation – excessive
Uterus – enlarged, tendered
Peritonitis
Septicemia.

Investigations   CBC
TLC and DLC
Endometrial curettage.

Management

Conservative treatment
    Antibiotics
    Analgesics
    Avoid instrumentation
    Removal of IUC device.

Surgical treatment: **Refer** the patient to the gynecology and obstetric team for:

Surgery   Hysterectomy – rarely and in extreme cases.

Acute Cervicitis

Definition   Inflammation of uterine cervix
Commonest of all gynecological disorders.

Etiology   Infective: Bacterial: Gonococci, streptococci, E. coli, claustridia
    Traumatic: Obstructed labor, instrumentation.

Diagnosis   Vaginal discharge (leukorrhea)
Low backache
Pain abdomen – in the hypogastrium.

Investigation   Hemogram – shows anemia
TLC and DLC – shows leukocytosis
Vaginal smear – for cytologic and bacteriologic study.

Management
Conservative treatment:

Antibiotics:
- Ampicillin 250–500 mg t.d.s.
- Cefazolin 25–100 mg/kg o.d. IM or IV
- Cefotaxime 1–2 g b.i.d. IM or IV
- Kanamycin 0.5–1 g o.d.
- Broad-spectrum antibiotics IV drip
- Metronidazole (flagyl) 400 mg b.i.d. PO for 1/52

Avoid instrumentation

Sulphonamide creme – locally for 5 days

Oestrogen therapy: Diethylstilbestrol 0.1 mg B.D. for 2/52, beginning 1st day of menstruation.

Surgical treatment: **Refer** the patient to the gynecology and obstetric team for:

Surgery
- Cauterization – with silver nitrate 5% sol or electric cautery
- Cryosurgery
- Hysterectomy – rarely and in extreme cases.

ACUTE INFECTIONS

Acute Influenza   Described in Pediatric Emergency Section

Chickenpox   Described in Pediatric Emergency Section

Rubella   Described in Pediatric Emergency Section

Measles   Described in Pediatric Emergency Section

Scarlet Fever   Described in Pediatric Emergency Section

Typhoid Fever   Described in Pediatric Emergency Section

Infective Hepatitis Described in Pediatric Emergency Section

Cholera   Described in Emerging and Re-emerging Emergency Section

Acute Poliomyelitis Described in Pediatric Emergency Section

Dengue Fever   Described in Emerging and Re-emerging Emergency Section

Acute Malaria   Described in Emerging and Re-emerging Emergency Section

Acute Gonorrhea

Definition	It is a venereal disease contracted during sexual intercourse and rarely by use of infected water bath, towels, or clothing.
Etiology	*Neisseria gonorrhoeae* – gram-negative diplococcus.
Transmission	Bacterial entry through the urethra.
Incubation	2–8 days.
Diagnosis	Infection contracting rate: Females/males – 3:1
S/S Male	Burning micturation, purulent discharge, prostatitis.
Female	Vaginal discharge – purulent, pruritis, dyspareunia, dysuria
	External genitalia – enlarged, tendered

External urinary meatus – erythmatic

Bartholinitis, vaginitis.

Complications	Urethritis, dysmenorrhea, dyspareunia, pelvic abscess, infertility.
Investigations	Smear (Gram-stained) examination of urethral discharge
	Culture – on blood agar, or on Thayer Martin medium.
Management	
Preventive	Sexual abstinence (avoid sex with unknown partner)
	Better use the condom – reduces the risk.
Specific	Antibiotics:

- Penicillin – procain G 4.8 million units IM + probenecid 1 g PO, or
- Ampicillin 250–500 mg t.d.s.
- Cefazolin 25–100 mg/kg o.d. IM or IV
- Cefotaxime 1–2 g b.i.d. IM or IV
- Kanamycin 0.5–1 g o.d.
- Broad-spectrum antibiotics IV drip
- Metronidazole (flagyl) 400 mg b.i.d. PO for 1/52

General	Bed-rest
	Hot sitz baths
	Short-wave diathermy
	Truss support to the scrotum
	Physiotherapy.

Puerperal Pyrexia

Definition	It is defined as maternal temperature > 38°C post-delivery, i.e. during two weeks after delivery.
Cause	Infective: Urinary tract infection (UTI)
	Genital tract infection (GTI)
	Chest infection
	Wounds infection – cesarean, perineal
	Causative bacteria: *E.coli, Proteus, Klebsiella, Streptococcus, Staphylococcus, Clostridium*
	Inflammatory: DVT, mastitis
Diagnosis	History of obstructed labor, operative delivery, prolonged rupture of membranes, leukorrhea
	Fever, malaise
	Tachycardia
	Hypertension/hypotension
	Breasts – engorged, tendered
	Legs – edematous, tendered
	Perineum – swollen, tendered.
P/V	Uterus – enlarged, tendered.

Investigation	Hemogram
	Blood culture
	Swabs for bacterial culture – from wounds, discharging nipples, cervix
	Urine – midstream urinalysis for bacteriuria, and culture
	CXR.

Management

Conservative treatment

Admit the patient

IV fluids

Antibiotics:

- Penicillin – procain G 4.8 million units IM + probenecid 1 g PO, or
- Ampicillin 250–500 mg t.d.s.
- Cefazolin 25–100 mg/kg o.d. IM or IV
- Cefotaxime 1–2 g b.i.d. IM or IV
- Kanamycin 0.5–1 g o.d.
- Broad-spectrum antibiotics IV drip
- Tetracyclines – avoid if breastfeeding
- Amoxycillin 500 mg t.d.s or q.d.s. PO
- Metronidazole 400 mg b.i.d. PO for 1/52
- Augmentin 1.2 g IV or intermittent infusion 6–8 hrly × 2/52

Surgical treatment: **Refer** the patient to the gynecology and obstetric team.

Surgery	Incision drainage of breast, pelvic, or wound abscess.

Backache in Pregnancy

Very common complaint during pregnancy.

Etiology	Postural changes – with advancing pregnancy.
Diagnosis	Local tenderness positive
	Movements painful and restricted.
Management	Bed-rest
	Avoid – forward bending, prolonged standing, high heeled shoes
	Corset wearing, massage, sleeping on a firm mattress
	Analgesics
	Physiotherapy.

Toxemias of Pregnancy

Definition	It is a group of disorders occurring commonly during last trimester of pregnancy or early in the puerperium. This group has 3 common clinical features, e.g. hypertension, edema, and albuminuria, and is responsible for high maternal mortality rate, and for large number of stillbirths, or neonatal deaths.
Types	Pre-eclampsia
	Eclampsia
	Essential hypertension
	Renal disease.

Pre-eclampsia and Eclampsia

Definition	Defined as different degrees of the same condition.
Pre-eclampsia	Defined as a multi-system disorder, characterised by hypertension, edema, and albuminuria.
Incidence	It is the commonest amongst toxemias (75%) of pregnancy.
Eclampsia	It is defined as pre-eclampsia complicated with convulsions and/or coma.
Etiology	Unknown.

Predisposing factors:

Malnutrition, CVS and renal disease, sodium retention

Primigravidae

Family history of hypertension, diabetes

Obesity

Hydatidiform mole.

Diagnosis	Mild degree of toxemia – mostly remains undetected
	Nausea, vomiting, headache, agitation, vertigo, malaise
	Visual impairment – blurring, blindness
	Hypertension
	Edema
	Albuminuria
	Convulsions, coma.
D/d	Primary hypertension
	Renal disease
	Neurological disease.
Investigation	Hemogram – hemoconcentration
	Blood uric acid – increased
	BUN – increased
	Ophthalmoscopic examination shows:

• Papilledema, retinal hemorrhages, retinal detachment.

Management of Pre-eclampsia

Aims
• To prevent development of eclampsia from pre-eclampsia
• To prevent permanent cardiovascular and renal damage
• To deliver a normal healthy baby.

Preventive treatment

Adequate antenatal care

Control of weight

Control of blood pressure

Control – prevention/treatment of anemia.

Specific treatment:

Admit the patient, bed-rest

Monitor – BP, pulse, respiration, urine analysis – proteins, serum electrolytes, input/output charting

Diet – salt restricted, low fat, high carbohydrate.

Drugs	Sedatives/tranquilizers/anticonvulsants:

Sedatives/tranquilizers/anticonvulsants:
- Diazepam 5–10 mg o.d. PO or IV

Others:
- Alprazolam 0.25–0.5 mg b.i.d.
- Chlordiazepoxide 10–30 mg PO
- Lorazepam 1–4 mg o.d. PO
- Phenobarbitone 60–180 mg t.d.s. PO
- Phenytoin sodium 100 mg b.i.d. PO

Diuretics:
- Frusemide 40 mg o.d. PO, Alt:
- Hydrochlorthiazide 25 mg o.d. PO

Antihypertensive drugs:
- Diazoxide (hyperstat) 300 mg IV. It is a fast acting vasodilator, without affecting (decreasing) cardiac output or renal circulation, used especially in toxemia of pregnancy

Others:
- Methyldopa (aldomet) 500 mg IV. Maint 250–500 mg b.i.d. PO
- Hydralazine 5–20 mg IM. Repeat – every 2–4 hrs
- Amlodipine besylate 5–10 mg o.d. PO

Obstetric care: **Refer** the patient to the obstetric team.

Mild pre-eclampsia: BP < 160/100 mm Hg

  Treatment: Bed-rest, normal safe delivery

Severe pre-eclampsia: BP > 160/100 mm Hg

  Treatment: Bed-rest, diuretics, hypotensive drugs, normal delivery

Very severe (imminent eclampsia) BP > 60/100 + headache, nausea, vomiting

  Treatment: Admit the patient

  Sedative – IV pentothal to control fits

  Hypotensive drugs

Obstetric treatment: Termination of pregnancy

Procedures	Rupture of membranes – patient at term
	Cesarean section – patient not at term.

Management of Eclampsia

Emergency care	Admit the patient and treatment given on top priority basis.

Turn her on her side, to prevent aspiration of saliva, vomitus

Airway maintenance – Endotrachial intubation

              – Ventilator – oxygen therapy

Aspiration of fluid and food, etc. from the trachea

Convulsive patient – nothing by mouth, IV fluids

Monitor input/output 24 hrly

Diet – if able to drink and eat, then give fluids and salt restricted diet

Drugs	Sedatives/tranquilizers/anticonvulsants:

- Pentothal 0.25 to 0.5 g in 10 ml 20 mg of 20% sol. IV infusion

Maint phenobarbitone 60–180 mg b.d.s. PO, Alt:
- Magnesium sulphate 10 ml of 20% sol IV. Rept 6 hrly, Alt:
- Diazepam 5–10 mg IV. Maint 5–10 mg o.d. PO,

Others:
- Alprazolam 0.25–0.5 mg t.d.s. PO
- Chlordiazepoxide 10–30 mg PO
- Lorazepam 1–4 mg o.d. PO
- Phenytoin sodium 100 mg b.i.d. PO

Diuretics:
- Frusemide 40 mg o.d. PO, Alt:
- Hydrochlorthiazide 25 mg o.d. PO

Antihypertensive drugs:
- Diazoxide (hyperstat) 300 mg IV. It is a fast-acting vasodilator, without affecting (decreasing) cardiac output or renal circulation, used especially in toxemia of pregnancy.

Others
- Methyldopa (aldomet) 500 mg IV. Maint 250–500 mg b.i.d. PO
- Hydralazine 5–20 mg IM. Repeat – every 2–4 hrs
- Amlodipine besylate 5–10 mg o.d. PO

Obstetric care	Termination of pregnancy.

Refer: The patient to the obstetric team for termination of pregnancy.

Procedures	Rupture of membranes – if patient at term.
	Cesarean section – if patient not at term
Prognosis	Fetal mortality:
	Etiology: Immaturity, asphyxia, intrauterine death
	Maternal mortality:
	Etiology: Eclampsia, accidental hemorrhage, renal failure

Essential Hypertension in Pregnancy

Definition	A condition characterized by a sustained hypertension, that contributes in toxemia of pregnancy.
Etiology	Unknown.
Diagnosis	Hypertension (BP 140/90), edema, albuminuria.
Investigation	Monitor: BP, pulse, respiration.
Management	In majority of patients as the disease is detectable in early pregnancy, it is easier to manage.
Treatment	
Emergency care	Admit the patient and treatment given on top priority basis.
	Turn her on her side, to prevent aspiration of saliva, vomitus
	Airway maintenance – Endotrachial intubation
	– Ventilator – oxygen therapy

Aspiration of fluid and food, etc. from the trachea

Convulsive patient – nothing by mouth, IV fluids

Monitor input/output 24 hrly

Monitor BP

Diet – if able to drink and eat, then give fluids and salt restricted diet

Adequate rest, sound sleep

Control of obesity

Monitor fetal growth: Failure of growth – poor prognosis for baby

Drugs Sedatives/tranquilizers/anticonvulsants:
- Pentothal 0.25 to 0.5 g in 10 ml 20 mg of 20% sol. IV infusion Maint phenobarbitone 60–180 mg b.d.s. PO, Alt:
- Magnesium sulphate 10 ml of 20% sol IV. Rept 6 hrly, Alt:
- Diazepam 5–10 mg IV. Maint 5–10 mg o.d. PO,

Others:
- Alprazolam 0.25–0.5 mg t.d.s. PO
- Chlordiazepoxide 10–30 mg PO
- Lorazepam 1–4 mg o.d. PO
- Phenytoin sodium 100 mg b.i.d. PO

Diuretics:
- Frusemide 40 mg o.d. PO, Alt:
- Hydrochlorthiazide 25 mg o.d. PO

Antihypertensive drugs:
- Diazoxide (hyperstat) 300 mg IV. It is a fast acting vasodilator, without affecting (decreasing) cardiac output or renal circulation, used especially in toxemia of pregnancy

Others
- Methyldopa (aldomet) 500 mg IV. Maint 250–500 mg b.i.d. PO
- Hydralazine 5–20 mg IM. Repeat – every 2–4 hrs
- Amlodipine besylate 5–10 mg o.d. PO

Obstetric care **Refer** the patient to the obstetric team.

Procedures Normal safe delivery – in majority of patients at term

Termination of pregnancy – associated pre-eclampsia, fetal mortality rate high.

Renal Disease (Nephritis) in Pregnancy

It is a rare complication of pregnancy.

Etiology Hypertension, eclampsia, infection.

Diagnosis Hypertension, edema, albuminuria.

Investigation Urine – for albumin.

Management Admit the patient, bed-rest

Sedatives

Monitor BP, pulse, input/output charting

Diuretics

Hypotensive drugs

Antibiotics.

Obstetric care	**Refer** the patient to the obstetric team.
Procedure	Termination of pregnancy
Prognosis	Poor.

Prolapse Uterus (Procidentia)

It is a common disorder seen in women of menopausal age and having born children.

Etiology   Trauma: Childbirth injury – commonest cause, and due to laxity of endopelvic fascial support

Laxity: Of abdominal and pelvic muscles especially at menopause.

Precipitating factors

Obstructed labor

Faulty use of forceps, before full dilatation of the cervix

Lacerated injury of perineal body

Multipara

Heavy weight lifting

Chronic constipation

Pelvic mass

Trauma – surgical, e.g. hysterectomy

Menopause – estrogen deficiency.

Diagnosis   Feeling of some mass (swelling) descending in the vagina or protruding beyond introitus

Low backache

Pain abdomen

Vaginal discharge

Uncontrolled micturition

Constipation.

P/V examination: With patient bearing down – show downward movement of prolapsed uterus and cervix.

Management

Preventive treatment

Active exercises during antenatal period

Proper care of bladder

Avoidance of obstetric trauma – as much as possible, an episiotomy should be preffered especially in primigravidae

Posterior vaginal wall and perineal tears must be sutured post-delivery

Postnatal exercises are helpful

Proper spacing between pregnancies.

Specific treatment

Conservative treatment

> Use of pessary – in those patients, where operative treatment is contraindicated. It has some reservations, e.g.
> - Never curative and can only be palliative
> - Chances of infection – vaginitis
> - Chances of bleeding
> - May be discomfortable
>
> Physiotherapy – Pelvic floor exercises
> - Electric stimulation of pelvic floor muscles
> - Hormone replacement therapy (HRT).

Surgical treatment: **Refer** the patient to the gynecology and obstetric team.

Preoperative care

> - Shave and prepare the external geitalia – an evening before the operation
> - An enema in the same evening
> - Catheterize the patient before start of operation
> - Patient in lithotomy position
> - Anesthesia – general

Surgery

> Type of operation depends upon the prolapsed structures, i.e.
> - Anterior and posterior colporrhaphy – for vaginal prolapse without prolapse of uterine vault
> - Anterior and posterior colporrhaphy with suburethral and bladder neck buttressing by the pubo-vesicocervical fascia – for vaginal prolapse with stress incontinence
> - Fothergill's (Manchester) operation – for vault prolapse descent
> - Mayo's vaginal hysterectomy, for uterovaginal prolapse with uterine symptoms
> - Posterior colporrhaphy – for rectocele.

After care

> Nursing care
> Physiotherapy.

Endometriosis and Adenomyosis

Definition

> Abnormal growth of endometrium outside the uterine cavity is called endometriosis, while infiltration of endometrium into the uterine muscles called adenomyosis.

Etiology

> Disorder of the childbearing period
> Implantation factor – reflux of menstrual endometrium
> Metastatic factor – embolization of menstrual fragments through vascular or lymphatic routes
> Metaplastic factor – metaplastic changes in the embryonic cell
> Hormonal factor – rarely seen in pre-puberty or post-menopausal

Risk factors

> Polymenorrhagia
> Retroverted uterus

Diagnosis	Uterine bleeding
	Dysmenorrhea
	Dyspareunia
	Rectal bleeding
	Pain abdomen
	Dysuria
	Hematuria

P/V examination: Tendered masses in the uterus

Investigation	Ultrasound – helpful in diagnosis
	Laparoscopy – confirms the diagnosis.
D/d	Pelvic inflammatory conditions
	Tuberculosis of genital tract.
Investigation	Hysterography – confirms of adenomyosis
	Diagnostic laparotomy – very helpful in diagnosis.
Management	Encourage young married women with endometriosis, to become pregnant at the earliest

Hormonal therapy – in case the patient does not want a child:
- Enovid 2.5 mg o.d. for 1/52, then 5.0 mg o.d. for 2/52 to control bleeding
- Danazol – androgenic steroid to attain amenorrhea
  Dose: 200–800 mg o.d. for 6/12
  S/E: Hirsutism, weight gain

Analgesics.

Surgical treatment: **Refer** the patient to the gynecology and obstetric team.

Surgery	Laparoscopic (operative) surgery:

- Myomectomy
- Salpingo-oophorectomy
- Hysterectomy – abdominal

Post-care	Hormonal replacement therapy (HRT) – estrogen.

Gynecologic Oncology
Uterine Fibroids

It is the commonest cancer of female genital tract. It is a round, firm, benign tumor.

Etiology	Unknown.

Predisposing factors: Cervicitis, cervical erosion, endometriosis.

Diagnosis	Pain abdomen – in the hypochondrium or pelvis
	Bleeding P/V: Hypermenorrhea, metrorrhagia, dysmenorrhea
	Vaginal discharge – leukorrhea
	Uterus – enlarged.
Investigation	Hemogram – polycythemia, anemia
	Plain X-ray abdomen – may show calcification.
D/d	Uterine gestation
	Uterine bleeding
	Cervicitis

Management

Emergency treatment

> IV fluids
> Blood transfusion
> Analgesics
> Antibiotics
> Myomectomy

Specific treatment

Surgical treatment

Refer: The patient to the obstetric and gynecology team for surgery:

Surgery   Indications: Large, rapidly growing, symptomatic fibromas

> Procedures: Myomectomy – during childbearing age
>> Hysterectomy – Abdominal or vaginal
>>> Total or subtotal
>> Subtotal – not of much value for leaving cervix

Radiotherapy   For non-surgical cases (surgery contraindicated).

Carcinoma Uterine Cervix

Etiology   One of the commonest cancer (2nd to breast and colon)

> More common in multipara
> More difficult to treat
> Mortality rate very high.

Type   Squamous cell carcinoma – 95%

> Adenocarcinoma   – 5%

Pathogenesis   Appears first in the epithelial layers. Then it penetrates the basement membrane and invade tissues (causing ulceration and spotting) resulting in vaginal discharge and excessive uterine bleeding.

Diagnosis   Bleeding per vaginum – especially in post-menopausal age

> Discharge per vaginum – blood-stained, and of foul smelling
> Pain – usually a late feature, due to infiltration of adjoining tissues
> Anemia – due to blood loss
> Anorexia, loss of weight

P/V   To examine cervix for bleeding, induration, infection.

Investigation   Vaginal smears: For cytological examination (Papanicolaou).

> Positive – suggestive of carcinoma
> Schiller's test: Helpful in diagnosis in early carcinoma of cervix and helpful in excluding carcinoma in case of cervical erosion
> Cervical biopsy: Confirms clinical diagnosis
> Colposcopic examination: May be helpful in the diagnosis
> CXR: May show metastases.

D/d   Cervicitis, cervical erosion, cervical polyp

> Endometriosis
> Ectopic gestation.

Management

Preventive treatment

Improved personal hygiene

Avoidance of sexual intercourse at an early age

Avoidance of extramarital intercourse especially with an unknown person

Regular cancer screening of all women

Prompt treatment of cervical lesions, i.e. epithelial anaplasia and dysplasia

Prompt treatment of vaginitis, cervicitis.

Vaccine   HPV (human papillomavirus vaccine)

Types   Bivalent and quadrivalent vaccines

Action
- Acts against 70% of cervical cancer and 90% of genital warts
- Acts against vaginal and vulva intraepithelial neoplasia
- Benefits women of all ages (sexually active)

Doses   3 doses given over a period of 6/12, e.g.:

1st dose at elected date, 2nd dose after 2/12, 3rd dose after 4/12.

Emergency treatment:

Admit the patient

Control of bleeding by:
- Vaginal packing
- Radiotherapy (irradiation therapy)
- Ligation/suturing – usually non-feasible, but ligation of uterine/ hypogastric arteries – life saving measure
- Local ablation methods: Cryocautery, electrodiathermy, cold- regulator, carbon dioxide laser vapourization

Specific treatment: Treatment is either surgical or radiotherapy.

Refer: The patient to the surgical and radiotherapy teams.

Factors   Advanced cancers are unsuitable for surgical treatment

Non-invasive carcinoma (Stage 0):
- Total hysterectomy – is treatment of choice. Alt:
- Radiotherapy – in poor surgical risk cases

Invasive carcinoma:
- Radiotherapy – is treatment of choice. Irradiation helps in:
- Destruction of carcinoma within pelvis
- Preservation of healthy tissues

All stages of cancer may be treated by the method, with the comparatively fewer complications than with surgical treatment.

Cases unsuitable for irradiation are better treated by surgery.

Prognosis   Early diagnosis – better results with treatment, i.e.:

Surgical treatment (ST)

Radiotherapy (RT)

Combination of surgery and radiotherapy

Late diagnosis – poor results with either of treatment.

Twisted (Torsion) Ovarian Cyst

Definition	It is a common serious complication, demands priority treatment.
Etiology	Unknown
Predisposing factors	Trauma
	Inflammation
	Cysts – parovarian and broad ligament cysts
	Tumors – ovarian
Pathogenesis	Due to rotation, the veins in the pedicle get compressed, the tumor gets congested, hemorrhagic, peritoneal irritation, pedicle necrosis peritoneal adhesions.
Diagnosis	Pain abdomen – severe, referred to loin, rigidity of abdominal wall
	Pulse rate – rising
	Temperature – unchanged
Investigation	Plain X-ray abdomen
	Ultrasonic scanning
	Laparoscopy (diagnostic).
Management	Surgery (laparotomy) is the treatment of choice.

Refer: The patient to the gynecology and obstetric team for surgery.

Surgery	Ovariectomy.

Practical Procedures

Obstetrics	Forceps
	Cesarean section
	Episiotomy
	Induction of labor: Medical, amniotomy, oxytocin drip infusion
	Induction of abortion: Rupture of membranes, hysterotomy
	Dilatation of cervix
	Dilatation and curettage (D&C)
	Dilatation and evacuation (D&E)
	Hysterotomy – abdominal and vaginal
Gynecology	D&C
	Cervical biopsy cauterization
	Endometrial biopsy
	Hysterectomy
	Endoscopy:
	• Hysteroscopy
	• Laparoscopy
	• Salpingoscopy
	• Colposcopy
	Imaging modalities:
	• Plain radiography
	• Plain X-ray abdomen

- CXR
- Hysterosalpingography
- Ultrasonography
- Transabdominal ultrasound
- Transvaginal ultrasound
- CT scan
- MRI

Forceps

Definition	It is a pair of instruments designed to extract the fetal head, in order to assist delivery of the fetus, in an obstructed labor.
Indications	• Faulty powers, e.g. uterine inertia • Faulty passages, e.g. cervix not fully dilated, rigid perineum, contracted pelvis • Faulty child, e.g. large head, malpositions such as face • Dangers to the mother, e.g. accidental hemorrhage, eclampsia, placenta previa, heart disease, tuberculosis • Dangers to the child, e.g. cord prolapse, fetal distress.
Essential conditions	• Cervix fully dilated • Suitable attitude and position of the head • Membranes must be ruptured • Bladder and rectum to be evacuated.
Operation varieties	• Low forceps: Forceps applied to the head lying on the perineum, with head's maximum circumference below the ischial spines. • Mid forceps: Forceps applied to the head lying in the cavity, with head's maximum circumference is at or near the ischial spines. • High forceps: Forceps applied to the head lying at the brim, with head's maximum circumference has not crossed the brim. Disadvantage: It is a difficult operation, dangerous to child/mother.
Technique	Cephalic application: The blades of the forceps to be applied over the sides of the fetal head. Much safer for the child. Pelvic application: The blades of the forceps lie parallel to the sides of the pelvis.
Anesthesia	General
Appliance	Simpson's long forceps – cephalic and pelvic curves. Used as the standard forceps for routine purpose. Simpson's short forceps – cephalic curve only. Wrigley's forceps – a short curved forceps, with reduced weight. Kielland's forceps – a short pelvic curve, and without lock.
MO action	Traction Head compression Head rotation

Leverage

Dilatation of the passages

Uterine contractions stimulation.

Complications   Trauma: Maternal – labial, vaginal, perineal tears

Fetal – facial bruising, facial nerve palsy.

Cesarean Section

Definition   It is defined as an operation, whereby the fetus by the end of 28th week is delivered by cutting through the abdominal and uterine walls.

Indications   Faulty cephalopelvic proportion

Faulty passages: Contracted pelvis, rigid cervix, cancer cervix, vaginal atresia, stenosis

Faulty powers – uterine inertia (faulty uterine contraction)

Malpresentations – cord prolapse, breech, brow, shoulder or transverse lie

Poor obstetric history

Previous cesarean section, hysterotomy, or myomectomy

Fetal distress

Postmortem cesarean – to save life of baby if it is still alive

APH – placenta previa

Toxemias – pre-eclampsia, eclampsia, hypertensive crises

Endocrinal – diabetes mellitus,

Elderly primigravidity

Infective – maternal infections, e.g. herpes, HIV

Investigation   Complete hemogram

Blood grouping and crossmatching

X-ray pelvis – AP view

Ultrasound – to localize the placenta in case of a repeat section, so as not to take risk of severe hemorrhage.

Anesthesia   General.

Types   Lower segment

Upper segment (classical operation).

Lower segment operation

Advantages   Extraperitoneal operation

Less bleeding

Postoperative infection – uncommon

Preoperative   Shave and prepare the part by painting the skin with iodine and spirit bladder emptied by a soft rubber catheter, kept till end of operation.

Technique
- Skin incision: Midline, between umbilicus and pubes
- A transverse incision through the uterovesical fold of peritoneum
- Exposure of the lower segment by retracting the bladder
- A small transverse incision through the lower segment down to the membranes

- Membranes perforated, and gushing out liquor aspirated
- Incision of lower segment extended laterally by scissors/fingers
- The child delivered, and the cord clamped in two places and cut between them
- Placenta removed manually
- Inj. ergometrine IV given
- Muscle of lower segment sutured by continuous no. 2 chromic catgut
- Uterovesicle fold of peritoneum sutured by continuous no. 0 catgut
- Skin sutured by interrupted silk.

Upper segment operation:

Indications	• Placenta previa
	• Transverse lie
	• Pre-eclampsia.
Technique	• Skin incision: Paramedian, beginning 5–7.5 cm above the umbilicus, extending downwards for about 15 cm
	• The incision placed high to save the bladder
	• The uterus opened by a midline longitudinal incision
	• The membranes perforated, and gushing out liquor aspirated
	• The child extracted, and the cord clamped and cut between clamps
	• Placenta removed manually
	• Inj. ergometrine IV given
	• Wounds closed in layers.

Episiotomy

Definition	It is defined as an operation, whereby the perineum and the posterior vaginal wall incised, during labor, so as to avoid stretching of the pelvic floor- resulting in tears. It is one of the commonest obstetric procedure performed.
Indications	Primigravidae
	Cephalopelvic disproportion
	Perineum – rigid
	Malpresentations – breech, face
	Forceps delivery.
Essential Conditions	Perineum – bulging
	Scalp – showing.
Technique	Anesthesia: Local
	Two fingers inserted into the vagina
	Incision: From mid-point of perineum, in a posterolateral direction
	Suturing of the wound, soon after delivery of placenta.

Induction of Labor

Definition	It is defined as initiation of uterine contractions by medical, surgical, or combined methods, to facilitate vaginal delivery.

Induction of Premature Labor

Indications
- Contracted pelvis
- APH – placenta previa and accidental hemorrhage
- Polyhydramnios
- Toxemias of pregnancy
- Medical disorders – diabetes, heart disease, nephritis, tuberculosis

Methods

Medical induction
- Oxytocin IV infusion 4 mU/min, with increase every 30 min, i.e. up to 32 mU/min
- Prostaglandins orally or intravaginally – more effective.

Surgical induction
- Rupture of membranes (amniotomy) – by a toothed artery forceps or by an induction catheter (Drew-Smythe's) with puncturing stylet followed by stimulation of uterus – by oxytocin infusion (pitocin/or syntocinon in dextrose)

Complications: Trauma: Maternal, fetus, placental.

Induction of Postmature Labor

Indications
- Contracted pelvis, uterine inertia
- Cephalopelvic disproportion
- Toxemias – pre-eclampsia, eclampsia, essential hypertension.

Induction of Abortion

Indications
- Abortion: Threatened abortion, missed abortion
- Hydatidiform mole
- Hydramnios
- Hyperemesis gravidarum
- Toxemias of pregnancy
- CHF
- Infective: Tuberculosis, HIV

Methods During first 12/52: Dilatation and evacuation (D&E)
Dilatation and curettage (D&C)
During 12–28/52: Hysterotomy (abdominal)
After 28th week: Induction of premature labor.

Dilatation of Cervix

Indications Dysmenorrhea

Method Anesthesia: General
- Position: Patient placed in the lithotomy position
- Toilet of the external genitalia and vagina
- Sims' speculum introduced into the vagina

- Cervix pulled down by a volsellum forceps applied to the anterior lip of cervix
- Uterine sound introduced into cervical canal, to assess the depth and direction of uterine canal
- The cervix dilated with Hegar dilators.

Dilatation and Evacuation (D&E)

Indications
- Termination of pregnancy (TOP)
- Abortion – Incomplete, inevitable
- Hydatidiform mole.

Method
Anesthesia: General
- Position: Patient placed in the lithotomy position
- Toilet of the external genitalia and vagina
- Sims' speculum introduced into the vagina
- Cervix pulled down by a volsellum forceps applied to the anterior lip of cervix
- Uterine sound introduced into cervical canal, to assess the depth and direction of uterine canal
- The cervix dilated with Hegar dilators
- A plastic aspiration cannula attached to a vacuum device is introduced into uterus through uterine canal, and oxytocin given to reduce blood loss. Uterus is evacuated of pregnancy
- Curette the uterine cavity with a curette
- Reintroduce the cannula to suck out any remnants
- Place a sterile vulval pad.

Dilatation and Curettage (D&C)

Indications
- Abnormal premenstrual uterine bleeding
- Post-menopausal bleeding
- Threatened abortion
- Inevitable abortion
- Septic abortion
- Hydatidiform mole
- APH
- To establish presence of ovulation
- To confirm a suspicion of endometrial cancer

Method
Anesthesia: General
- Position: Patient placed in the lithotomy position
- Toilet of the external genitalia and vagina
- Sims' speculum introduced into the vagina
- Cervix pulled down by a volsellum forceps applied to the anterior lip of cervix

- Uterine sound introduced into cervical canal, to assess the depth and direction of uterine canal
- Cervix dilated with Hegar dilators, starting with smaller no. until it admits no. 12–14
- Inj. methergin 0.2 mg IV
- Curette introduced (with sharp pointed and blunt border ends) and the uterine cavity curetted with care not to perforate uterus
- Ovum forceps introduced to remove the conception product
- Packing forceps introduced for packing sterilized gauze to control any excessive bleeding.

Complications Traumatic – uterine perforation.

Hysterotomy (Abdominal)

Definition   It is a miniature cesarean section, and now is rarely used for TOP

Indications
- Termination of pregnancy (TOP)
- Abortion – incomplete, inevitable
- Hydatidiform mole
- Severe hyperemesis gravidarum
- Toxemias of pregnancy
- CHF.

Cervical Cauterization

Indication
- Cervical erosion
- Cervical polyp
- Uterine bleeding.

Method   Anesthesia: General
- Patient placed in the lithotomy position
- Toilet of external genitalia and vagina
- Sims' speculum introduced into the vagina
- Cervix pulled down by a volsellum forceps
- Cauterization of the affected part.

Cervical Biopsy

Indications   Suspicious areas felt or seen on the cervix.

Method   Anesthesia: General
- Patient placed in the lithotomy position
- Toilet of external genitalia and vagina
- Sims' speculum introduced into the vagina
- Cervix pulled down by a volsellum forceps
- Excise a piece of suspected tissue
- Histopathological examination of the excised tissue.

Endometrial Biopsy

Indications	To establish the presence of ovulation
Method	Anesthesia: General

- Position: Patient placed in the lithotomy position
- Toilet of the external genitalia and vagina
- Sims' speculum introduced into the vagina
- Cervix pulled down by a volsellum forceps
- Cervix dilated with Hegar's dilators
- Endoscope (fibreoptic telescope) introduced into the uterine cavity
- Strips of endometrium removed from body of uterus
- Examination of endometrium removed and aspirated materials.

Hysterectomy

Indications

- Dysfunctional uterine bleeding (DUB)
- Uterine fibroids.

Method   Anesthesia: General or spinal

Preoperative: Catheterize the bladder

- Position: Patient placed in Trendelenburg position
- Skin incision: Midline or paramedian
- Uterus drawn out of the wound
- In case of healthy Fallopian tubes and ovaries: Ovarian ligament, fallopian tube and round ligament, exposed, and divided between clamps, placed near cornu of uterus.
- Same procedure carried out on the opposite side. Uterovesical pouch of peritoneum exposed by pulling uterus upwards and backwards.
- A transverse incision into uterovesical pouch, extending from the round ligament of one side to round ligament of opposite side, thus opening up of the broad ligaments of two sides, facilitating separation of the bladder from the front of cervix.
- Uterine vessels along the lateral borders of uterus exposed and divided between clamps.
- Vagina opened up from lateral sides
- Cervix separated from the vagina
- Uterus removed, and vagina packed from above with gauze
- Wound closed in layers.

Complications Hemorrhage; wound infection; UTI; prolapse uterus

Hysteroscopy

Indications

- Viewing the cavity of uterus
- Endometrial biopsy
- Fibroids (submucous) – resection.

Method   Anesthesia – local/general

Preoperative: Catheterize the bladder
- Position: Patient placed in Trendelenburg position
- Toilet of the external genitalia and vagina
- Sims' speculum introduced into the vagina
- Cervix pulled down by a volsellum forceps
- Cervix dilated with Hegar's dilators
- Endoscope (fibreoptic telescope) introduced into the uterine cavity.

Laparoscopy

Indications
- Diagnostic – Pelvic pain
  - – Infertility
- Therapeutic – Sterilization
  - – Pelvic lesions treatment
  - – Ectopic gestation
  - – Hysterectomy.

Imaging Modalities

Plain X-ray Abdomen and Pelvis: Currently have a minor role

Indications
- Foreign body – to confirm its presence and exact location
- IUCD – to locate a misplaced IUCD.

CXR

Indications
- Tuberculosis – for diagnostic purpose
- Metastatic – for diagnostic purpose
- Preoperatively.

Hysterosalpingography

Indications
- Infertility – to test the tubal patency
- Uterine abnormalities – to detect fibroids, polyps, septate uterus
- Abortions (habitual) – to study the status of internal os

Method
Anesthesia: General
- Toilet of the external ganitalia and vagina
- A radiopaque dye (50% diodone + polyvinyl alcohol in water)
  Injected through a cannula into cervical canal under direct vision with the X-ray screen

Note
Hysterosalpingography is being replaced by hysterosonography (ultrasound).

Hysterosonography/Ultrasonography (Ultrasound)

Indications
- Obstetrical: Assessment of gestational age, fetal status, multiple pregnancy, placental status
- Gynecological: Assessment of swellings, bladder status, anal status.

Types
Transabdominal, transvaginal, transperitoneal or transrectal.

Transabdominal Ultrasound

Method	Performed on a patient with a full bladder, as the distended bladder displaces the bowel loops and thereby provides a window for clear visibility of the pelvic structures.

Transvaginal Ultrasound

Method	Vaginal ultrasound visualization, while the uterine cavity is filled with saline, to obtain views
Advantages	Full bladder – not required
	Better imaging.

Computed Tomography (CT) Scan

Indications
- Abscess – to diagnose an intra-abdominal abscess
- Thrombophlebitis – to diagnose pelvic vein thrombophlebitis
- Metastatic – to study myometrial infiltration in endometrial cancer
  - to identify local recurrence and parametrial infiltration in cervical cancer
  - to identify intrahepatic metastasis and regional lymph nodes in ovarian cancer.

Magnetic Resonance Imaging (MRI)

Indications
- Pregnancy– to differentiate maternal and fetal tissues
  - to study fetal physiology and pathology
- Infertility – to assess the pelvic structures
- Fibroids – to confirm the position and size
- Cervical Cx – staging and assessment of pelvic neoplastic disorders
- Uterus Cx – staging.

References

1. Silen W: Cope's Early Diagnosis of the Acute Abdomen. 17th ed. London, Oxford, 1987.
2. Steer ML, Silen W: Diagnostic procedures in gastrointestinal hemorrhage. N Engl J Med 309:646; 1983.
3. Valman HB: Acute abdominal pain. Br Med J 282:1858;1961.
4. Cope E: Physiology of abnormal bleeding. Brit Med J 2:573;1971.
5. Procope BJ: Etiology of postmenopausal bleeding. Acta Obstet Gynec Scandinav 50:311;1971.
6. Barchet S: A new look at vaginal discharges. Obst Gynec 40:615;1972.
7. Kelso JW, Funnell JD: Combined surgical and radiation treatment of invasive carcinoma of the cervix. Am J Obst Gynec 116:205;1973.
8. Whetham JCG, Bean JLM: Carcinoma of the endometrium. Am J Obst Gynec 112:339;1972.
9. Overstreet EW: Clinical aspects of endometrial polyps. S Clin North America 42:1013;1962.
10. Stearns HC: Uterine myomas: Clinical and pathologic aspects. Postgrad Med 51:165;1972.
11. Molitor JJ: Adenomyosis: A clinical and pathologic appraisal. Am J Obst Gynec 40:28;1972.
12. Myerscough PR: Genital Prolapse. Practitioner 208:470;1972.
13. Fraser AC: Surgical treatment of acute pelvic sepsis. J Obstet Gynec Brit Common 79:560, 1972.

14. Fullerton WT: Dyspareunia. Brit Med J 2:31;1971.
15. Herzberg BN, et al: Oral contraception, depression and libido. Brit Med J 3:495;1971.
16. Richards MT: Uterine curettage as an office procedure. Canad MAJ 107:133;1972.
17. Andras EJ, et al: Radiotherapy of carcinoma of the cervix following simple hysterectomy. Am J Obst Gynec 115:647;1973.
18. Samuelsson S, Sjovall A: Laparoscopy in suspected ectopic pregnancy. Acta Obst Gynec Scandinav 51:31;1972.
19. Pahe EW: On the pathogenesis of pre-eclampsia and eclampsia. J Obstet Gynaec Brit Common 79:883;1972.
20. Marshall BR: Emergency room vacuum curettage for incomplete abortion. Reprod Med 6:177;1971.
21. Li MC: Trophoblastic disease: Natural history, diagnosis and treatment. Ann Int Med 74:102;1971.
22. Jacob SJ: Rupture of the uterus: A study of 52 cases. J Obstet Gynaec India 21:22;1971.
23. Gaither D, Clark JFJ: Pregnancy and latent diabetes. J Nat Med A 65:139;1973.
24. Wallace JF, Petersdorf RG: Urinary tract infections. Postgrad Med 50:138;1971.

Bibliography

1. Johnstone RW: Operative Obstetrics. A Text Book Of Midwifery. Adam And Charles Black London 527–79;1965.
2. Howkins J: Shaw's Textbook of Gynaecology. 8th ed. J & A. Churchill Ltd. London, 1962.
3. Arulkumaran S, Symonds IM, Fowlie A: Oxford Handbook of Obstetrics and Gynaecology. Oxford University Press, New Delhi, 2004.
4. Swash M: Hutchison's Clinical Methods. 21st ed. Saunders London, 2002.

Eye (Ocular) Emergencies

Symptoms and signs (non-specific manifestations)
Eye emergencies:
- Traumatic – contusions (syn. black eye)
  - Lacerations
  - Burns and chemical injuries
  - Retinal detachment
  - Foreign bodies

- Inflammatory
  - Acute conjunctivitis
  - Acute corneal ulcer (purulent keratitis)
  - Acute glaucoma (angle-closure)
  - Sympathetic ophthalmitis (sympathetic uveitis)
  - Practical procedures

Symptoms and Signs (Non-specific manifestations)

Vision – any disturbance of vision, e.g. blurred vision
– any complaint of halos around lights, flashes
Eye-strain (pain) – irritable, dullache, or severe headache
Discharge from eye(s) – watery, or purulent
Diplopia – traumatic, inflammatory or infective.

Contusions (syn. Black Eye)

MOI   Direct violence: Hit by a stick
                Sports injury: Boxing
                             Hit by a flying cricket/hockey ball
                Mine injury: Hit by a flying stone
                RSA.
Lesions   Simple abrasion to rupture of the globe.
Diagnosis   Pain
                Swelling
                Subconjunctival hemorrhage
                Injured cornea, sclera, iris and ciliary body, lens, vitreal hemorrhage, retinal
                hemorrhage.
Management
Conservative treatment
                Bed-rest
                Bandaging of injured eye, analgesics.

Surgical treatment: **Refer** the patient to an ophthalmologist for surgery.
Surgery: Suturing of the ruptured globe.

Lacerations (Perforating Injuries)

These are potentially serious emergencies, thereby demand priority treatment.

MOI	Direct violence: Hit by a stick, sharp instrument, foreign bodies
	Sports injury: Boxing
	Hit by a flying cricket/hockey ball
	Mine injury: Hit by a flying stone
	RSA.
Site	Usually eyelids, conjunctiva, cornea, sclera, lens, vitreous or retina.
Diagnosis	Lacerated wound
	Pain
	Discharge.
Investigation	Slit-lamp examination – especially of the anterior segment
	X-ray – for radiopaque foreign bodies location

Management

Conservative treatment

Conjunctival wounds heal readily

Toilet of wound with warm water

Instill antibiotic ointment, e.g. achromycin eye ointment

Bandage the eye.

Surgical treatment: **Refer** the patient to an ophthalmologist for surgery, so as to avoid permanent notching.

Surgery   Removal of foreign body.

Suturing of:
- Lid lacerations (except lacerations of margin).
- Corneoscleral wounds.

Excision of the eye – for vitreous, iris and cilliary body, in order to avoid risk of sympathetic ophthalmitis.

Burns and Chemical Injuries

MOI	Burns: Due to steam, boiling water, hot ashes, caustics, acids, alkalies.
Diagnosis	Acute conjunctivitis
	Cornea – may be normal or opaque.
Investigation	Instill a drop of fluorescein solution – reveals the extent of injured area.
Management	• Caustics injury: Remove deleterious material, at the earliest possible

- Acids injury: Wash with dilute alkalies, e.g. sodium bicarbonate 3% solution
- Alkalies injury: Wash with weak acids, e.g. boric acid or milk or wash with water, abovesaid chemicals, if nothing available at hand
- Instill an antibiotic ointment, e.g. achromycin eye ointment
- Instill corticosteroid ointment/drops – to reduce acute inflammation.

Refer: The patient to an ophthalmologist, until and unless fluorescein staining reveals no corneal damage and the surrounding conjunctiva appears normal and painless.

Retinal Detachment

Etiology	Direct trauma
	Hemorrhage – vitreous.
Diagnosis	Flashes of light – initially
	A cloud in front of *eye*
	Diminution in vision.
Investigation	Ophthalmoscopy – indirect
Management	

Refer: The patient to an ophthalmologist for surgical treatment.

Surgery
- Approximating the torn retina to choroid by diathermy or laser, or
- Approximating the choroids to retina by scleral resection.

Foreign Bodies

Types	Conjunctival and corneal.

Conjunctival Foreign Body

Diagnosis	Pain
	Irritation.
Management	Under local anesthesia
	Evert the eyelid
	Remove the foreign body with the help of a wet cotton swab
	Instill antibiotic ointment, e.g. achromycin eye ointment.

Corneal Foreign Bodies

Diagnosis	Pain
	Irritation.
Investigation	When foreign body not visible, then instill a drop of fluorescein into conjunctival sac.
Management	Under local anesthesia
	Remove the foreign body with a wet cotton applicator
	Instill antibiotic ointment, e.g. achromycin eye ointment
	Corneal opacity if formed then:

Refer: The patient to an ophthalmologist.

Acute Conjunctivitis

Etiology   Infection:
- Bacterial: *Staphylococcus aureus, Streptococcus pneumoniae, Haemophilus influenzae, Neisseria gonorrhoeae,* Ps. pyocyanea, E. coli
- Viral: Adenoviruses, herpes virus, *Lymphogranuloma venereum*
- Fungal – actinomycosis, rhinosporidosis, etc.

Unhygienic

Allergy

Foreign body.

Mode of transmission: Contaminated fingers, handkerchiefs, towel.

Diagnosis	Eye – Red, inflamed
	– Painful
	– Discharge of water or pus
	– Feel – a sandy, gritty feel in the eye.
Investigation	Culture sensitivity test.
Management	Self-limiting disorder
	Washing of eye with warm water
	Instil antibiotic eye drops/ointment – achromycin eye ointment
	Antibiotics – systemic
	Analgesics
	Use goggles while moving outdoors.

Refer: The patient to the next ophthalmology clinic.

Acute Corneal Ulcer (Purulent Keratitis)

Definition	It is an emergency that requires prompt treatment
Etiology	Traumatic – direct trauma, fall from height, foreign body
	Infective:

- Bacterial, e.g. gonococcal, pneumococcal, diphtheria, pseudomonas and staphylococcal
- Viral, e.g. herpes simplex
- Fungal, e.g. actinomycosis
- Allergic – hay fever.

Diagnosis	Eye – red, inflamed, painful,
	– lacrimation – watery or purulent discharge
	– feel – a sandy, gritty feel in the eye
	– vision -- blurred
	– photophobia.
Complications	Perforation of ulcer, hemorrhage, prolapsed of iris, lens dislocation, corneal opacity (scar) – nebula, macula or leucoma
Investigation	Culture sensitivity test
Management	

Conservative treatment

	Washing of eye with warm water
	Instill antibiotic eye drops/ointment (achromycin eye ointment)
	Atropine drops/ointment t.d.s/or q.d.s.
	Cortisone drops/ointment – to control severe reaction
	Antibiotics – systemic
	Analgesics
	Rest and protection – by use of a pad and bandage.
Cauterization	To control ulcer's progress
Method	By use of carbolic acid/trichloracetic acid (10–20%)

Surgical treatment: **Refer** the patient to an Ophthalmologist

Surgery
- Paracentesis – aqueous evacuation to prevent perforation
- Optical iridectomy – to improve vision in case of dense leucoma
- Keratectomy – to shave off a superficial scar
- Keratoplasty (corneal grafting) – to fill up defect with corneal graft
- Prolapse iris – to be abscised.

Acute Glaucoma (Closed Angle)

Definition
: Defined as a type of optic neuropathy characterized by increased intra-ocular pressure, with decrease in the visual field.

Etiology
: Primary: Cause is unknown
Secondary: Causes are:
- Traumatic – blockage by intraocular hemorrhage
- Inflammatory – blockage of circulation by synechie
- Lens disorders – blockage by cataract, injured swollen lens
- Metabolic – venous engorgement by IO tumors

Precipitating factors: Pupil dilatation by:
- Misuse of mydriatics, by the patient or physician
- Misuse of cycloplegics (atropine or scopolamine) by the anesthetist.
- Stress, anxiety, overexcitement, over-work

Pathogenesis
- An obstruction to the drainage of aqueous through the angle of anterior chamber
- An increased hydrostatic pressure in the ocular capillaries
- An increased aqueous humor protein.

Diagnosis
: Pain – severe pain in the eye, headache, nausea, vomiting
Blurring of vision, appearance of halos around lights due to accumulation of fluid in the cornea
Eye – highly congested
- Lids, conjunctiva, ciliary, iris – congested, red, edematous
- Cornea – hazy
- Anterior chamber – shallow
- Pupil – moderately dilated
- Reaction to light and accommodation – absent
- Intraocular pressure – raised (tested manually and by tonometre)
- Loss of vision
- Pulse – irregular

D/d
: Acute conjunctivitis, acute iritis, corneal abrasion and cataract

Investigation
: Tonometry – to test intraocular pressure
Slit lamp examination – to assess the state of angle
Stress tests:
- Dark room test: Patient kept in a dark room for ½ hr. He must remain awake so the pupils dilate.

Interpretation: Measuring of tension before and after may show
Rise > 8 mm is pathological
- Water drinking test: Patient drinks 1 litre of water, before meals.
Interpretation: Rise > 6 mm is pathological
- Mydriatic test: Pupil dilated by a mydriatic agent.
Interpretation: Pupil dilatation and raised IOP within 2 hrs.

Management   It is an emergency and needs priority treatment.
Medical treatment
Drugs   Parasympathomimetics: To constrict pupil (miosis):
- Eserine (anticholinesterase) 1–2% sol. To be instilled with:
  – Pilocarpine (acetylcholine-like drug) 1% to be instilled at 5 mts intervals for ½ hr and then ½ hrly until miosis is achieved, e.g. the corneal clearance and reduced intraocular pressure
- Beta-blockers: To decrease intraocular pressure (IOP):
  – Timolol 0.5% eyedrops. 1 drop b.i.d.
  – Others: Betaxolol, levobunolol
- Carbonic anhydrase inhibitors: To decrease IOP by reducing sodium bicarbonate and fluid in the aqueous humor
- Acetazolamide 250–500 mg o.d. PO

Dehydration   IV mannitol 1.5 g/kg PO – to lower intraocular pressure, or measures
- Glycerol 1.5 g/kg PO – to lower intraocular pressure
Analgesics – morphine 2.5 mg IV or tramadol HCl 100 mg IV/IM

Surgical treatment: **Refer** the patient to an ophthalmologist for surgery.

Preoperatively   Inj procain 4% plus adrenaline injected into ciliary ganglion, lowers tension as well as relieves pain and anxiety

Surgery   Iridectomy – surgical and laser types

Laser   Yag laser used, iridectomy of other eye also done in the same sitting
iridectomy

Surgical iridectomy: In case of failure of laser iridectomy

Trabeculectomy: Indicated in chronic angle glaucoma with presence of posterior synechiae

Sympathetic Ophthalmitis (Sympathetic Uveitis)

Definition   It is the much dreaded disorder in which serious inflammation attacks the sound eye after injury of the other one.

Etiology   Unknown

Risk factors   Trauma – perforating injury especially of ciliary body, iris and lens
Foreign body (lodged within the eye), e.g. gunshot, stone, glass
Infection
Allergy.

Diagnosis   Age – common in children but may occur at any age
Onset – 4–8/52 post-trauma to the 1st eye.

S/S	Sensitivity to light
	Blurred vision
	Lacrimation
	Ciliary injection
	Local tenderness of eyeball
	Vitreous opacities
	Blindness – bilateral.
Management	It is one of the most difficult problem and demands priority care.
Preventive	Enucleation (removal) of the damaged (injured) eye
	Cortisone drops or ointment
	Systemic corticosteroids – to control inflammation
	Drugs – prednisone and prednisolone.

Practical Procedures

Visual acuity:
- Testing distal vision – by Snellen's test
  Patient sitting at 6 meter distance
  Patient to read letters from illuminated view box
  Normal distal vision 6/6 (can read all letters)
- Testing near vision – by reading test types

Visual fields:
- Testing by a perimeter

Color vision:
- Testing by plates having multicolored dots

Refraction test for ascertaining optical power of an eye:
- Testing by neutralizing lenses with a retinoscope

Ophthalmoscopy:
Direct and indirect ophthalmoscopy
- Testing by examiner's head light source, focussed on a lens held in front of patient's eye

Slit lamp
- Testing an optical section of eye's structures and to detect foreign bodies in the anterior segment

Fundus: Testing optic disc and choroid status

Tonometry: Testing the intraocular pressure – with fingers and by a tonometer

Ultrasonography: Testing retinal detachment and tumors

CT scan and MRI

References

1. Percival SPB: A decade of intraocular foreign bodies. Brit J Ophth 56:454;1972.
2. Paton D, Goldberg MF: Injuries of the Eye, the Lids, and the Orbit: Diagnosis and Management. Saunders, 1970.
3. Tredici TJ: Management of ophthalmic casualties in Southeast Asia. Mil Med 133:35;1968.
4. Thygeson P, Dawson CR: Trachoma and follicular conjunctivitis in children. Arch Ophth 75:3;1966.

Bibliography

1. Duke Elder S: Parson's Diseases of the Eye. 15th ed. Williams and Wilkin.

Ear, Nose and Throat (ENT) Emergencies

Symptoms and signs (non-specific manifestations)
ENT emergencies
- Traumatic
  - Nasal fracture
  - Epistaxis (syn. nosebleed)
  - Ruptured drum
- Allergic – allergic rhinitis (syn. hay fever)
- Inflammatory
  - Acute sinusitis
- Acute tonsillitis
  - Peritonsillar abscess (syn. quinsy)
  - Ludwig's angina
  - Acute otitis media
  - Acute mastoiditis
- Foreign bodies – in the air and food passages

Practical procedures
- Tracheostomy

Symptoms and Signs (Non-specific manifestations)

Ear	Earache
	Discharge – watery/purulent
	Deafness
	Any hearing loss
	Tinnitus – any ringing sensation
	Vertigo – any hallucination of movement
Nose	Sneezing
	Discharge – watery
	Stuffiness
Throat	Sore throat, cough, expectoration

Emergencies
Nasal Fracture

Prone to injury due to prominent exposed nasal position

Etiology	Direct trauma – direct blow
	Fall on to the face.
Diagnosis	History of injury
	Swelling
	Local tenderness
	Deformity – nasal deviation

	Difficulty in breathing
	Epistaxis
Investigation	X-ray face – to rule out other bony injuries
	CT scan.
Management	Resuscitate and treat the associated head injury
	Toilet of the skin wounds
	Analgesics

Refer: The patient to ENT surgeon – if there is continuing hemorrhage, septal hematoma, or deviated nose.

Epistaxis (syn. Nosebleed)

Site	Little's area.
Etiology	Trauma
	Infection
	Hypertension
	Blood dyscrasias
	Nasal tumor.
Diagnosis	Nasal bleeding
	Signs/symptoms of underlying cause.
Management	Make the patient sit up, with head bent, e.g. chin touching chest
	Pinching of the nose
	Packing of nose with cotton moistened with hydrogen peroxide, phenylepherine
	Cauterization.

Ruptured Drum

MOI	Direct trauma – hard slap on the ear, syringing
	Foreign body.
Diagnosis	Pain
	Bleeding from ear
	Tinnitus
	Deafness.
Investigation	Examination – shows subtotal or attic perforations
Management	Toilet of the ear – clear the blood clots, etc. gently with ear bud
	Avoid syringing of ear and eardrops
	Watch the patient's condition daily
	Analgesics
	Antibiotics – in case of infection.

Refer: The patient to ENT surgeon for surgery.

Surgery	Tympanoplasty.

Allergic Rhinitis (syn. Hay Fever)

Etiology	History of allergy, mostly dust, pets, especially in children having repeated colds.
Diagnosis	Nasal discharge (watery)
	Sneezing
	Nasal congestion (blocking)
	Difficulty in breathing
	Eyes – red and discharging
	Headache, fever, malaise.
Investigation	TLC and DLC – eosinophilia.
Management	Shift the patient to a dustproof room
	Isolation from pets, e.g. dogs, cats, rabbits.
	Analgesics, e.g. disprin or paracetamol orally
	Sedatives – to relieve tension
	Antihistaminics
	Corticoids – required in severe hay fever.

Acute Sinusitis

Etiology	History of upper respiratory catarrh (URC)
	Allergy.
Diagnosis	Pain, headache, fever, malaise
	Nasal stuffiness
	Nasal congestion.
Investigation	X-ray sinus – shows cloudiness
	TLC: Leukocytosis
Management	Bed-rest
	Steam inhalation
	Analgesics, sedatives
	Antihistaminics
	Nasal decongestants
	Antibiotics.

Surgical treatment: **Refer** the patient to the ENT team for surgery.

Surgery	Drainage.

Acute Tonsillitis

Etiology	Infection, e.g. streptococcal infection (air-borne).
Diagnosis	Sore throat, pain, headache, fever, anorexia, malaise
	Tonsils – red, edematous, pus over tonsils
	Cervical lymph nodes – enlarged, tendered.
Investigation	TLC and DLC – leukocytosis
	Throat swab for culture sensitivity test.

Management   Bed-rest, semi-liquid diet
              Warm saline water gargles, lozenges
              Analgesics
              Antibiotics.
Spontaneous resolution within 5–7 days.

Chronic Tonsillitis

Definition   Repeated attacks of tonsillitis.
Diagnosis   Sore throat, pain, headache, malaise
                 Tonsils – red, edematous, pus over tonsils
                 Cervical nodes – enlarged
Investigation   TLC and DLC – leukocytosis
                 Throat swab for culture sensitivity test.
Management
Surgical treatment: **Refer** the patient to the ENT team for surgery.
Surgery   Tonsillectomy.
Indications   Repeated attacks of tonsillitis
                 Systemic diseases, e.g. cardiac disease, rheumatism, nephritis, diabetes,
                 allergic throat, asthma, hemophilia.

Peritonsillar Abscess (syn. Quinsy)

Etiology   It is a complication of acute tonsillitis due to local spread of infection.
Bacteria   Streptococci, staphylococci, pneumococci.
Diagnosis   Sore throat, pain, headache, dysphagia, fever, malaise, swelling.
Investigation   TLC and DLC – leukocytosis
                 Throat swab for culture sensitivity test.
Management
Conservative treatment
                 Bed-rest
                 Analgesics
                 Antibiotics.
Surgical treatment: **Refer** the patient to the ENT team for surgery.
Surgery   Incision drainage
                 Tonsillectomy – after few days to prevent recurrences.

Ludwig's Angina

Definition   It is a severe life-threatening emergency due to cellulites of the sublingual
                 and submandibular regions.
Etiology   Infection of cellular tissues surrounding submandibular gland.
Bacteria   Streptococci, staphylococci, pneumococci, *Haemophilus influenzae*.
Diagnosis   Airway obstruction – tongue pushed upwards against the roof of the mouth
                 Pain neck, swelling, tenderness, difficulty in breathing

	Fever
	Death – may occur due to edema of glottis.
Investigation	TLC and DLC – leukocytosis.
Management	Airway maintenance
	Antibiotics
	Analgesics.
	Bed-rest

Surgical treatment: **Refer** the patient to the ENT team.

Surgery	Incision drainage of abscess.
Anesthesia	Local.
Method	Skin incision: A curved incision below the jaw
	Deepen the incision and displace the superficial lobe of submandibular gland
	Divide the mylohyoid muscles
	Decompress the closed fascial space
	Drain and suture the wound
	A tracheostomy may be necessary.

Acute Otitis Media

Definition	It is defined as the inflammation of middle ear
Etiology	Upper respiratory catarrh (URC)
Bacteria	Streptococci, staphylococci, pneumococci, *Haemophilus influenzae*.
Diagnosis	Age: Common in infants and children.
	Site: Common in middle ear.
	Earache, discharge from ear, deafness, fever.
Complications	Acute mastoiditis, subperiosteal abscess, meningitis, deafness
Investigation	TLC and DLC – leukocytosis
	Culture sensitivity testing of discharged fluid
	Hearing tests – show loss of hearing
Management	Bed-rest
	Analgesics
	Antibiotics – penicillin, ampicillin, BSA, for 1–2/52
	Eardrops:
	Chloramphenicol 2–3 drops t.d.s. Children 1–2 dropst.d.s.
	• Norfloxacin 2–3 drops t.d.s.

Surgical treatment: **Refer** the patient to the ENT team for surgery.

Surgery	Myringotomy.

Acute Mastoiditis

Definition	It is a complication of acute otitis media due to local spread of infection.
Etiology	Age – common in infants and children.

Bacteria	Streptococci, staphylococci, pneumococci, *Haemophilus influenzae*
Diagnosis	Earache, discharge from ear, tenderness over mastoid, deafness, fever, headache.
Complications	Extradural abscess, cererbral/cerebellar abscess, meningitis, deafness.
Investigation	TLC and DLC – leukocytosis
	Culture sensitivity testing of discharged fluid
	Hearing tests – show loss of hearing.
Management	Bed-rest
	Analgesics
	Antibiotics – penicillin, ampicillin, BSA, for 1–2/52
	Eardrops:

- Chloramphenicol 2–3 drops t.d.s. Children 1–2 dropst.d.s.
- Norfloxacin 2–3 drops t.d.s.

Surgical treatment: **Refer** the patient to the ENT team for surgery

Surgery	Mastoidectomy.

Foreign Bodies – in the air and food passages

Site	Larynx, esophagus or bronchi
Etiology	Accidental – holding something in the mouth,
	– sudden inspiration while eating
	Unconsciousness.
Diagnosis	Laryngeal foreign bodies:

- Cough, stridor, hoarseness, gagging, asphyxia, dyspnea, pain, swelling, tenderness, fever

Bronchial foreign bodies:
- Cough, wheezing, dyspnea, chest pain

Esophageal foreign bodies:
- Cough, gagging, pain in the neck, feeling of something stuck in the throat, dysphagia.

Investigation	X-ray – shows the foreign body
	Bronchoscopy
	Esophagoscopy
Management	Laryngeal foreign bodies: Removed with a grasping forceps through a direct laryngoscope under local/general anesthesia.
	Bronchial foreign bodies: Removed with a grasping forceps through a bronchoscope under general anesthesia.
	Esophageal foreign bodies: Removed with a grasping forceps through an esophagoscope/endoscope.

Practical Procedures
Tracheostomy   **Refer** the patient to the anesthetist/surgical team

Indications	Acute airway obstruction due to: Acute laryngeal obstruction – e.g.

- Foreign bodies in glottis
- Trauma – cut throat injury, head/spinal injury, spinal cord injury
- Vocal cords paralysis – by injury to recurrent laryngeal nerves
- Acute laryngotracheobronchitis
- Acute epiglossitis –due to viral or *Haemophilus influenzae*, sedema glottis, diphtheria laryngae, tetanus

Anesthesia induction

Removal of secretions – from trachea and bronchi.

Types	Emergency tracheostomy – required immediately, e.g.

- Cricothyrotomy

Elective tracheostomy – indicated while airway is still adequate or re-established, e.g.

- Endotracheal intubation.

Method

Cricothyrotomy

Anesthesia	Local or general
Skin incision	• Midline – with a sharp knife or scissors, a vertical skin incision is made over the cricothyroid membrane.
Dissection	• A transverse incision in the membrane.
	• Spread the wound with the help of knife handle or a dilator. Airway established with an endotracheal tube

Elective tracheostomy

Anaesthesia	Local or general
Skin incision	• Midline or horizontal
Dissection	• Sharp or blunt, division of thyroid isthmus
	• A cricoid hook inserted under cricoid cartilage, the hook steadies the trachea
	• Trachea incised with a scalpel – dividing 2nd, 3rd, 4th rings
	• A tracheal dilator inserted
	• Cricoid hook removed
	• A tracheostomy tube on a pilot, inserted into trachea
	• Tracheal dilator removed, and attached tapes tied around the neck
	• The inner tube fixed in position.
Note	The tracheostomy opening should be round in shape, to facilitate the introduction and changing of tube later on, and the wound heals well after removal of tube.
Postoperative care	Place over the bedside trolley, a tracheal dilator, retractors, cannulae, rubber catheter attached to a syringe, to remove the secretions, dressings, oxygen apparatus, suction apparatus.
	A special nurse in constant attendance.

Audiometery

Indication	Assessment of hearing.
Method	Pure tone sounds introduced into each ear at different frequencies Standardized sound levels being used, in comparison to a hearing level of 0 dB.
Threshold	Testing frequencies from 250 to 8000 Hz, to find out the threshold in decibels.
	The sound level is increased > threshold, and patient responds, when sound is heard.
	The sound level is then reduced in 10 dB steps, until no response.
	The sound level is then increased in 5 dB steps, until threshold is achieved.

References

1. Beales PH: Acute otitis media. Practitioner 199:752;1967.
2. Stroh JE: Allergic rhinitis. Postgrad Med 45:151;1969.
3. Mills CP: Acute sinusitis. Practitioner 199:757;1966.
4. Call WH: Control of epistaxis. S Clin North America 49:1235;1969.
5. Malcomson KG: Tonsillitis: Acute and chronic. Practitioner 199:777;1967.
6. Hora JF: Deep-neck infections. Arch Otolaryng 77:129;1963.
7. Goff WF: What to do when foreign bodies are inhaled or ingested. Postgrad Med 44:135;1968.
8. McConnell F: A new approach to the management of childhood deafness. P Clin North America 17:347;1970.

Maxillofacial and Dental Emergencies

Traumatic
- Wounds of the face
- Injuries of upper jaw (maxilla)
- Injuries of lower jaw (mandible)
- Dislocation of mandible (syn. temporomandibular joint)
- Fracture of zygomatic arch
- Fracture of orbit
- Tooth injuries

Inflammatory
- Impacted tooth
- Acute alveolar abscess
- Acute gingivitis and pyorrhea alveolaris
- Trgeminal neuralgia

Wounds of the Face

Types	Contusions and lacetared wounds.
MOI	Direct violence
	RSA
	Fall from a height.
Diagnosis	Contusion: Swelling, local tenderness
	Lacerated: Superficial or deeper wound
	Oozing of blood/serous from the wound
	Wound – clean or contaminated.
Investigation	X-ray face.
Management	Contusion: Cold (ice) fomentation
	Analgesics
	Lacerated: Toilet of wound with antiseptic solution
	Debridement of wound
	Suturing of wound
	Deeper wound: Repair of each layer – meticulously
	Stitches passed through muscular layers in an inverted manner
	Skin sutures inserted by an eyeless needle
	Dressing: Place a gauze moistened with saline solution to absorb exudate
	Place over this a petroleum-jelly gauz.

Refer: The patient to next (visit) maxillofacial surgical team for consultation and removal of stitches on 4th day.

Injuries of Upper Jaw (Maxilla)

MOI	Direct violence
	RSA
	Fall from a height.
Diagnosis	Swelling
	Local tenderness
	Epistaxis
	Movements – of face painful.
Investigation	X-ray face.
Management	Airway maintenance
	Packing of nose – for epistaxis
	Analgesics.

Refer: The patient to the maxillofacial surgical team for further necessary treatment, e.g. treatment of fracture.

Injuries of Lower Jaw (Mandible)

MOI	Direct violence
	RSA
	Fall from a height.
Site of injury	Ramus, angle, body, symphyseal, condyle.
Diagnosis	Swelling of lower jaw
	Local tenderness
	Bone irregularity,
	Laceration of gum – at site of irregularity
	Teeth – may be loosened/broken
	Movements – painful.
Investigation	X-ray mandible: AP and lateral views.
Management	

Conservative treatment

Support the mandible with a barrel bandage

Analgesics

Nothing by mouth, IV fluids given.

Refer: The patient immediately to the maxillofacial surgeon for unstable/displaced fracture, otherwise refer the patient to the next (visit) maxillofacial surgical clinic.

Surgical treatment:

Surgery	ORIF – Wiring of the fractured mandible (circumdental wire)
	– Repair of lacerated gum.
After care	Support with a bandage.

Dislocation of Mandible (syn. Temporomandibular Joint)

MOI	Direct violence
	Exposure to cold
	Yawning – sudden, forced.

Type	Unilateral or bilateral.
Diagnosis	Deformity – mouth open
	Local tenderness
	Crepitus/clicking – produced by the movement of mandibular's condyle, by asking the patient to open and close the mouth, while the physician places his fingers over the joint, below and in front of the tragus.
Investigation	X-ray temporomandibular joints – AP and lateral views.
Management	Anesthesia: Short general.
Method	Grasp mandible with thumbs inside the mouth and fingers over chin apply pressure downwards with thumbs, followed by pushing backwards to reduce the condyle back in the fossa.
	Check X-ray to confirm reduction.
	Apply a barrel bandage to prevent wide opening of mouth.

Refer: The patient to the next (visit) maxillofacial surgical clinic.

Fracture of Zygomatic Arch

MOI	Direct violence – boxing.
Diagnosis	Swelling
	Local tenderness
	Bone irregularity
	Crepitus
	Movements of jaw – painful and restricted
	Epistaxis, subconjunctival hemorrhage.
Investigation	X-ray face.
Management	Packing of nose – for epistaxis
	Analgesics
	Antibiotic.

Refer: The patient to the maxillofacial surgical clinic, for further necessary treatment, e.g. surgical lifting of depressed cheekbone.

Fracture of Orbit (Blow-out Fractures)

MOI	Direct violence – direct blow from a squash/cricket ball
	RSA
	Foreign body.
Diagnosis	Swelling
	Subconjunctival/orbital hemorrhage
	Eyeball – contused/perforated/dislocated outside the lids
	Local tenderness
	Crepitus
	Enophthalmos
	Diplopia.
Investigation	X-ray orbit – AP and LAT – for foreign body.

Management	Toilet of the wound
	Antibiotics
	Analgesics.

Refer: The patient to the ophthalmology team immediately.

Foreign body – extraction by ophthalmology team.

The patient to the maxillofacial surgical team for further necessary treatment.

Ludwig's Angina

Described in Section of Ear, Nose and Throat Emergencies

Tooth Injuries

MOI	Direct violence
	RSA.
Diagnosis	Undisplaced/displaced tooth
	Bleeding from gums
	Toothache.
Investigation	X-ray (dental) of affected tooth.
Management	Rinse the mouth with saline solution or chlorhexidine mouthwash
	Bleeding – infiltrate with 1% xylocain with adrenaline 1:200000
	Analgesics
	Antibiotics.

Refer: The patient to a dental surgeon for:

- Reduction and immobilization of mobile teeth
- Extraction of tooth
- Suturing of soft tissue lacerations.

Impacted Tooth

Etiology	Infection: The tooth most often to be affected is the third lower molar (wisdom tooth). It is prevented from eruption by an adjacent tooth. The unerupted part of the crown is covered by a flap of the gum, underneath that collection of food debris occurs, resulting in infection, clenching.
Diagnosis	Swelling
	Pain – very severe, throbbing type
	Difficulty in chewing food
	Fever
	Malaise.
Investigation	X-ray (dental) of affected tooth.
Management	Antibiotics
	Analgesics.

Refer: The patient to a dental surgeon for extraction of tooth.

Acute Alveolar Abscess

Common during childhood and young adults.

Etiology	Infection.
Diagnosis	Pain – dull and constant
	Swelling of the cheek
	Edema of the gum
	Difficulty in chewing food.
Investigation	X-ray (dental) of the affected tooth.
Management	Antibiotics
	Analgesics
	Incision drainage of abscess.

Refer: The patient to a dental surgeon.

Acute Gingivitis and Pyorrhea Alveolaris

The periodontal membrane is the periosteum lining the tooth socket. It forms a sling for the root of a tooth in its bed of bone.

Etiology	Infection.
Predisposing	Gum recession
	Tartar deposit
	Accumulation of food particles between gum and the teeth
	Inflammation (gingivitis)
	Suppuration (pyorrhea)
	Discharge of pus
	Loosening of teeth
Diagnosis	Pain – toothache
	Fowl smell
	Gums – swollen, bleeding gums
	Loosened teeth.
Investigation	X-ray (dental) affected teeth.
Management	

Conservative treatment: Successful in early cases:

> Regular scaling
> Massaging of gums with fingers
> Mouth washes – with astringents
> Local application of clove oil.

Surgical treatment: **Refer** the patient to a dental surgeon for:

> Extraction of tooth
> Gingivectomy – to eradicate the periodontal pockets.

Trigeminal Neuralgia

Etiology	Unknown
Precipitating	Viral (herpes simplex) infection.
Diagnosis	Common in females
	Pain – very severe, e.g. sharp, stabbing, intermittent pains in the distribution of one or more branches of the nerve.

Management

Conservative treatment

       Carbamazepine (tegretol) is drug of choice

       Dose: 0.2–2 g/day

       S/E: Hematologic and cutaneous reactions

       Anticonvulsants: Diphenylhydantoin sodium (dilantin)

       Dose: 0.1 g q.d.s.

       Alcohol injection: Into Gasserian ganglion may produce analgesia.

       Surgical treatment: **Refer** the patient to maxillofacial surgical team.

Indications   Failure of conservative measures

Method   Percutaneous electrocoagulation of the preganglionic roots under local anesthesia.

References

1. Robert G, Scully C, Shotts R: ABC of oral health: Dental emergencies. BMJ 321:559–62;2000.
2. Benjamin William Fickling, Contemporary. Dental Surgeon, St. George's Hospital, London.
3. Singh G, Joshi JL: Dental problems of the handicapped child. In: Gupte S (ed). Recent Advances in Pediatrics. Vol. 7. New Delhi : Jaypee Brothers. 265–280;1997.
4. Mitchell L, Mitchell DA: Oxford Handbook of Clinical Dentistry, 3rd ed. Maxillofacial Surgery. 492–520;2004.

Part V

Administrative and Legal Considerations

Clinical Audit

Definition

It is defined as the systematic approach to quality improved clinical care, by reviewing patient's care against standard criteria and the implementation of changing and strengthening many aspects of hospital practice and administration. Any departures from the best practice can then be reviewed, in order to remove the causes, i.e. clinical audit compares current practice to the standard practice. It should not be linked to the research which determines the constitution of best practice. Research involves new diagnostic and therapeutic parameters.

Aims of Audit

1. To assess the clinical performance of medical professionals.
2. To play an important role in continuing professional development (CPD).
3. To enhance management and communication skills.
4. To improve learning, assessment and teaching skills.
5. To help medical professionals, health service managers, patients and public.
6. To encourage medical professionals for providing the best available care to their patients.
7. To inform the health service managers about requirement for any change or new investment to upgrade medical professionals' practice.
8. To ensure the patients being given the best possible medical care.
9. To aware the public about being provided a quality-based service.

Characteristics of a Good Audit

A good audit constitutes:
1. Good planning.
2. Systematic and adequate collection of the data.
3. Participation of all people in the audit process in the unit.
4. Coordination between the individuals involved in the audit.
5. Presenting the conclusions of the work to the audit board, consisting of the surgeon, practitioners, nurses, social services and local health authorities and managers. They all should be collectively responsible for delivery of good quality of medical care to the population in question by reducing health inequalities.

Perspective of Clinical Audit in Practice

Clinical practice has seen major advancement in every field, due to refinements and improvements in skills, knowledge and technology. The true essence of surgical innovation and improvement has come through individual medical/surgical experiences and new techniques with little evidence of clinical trials. The physician/surgeon relies on multidisciplinary approach for developing a new technique or method of the treatment. These refinements need to be evidence-based and accountable. The medical/surgical trials are often expensive and difficult to run. Without sponsorship and financial support, surgical trials are impracticable.

Uses of Clinical Audit

1. Maintaining good medical practice.
2. Providing good clinical care.
3. Teaching and training, appraising and assessing.
4. Maintaining good relationships with patients.
5. Working with/treating colleagues fairly – need to work in teams.
6. Probity (being honest and trustworthy).
7. Keeping oneself healthy.
8. To be constantly and constructively self-critical.
9. To be committed to continuous professional development.
10. To know how to avail themselves of and apply relevant best evidence.
11. To meet the responsibility set out in good medical practice.
12. Supports a legal claim.
13. Supports an application for a funding allocation.
14. Enhances management and communication skills.
15. Improves in their learning, assessment and teaching skills.
16. Able to effectively use information technology.

References

1. Baker R, Hearnshaw H, Robertson N. Implementing Change with Clinical Audit. John Wiley and sons. Chichester. 1999.
2. Clinical Governance Support Team. A Practical Handbook for Clinical Audit. London. 2004.
3. Department of health. The evolution of clinical audit. Leeds:NHS executive. 1994.
4. Debnath UK, Subramanian KN. Clinical audit in orthopaedics. Current concept review. Indian Journal of Orthopaedics. Vol 40:2:63–69;2006.
5. Fraser RC. Medical audit in general practice. Trainee. 2:113–115;1982. General Medical Council. Good Medical Practice. London. 2006.
6. Grimshaw J, Freemantie N et al. Developing and implementing clinical practice guidelines. Quality in Health Care. 4:55–64;1995.
7. National institute of clinical excellence/commission for health. Improvement Principles for best practice in clinical audit. London: NICE 2002.
8. Royal college of Surgeon. Guidelines to clinical audit in surgical practice. London: Royal College of Surgeons. 1989.
9. Secretaries of State for Health, Social services, Wales, Northern Ireland and Scotland. Working for patients (Cmn 555) London: HMSO. 1989.

Medical Records Keeping

Definition

It is defined as clinical, scientific, administrative and medicolegal document relating to medical care. The medical defence organizations constantly stress the importance of good medical records.

Aims

- Monitoring of the patient
- Medical audit and statistical studies
- Medical education and research
- Medical insurance/reimbursement claims
- Medicolegal purpose

Advantages

These records serve as basis for well-defined indicators.
- These records keep the managers/administration in touch with the pulse of the hospital administration (service).
- These records keep a watchful survey of hospital administration.

Instructions while Issuing Medical Records

- All medical records/documents should be neat, comprehensive and chronologically correct. Do not overwrite while writing the notes.
- Reports: X-ray, US, MRI, CT scan, ECG, laboratory reports, should be issued only by a qualified/responsible person, retaining the original/xerox copy.
- Prescription: Preferably on the doctor's letter pad. Should mention: Patient's name, age, sex, date, doctor's name, qualification, registration no., prescribed drugs, investigations advise, any instructions and follow up (next appointment).
- Discharge slip: Filled up/supervised by the doctor incharge. Should mention condition of the patient at time of admission, clinical diagnosis, investigations done, treatment given, operation notes, and mention condition of the patient, any advice, instructions to referring GP, and follow up date, at time of discharge.
- Referral notes: Should mention date and time of writing the notes, medicines and treatment given, and any particular instruction.

- Certificates: Medical certificate is an important document of written evidence vouching for the truth of a fact, determined by the issuing doctor. It is admitted in a court of law as an evident evidence, and if proved to be false, the issuing doctor is liable for punishment (fine or imprisonment or both).
- Types: Birth, illness, temporary/permanent disability, mental illness, permanent illness–impotence, recovery, pre-employment fitness, fitness certificate for admission to school, and death certificate.

Analytic Indicators

Uses   These are used for evaluation of day to day performance of the hospital management/administration.

Types
- Average no. of out-patients/day.
- Average number of in-patients
- Percentage of bed occupancy
- Bed turnover rate
- Average length of stay
- Birth rate
- Mortality/death rate

References

1. Hill G. A&E risk management. Medical Defence Union, London. 1991.
2. MDU (Medical Defence Union). Medical records. Medical Defence Union, London 1992.
3. Dhamija TD. Managerial/Management information system related to medical record. Niramayam. Vol 2006-issue 4:10–12.
4. Behere SB. Medical Documents and Records: The most important aspect of your professional life. The Doctor's People. Vol II-Issue 5:12–14.

Legal Considerations

Medical Negligence

Definition It is defined as perceived and actual dereliction of duty, e.g. deficient care/attention, by a medical professional, causing injury or death of a patient. Medical negligence or medical malpractice comes under the purview of claw of contracts.

Types Criminal:
- Wrong diagnosis despite due diligence
- Wrong treatment: Amputating a wrong limb
- Delayed treatment: Not providing priority treatment in time
- Gross negligence: Leaving a sponge, instrument inside body
- Non-compliance of prescribed investigations.

Vicarious Held responsible for the wrong-doings of his staff, e.g. assistants, HOs, paramedical staff.

Contributory Unreasonable conduct on the part of the patient, resulting in injury or damage as complained, e.g. the patient does not comply with doctor's suggestions/advice, regarding his/her treatment.

Onus of proof Caught to be on the complainant (patient) alleging negligence, but this burden shifts to the defendant doctor/hospital, to prove non-negligence.

Prevention (precautions taken by the doctor) of negligence:
- Make the patient's care – a first concern
- Protect and promote the health of patients
- Behavior – avoid provoking the patient/attendants
- Avoid criticizing colleagues/have respect for colleagues
- Taking of additional opinions – especially in doubtful cases.
- Never try to over do – remain within one's knowledge and facilities
- Taking of informed consent of the patient/attendant
- Avoid change of records
- Avoid issuing bogus certificates
- Avoid disclosing privileged information of the patient to anyone
- Be honest and trustworthy
- Maintain good communication

- Provide a good standard of practice and clinical care
- Provide priority care to serious emergency case
- Keep professional knowledge and skills up-to-date
- To opt for professional indemnity insurance.

Legal   The law expects a standard reasonable care of an average but prudent doctor and not cure (Tindal J).

One must remember: **'Ignorance of law' is un-excusable'**

Prenatal Diagnostic Techniques (PNDT): Act and Rules

Definition   The act prohibits determination and disclosure of the sex of the fetus. Also prohibits advertisements related to prenatal determination of sex.

Indications
- To detect genetic, metabolic or chromosomal disorders of the fetus.
- To detect congenital malformations or sexual disorders.

Offence   Misuse of the test for the purpose of prenatal sex determination, thereby opting for female feticide.

Punishment   Imprisonment and fine.

Medical Termination of Pregnancy (MTP) Act

Definition   The act prohibits termination of pregnancy by an unauthorized person who is not an RMP for doing MTP.

Indication   MTP under following circumstances by an RMP at a registered place:
- Medical: Continuance of pregnancy would endanger the life of the pregnant woman.
- Psychological: Grave injury to her mental health – that if the child was born, it would suffer from serious mental or physical abnormalities.
- Pregnancy caused by rape – the agony caused by such pregnancy shall be presumed to constitute a grave mental injury.
- Pregnancy caused by failure of any device/contraceptive – used for the purpose of family planning (limiting no. of children).
- Pregnancy of a minor girl.

Offence   Misuse of the test for the purpose of terminating pregnancy (ulterior motives), e.g. opting for female feticide.

Punishment   Rigorous imprisonment for a term of 2 to 7 years.

Torture

Definition   An act of deliberate hurting someone in order to compel them to confess: "Deliberate systematic or wanton infliction of physical/mental injury or damage by one or more persons acting alone or on the orders of the higher authority, to force another person to disclose information/to make a forced confession, or for any other reason."
(Source: World Medical Association in its Tokyo Declaration, 1975)

Violation   Global issue of concern – Human rights violation: Torture is considered as an important human rights violation – a worldwide misuse of power.

"Any act by which severe pain or suffering (physical or mental) inflicted intentionally on a person for purposes, e.g. obtaining information or a confession, punishing him for an act he/she or a third person has committed or is suspected of having committed, or intimidating or coercing him for any reason based on discrimination of any kind, when such pain or suffering is inflicted by/or at the instigation of or with the consent or acquiescence of a public official/or another person acting in an official capacity, excluding pain of suffering inflicted from, inherent in or incidentals to lawful sanctions."

(Source: United Nations Convention, December 1991).

Motives
- To extort a confession – misused as legal proof.
- To extract information.
- To punish a person.
- To suppress persons associated with tortured person (violent distortion).
- To torture/torment – prisoners, political opponents, by methods include water boarding, etc.

Rehabilitation Antitorture and rehabilitation centre is in Copenhagen, Denmark, where torture victims are rehabilitated and studies are carried out on the effects of torture. So many works are done but many objectives are still to be fulfilled.

Sexual Torture
Sexual torture/assault is as old as human civilization and has been prevalent since ancient times in one form or other.

Types
- Mental: Forced nakedness, humiliations, abuses, threats and forced to witness others being sexually tortured/assaulted.
- Physical: Molestation/assault of victim by the tormentor or by using an animal for physical contact with the victim.

Objectives/motives
- Forceful confession – misused as legal proof.
- Personal vendetta – by torturing individual or his family members.
- To pollute (defile) the race.
- To satiate – sexual starvation of soldiers at war by assaulting women of enemy.
- Ethnic conflicts.
- Personality disorder – sexual assault of men/women in custody by a mentally deranged person.
- Misuse of custodial power – by sexual assault of victims in custody.
- Distortion of the personality – victim tortured to develop helplessness, loss of self-confidence, and worthlessness.
- To extract information
- Family violence (domestic/marital violence), child abuse, sexual harassment, rape, kidnapping, hostage taking and terrorist act and pornography, etc. Should also be viewed as human right violation as its repercussions are far reaching in society.

Modus operandi

Psychological:
- Verbal abuses, threats, and humiliation, publically
- Undressing (nudity) in front of opposite sex especially fair sex
- Being photographed in compromising positions.
- Forced to masturbate in front of others.
- Forced to watch sexual torture/assault of others.
- Forced to perform sexual torture/assault on other collegue victims.

Physical:
- Introduction of chillies, irritants, etc. into eyes, mouth, vagina, or anus.
- Introduction of ants, rats, insects, etc. into vagina, or anus.
- Penetration of vagina, anus by batons, rods, handle bars, candles, etc
- Plucking of nails, fingers, teeth, toes by instruments.
- Use of burning cigarettes on sensitive parts (genitals, breasts, etc.).
- Electrical shocks – given to sensitive parts.
- Mutilation of breasts, genitals, buttocks, etc.

Sexual:
- Fondling, squeezing, kissing/sucking of breasts, buttocks, genitalia
- Raped by person of same/opposite sex.
- Sexual assault (rape, etc.) by animals, e.g. trained dogs, monkeys.

Prevention:
- Public awareness – to condemn these barbarous, uncivilized acts and fight against torture.
- Media support – especially for women's rights, curbing domestic violence.
- Police and administration's support – for implementation of law strictly.
- Motivation of National Commission for Women and ILO.
- Medical organizations participation should spread the ethical principles that address human right and their violations.
- Motivation of employers (public and private) – to set up women cells in order to curb sexual exploitation at their working places.
- Motivation of every physician to realize his/her duty to protest his/her fellow citizen against violation of his right.

(Source: Tokyo Declaration, 1975)

Doctors and Torture

Definition   A doctor may be involved illegally in the process of torture/assault directly or indirectly, either voluntarily (a human right activist) or under compulsion from the society, government or terrorists. He may participate unwillingly or unintentionally or may participate directly with malafide intentions.

Motives
- To assess victim's threshold to tolerate pain/suffering.
- To provide professional knowledge and skill to the tormentor

- To monitor torture/assault by means of medical therapy
- To suppress medical information deliberately while issuing medical certificates especially death certificates, surgical or autopsy reports, etc.
- To conceal/withhold information about incidence of abuses.
- To participate actively in administering torture/assault.

Role of doctors

Ethical: Doctors in the government and military services are most vulnerable (under compulsions) to pressure from seniors, for these illegal acts.

Criminal Liability of Doctors

Definition   During the last decade doctor – patient relationship has deteriorated and criminal complaints against doctors especially medical negligence have increased alarmingly.

Factors

- Medical negligence
- Behavior of doctors/staff – rude, rough and unbearable
- Cost factor – exorbitant rates of treatment
- Lack of awareness among the masses about inherent risk

Liability   Criminal law (u/s 304 and 304-A) is applicable to all. Doctors are no exception to it.

Sections 304 and 304-A (related to professional negligency)

Section 304   Non-bailable offence

Offence   Professional negligency causing patient's death. Criminal negligence is the gross and culpable neglect/failure to exercise reasonable care and precautions to guard against injury or mishap.

Effects   Causes lot of embarrassment, harassment, hardship, bad reputation and mental agony to the doctors.

Section 304-A: Bailable Offence

Offence   Professional negligency causing death of a patient.

Mere inadvertence or some degree of want of adequate care and caution might create civil liability, but would not suffice to hold him criminally liable.

When Doctors Should Inform Police

Duty   Police must be informed in following cases, and failure to inform may result in legal penalities.

Cases

- Of homicidal death
- Of suicidal death
- Of operational death (during or postoperative)
- Of unnatural death
- Of sudden, unexpected death

- Of instant death post-treatment/medicine reaction
- Of undiagnosed death within 24 hrs of admission
- Of accidental deaths
- Of poisoning, burns, tetanus, AIDS death
- Of married woman dying within 7 yrs of marriage
- Of sexual offences:
  - Rape
  - Marriage related offences, e.g. mock marriage, bigamy, adultery, criminal elopement, husband/relatives subjecting wife to cruelty.

Procedure Information to police should preferably be in writing, and a written acknowledgment to be obtained. If the information is telephonic, then note down name, belt no. and designation of the police.

Can a Doctor be Arrested and Bailed

Doctors have no immunity against arrest for the various criminal acts.

Offence Cognizable (non-bailable under section 304)

Examples
- Criminal negligence in treating, causing grievous injury/death, as per an FIR filed by the patient/relatives in the police station
- Dealing in illegal organ trading
- Dealing in un'awful sex-determination test (PNDT)

Offence Non-cognizable (bailable under section 304-A).

Examples
- Criminal negligence in treating, causing simple injury
- The police are reluctant/refuse to register an FIR. The complaint has to be filed in the court of judicial magistrate.

Bail Doctor is entitled to be released at the police level, by executing a personal release bond of sureties, or by orders of the magistrate.

Anticipatory Bail

In case of likelihood of a criminal complaint being filed against a doctor, he/she can apply for a anticipatory bail under section 438(1), in order to avoid arrest by the police.

Limitation of Each Pathy and Speciality

- Graduates/GP (MBBS) cannot perform major surgeries.
- General surgeons cannot perform CS and hysterectomies.
- Gynecologist cannot perform ultrasonographies.
- Physician/surgeons cannot give general/spinal anesthesia.
- Specialist to restrict to his/her speciality.
- Dentist cannot issue death certificate.
- Homeopath cannot prescribe allopathic drugs.

Consent An agreement between doctor/hospital and the patient/parents of a young child or an unconscious patient, for medical care.

Informed Consent

Definition   It is defined as an agreement between doctor and patient (parents in case of young child), whereby information in details, to be provided by the doctor the nature of disease/disorder, necessary investigations, treatment include type of surgery required, cost of treatment, any complication, e.g. drug reaction, anesthesia or surgical complication, prospects of success, alternative treatment and prognosis.

Caution   Consent should not be given by a person under threat, misconception, mis-representation, unsoundness of mind and minors.

Offence   Negligence and doctor/hospital is charged under negligence Act.

Implied Consent

Definition   It is defined as assumed consent, e.g. the visit of a patient to a doctor's clinic, or hospital may be taken as agreeable to medical examination.

Express Consent

Definition   It is defined as an oral or written permission, obtained for specific examination, e.g. P/V or P/R, and specific investigations/diagnostic procedures.

Laws Governing, Controlling and Regulating Medical Profession

Classification   • Registration Act: Applicable to all doctors. MCI is the monitoring body, empowered to approve, recognize, inspect and monitor the medical education. It has clearly defined the code of conduct and medical ethics
                  • Nursing Home Registration Act
                  • Shop and Establishment Act
                  • Labor laws
                  • Special acts: MTP Act, PNDT Act, Organ Transplant Act, Lunacy Act.
                  • Medical evidence Act: In accidental cases, sexual offences, suicides and homicides.

References

1. Navarange JR: Medical negligence.The Doctor's People. Vol.-II, Issue-4, New Delhi.
2. Halder S: Medical negligence – Indian Penal Code and CPA vis-a-vis medical profession.
3. Gupta P: Doctor's vis-a-vis CPA. The Doctor People. Vol.-II, Issue-4, New Delhi.
4. Baldwa M: Criminal liability of doctors and when doctors should inform police. The Doctor People. Vol.-II, Issue-5, New Delhi.
5. Baldwa M, Navarange J: Law of Consent. The Doctor People. Vol.-II, Issue-6, New Delhi.
6. Behere SB: Doctor and Law. The Doctor People. Vol.-II, Issue-6, New Delhi.
7. Basu R: Torture – Global Issue of Concern. JIMA 97:11:449;1999.
8. Amnesty International – Torture in the Eighties. London. Amnesty International, 1984.
9. Fimate L: Medical Ethics and Torture. JIMA 97:11:453–56.
10. Sobti JC, et al: Role of Doctors in Prevention of Torture JIMA 97:11:466–68;1999.
11. Dogra TD: Sex Oriented Torture – An Overview. JMA 97:11:450–52;1999.

Appendices

Laboratory Procedures

Laboratory Procedures

Laboratory tests (procedures) contribute vital information about a patient's health. Correct diagnostic and therapeutic decisions rely, in part, on the accuracy of test results.

Principles

1. Adequate patient's preparation, specimen collection, and specimen handling are essential prerequisites for accurate testing.
2. Safety and disposal: Laboratory and healthcare personnel should follow current recommended sterile techniques, including precautions regarding the use of needles and other sterile equipment, as well as guidelines for the responsible disposal of all biological material and contaminated specimen collection supplies.
3. Collection of specimens:
   i. All specimens should be legibly labelled with the patient's name, age, sex. Also indicate the material sent, its source and the investigations requested.
   ii. All specimens should reach the laboratory fresh and correctly transported into the correct kind of containers, having properly fitting lids or caps.
   iii. Particular anticoagulants are necessary for particular chemical or other tests on blood.

Blood Chemistry and Hematology

Blood components: Blood volume (in adult male) = 5 quarts (4.75 L)

Plasma (fluid) = 3 quarts (2.85 L)

Cells (solid) = 2 quarts (1.90 L)

Cells are suspended in the plasma, which is made up of water and dissolved materials, including hormones, antibodies, and enzymes.

Cells: Erythrocytes (red cells), leukocytes (white cells), and thrombocytes (platelets) Red cells are round, biconcave, flexible discs, containing hemoglobin, a complex chemical that transports oxygen and carbon dioxide.

Hemolysis occurs due to rupture of cell membrane (due to rough handling of a blood specimen, dilution, exposure to contaminants, extreme in temperature, poisons, or pathological conditions) allowing hemoglobin to escape into plasma White cells – primarily control infection.

Platelets – primarily help in blood clotting

Plasma or serum may be separated from blood cells by centrifugation.

Plasma retains fibrinogen (clotting component), which is removed from serum.

Plasma is obtained by centrifugation of blood mixed with an anticoagulant in the collection tube. Specified anticoagulant/preservative must be used for the required test procedure.

Serum is obtained by centrifugation of clotted blood that has not been mixed with an anticoagulant.

Specimen Containers

i. Red-stopper tube: Contains no anticoagulant/preservative.
   Use: Serum or clotted whole blood. Serum must be separated from cells within 45 mts of venepuncture.

ii. Lavender-stopper tube: Containing liquid K3 EDTA
   Use: Plasma or EDTA whole blood

iii. Gray-stopper tube: Contains sodium fluoride – a preservative and potassium oxalate – an anticoagulant.
   Use: Plasma or sodium fluoride whole blood

iv. Blue-stopper tube: Contains 3.2% sodium citrate (yellow stripes on label)
   Use: Sodium citrate plasma or whole blood

v. Green-stopper tube: Contains sodium heparin or lithium heparin
   Use: Heparinized whole blood or plasma

vi. Yellow-stopper tube: Contains 1 ml acid citrate dextrose (ACD) solution
   Use: ACD whole blood

vii. Royal blue-stopper tube: May contain sodium heparin for trace metal studies
   Use: Heparinized whole blood

Venepuncture

Method   Apply a tourniquet (a piece of rubber tubing or a strap)
           Select the best vein – by inspection and palpation
           Sterile the site with spirit or alcohol
           Allow the puncture site to air dry. Hold the syringe with the needle, almost parallel with the patient's arm. Ask the patient to make a fist, and then insert the needle into the selected vein.

Draw up the required amount of blood into the syringe.

Place a piece of dry gauze over the needle and withdraw the needle carefully.

Note: For pediatric and geriatric patients, the total volume of blood collected should be noted on the test request form.

Blood Film (Blood Smear) Slide Preparation

Indication   RBC and WBC– physical appearance, morphology (size, shape, structure) presence of abnormal cells

Platelets – size and number

Malarial parasite – detection

Method   A clean dry slide is touched to a newly formed drop of blood from finger prick. One edge of a spreader slide is placed over the drop of blood smearing across the first slide to be done. Allow the smear to dry.

Staining   For **RBC** and **WBC**, staining is done either with Leishman stain or Wright stain.

For malarial parasite, both thick and thin smears to be prepared. Staining is done by Giemsa stain.

Hemoglobin Estimation

Low hemoglobin In anemia.

Method   1. Sahli's hemoglobinometer method

2. Haldane's hemoglobinometer method

3. Photoelectric method

Sahli's hemoglobinometer:

Place N/10 HCl in the hemoglobinometer diluting tube up to mark 10%.

A puncture made in the finger or an ear's lobe.

Draw blood in a hemoglobin pipette up to 20 cu mm mark, and transfer it into diluting tube. Rinse well the mixture.

After 10–20 mts, distilled water is added drop by drop, mixing with a glass rod. Continue adding water, until color of diluting tube matches that of standard provided with hemoglobinometer

Reading   Reading against the lower level of meniscus of the fluid in the diluting tube. Accuracy is doubtful.

Method   Haldane's hemoglobinometer:

Ammonia solution (4%) placed in the diluting tube up to 20 cm mark

A puncture made in the finger or an ear's lobe, and the pipette filled up to 20 cm mark, and transfer it into diluting tube. Saturate the solution with carbon monoxide gas with a pipette attached to gas mains. Distilled water is added drop by drop, until color of diluting tube matches that of standard tube.

Reading   Reading noted 1 mt after adding last drop of water. Accuracy is doubtful.

Method   Photoelectric method:

Most accurate method of hemoglobin estimation, which eliminates error due to matching colors with the eye.

Hematocrit (PCV) It is a measurement of cells in blood, expressed as %.

Low PCV	In iron deficiency anemia, cirrhosis liver, malignancies.
High PCV	In dehydration, polycythemia vera
Method	By using a capillary pipette, fill the Wintrobe tube – up to 100 mark, with blood, already treated with an anticoagulant, and centrifuged for 30 mts @ 2500 rpm in a 15 cm radius centrifuge
Reading	Reading by the upper level of the red cell column in %

Red Cell Count

Method	Blood is drawn up to 0.5 mark in the RBC pipette, followed by drawing in up to 101 mark, the RBC diluting fluid. Material mixed by rotating the pipette. Charge the Neubauer counting chamber with the mixture.
	Count RBC in 80 smallest squares in the 4 corners and one central big square

$$RBC \text{ count} = 200 \times No \text{ of corpuscles counted} = 10,000 \text{ 'x' } /cmm$$
$$= 0.02$$

Total Leukocyte Count (TLC)

Method	Blood sucked up to the 0.5 mark in the WBC pipette, followed by drawing in up to 11 mark, the WBC diluting fluid. The material is mixed by rotating the pipette
	Charge the WBC counting chamber with mixture
	Count WBC in 4 large corner squares
Reading	Counted in 4 large corner squares, i.e.
	TLC = 50 × No. of cells counted/cmm

Differential Leukocyte Count (DLC)

Method	A well-stained peripheral blood film is examined under the oil immersion lens. Count at least 100 white cells with individual identification, proceeding from one end to other.
Reading	Individual cells expressed as a %.

Platelet Count

Indications	Bleeding disorders, bone marrow disorders, e.g. leukemia.
Method	Cell counter
	Platelet solution is drawn up to 0.5 mark in red cell pipette, followed by drawing in up to 0.5 mark, blood, so that platelet solution reaches up to 1.0 mark. The pipette is further filled up to 101 mark with platelet solution. The material is mixed by rotating the pipette.
Reading	Counted directly in a Neubauer counting chamber using a diluting fluid containing urea, which hemolyses red cells.

Urine Analysis

Collection	Collected as routine into a clean glass vessel.

Avoid catheterization, unless urgently required, to combat introducing infection.

For bacteriological testing, a mid-term specimen to be collected with sterile precautions.

Physical examination

Quantity:

Normal: 700–2500 ml/day

Polyuria: Diabetes, chronic renal failure

Oliguria: Shock, acute nephritis, dehydration

Anuria: Renal circulation impairment

Color:

Colorless: Diabetes mellitus or insipidus, drinking

Brown: Jaundice

Specific gravity:

Measured by a urinometer

Normal specific gravity 1001–1025 at 15°

Increased specific gravity: By cooling

Naked eye characters of deposit:

Normal: Clear and transparent

White deposit on heating: Phosphates

Chemical examination

Reaction: Test with litmus paper

Normal: Acidic, rarely neutral or alkaline

Chlorides: NaCl: Tested with 20% potassium chromate and 2.9% silver nitrate solution

Proteins: Filtered and centrifuged urine is tested with:

Boiling test

Dipstick test (Uristix, Albustix)

Bence Jones proteose: Multiple myeloma

Blood: Confirm microscopically by Guaiac test or by use of Occul test tablets

Hematuria, haemoglobinuria

Sugar: Benedict qualitative test:

To 5 ml of Benedict's reagent in a test tube, add 0.5 ml (8 drops) of urine and shake well

Boil over naked spirit lamp flame for 2 mts and allow to cool for 5–10 mts

Reading

Blue color: No sugar

Light green: Negligible 0.1–0.5%

Green: Traces   0.5–1.0%

Yellow   1.0–1.5%

Orange   1.5–2.0%

Brick-red   2.0% or over

Ketones:

Acetone, hydroxybutyric acid and acetoacetic acid may all appear in the urine (ketosis) – Occurs in diabetes, starvation.

Test:

Rothera's test: 10 ml of urine in a test tube is saturated with Rothera's mixture (99 parts of ammonium sulfate + 1 part of sodium nitroprusside) Pour 2 ml of strong ammonia along side of tube. Make it stand for 5 mts

Reading:

Positive reaction: Purple color at the junction of urine and ammonia solution

Bile salts: To 10 ml of urine in a beaker, add finely powdered dry sulfur

Reading: Positive test: Sinking of sulfur particles

              Negative test : Floating of sulfur particles

Bile pigments: Fouchest test: Add 5.0 ml barium chloride solution

                    To 5–10 ml of urine. Filter the resulting mixture

                    To the precipitate on the filter paper add 1–2 drops of

                    Fouchet reagent

Reading: Color: Green – biliverdin, blue – cholecyamin

Microscopical examination:

10 ml of urine is centrifuged for 5 mts @ 1000 rpm

Supernatant is poured off, leaving behind 0.5 ml stuff in which sediment is resuspended by brisk agitation. Drops of sediment placed over a slide and examined microscopically with/without cover slip for:

RBC, WBC, epithelial cells, casts (red cell, white cell, granular) crystals (calcium oxalate, uric acid, urate, phosphate, cystine), bacteria, protozoa and yeasts.

Results expressed in terms of number/high power field.

Stool Examination

It is an investigation of great importance, too frequently omitted. White surface of a bedpan makes an ideal background for detection of blood, pus and mucous.

Naked eye examination:

Amount: Copious or scanty

Form: Hard, drier, or friable – constipation

      Watery – cholera (rice-water), diarrhea

      Purulent – dysentery, ulcerative colitis

      Blood and pus – bacillary dysentery

Color: Black – ingestion of iron or bismuth

      Dark tarry – haemorrhage in upper GI Tract

      Pale – obstructive jaundice due to absence of bile

Odor: Offensive – jaundice

Odorless – cholera, acute bacillary dysentery

Chemical examination

Test for blood   Benzidine test : Emulsify 1 ml of stool sample in 10 ml of water containing 5 drops of glacial acetic acid and centrifuging for 1 mt to separate large stool particles. Add 0.5 ml of 0.6% H_2O_2 to 1 ml benzidine solution in a test tube. Allow it to stand for 5–15 mts.

Reading: Blue color – positive reaction

Orthotolidine test: Boil a portion of feces in 5 ml of water.

Prepare 4% solution of orthotolidine in 95% ethyl alcohol. For use a 1-in-5 solution is made in glacial acetic acid. 1 ml of this reagent, 0.25 ml of fecal suspension, and 0.25 ml of H_2O_2, are mixed in a test tube, wait for 3 mts.

Reading: Dark green – positive reaction

Test for fats   Add alcoholic solution of dye – Sudan III/IV, to a 1–2 ml pellet of stool sample on a glass slide, and mixed with an applicator stick. Add 1 drop of 0.9% saline solution. Cover the preparation with a cover slip and examine under the microscope

Reading: Fat globules appear pink

Test for sugar   Take a small amount of stool sample in a test tube and to it add four times the volume of water, mixed well, and then to be centrifuged. Transfer the supernatant fluid to a test tube.

Add 5 ml of Benedict's qualitative reagent. After shaking, the mixture is boiled over a spirit lamp flame for few mts.

Reading: Changes in color, e.g. green: traces, brick red: +++

Microscopical examination: Done under high as well as low power.

Direct   Place a drop of NaCl solution at one end of a slide and a drop of Lugol iodine at the other end. To each, add a small portion of stool sample, each covered with a cover slip.

Concentration   One of following concentration techniques may be employed, as direct microscopy may miss ova and cysts, i.e.

- Formalin-ether sedimentation technique: Emulsify a portion of stools in 30 ml of saline. Strain 10 ml of emulsion through wet gauze, into a 15 ml centrifuge tube with a conical tip. Centrifuge at a moderate speed for few minutes and the supernatant decanted. The sediment resuspended in fresh saline, centrifuged and decanted as before. Add 10 ml of 10% formalin to the sediment. After mixing, allow it to stand for 5 mts. Add 3 ml of ether to it, and seal the tube and shake, then centrifuge at low speed.

Reading: 4 layers result, e.g.

At the bottom, a small amount of sediment containing most of parasites

Above that a layer of formalin

Above that a plug of fecal debris

At top a layer of ether
- Zinc sulfate centrifugal floatation technique: Emulsify 1 ml of stool sample in 10 ml of tap water. Filter the emulsion through wet gauze. The mixture centrifuged for 1 mt @ 26000 rpm, and the supernatant fluid poured off. Add fresh water, mix, and centrifuged again. Repeat process 3–4 times.

Reading: Eggs and cysts rise to surface, whereas trophozoites destroyed.

CSF examination: Refer to Pediatric Section

References

1. King AWE: Pediatric laboratory tests in developing countries. Asian J Lab Invest 234–242;2000:8.
2. Morley JKS: Pediatric Laboratory Techniques, 6th ed. Tokyo: United Publishers, 2003.
3. Gupte S, Chowdhary BB: Pediatric Laboratory Procedures, 10th ed. The Short Textbook of Pediatrics. Jaypee Brothers, New Delhi.
4. Directory of Services, 2nd version. SRL Ranbaxy, Clinical Reference Laboratories, Mumbai, 2002.
5. Hunter D, Bomford RR: Hutchison's Clinical Methods, 14th ed. Cassell London, 1964.

Important Conversions

Milliequivalents

$$\text{Milliequivalents (mEq) per litre} = \frac{\text{Milligrams \% + 10}}{\text{Atomic weight}} \times \text{Valency}$$

With this formula, number of reacting particles in a litre of solution can be determined by dividing the atomic weight of each ion into the total quantity (in milligrams) of that particular ion on one litre of solution (Table AII.1).

Conversion of milligrams per 100 mL to milliequivalents per litre of plasma (Table AII.1):

$$\text{Sodium (Na)} = \frac{\text{mg/100 mL} \times 10}{23 \text{ (atomic weight)}} \times 1 \text{ (valency)} = \text{mEq/litre}$$

$$\text{Potassium (K)} = \frac{\text{mg/100 mL} \times 10}{39} \times 1 \text{ (valency)} = \text{mEq/litre}$$

$$\text{Calcium (Ca)} = \frac{\text{mg/100 mL} \times 10}{40} \times 2 \text{ (valency)} = \text{mEq/litre}$$

$$\text{Chloride (Cl)} = \frac{\text{mg/100 mL} \times 10}{35.5} \times 1 \text{ (valency)} = \text{mEq/litre}$$

Table AII.1: Factors for rapid conversion of mg/dL to mEq/L

Cations	Factors	Anions	Factors
Sodium (Na)	0.435	Bicarbonate (HCO_3)	0.455
Potassium (K)	0.257	Chloride (as NaCl)	0.150
Calcium (Ca)	0.5	Phosphate (HPO_4)	0.58
Magnesium (Mg)	0.833	Sulphate (SO_4)	0.625

SI Unit Conversion

The SI system (System International d' Units) is an international version of the metric system of units now generally employed in the basic sciences, and has now been adopted in clinical biochemistry in the United Kingdom and many other countries, since 1960. It has replaced the empirical range of units, e.g. mg/100 mL, mEq/litre, which has varied from one laboratory to another. Administration of medicines and the reports of chemical analysis are now expressed in SI units (Table A II.2):

Length	Metre is the basic (SI) unit of length
	Decimetre (dm) = 0.1 metre
	Centimetre = 0.01 metre
Weight (mass)	Kilogram (kg) is the basic (SI) unit of weight (mass)
	Gram (g) = 0.001 kg
	Milligram (mg) = 0.001 g
	Microgram (μg) = 0.001 mg
Volume	Litre is the accepted basic unit of volume, although a non-SI unit
	Liquids are expressed in millilitre (mL) and litres (L)
Amount of substance	Mole is the basic (SI) unit, where the molecular weight (MW) of the substance measured is expressed in grams.
	Reports of chemical analysis are prepared in millimoles/litre (mmol/L) inplace of mg/100 mL

Conversion   No. of moles (mol)/L = $\dfrac{\text{mg}/100 \text{ mL}}{\text{mol. Wt.}} \times 10$

Table AII.2: SI Units

Physical quantity	SI unit	Symbol
Length	Metre	m
Weight (mass)	Kilogram	kg
Volume (dry and liquid)	Litre	L
Amount of substance	Mole	mol

Conversion of Units: Table A II.3 illustrates SI Unit conversion.

Table AII.3: Conversion of units

Analyte	Conventional Units	Conventional to SI (x)	SI Units	SI to Conventional (x)
Acid phosphatase	units/L	NA	units/L	NA
Albumin (S)	g/dL	10	g/L	1
Alkaline phosphatase	units/L	NA	units/L	NA
Ammonia (P)	Mug/dL	0.59	MUmol/L	1.69
Amylase (S)	units/L	NA	units/L	NA
ACE	units/L	1	units/L	1
ADH	pg/mL	1	ng/L	1
Bilirubin (S)	mg/dL	17.1	MUmol/L	0.0584
Bromide (P)	Mug/mL	0.0125	mmol/L	799
Calcitonin	pg/mL	1	ng/L	1
Calcium (S)	mg/dL	0.25	mmol/L	4
Chloride (S)	mEq/L	1	mmol/L	1

Contd...

Contd...

Analyte	Conventional Units	Conventional to SI (x)	SI Units	SI to Conventional (x)
Cholesterol	mg/dL	0.0259	mmol/L	38.61
HDL	mg/dL	0.0259	mmol/L	38.61
LDL	mg/dL	0.0259	mmol/L	38.61
Cholinesterase (S)	units/L	1000	kU/L	0.001
Copper (S)	Mug/L	0.0157	MUmol	63.7
Creatine kinase	units/L	NA	units/L	NA
Creatinine (S)	mg/dL	88.4	MUmol/L	0.0113
Estradiol (S)	pg/mL	3.67	pmol/L	0.272
Ferritin (S)	ng/mL	1	MUg/L	1
Glucose				
Blood	mg/dL	0.0555	mmol/L	18.02
CSF	mg/dL	0.0555	mmol/L	18.02
Urine	mg/dL	0.0555	mmol/L	18.02
Insulin (B)	MUIU/mL	1	mIU/L	1
Lipids (total)	mg/dL	0.01	g/L	100
Potassium (B)	mEq	1	mmol/L	1
Sodium (B)	mEq/	1	mmol/L	1
Testosterone	ng/dL	0.0347	nmol/L	28.8
TSH	MUIU/mL	1	mIU/L	1
Urea, nitrogen, blood (BUN)	mg/dL	0.357	mmol	2.8
Uric acid (S)	mg/dL	0.059	mmol/L	16.9

Units of energy – Joules (kJ) × 0.238=calories, calories × 4.2=Joules (kJ)
(Specimen used : Blood (B), plasma (P), serum (S).
(Source : SRL RANBAXY, Clinical Reference Laboratories)

Table AII.4 Illustrates Prefixes

Table AII.4: Prefixes					
Prefix	Symbol	Multiple	Prefix	Symbol	Fraction
mega	M	$(10)^6$	deci	d	$(10)^{-1}$
kilo	k	$(10)^3$	centi	c	$(10)^{-2}$
deca	da	$(10)^1$	milli	m	$(10)^{-3}$
			micro	u	$(10)^{-6}$
			nano	n	$(10)^{-9}$
			pico	p	$(10)^{-12}$

Conversion of Centigrade and Fahrenheit scales:
To convert Fahrenheit into Centigrade – substract 32, multiply by 5, and divide by 9
To convert Centigrade into Fahrenheit – multiply by 9, divide by 5, and add 32.

Index

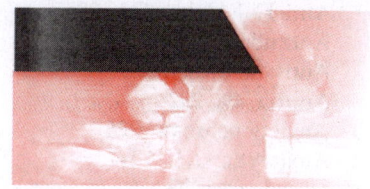

Reader's Notes

Reader's Notes

Reader's Notes